MANUAL OF

High Risk Pregnancy
Delivery

&

MANUAL OF

High Risk Pregnancy

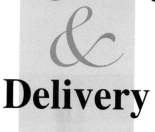

Delivery

Elizabeth Stepp Gilbert, RNC, MS, FNP

Family Nurse Practitioner in private practice
Associate Professor
Grand Canyon University
Phoenix, Arizona

Judith Smith Harmon, RN, MS, FNP

Certified Family Nurse Practitioner
Samaritan Family Health Center
Payson, Arizona

Resolve Through Sharing
LaCrosse Lutheran Hospital
LaCrosse, Wisconsin

Second Edition
with 108 illustrations

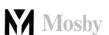

St. Louis Baltimore Boston Carlsbad
Chicago Minneapolis New York Philadelphia Portland
London Milan Sydney Tokyo Toronto

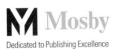

Dedicated to Publishing Excellence

Publisher: Nancy L. Coon
Editor: Michael S. Ledbetter
Developmental Editor: Laurie K. Muench
Project Manager: John Rogers
Project Specialist: Betty Hazelwood
Designer: Yael Kats
Manufacturing Supervisor: Donald Carlisle

Second Edition
Copyright © 1998 by Mosby, Inc.

Previous edition copyrighted 1993

Printed in the United States of America
Composition by Graphic World, Inc.
Printing/binding by R.R. Donnelley & Sons Company

Mosby, Inc.
11830 Westline Industrial Drive
St. Louis, Missouri 63146

Library of Congress Cataloging in Publication Data
Gilbert, Elizabeth Stepp.
    Manual of high risk pregnancy & delivery / Elizabeth Stepp
Gilbert, Judith Smith Harmon.—2nd ed.
        p.   cm.
    Includes bibliographical references and index.
    ISBN 0-8151-4462-8
    1. Maternity nursing—Handbooks, manuals, etc.   2. Pregnancy—
Complications—Nursing—Handbooks, manuals, etc.   3. Labor
(Obstetrics)—Complications—Nursing—Handbooks, manuals, etc.
I. Harmon, Judith Smith.   II. Title.
    [DNLM: 1. Obstetrical Nursing.   2. Neonatal Nursing.
3. Pregnancy, High Risk—nurses' instruction.   4. Pregnancy
Complications—nurses' instruction.   WY 157 G464m 1998]
RG951.G543   1998
610.73'678—dc21
DNLM/DLC
for Library of Congress   97-46588
                                                          CIP

99 00 01 02 / 9 8 7 6 5 4 3 2

To my husband Robert, who confidently supports all my professional endeavors, and to my son Michael, who has grown from a fetus to a teenager during the writing of two books and a revision.

Elizabeth Gilbert

To all three of my daughters, who have lived through two books and a revision. I am most appreciative of their support, encouragement, and assistance. Elizabeth gave of her time to do some preliminary editing and to input professionally at least half of this book. In the process, she learned more about pregnancy than she expected or needed to be the mother of my very healthy grandchildren. To Kathleen, who has listened to my complaints about the time this has taken. To Jennifer, who is an RN, BSN, and is following in my footsteps, and who has complimented me at all the right times. Finally, to my husband Loren, who has always been there for me and is the father of three wonderful daughters.

Judith Harmon

REVIEWERS

Patricia M. Sauer, RNC, MSN
Clinical Nurse Specialist
Labor and Delivery/High Risk Obstetrics
Northside Hospital
Atlanta, Georgia

Kathleen Rice Simpson, RNC, MSN
Perinatal Clinical Nurse Specialist
St. John's Mercy Medical Center
St. Louis, Missouri

PREFACE

Today's technologic advances make it possible to offer the woman and family experiencing a high risk pregnancy and delivery a good chance of a positive outcome. Nurses can play a key role in ensuring that these women and their fetuses receive the best care possible. Perinatal nurses in all obstetric facilities must be knowledgeable about screening for risk factors, providing preventive management, and intervening appropriately when problems develop. Many women, unfortunately, do not receive adequate prenatal care and enter the health care system only after complications occur. Because these women may seek assistance from various types of facilities, nurses practicing in clinics, emergency rooms, and primary care settings must also be alert to perinatal complications and be prepared to provide immediate stabilizing care.

Manual of High Risk Pregnancy and Delivery is designed to provide comprehensive information in a concise, portable, accessible format. Clearly written narrative and numerous tables and boxes enhance comprehension and facilitate retrieval of information. The nursing process serves as the organizational framework for discussions of both preventive and emergent care for a wide range of topics. Nursing interventions are based on NANDA diagnoses, AWHONN Standards of Practice, and ACOG Guidelines.

The coverage of the various problems includes incidence, etiology, physiology, pathophysiology, and usual medical management with protocols for nurse practitioners. Collaborative problems and desired outcomes are also addressed. Psychosocial implications and family considerations are incorporated throughout.

Manual of High Risk Pregnancy and Delivery is organized into seven units to facilitate easy retrieval of critical content. Unit I presents physiologic considerations and identification of a high risk pregnancy, fetal assessment and monitoring, and technologic advances in perinatal nursing. Unit II addresses the psychologic implications and adaptation to a high risk pregnancy. A separate chapter covers pregnancy loss and grief. Unit III discusses ethical dilemmas and legal considerations in perinatal nursing. Separate chapters in Unit IV focus on the effects of diabetes and cardiac, renal, connective tissue, and pulmonary diseases on pregnancy. Unit V deals with spontaneous abortion, ectopic pregnancy, gestational trophoblastic disease, placental abnormalities, disseminated intravascular coagulopathy, hemolytic incompatibility, hypertensive disorders of pregnancy, preterm labor, premature rupture of membranes, and trauma during pregnancy. Unit VI discusses the impact of sexually transmitted diseases and substance abuse on both mother and fetus. Unit VII focuses on alterations in the mechanics of labor and delivery with a strong emphasis on prevention of complications.

It is our conviction that thorough, knowledgeable care of the mother and fetus can considerably decrease neonatal morbidity and mortality and lessen complications for the mother. It is our intent and hope that this text will enable health care professionals to provide optimal care for mother, infant, and family.

Elizabeth Stepp Gilbert
Judith Smith Harmon

CONTENTS

UNIT

I

Physiologic Considerations of a High Risk Pregnancy

Significant physiologic changes occur during pregnancy. Within a very few weeks, alterations are measurable in many body systems. The mother must acquire and circulate increased quantities of nutrients to herself and the fetus. Her body must form and maintain a new organ, the placenta. Through the placenta, her body must dispose of fetal waste products and provide for fetal nutrition and respiration. Throughout the pregnancy, homeostatic mechanisms must adapt to provide protection of the fetus and to guard against its rejection as a foreign substance.

When caring for the high risk pregnant woman, the nurse must consider numerous physiologic aspects of pregnancy, such as adaptations in maternal body functions and the development of the maternal-fetal unit. Through analysis of these physiologic aspects, specific antenatal assessments can be made and high risk pregnancies can be identified. Special antepartum and intrapartum assessments of fetal well-being, including fetal monitoring and other surveillance modes, can also be used.

CHAPTER

1

Physiologic Adaptations to Pregnancy

The following sections describe adaptations as they relate to cardiovascular, respiratory, metabolic, endocrine, renal, hepatic, hematologic, gastrointestinal, and reproductive physiology. Descriptions of development of the fetus, beginning as an embryo, and the formation of the placenta follow. Antepartum nursing assessments directed at promotion and maintenance of health are described as they relate to laboratory studies, physical assessment, and nutritional requirements.

ADAPTATIONS
Cardiovascular

Body fluid is compartmentalized into cellular space, interstitial space, and blood space. Water and solutes exit from the capillaries into the interstitial space, where they are continually exchanged with water and solutes in the cellular space.

Blood, which consists of a suspension of various specialized cells in plasma, exerts a pressure on vessel walls. The pressure exerted depends on blood volume and distensibility of the vessel walls. Blood flow is related to the pressure gradient and the resistance of the vessel walls. Flow is measured as cardiac output, and the pressure gradient is measured as arterial blood pressure. During pregnancy specific adaptations, ultimately aimed at fetal sustenance, occur in these functions.

Total body fluid increases during pregnancy, but blood volume, in particular, increases by approximately 45% over prepregnant levels. The increase occurs in the cells and in the plasma of the blood. Plasma volume expands roughly 2.5 L to a total of 3.7 L. This increase in plasma volume results in increased intracapillary pressure and decreased oncotic pressure. The red blood cell mass may not increase in as great a proportion as the plasma.

To respond to the enlargement of the vascular volume, greater demands are placed on the heart to promote increased blood flow. Cardiac output rises from 4.5 to 5.5 L/min to 6 to 7 L/min. Heart rate during pregnancy increases by 10 to 15 beats per minute (bpm). Cardiac output increase is a product of heart rate and stroke volume.

In theory it might be assumed that arterial pressure would increase, but it does not because of hormonal and neurogenic influences. Both estrogen and the autonomic nervous system (ANS) promote vasodilation. Therefore arterial pressure actually decreases, with the diastolic pressure decreasing more than the systolic pressure. Venous pressure, however, increases as a reflection of resistance to blood return from the lower limbs because of partial obstruction of femoral veins.

If diseases or pregnancy complications do not affect cardiac function, blood volume changes, or peripheral vascular resistance, the uteroplacental unit serves as a reservoir for the additional volume. Estimates of uterine blood flow are from 500 to 750 ml/min by term. During labor, contractions force some of that volume into maternal circulation. Conditions such as cardiac disease, anemia, or hypertension can cause profound deficiencies in adaptive responses of the circulatory system. Influences such as changes in the autonomic nervous system can also have profound effects on vasoconstrictive factors. Such changes may be seen with anesthesia. Simple changes in posture can reduce cardiac output. Obstruction of the inferior vena cava occurs when the pregnant woman is placed in a supine position.

At all times of physiologic circulatory crisis, the uteroplacental unit is considered expendable to the mother. Any force competing against the cardiovascular adaptations will surely reduce blood flow to the uteroplacental unit and thus the fetus.

Respiratory

Respirations occur so that oxygen can be used in chemical processes for cellular proliferation and maintenance. This is accomplished through the processes of ventilation and gas transport and exchange among lungs, blood, and tissues.

Blood gases, primarily carbon dioxide (CO_2) and oxygen (O_2), remain in solution because of their individual or partial pressures. The partial pressures of each are changed in the alveoli of the lungs during inspiration and expiration. The gases move from the side of greater concentration to the side of lesser concentration. This exchange occurs again between blood and tissues. Normal partial pressure of oxygen (pO_2) is 80 to 100 mm Hg and that of carbon dioxide (pCO_2) is 40 mm Hg. O_2, because of its low solubility, is carried by hemoglobin. Most CO_2 is carried in the plasma, becoming carbonic acid and increasing free hydrogen ions.

Because pregnancy increases cell numbers, requiring increased O_2, changes are directed at facilitating O_2 availability. Hormonal influences and anatomic changes accomplish this. Progesterone stimulates respiratory rate. The mother, however, increases her rate in excess of O_2 demand. In the process, excess CO_2 is blown off. The resulting decrease in carbonic acid creates a pH difference in pregnancy. Normal pH is 7.38 to 7.42; although the normal range of pH is still 7.38 to 7.42 in pregnancy, the pH tends toward the upper range of 7.40 to 7.42.

Anatomic changes also influence respiration. Upward displacement of the diaphragm by the gravid uterus causes a lateral expansion of the chest wall. Hormonal influences are thought to dilate the airways and cause increased chest wall elasticity, promoting these anatomic changes.

Metabolic

Substrates for cellular metabolism are derived from ingested foods. They consist of carbohydrates, lipids, proteins, vitamins, and inorganic substances. These substrates are used to form new cells, to synthesize new substances, or to be burned as fuel for energy.

Carbohydrate is normally present in the blood, primarily in the form of galactose and fructose. Galactose is converted to glucose, and fructose goes directly through the same pathways as glucose. Glucose can be used directly or can be converted and stored as glycogen. When glucose is not available, amino acids are the main source of glucose.

Glucose can be oxidized to CO_2 and water. Glucose can also be changed to glucose-6-phosphate and then channeled into glycogen formation or synthesized into other metabolites through degradation to pyruvate. Pyruvate enters the tricarboxylic Krebs cycle, in the presence of O_2, and is converted to acetyl-CoA. Acetyl-CoA can also be formed by amino acids and fatty acids. Thus the Krebs cycle is a common junction in the metabolism of fats, proteins, and carbohydrates.

Lipids are hydrolyzed to form glycerol and fatty acids. Fatty acids are also synthesized from glucose and keto acids and can be stored as depot fat in the adipose tissue. When carbohydrates are not available, depot fat is mobilized so that fatty acids, easily oxidized, can be used as energy by cells. Fatty acids can also enter the Krebs cycle. In the liver, fatty acids may be used, in the absence of glucose, to spare amino acids. When this occurs, ketones are produced by fatty acid breakdown and are used as an alternative energy source.

Proteins are hydrolyzed to form amino acids. Amino acids are used for building new protein or for forming other nitrogen compounds. To supply energy, amino acids must be converted to carbohydrates or fats. Liver cells provide their own energy by converting amino acids into a carbohydrate form, keto acids, for entry into the Krebs cycle.

Insulin is necessary for utilization of glucose in oxidation and for the formation of glycogen and fats. It provides a carrier system for taking glucose into the cells and across the cellular membrane. During pregnancy, an acceleration in the use of glucose occurs because of rapid fetal cell and organ growth requiring a rapid source of energy in the first half of pregnancy. Complicating this is a diminished maternal sensitivity to insulin. As a result, pregnancy has been said to produce a diabetogenic state. Because the fetus is a continuous feeder from the mother, who is a periodic feeder, a starvation-like situation increases the potential for ketonemia. Placental hormones contribute to this by promoting insulin resistance and forcing the woman to use fats for energy needs. The entire metabolic rate increases in pregnancy, as does the need for increased caloric intake to supply the fetus while maintaining maternal needs.

Endocrine

Pituitary

The pituitary gland enlarges during pregnancy. This is presumably a result of its function as the master for all other glandular functions. It must aid in stimulating each of the following:

1. Thyroid function to meet the increased metabolic demands of pregnancy
2. Pancreatic function in the production of increased insulin

3. Ovarian function to aid in hormonal maintenance of the pregnancy
4. Adrenal function to increase cortisol

In addition, the pituitary produces oxytocin and antidiuretic hormone (ADH). Oxytocin improves uterine contractility in labor. ADH aids in increasing fluid volume in pregnancy.

Thyroid Gland

The thyroid gland also enlarges during pregnancy and produces a physiologic goiter. This is a response to the need for increased metabolism. Initially there is increased thyroid-binding globulin. Then T_4 uptake increases and T_3 uptake decreases.

Adrenals

Increased cortisol and catecholamine production occurs. Cortisol contributes to the increase in catecholamines (epinephrine and norepinephrine), which serve to increase maternal cardiac rate. Cortisol also mobilizes glucose and free fatty acids, thereby contributing to improved metabolism. To counteract some of the effects of vasodilation, the adrenals produce increased amounts of renin and angiotensin. To aid in blood volume expansion, aldosterone levels are also increased, contributing to sodium retention.

Renal

Increased blood volume circulates through the kidneys. This forces glomerular filtration of waste substances to increase. Renal blood flow constitutes about one fifth of the cardiac output. The entire plasma volume is filtered about 60 times per day. Substances to be retained by the body are first filtered and then reabsorbed in the tubules. Substances to be excreted are added to the fluid and flow to the distal portion of the tubule. In pregnancy, larger quantities are filtered in the glomerulus because of the greater capillary pressures associated with the increased blood flow.

In pregnancy, the glomerular filtration rate rises about 50%. Glucose and nitrogenous waste products of metabolism are therefore excreted in the urine in greater quantities. In turn, blood levels of nitrogenous waste products decrease. During pregnancy, normal laboratory values indicating renal function must be adjusted. A blood urea nitrogen (BUN) more than 13 mg/dl is abnormal even though it is within the nonpregnant normal range. Serum creatinine levels more than 0.8 mg/dl also require further investigation of renal function.

Renal function is affected, too, by anatomic changes. As the gravid uterus displaces other organs in the abdomen, it causes a physiologic hydroureter and hydronephrosis. This is usually more pronounced on the right side than on the left. The dilation of the ureters is further facilitated by estrogen. During pregnancy, the bladder has decreased tone because of hormonal influences. This factor and the distended ureters cause the pregnant woman to be more vulnerable to urinary tract infections. The increased glucose excretion into the urine also promotes bacterial growth.

Hepatic

In pregnancy, no change in hepatic size or blood flow occurs. However, the changes in metabolism during pregnancy lead to liver storage and conversion changes. Serum albumin is lower, cholesterol increases 40% to 50%, free fatty acids increase 60%, and phospholipids increase 35% to provide for the nutritional needs of the fetus.

Liver enzymes also reflect changes. Although serum aspartate aminotransferase (AST; formerly serum glutamic-oxaloacetic transaminase [SGOT]) and serum alanine aminotransferase (ALT; formerly serum glutamic-pyruvic transaminase [SGPT]) do not change, alkaline phosphatase and leukocyte alkaline phosphatase (LAP) markedly increase.

Hematologic

White blood cells, or leukocytes, are primarily responsible for fighting infections. Leukocytes are described as either granulocytes or nongranulocytes. When infection occurs, granulocytes increase and nongranulocytes migrate to inflammatory areas through the circulatory system. During pregnancy, the number of neutrophils that are granulocytes increases. This increase is stimulated by estrogen and plasma cortisol.

Normally there is a coexisting potential for coagulation and fibrinolysis. This might also be described as clotting and lysis of clots simultaneously. Coagulation begins when a platelet comes in contact with a damaged vessel surface. This contact triggers a cascade of events. First, prothrombin activator causes prothrombin to be released in the liver and converted to thrombin. Then thrombin is converted to fibrinogen, which forms fibrin, causing the red blood cells and plasma to mesh. A clot is thus formed. The clot triggers release of activators for plasminogen formation. Plasminogen converts to plasmin, and the clot is lysed.

In pregnancy, the equilibrium for coagulation-fibrinolysis is skewed toward coagulation. Plasma fibrinogen rises throughout pregnancy. Platelet count can remain normal or can be reduced insignificantly. Circulating activators of plasminogen, however, are reduced, and therefore fibrinolytic activity is diminished. What cannot be explained, however, is the rise in fibrin breakdown products despite apparent diminished fibrinolytic activity in the normal pathways. Factors in pregnancy promoting the increased fibrin breakdown include entry of placental thrombin into maternal circulation, increased amounts of fetoplacental hormones, and perhaps the effect of immunologic complexes present for the fetus.

Gastrointestinal

Gastrointestinal changes, such as decreased gastric motility and prolonged stomach-emptying time, result primarily from the anatomic shifting of abdominal contents. Constipation is frequently a problem in pregnancy.

The gallbladder is influenced by estrogen and becomes hypotonic. This causes an increased concentration of bile. An increased incidence of gallstones can result.

Reproductive

Changes in the reproductive system during pregnancy are the result of increased vascularity and increased hormone production. The vulva and vagina become more vascular during pregnancy. Increased estrogen promotes elasticity. The increased vascularity and elasticity can result in vulvar varicosities. Increased estrogen also increases vaginal secretions and promotes a more alkaline pH, which can predispose to increased vaginal infections.

The cervix becomes softer and shorter and appears cyanotic (Goodell sign). Near term, the cervix becomes even softer and shortens because of the influence of prostaglandins released from the stretching uterine musculature.

The muscle of the uterus increases in weight from approximately 60 to 800 g. It does this through hyperplasia, hypertrophy, and stretching. A marked increase in uterine vasculature occurs. Vascular resistance is considerably reduced, and uterine blood flow increases in the absence of disease. The increased uterine blood flow occurs because of the influences of progesterone, estrogen, and prostaglandins. It is also influenced by vasodilation from the autonomic nervous system and by the trophoblastic replacement of the muscular and elastic elements in the placental vessel walls.

The ovaries may be enlarged in early pregnancy. The corpus luteum becomes cystic and begins an increased production of progesterone and estrogen to maintain the nutritive lining in the myometrium of the uterus. As the placenta assumes the role of hormone production, by 14 to 16 weeks, the ovaries and corpus luteum return to normal size.

Breast tissue also responds to increased hormonal production of estrogen and progesterone. Increased vascularity occurs, and veins become more prominent. There is usually an increase in pigmentation and in the size of the areolae. The periareolar glands enlarge to provide greater lubrication during lactation.

DEVELOPMENT OF THE MATERNAL-FETAL UNIT

Knowledge of the growth and development of the maternal-fetal unit provides a basis for the care of the mother and fetus at risk for disease or pregnancy complications. This knowledge can provide a basis for early detection of maternal or fetal problems; therefore more serious complications can be prevented.

Embryo

During the luteal phase of the menstrual cycle, cervical mucus becomes receptive to spermatozoa. Ejaculation of sperm into the vagina is aided by mucoid receptivity, which allows rapid migration of spermatozoa through the cervix, into the uterine cavity, and into the fallopian tube.

Active spermatozoa can reach the outer portion of the fallopian tube within 75 minutes. The sperm and ovum meet in the distal portion of the fallopian tube. Fertilization occurs when the sperm penetrates the vitelline membrane of the ovum. Cell division begins, forming a small cell mass called the *morula.*

The morula is passed through the fallopian tube by tubal peristalsis and ciliary propulsion. The outer cell layer of the morula secretes a fluid, which pools in a segmentation cavity. Now the cell mass is called a *blastocyst.*

The blastocyst takes approximately 6 to 7 days to form. Implantation takes place at the blastocyst stage, usually occurring high in the uterine fundus. At this time the outer cells on the blastocyst are called *trophoblasts.*

The trophoblasts then invade the endometrium. It is thought that the reason the trophoblast cells are not treated as foreign and rejected by the mother is an exchange of fetal and maternal cytoplasmic and nuclear material from the trophoblastic cells. This allows the maternal immunologic system to tolerate the fetus as a part of the body rather than as foreign to it.

Progesterone from the corpus luteum provides stored nutritive substances in the endometrium, now called the *decidua.* The trophoblasts secrete proteolytic and cytolytic enzymes, permitting them to destroy vessels, glands, and stroma in the endometrium.

Placenta

The trophoblasts proliferate rapidly after implantation, and three layers of cells appear. These send out fingerlike projections called *villi.* The outer layer of cells, or the *syncytiotrophoblast;* the inner layer, or *cytotrophoblast;* and the dividing layer of thin connective tissue, the *mesotrophoblast,* are formed within these fingerlike projections. The mesotrophoblast forms the support for the villi and fetal vascular tissue. The syncytial cells then synthesize proteins, glucose, and hormones for use by the embryo.

After 2 or 3 weeks, the chorion begins to develop within the villi. While the chorion is developing, the amnion and its cavity are forming. Two cavities form in the embryonic pole. The ventral cavity is the yolk sac. The dorsal cavity becomes the amniotic cavity. As it enlarges, it forces the formation of the body stalk, the allantois, the blood vessels, and the beginning of the umbilical cord.

The decidua basilis, the layer beneath the embryoblast tissue, comes into contact with the villi, which then multiply rapidly. During villi multiplication, the decidua basilis is called the *chorion frondosum.*

By 14 weeks the chorion frondosum organizes into the discrete organ called the *placenta.* The placenta has segments, called *cotyledons,* which are connected by vascular channels to the umbilical cord. The placental surface is exposed to the maternal blood in the intervillous space and thins to a single layer of cells called the *placental membrane.* The exposure of fetal blood to maternal blood across this membrane provides for fetal oxygenation, nutrition, and excretion of fetal wastes. The two umbilical arteries carry CO_2 and other wastes from the fetus to the mother. The vein carries nutrition and oxygen to the fetus.

Transfer of O_2, CO_2, nutrition, and wastes depends on molecular size. Smaller molecules, such as O_2, CO_2, electrolytes, and water, transfer by simple diffusion, moving passively from the side of greater molecular concentration to the side of lesser molecular concentration. Their transfer largely depends on the adequacy of uterine blood flow into the intervillous space.

Larger molecules, such as glucose, are selectively transferred by a more complex process called *facilitated diffusion.* This process occurs against a large concentration gradient and requires a carrier system. Energy expenditure can also provide for selective transfer. Both depend more on placental surface area and thickness for their diffusion.

In addition to simple and complex diffusion, the placenta also assumes an endocrine function. Early in the pregnancy it assumes responsibility for maintenance of the pregnancy. The principal hormones produced are estrogen, progesterone, human chorionic gonadotropin, and human placental lactogen.

Amniotic Fluid

Origin

Initially the amnion fetal membrane primarily produces the amniotic fluid by actively transporting solute and passively transporting water from maternal serum to the amniotic fluid space. As the fetus develops, it makes a significant contribution by excreting urine into the amniotic fluid.

Functions

Amniotic fluid is normally swallowed by the fetus and absorbed in the gastrointestinal tract. If there are abnormalities of the fetal gastrointestinal tract or renal system, neurotube defects, or ruptured membranes, amniotic fluid may be excessive, deficient, or absent. Sufficient amounts of amniotic fluid provide a buoyant medium, which does the following:

1. Permits symmetric growth and development
2. Prevents adherence of the amnion to embryo or fetal parts
3. Cushions the baby against jolts by distributing impacts the mother may receive
4. Assists in control of the fetal body temperature by maintaining a relatively constant temperature
5. Enables the fetus to flex, extend, and move freely, thus aiding musculoskeletal development
6. Provides nutritional development
7. Allows the umbilical cord to be relatively free of compression

Fetus

The first trimester is a period of tremendous growth and organogenesis from an embryo into a fetus. By the end of the second week, the three embryologic germ layers develop to form body organs and systems. The formation of these layers is called *gastrulation.*

The ectoderm gives rise to the skin, hair, and nails; the epithelium of the internal and external ear, nasal cavity, mouth, and anus; the nervous system tissues; and the glands. The mesoderm forms connective tissue, blood vessels, lymphatic tissue, kidneys, pleura, peritoneum, pericardium, muscles, and skeleton. The endoderm forms the respiratory tract, bladder, liver, pancreas, and digestive tract.

By 6 weeks, a single-chamber heart is functioning and lung buds appear, as do a rudimentary kidney and gut. By the end of the first trimester, the heart has compartmentalized into four chambers; the lungs have bronchi; the gut, liver, pancreas, and spleen have developed; and the gender can be distinguished.

During the second trimester, facial features become defined. Fine body hair, called *lanugo,* appears, and vernix is produced to protect fetal skin. Meconium begins to appear in the gut. Maturation of organs allows some immature functioning.

In the third trimester, the fetus rapidly gains weight and final maturation of the organs for extrauterine life occurs. Subcutaneous fat deposits appear, and the body has a rounded appearance.

Assessments of fetal well-being have become more sophisticated. In addition to estimating fetal well-being by maternal well-being, fetal assessment can be made biochemically through laboratory studies and physically through observation of fetal heart activity on the fetal monitor. Visual examination of the fetus can be provided by ultrasound techniques.

ANTEPARTUM MATERNAL ASSESSMENTS
Laboratory Studies

Initial laboratory studies give baseline data about previous maternal disease, existing maternal disease, or a predisposition to disease or complications in pregnancy. A typical prenatal profile includes a number of laboratory studies.

Complete Blood Count

A complete blood count (CBC) gives information regarding leukocyte and erythrocyte levels and plasma/volume ratio. It also provides information regarding platelets and erythrocyte formation. If leukocytes are high, infection may be present and thus can be treated early. Shifts in the granular and nongranular leukocyte counts can aid in determining whether viral or bacterial infections are present. If the erythrocyte count is low or hemoglobin and hematocrit levels are low, anemia may be a problem; it should be treated vigorously with nutritive and iron supplements. If the woman is from the African or Mediterranean race, further screening for sickle cell disease or thalassemia may be needed. All women should have repeat hemoglobin and hematocrit determinations at 28 to 32 weeks. Although serum volume increases slightly more than the proportion of erythrocytes, anemia should not occur if red blood cells (RBCs) are normal to start and iron and folic acid intake are increased in pregnancy.

Urinalysis

A urinalysis and culture and sensitivity of the urine can offer information about renal function and urinary tract infection. If renal function is in question, further evaluation for creatinine, protein, and uric acid in the urine and serum may be done. If infection is present, appropriate treatment can be instituted before renal function is impaired or the pregnancy is threatened by premature labor.

Blood Type and Rh

Blood type and Rh are important for prevention or treatment of erythroblastosis in the fetus. If the mother is Rh negative and unsensitized, preventive Rh immune globulin should be given at 28 weeks.

Antibody Screen

Screening should be done regardless of the Rh type because other hemolytic incompatibilities may be present.

Rubella Screen

A rubella screen gives information about immunity against the disease rubella. A titer of less than 1:16 indicates that the mother has insufficient immunity against the disease. She cannot be vaccinated during pregnancy because the vaccine contains a live virus and could cause fetal anomalies. She should be instructed to avoid contact with groups who could potentially infect her.

Venereal Disease Research Laboratory (VDRL)

A serologic test to screen for syphilis should be done on all mothers because this has implications for the treatment of the mother and for potential congenital syphilis in the fetus caused by maternal infection. The prenatal health examination may be the first opportunity for the woman to realize that she is infected. Treatment with antibiotics and follow-up serology must be undertaken.

Infections

All patients should be screened for beta-streptococcus group A and for chlamydia at the first prenatal visit. See Chapter 24 for treatment of these if the patient is positive. All patients should also be screened for venereal gonococcus (GC).

Hepatitis B Virus (HBV) Screen

The Centers for Disease Control and Prevention and the American College of Obstetricians and Gynecologists (ACOG) recommend that all pregnant women be screened for hepatitis B surface antigen (HBsAg) at the initial prenatal visit (see Chapter 24).

Human Immune Deficiency (HIV) Screening

HIV testing is recommended routinely. Pregnant women should be offered testing and a statement with explanations of confidentiality of test results. If test results are positive, the woman can be treated with azidothymidine (AZT) to prevent the transfer of HIV status to the fetus (see Chapter 24).

Glucose Challenge Test

All pregnant women between 24 and 28 weeks of gestation should have a 1-hour postprandial blood sugar to screen for gestational diabetes. This is done by drawing a plasma glucose sample 1 hour after a 50-g glucose load. A value of 140 mg/dl or greater indicates the need for a 3-hour, 100-g glucose tolerance test (Cousins and others, 1991; Reece and others, 1991). If the woman has a family history of diabetes, is extremely obese, has had a previous infant weighing more than 9 pounds, has had a previous unexplained stillbirth, or has had recurrent spontaneous abortions, a glucose challenge test will be done on the first prenatal visit, as well as between 24 and 28 weeks of gestation.

Renal Function Laboratory Studies

Renal function laboratory studies are usually ordered if collagen diseases, diabetes, or chronic hypertension is present. These studies include serum and urinary determinations of creatinine, uric acid, and total protein. Urinary determinations must be 24-hour collections but can be done on an outpatient basis.

Plasma Progesterone

Plasma progesterone determinations can be done serially during the first 16 weeks when the woman has a history of frequent first-trimester spontaneous abortions. The laboratory must adjust usual normal values to fit early pregnancy, and values vary among laboratories. The tests are done weekly and must be compared with the normal range, as well as with each other. If low or falling levels are found, natural progesterone in vaginal suppositories may be used to maintain the pregnancy until placental production is sufficient.

Papanicolaou Smear

A Pap smear should be done on all pregnant women at the time of their first prenatal visit if one was not done in the previous year. If third-trimester bleeding develops, a Pap smear can be repeated to rule out bleeding caused by carcinoma. Pregnancy may increase cervical cancerous growth because of hormonal influences. In the presence of cervical cancer, pregnancy might need to be terminated for the treatment of the mother.

Other diseases, such as *Monilia* infection, may be detected on the Pap smear. These should be treated even if the woman is asymptomatic. Organism proliferation, if found on the Pap smear, may become great enough to cause pregnancy loss or premature rupture of membranes if left untreated.

Antepartum Physical Assessments

Ongoing assessment of a high risk pregnancy demands more frequent prenatal visits. An in-depth physical assessment should be done at each prenatal visit, along with an evaluation for complication-related parameters. Various parameters to be evaluated follow.

Maternal Weight

See the section on nutrition (beginning on p. 20).

Fundal Height

Fundal height should be measured each visit after the twentieth week. It is measured in centimeters from the top of the symphysis pubis to the top of the fundus of the uterus. It is roughly equal in centimeters to the weeks of gestation. Thus at 28 weeks, fundal height would be expected to be 28 cm. Because of varying techniques by care providers, it is important to use a consistent method and to know how each staff member does this measurement. It is acceptable to find variations of 1 to 3 cm. Variations more than 3 cm should lead to further investigation of possible estimated date of delivery (EDD) inaccuracies or growth abnormalities.

Blood Pressure

Blood pressure assessment should be done at each visit in the same arm and in the same position. The diastolic blood pressure normally drops 7 to 10 mm Hg during the first and second trimesters, followed by a return to nonpregnant baseline during the third trimester. A blood pressure of 140/90 or greater may warn of a hypertensive disorder of pregnancy and should be evaluated.

Physiologic/Pathologic Edema

Assessment of edema includes an inspection of the lower extremities and questions regarding facial or other edema. Pathologic edema does not lessen with rest and may warn of a hypertensive disorder of pregnancy or a cardiovascular complication.

Urine

The urine should be evaluated for presence of glucose, protein, ketones, and leukocyte esterase. This facilitates screening for complications such as diabetes, renal problems, a hypertensive disorder of pregnancy, or urinary tract infection.

Fetal Heart Rate

The fetal heart rate (FHR) should be auscultated by Doppler device beginning at 10 to 12 weeks of gestation and at each visit thereafter. The technique for calculating rate is to listen for a full 60 seconds. The FHR is usually not detectable by fetoscope until 16 to 18 weeks. FHR documentation assists in confirmation of early dating, as well as documentation of fetal life.

Fetal Movement

After 18 weeks the woman should be questioned regarding fetal movement. After 24 weeks she should be instructed to count at least once daily as a simple means of facilitating a dependable report of expected fetal well-being. See Chapter 3 for further discussion.

Risk Evaluation

Special physical assessment and laboratory analyses may be necessary depending on the risk of a specific complication or complications, such as the following:

- Alpha-fetoprotein screening
- Blood glucose determinations
- Preeclamptic profiles, cardiac laboratory studies, respiratory

blood gas studies, or bleeding and coagulation studies (Refer to various chapters related to health disorders or pregnancy complications.)

- Assessment of lung fields, cardiac rate, and heart sounds, or renal function
- Inquiry regarding possible signs of preterm labor
- Evaluation of special education needs related to specific complicating disorders or to activity restrictions

ACTIVITY/EXERCISE AND BED REST IN PREGNANCY

Changing life-styles have led to increased participation by pregnant women in exercise and sports. Many pregnant women also continue employment outside the home, and this may affect high risk pregnancy management. At the same time, bed rest or modified activities remain common management issues for the high risk pregnancy.

Aerobic exercise in pregnancy poses special concerns and controversy. Health care providers are particularly concerned with the effects of aerobic exercise secondary to the considerable increase in cardiovascular demands and fetal adaptation. Because exercise normally diverts blood from the visceral organs to the working muscles, uteroplacental blood flow may be insufficient.

As pregnancy progresses, oxygen consumption in the pregnant woman increases, even at rest. Some sources dispute the explanation that this is because of the increased demands of pregnancy but, rather, describe it as needed because of increased weight and body fat stores (American College of Obstetricians and Gynecologists, 1994; Fishbein, Phillips, 1990; Shangold, 1988). The effect of exercise during pregnancy on respirations is also in question. Although few differences are seen in the overall effects of exercise on the pregnant woman compared with the nonpregnant woman, a 30% increase in tidal volume occurs near term when a pregnant woman exercises. Pregnant women, however, have a decreased pulmonary reserve when compared with nonpregnant women (Fishbein, Phillips, 1990).

Maternal thermoregulation is also in question when exercise is added to her needs to adapt. However, regulatory mechanisms appear capable of dissipating heat produced by exercise (Fishbein, Phillips, 1990). Epinephrine and norepinephrine increase during exercise. Because norepinephrine increases the frequency and intensity of contractions, it may enhance contractility in women susceptible to preterm labor (Creasy, 1994). Increased exercise may have injury potential in pregnant women. Injury is possible because of the hormonal influences that increase connective tissue laxity. Additional strain on joints and the altered center of gravity tend to make a pregnant woman relatively unstable in certain activities (American College of Obstetricians and Gynecologists, 1994).

Studies of the effects of maternal exercise on the fetal response present varied and conflicting data (Fishbein, Phillips, 1990). Concerns are directed at the fetal ability to maintain its heart rate in the normal range and dissipate heat. As the fetus is unable to cool down by respiration or perspiration, caution related to increased temperature in exercise is advised.

In a study of the effect of exercise on uteroplacental Doppler waveforms in normal and complicated pregnancies, Hackett and others (1992) found that exercise appeared to increase vascular resistance in complicated pregnancies. Therefore it is suggested that physical exertion has a deleterious effect in the third trimester, particularly in the presence of hypertension or a small-for-gestational age (SGA) fetus (Hackett and others, 1992).

In studies in healthy pregnant humans, the hemodynamic changes of increased resistance during short-term exercise do not seem to jeopardize fetal well-being (Erkkola and others, 1992). This, however, should not suggest that exercise outside normal activities of daily living should be encouraged in the third trimester, even in women who are experiencing healthy, uncomplicated pregnancies.

Study and review of the effects of bed rest have also recently begun. It is estimated that nearly 20% of all women who deliver each year in the United States have bed rest prescribed by their physicians for some period during their pregnancy after the twentieth week of gestation (Shroeder, 1996). In all the studies reviewed by these authors, no statistical differences existed when comparing newborn outcomes between groups who complied with bed rest and those who did not. In fact, there were some physical and psychosocial adverse effects in both the woman and her family when there was reported compliance with bed rest.

Physical effects include the following (Maloni and others, 1993):

1. Skeletal muscle atrophy within 6 hours with greatest progression of atrophy in 3 to 7 days

2. Muscle volume losses of more than 25% to 30% in 5 weeks of bed rest
3. Weight loss despite reduced activities and controlled calorie intake
4. Plasma and blood volume decrease by approximately 7% of body weight
5. Increased blood coagulation
6. Heartburn and reflux
7. Decreased cardiac output and stroke volume
8. Glucose intolerance and insulin resistance
9. Prolonged postpartum physical recovery, including symptoms of muscular and cardiovascular deconditioning

Negative psychosocial effects on pregnant women and their families include the following (Maloni and others, 1993):

1. Increased stress, which occurs with separation from family by prolonged antepartum hospitalization
2. Specific concerns increased about family status, emotional changes, health and body image
3. Loss of financial support

Because studies of outcomes for the newborn do not show improvement in outcomes and some studies suggest deleterious physical and psychosocial effects, we must reevaluate the frequent recommendations for expensive, prolonged antenatal home or hospital bed rest, especially for otherwise healthy women who experience preterm labor or are pregnant with multiples.

In general, the following guidelines are recommended by the American College of Obstetricians and Gynecologists (ACOG) (Fishbein, Phillips, 1990):

1. Maternal heart rate should not exceed 140 bpm.
2. Strenuous exercise should not exceed 15 minutes in duration.
3. No exercise should be performed in a supine position after the fourth month. Rather, exercise positions should be modified by support under head, neck, and shoulders and by tilting the abdomen to the left.
4. Breathing should be regular at all time during the exercise. The Valsalva maneuver should be avoided.
5. Caloric intake should be adequate to meet demands of pregnancy and the exercise employed.
6. Maternal core temperature should not exceed 38° C.
7. Dehydration should be prevented by frequent fluid intake.
8. Movements should be smooth at all times, and jerky, bouncy motions should be avoided.

Lack of normal exercise may also take its toll on the pregnant woman's body. Although specific research has not been done on the effects of long-term bed rest on the pregnant woman, it probably disposes her to joint pains, increased calcium loss, urine stasis, increased constipation, muscle atrophy, glucose intolerance, decreased lung expansion, and decreased ability to concentrate urine. It may also predispose her to the effects of sluggish circulation in the lower extremities, resulting in thrombosis. The isometric exercises in Box 1-1 can assist in preventing some of these problems for women who must have long-term bed rest or severely curtailed exercise. These exercises are not aerobic but do maintain conditioning and provide a sense of physical well-being.

ANTEPARTUM NUTRITION

Nutrition plays a significant role in fetal well-being and in the prevention and treatment of a high risk pregnancy. To give adequate counseling the nurse caring for high risk patients must have knowledge of nutrition needs, modifications, and risks of potential deficiencies.

Nutrient Needs

Adequate nutrients are critical for cell growth to take place during pregnancy. A 25% deficit in needed calories and protein can interfere with the synthesis of deoxyribonucleic acid (DNA). The cells that are undergoing rapid division at the time of insult will be most damaged (Luke, 1994; Worthington-Roberts, Williams, 1997). During the first 2 months of pregnancy a deficit in adequate nutrients can have teratogenic effects or cause a spontaneous abortion. After the second month a nutritional deficit can impede fetal growth, causing an SGA infant or a small-brain-growth infant (Kretchmer, Zimmermann, 1997). These infants may be unable to attain their potential in stature, intellect, and future health (Kretchmer, Zimmermann, 1997; Luke and others, 1993; Perez-Escamilla and Pollitt, 1992). After 24 weeks of gestation, a nutritional deficit is associated with a significant increase in preterm delivery and decreased fetal stores of nutrients, especially calcium, magnesium, and iron (Kretchmer and Zimmermann, 1997). Cell division occurs by two processes: (1) hyperplasia, or an increase in cell number, and (2) hypertrophy, or an increase in the size of the cell. If the insult occurs during hyperplastic cell division, the number of cells will be permanently reduced. This can cause mental retardation, even in the United States, where

Box 1-1

Exercises for Pregnant Women on Therapeutic Bed Rest

1. **Kegel exercise**

   Lying on your back at a left tilt or sitting up, tighten your pelvic floor muscles (as if stopping and starting your urine). Hold for three counts and then relax.

2. **Abdominal breathing**

   Lying on your back at a left tilt with knees bent, breathe in deeply, letting your abdominal wall rise. Exhale slowly through your mouth as you tighten your stomach muscles.

3. **Bridging**

   Lying on your back at a left tilt with knees bent, raise your hips off the bed while keeping your shoulders down *(see figure below).*

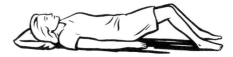

4. **Curl-ups**

   Lying on your back at a left tilt with knees bent, put your hands on your stomach. Lift head and shoulders up (tuck your chin); keep small of back against bed *(see figure below).*

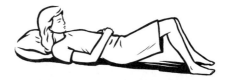

5. **Leg sliding**

   Lying on your back at a left tilt with knees bent, slide your leg out slowly, straightening your knees. Keep small of your back flat against the bed. Slowly pull both knees back up *(see figure below).*

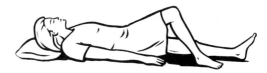

6. **Modified leg raises**

   Lying on your back at a left tilt with one knee bent, bend opposite knee up toward your chest; then straighten leg by kicking up toward ceiling and lower to bed. Repeat with first bent knee.

Continued

Box 1-1

Exercises for Pregnant Women on Therapeutic Bed Rest—cont'd

7. **Abduction**
   Lying on your back at a left tilt with knees bent, let your knees come apart and then squeeze them back together.
8. **Ankle circles**
   Pump ankles up and down. Circle in both directions while resting right ankle on left knee. Repeat with left ankle on right knee.
9. **Arm lifts**
   Exhale deeply through your nose as you lift one arm up to the side over your head. The sides of your chest should expand. Exhale as you bring your arm down. Repeat with opposite arm.

nutritional concerns are frequently overlooked. Malnutrition during pregnancy can also increase the risk for preeclampsia, premature rupture of membranes, and preterm labor (Worthington-Roberts, Williams, 1997). Excessive weight gain can have deleterious effects as well. Labor dystocia and birth trauma are two such deleterious effects related to high birth weight. These infants tend to be at greater risk of obesity in later life (Johnson and others, 1992; Kretchmer, Zimmerman, 1997).

Protein

Protein, 60 to 70 g daily or about 1 g/kg/day (National Research Council, 1989), is very important in supporting the increased embryonic-fetal cellular growth, in promoting the increased maternal blood volume, and possibly in facilitating the prevention of preeclampsia. To prevent the development of anemia, an adequate intake of iron, folic acid, and vitamins B_6 and B_{12}, as well as protein, is needed.

Iron

To prevent iron deficiency during pregnancy, 30 mg of iron is needed per day (National Research Council, 1989). Foods high in iron include meat and plant foods, such as legumes, dried fruits, whole grains, and green leafy vegetables. Iron from plant foods is less well absorbed by the body, but absorption can be improved by eating these foods with a food high in vitamin C. Caffeine beverages should be avoided or drunk between meals, since they interfere with iron absorption. Routine supplemental iron is being questioned for well-nourished pregnant women for the following reasons (Allen, 1994; Barrett and others, 1994; Hemminki, Meriläinen, 1995; Long, 1995):

1. As gestational age progresses, iron absorption correspondingly increases, averaging 7% at 12 gestational weeks, 36% at 24 gestational weeks, and 66% at 36 gestational weeks.
2. There is a normal drop in hemoglobin (normal levels are 10.4 to 13.2 g/ml) during pregnancy related to normal hemodilution.
3. Research studies have failed to provide conclusive evidence that routine supplemental iron benefits fetal growth or pregnancy.
4. Iron supplements increase the red blood cell mass and size of the red blood cell, which can increase blood viscosity and the risk of placental infarct.
5. Supplemental iron has been shown to lower zinc absorption.

To determine who should receive iron supplementation, the Institute of Medicine's *Iron Deficiency Anemia 1993* report (Earl, Woteki, 1993) encourages the use of hemoglobin, hematocrit, and serum ferritin values. The serum ferritin value reflects iron reserves. A ferritin value less than 12 µg/dl in the presence of a low hemoglobin value (<11.0 g/dl in the first trimester, <10.5 g/dl in the second, and <11 g/dl in the third) indicates iron deficiency anemia. Supplemental iron would be appropriate. In the presence of a low hemoglobin value, a normal serum ferritin value (>12 µg/dl) suggests that the anemia is not caused by iron deficiency and iron supplementation is less likely to be therapeutic (Allen, 1994; Engstrom, Sittler, 1994; Suitor, 1994).

When prophylactic iron supplementation is used, 30 mg of ferrous iron in the form of ferrous gluconate, 300 mg daily, or ferrous sulfate, 150 mg daily, should be given after 12 weeks of gestation (Niebyl, 1996). For best absorption, instruct the woman to take the supplemental iron between meals. Ascorbic acid does not increase absorption of iron supplements in ferrous form.

Folate

Folic acid is intimately involved in all DNA synthesis and functions as a coenzyme in amino acid metabolism. Therefore this vitamin is essential to all cell division such as the fetus, placenta, and maternal red blood and protein synthesis. Folic acid deficiency has been associated with an increased occurrence of neural tube defects (Glanville and Cook, 1992; Medical Research Council Vitamin Study Research Group, 1991; Romanczuk, Brown, 1994). The Committee on Genetics, American Academy of Pediatrics (1993), recommends all women of childbearing age capable of becoming pregnant consume 400 μg of folic acid daily. Folic acid is commonly found in dark-green, leafy vegetables, citrus fruits, eggs, legumes, and whole grains. The U.S. Food and Drug Administration (FDA) has established new rules under which specified grain products are fortified with approximately 140 μg of folic acid, effective January 1998.

Therefore if the woman is eating at least five servings of fruits and vegetables and includes whole or fortified grains in her diet, supplementation is not necessary. If the diet is inadequate or the patient is at risk of folic acid deficiency because of cigarette smoking or drug or alcohol abuse, a folic acid supplement of 400 μg/day (0.4 mg/day) is recommended throughout the childbearing years (American College of Obstetricians and Gynecologists, 1993; Centers for Disease Control and Prevention, 1992). If the mother has a personal obstetric history of a major central nervous system anomaly, such as a neural tube defect, a 4 mg/day dosage of folate is recommended. This should start before conception and continue through the first 3 gestational months (Committee on Genetics, American Academy of Pediatrics, 1993). Such supplementation can be met by prescribing one prenatal vitamin per day, containing 1 mg of folic acid, plus three 1-mg folate tablets per day (Rose, Mennuti, 1994).

Zinc

During pregnancy the diet should contain 15 mg of zinc each day. Zinc is commonly found in nuts, meats, whole grains, legumes, and dairy products. A deficiency of zinc during pregnancy increases the risk of intrauterine growth retardation, premature rupture of membranes, and preterm labor (Long, 1995; Worthington-Roberts, Williams, 1997). This deficiency may be the result of various cell-mediated immunologic dysfunctions (Luke and others, 1993). Other risks that increase when a zinc deficiency is present in the mother are a postdate pregnancy, bleeding disorders, protracted labor related to incoordinated uterine activity, and increased cervical and vaginal lacerations.

Sodium

Restricted sodium intake, as well as excessive intake, can cause problems during pregnancy. A restricted sodium intake can interfere with adequate maternal blood volume increase. An excessive sodium intake can increase the sensitivity of the blood vessel wall to angiotensin, causing vasoconstriction. Thus an average sodium intake of 2 to 3 g/day is considered therapeutic during pregnancy (Sullivan, Martin, 1994; Worthington-Roberts, Williams, 1997).

Minerals

According to the 1989 U.S. Recommended Daily Allowances (RDAs), the pregnant woman needs 1200 mg of calcium, 1200 mg of phosphorus, and 320 mg of magnesium. A significant correlation between adequate calcium and a decreased risk of preeclampsia and preterm labor has been demonstrated (Repke, 1994). Tetany or leg cramps, which occur in 5% to 30% of all pregnant women, have been associated with decreased calcium or magnesium (Worthington-Roberts, Williams, 1997). Excessive phosphorus, as opposed to a phosphorous deficiency, is more often a problem because of its presence in many foods, including processed foods and soft drinks. A high intake of phosphorus can upset the calcium/phosphorus balance and subsequently contribute to a calcium deficiency.

Assessment

To determine if the pregnant woman is obtaining adequate nutrition and to prevent nutrition-related complications, the nurse must conduct an ongoing assessment. To assess the nutritional needs and status of the pregnant woman, her pattern of weight gain, prepregnancy weight, daily activities, and dietary intake should be evaluated throughout the pregnancy. The formation of fatty and lean body tissues is important. These act as a reserve for energy that the fetus can draw on during the last part of pregnancy and provide a source of energy for labor and delivery and during lactation.

Weight Gain

An average weight gain during pregnancy (Table 1-1) should be between 25 and 35 pounds according to the Food and Nutrition Board of the National Academy of Science (Institute of Medicine, 1990, 1992). During the first 2 months, a 2- to 4-pound weight gain is considered average, with a gain of about 1 pound per week during the remainder of the pregnancy. Differences in fat deposition and water retention, as well as in body frame, influence the amount and rate of gain. Tall, thin women tend to gain more fat. Overweight women tend to gain fluid. According to the Food

TABLE 1-1   Weight gain during pregnancy

Weight before pregnancy	Recommended weight gain during pregnancy (pounds)
Underweight	28-40
Normal weight	25-35
Moderate overweight (120%-135% of standard)	15-25
Severe overweight (more than 135% of standard)	15

and Nutrition Board of the National Academy of Science (Institute of Medicine, 1990, 1992), a woman whose prepregnancy weight is 90% of the standard weight for her height and age should gain more than the average (28 to 40 pounds) to offset the increased risk of fetal mortality and maternal complications of pregnancy. During the first 2 months, the woman should gain the pounds she is underweight, with a gain of 1 pound or more per week during the remainder of the pregnancy. A woman whose prepregnancy weight is 120% to 135% of standard weight for her height and age needs to gain less than average (15 to 25 pounds). She will need to gain only a couple of pounds during the first trimester and then approximately ⅔ pound per week for the remainder of the pregnancy. If she is more than 135% of standard weight, a gain of approximately 15 pounds is recommended by the Food and Nutrition Board of the National Academy of Science (Institute of Medicine, 1990, 1992). However, because of the increased risk of macrosomia related to a prepregnancy maternal overweight state (more than 135% of standard weight for height), some health care providers recommend for these women a nutritious diet that maintains their prepregnancy weight instead of a weight gain. In a multiple-gestation pregnancy, a weight gain of more than 40 pounds has been associated with improved outcome (Keppel, Taffel, 1993).

Food Groups

To ensure that the body receives the needed additional nutrients, a pregnant woman should be encouraged to select high-nutrient foods using the guide to daily food choices given in Table 1-2. She should select servings from each of the food groups: protein, grains, milk and milk products, fruits, and vegetables (Table 1-2).

TABLE 1-2 Guide to daily food choices

Food groups	Adolescents (≤17 yr)	Adults (≥18 yr)
Protein	6 oz	6 oz
Grains	6-11 servings	6-11 servings
Fruits and vegetables	5-9 servings	5-9 servings
1 yellow fruit or vegetable		
1 vitamin C fruit or vegetable		
1 green leafy vegetable		
Dairy	5 servings	4 servings
Fats and sweets	Cautious use	Cautious use

Examples of servings from the protein group are a 1-ounce serving of meat, one egg, ½ cup of cooked legumes, 2 teaspoons of peanut butter, or ¼ cup of nuts or seeds. In the grain group at least three servings should be of whole grains. Calorie-laden foods, void of nutrients, and fried foods should be avoided. These foods increase the number of calories but do not supply the body with any nutrients. Thus they promote an abnormal weight gain. In addition, social habits such as alcohol intake, smoking, and drug abuse, if continued during pregnancy, will interfere with adequate absorption and intake of various nutrients (refer to Chapter 25).

Referrals

When obvious deficiencies cannot be met using a balanced meal plan, arrange a consultation with a registered dietitian. Cultural or religious practices can also influence and complicate nutritional intake. Careful planning in such situations may allow for alternative selections of foods that provide adequate nutrition while still meeting cultural and religious practices. Financial aid agencies, such as the Special Supplementary Food Program for Women, Infants, and Children (WIC), can be used if income is inadequate for purchase of healthful foods.

Caffeine

Caffeine is found widely in such sources as coffee, teas, colas, and chocolate. It does cross the placenta and reach the developing fetus. Some studies have reported an increased incidence of lowered infant birth weight and spontaneous abortions (Narod and others, 1991). However, the data from other studies have not been consistent in demonstrating these increased risks (McKim, 1991; Mills and others, 1993). Although the research data are inconsistent, the FDA advises that pregnant women eliminate or limit consumption of caffeine-containing beverages (Worthington-Roberts, Williams, 1997).

Hyperemesis Gravidarum

Hyperemesis is a condition characterized by severe nausea and vomiting with weight loss and dehydration. It may be seen more frequently in patients with hydatidiform mole, advanced diabetes, anorexia nervosa/bulimia, or gastrointestinal diseases such as peptic ulcers. Many explanations have been postulated in the literature, including the following:

1. High levels of human chorionic gonadotropin (HCG)
2. High levels of hydrochloric acid (HCl)
3. Increased glucose drain on maternal metabolism
4. Psychogenic factors

Thus far, these have not proven to be causes, because these same factors are present in women without hyperemesis and in women who have mild early pregnancy nausea with or without vomiting.

One major nutritional concern with severe nausea and vomiting is the vitamin B complex and protein deficiency. Various therapies have been tried. Therapies that correlate with supportive therapy seem to be the most effective (Box 1-2). The few women who experience intractable vomiting need close nutritional supervision. Therapy involves life-style change and the following stepwise approach:

1. Prevention
2. Remedies
3. Increased dietary sources of potassium and magnesium (Boxes 1-3 and 1-4)
4. Pharmacologic management, including pyridoxine, promethamine (Phenergan), prochlorperazine (Compazine), diphenhydramine (Benadryl), meclizine, thiethylperazine (Torecan), metoclopramide (Reglan), doxylamine (Unisom), and dimenhydrinate (Dramamine), although none of these have FDA approval for any use in pregnancy
5. Intravenous formula for nutrients and supplementation as follows: add one multivitamin injection, 10 mg pyridoxine, and 2 g magnesium sulfate (192 elemental magnesium) to 1 L of lactated Ringer's solution; administered for 2 hours (Table 1-3)

Box 1-2
Suggested Interventions for Nausea and Vomiting

Prevention
- Eat small amounts of food every 2-3 hours
- Eat low-fat protein foods, such as lean meat, broiled or canned fish, skinless chicken, eggs, and boiled beans
- Drink soups and other liquids between meals, rather than with meals, which may overly distend the stomach and trigger vomiting
- Avoid greasy or fried foods, which can produce nausea because they are hard to digest
- Eat lightly seasoned foods
- Sit upright after meals to reduce gastric reflux
- Have a snack before going to bed or during the night
- Eat a piece of bread or a few crackers before getting out of bed in the morning or whenever nauseated
- Get out of bed slowly and avoid sudden movements
- Avoid brushing teeth immediately after eating

Remedies
- Rest as needed, with feet up and head slightly elevated
- Sometimes fresh air can help (e.g., take a short walk or open windows)
- Drink herbal teas such as raspberry leaf and chamomile

Data from Newman V, Fullerton J, Anderson P: JOGNN 22(6): 483-490, 1993.

Box 1-3
Foods Rich in Potassium

Fruits	**Fruit juices**	**Vegetables**
Avocado	Apricot nectar	Broccoli
Bananas	Grapefruit	Cooked dry beans
Cantaloupe	Orange	Peanuts
Dates	Pineapple	Potatoes
Dried figs	Prune	Spinach
Prunes	Tomato	Dark yellow or orange
Raisins		squash
Watermelon		Yams
Dried apricots		

Box 1-4
Food Sources of Magnesium

Foods rich in magnesium
Vegetables
Spinach
Swiss chard
Nuts and seeds
Nuts
Pumpkin seeds
Sunflower seeds

Foods moderately rich in magnesium
Fruits
Avocado
Vegetables
Beans, including garbanzo, kidney, navy, pinto, or soy
Beet greens
Broccoli
Lima beans
Tofu
Cereals and grains
Cereal: bran or whole wheat
Wheat germ
Whole wheat bread or muffin
Nuts and seeds
Peanuts
Peanut butter

TABLE 1-3 Nutrient composition of one suggested formula for intravenous supplementation

Nutrients	Pregnancy RDA	Actual intake using D_5 lactated Ringer's solution
Vitamin A (IU)	4000	3300
Vitamin B_{12} (μg)	2.2	5
Vitamin C (mg)	70	100
Vitamin D (IU)	400	200
Vitamin E (IU)	15	10
Calcium (mg)	1200	80
Niacinamide (mg)	17	40
Potassium (mg)	2000	156
Magnesium (mg)	320	192
Thiamine (mg)	1.5	3.0
Riboflavin (mg)	1.6	3.6
Folic acid (μg)	400	400
Sodium (mg)	500	3381
Biotin (μg)	30-100	60
Pantothenic acid (mg)	447	15
Pyridoxine (mg)	2.2	14
Dextrose (kcal)		170
Chloride (mg)	750	5538

Data from Newman V, Fullerton J, Anderson P: JOGNN 22(6): 483-490, 1993.
RDA, Recommended daily allowance.

6. Enteral feeding

With any of these therapies or interventions, the goal is for the woman to obtain food, nutrients, vitamins, and protein from oral intake.

BIBLIOGRAPHY

General

Brinkman C: Biological adaptation to pregnancy. In Creasy R, Resnik R: *Maternal-fetal medicine: principles and practice,* ed 3, Philadelphia, 1994, Saunders.

Connon J: Gastrointestinal complications. In Burrow G, Ferris T, editors: *Medical complications during pregnancy,* Philadelphia, 1988, Saunders.

Cousins L and others: Screening recommendations for gestational diabetes mellitus, *Am J Obstet Gynecol* 165:493-496, 1991.

Creasy R: Preterm labor and delivery. In Creasy R, Resnik R, editors: *Maternal-fetal medicine: principles and practice,* ed 3, Philadelphia, 1994, Saunders.

Cunningham F, MacDonald P, Gant N: *Williams obstetrics,* ed 18, Norwalk, Conn, 1989, Appleton & Lange.

Reece E and others: Assessment of carbohydrate tolerance in pregnancy, *Obstet Gynecol* 46(1):1-14, 1991.

Scott J and others: *Danforth's obstetrics and gynecology,* ed 6, Philadelphia, 1990, Lippincott.

Varney H: *Nurse midwifery,* Boston, 1987, Blackwell Scientific Publications.

Working Group on High Blood Pressure in Pregnancy: National high blood pressure education program working group report on high blood pressure in pregnancy, *Am J Obstet Gynecol* 163:1689-1712, 1990.

Yen S: Endocrinology of pregnancy. In Creasy R, Resnik R, editors: *Maternal-fetal medicine: principles and practice,* ed 3, Philadelphia, 1994, Saunders.

Exercise

Abrams B, Salvin S: Maternal weight gain pattern and birth weight, *Obstet Gynecol* 86(2):162-169, 1995.

American Academy of Pediatrics & American College of Obstetricians and Gynecologists: *Guidelines for perinatal care,* ed 3, Elk Grove Village, Ill, 1994, The Academy.

American College of Obstetricians and Gynecologists (ACOG): *Exercise during pregnancy and the postpartum period.* Tech Bull no. 189, Washington, DC, 1994, Author.

Creasy R: Preterm labor and delivery. In Creasy R, Resnik R, editors: *Maternal-fetal medicine: principles and practice,* ed 3, Philadelphia, 1994, Saunders.

Erkklola R and others: Flow velocity waveforms in uterine and umbilical arteries during submaximal bicycle exercise in normal pregnancy, *Obstet Gynecol* 79(4):611-615, 1992.

Fishbein E, Phillips M: How safe is exercise during pregnancy? *Obstet Gynecol Neonatal Nurs* 19(1):45-48, 1990.

Goldenberg R and others: Bedrest in pregnancy, *Obstet Gynecol* 84(1):131-136, 1994.

Hackett G and others: The effect of exercise on the uteroplacental Doppler waveform in normal and complicated pregnancies, *Obstet Gynecol* 79(6):919-944, 1992.

Josten L and others: Bedrest compliance for women with pregnancy problems, *Birth* 22(1):1-12, 1995.

Maloni J: Bedrest during pregnancy: implications for nursing, *J Obstet Gynecol Neonatal Nurs* 22(5):422-426, 1993.

Maloni J: Home care of the high risk pregnancy woman requiring bedrest, *J Obstet Gynecol Neonatal Nurs* 23(8):696-706, 1994.

Maloni J: Bedrest and high risk pregnancy, *Nurs Clin North Am* 31(2):313-325, 1996.

Maloni J and others: Physical and psychosocial side effects of antepartum hospital bedrest, *Nurs Res* 42(4):197-203, 1993.

Shangold M: Exercise induced changes in uterine artery blood flow, as measured by Doppler ultrasound, in pregnant subjects, *Am J Perinatol* 4(2):187-188, 1988.

Shroeder C: Women's experience of bedrest in high risk pregnancy, *Image J Nurs* 28(3):253-258, 1996.

Nutrition

Allen L: Nutritional supplementation of the pregnant woman, *Clin Obstet Gynecol* 37(3):587-595, 1994.

American College of Obstetricians and Gynecologists (ACOG): *ACOG Committee Opinion: folic acid for the prevention of recurrent neural tube defects,* no. 120, Washington, DC, 1993, The College.

American College of Obstetricians and Gynecologists (ACOG): *ACOG educational bulletin: nutrition and women,* no. 229, Washington, DC, 1996, The College.

Barrett J and others: Absorption of non-haem iron from food during normal pregnancy, *Br Med J* 309:79-82, 1994.

Centers for Disease Control and Prevention: Recommendations for the use of folic acid to reduce the number of cases of spina bifida and other neural tube defects, *MMWR Morb Mortal Wkly Rep* 41(RR-14):1-7, 1992.

Committee on Genetics, American Academy of Pediatrics: Folic acid for the prevention of neural tube defects, *Pediatrics* 93:408, 1993.

Earl R, Woteki E, editors: *Iron deficiency anemia recommended guidelines for the prevention, detection, and management among US children and women of childbearing age,* Washington, DC, 1993, National Academy Press.

Engstrom J, Sittler C: Nurse-midwifery management of iron-deficiency anemia during pregnancy, *J Nurse Midwifery* 39(suppl):29-34, 1994.

Glanville N, Cook H: Folic acid and prevention of neural tube defects, *Can Med Assoc J* 146(1): 39, 1992.

Hemminki E, Meriläinen J: Long-term follow-up of mothers and their infants in a randomized trial on iron prophylaxis during pregnancy, *Am J Obstet Gynecol* 173:205-209, 1995.

Institute of Medicine, Subcommittee on Nutritional Status and Weight Gain During Pregnancy: *Nutrition during pregnancy,* Washington, DC, 1990, National Academy Press.

Institute of Medicine, Subcommittee for a Clinical Application Guide, Committee on Nutritional Status during Pregnancy and Lactation, Food and Nutrition Board: *Nutrition during pregnancy and lactation: an implementation guide,* Washington, DC, 1992, National Academy Press.

Johnson J, Longmate J, Frentzen B: Excessive maternal weight and pregnancy outcome, *Am J Obstet Gynecol* 167:353-372, 1992.

Keppel K, Taffel S: Pregnancy-related weight gain and retention: implications of the 1990 Institute of Medicine guidelines, *Am J Public Health* 83:1100, 1993.

Kretchmer N, Zimmermann M: *Developmental nutrition,* Boston, 1997, Allyn and Bacon.

Long P: Rethinking iron supplementation during pregnancy, *J Nurse Midwifery* 40(1):36-39, 1995.

Luke B: Nutritional influences on fetal growth, *Clin Obstet Gynecol* 37(3):538-549, 1994.

Luke B, Johnson T, Petrie R: *Clinical maternal-fetal nutrition,* Boston, 1993, Little, Brown.

McKim E: Caffeine and its effects on pregnancy and the neonate, *J Nurse Midwifery* 36(4):226-231, 1991.

Medical Research Council Vitamin Study Research Group: Prevention of neural tube defects: results of the Medical Research Council Vitamin Study, *Lancet* 338:131-137, 1991.

Mills J and others: Moderate caffeine use and the risk of spontaneous abortion and intrauterine growth retardation, *JAMA* 269:593, 1993.

Narod S, de Sanjose S, Victora C: Coffee during pregnancy: a reproductive hazard, *Am J Obstet Gynecol* 164:1109-1114, 1991.

National Research Council: *Report of the subcommittee on the tenth edition of the RDSs, Food and Nutrition Board, Commission of Life Sciences, Recommended Dietary Allowances,* Washington, DC, 1989, National Academy Press.

Newman V, Fullerton J, Anderson P: Clinical advances in the management of severe nausea and vomiting during pregnancy, JOGNN 22(6): 483-490, 1993.

Niebyl J: Iron therapy in pregnancy, *Contemp OB/GYN* 41(3):146-150, 1996.

Perez-Escamilla R, Pollitt E: Causes and consequences of IUGR in Latin America, *Bull Pan Am Health Organ* 26:128-148, 1992.

Repke J: Calcium and vitamin D, *Clin Obstet Gynecol* 37(3):550-557, 1994.

Romanczuk A, Brown J: Folic acid will reduce risk of neural tube defects, *MCN Am J Matern Child Nurs* 19(6):331-334, 1994.

Rose N, Mennuti M: Periconceptional folate supplementation and neural tube defects, *Clin Obstet Gynecol* 37(3):605-620, 1994.

Suitor C: Nutritional assessment of the pregnant woman, *Clin Obstet Gynecol* 37(3):501-514, 1994.

Sullivan C, Martin J: Sodium and pregnancy, *Clin Obstet Gynecol* 37(3):558-573, 1994.

Worthington-Roberts B, Williams S: *Nutrition in pregnancy and lactation,* ed 6, Madison, 1997, Brown & Benchmark.

CHAPTER

2

General Nursing Assessment of the High Risk Expectant Family

A pregnancy becomes high risk when the mother or fetus has a significantly increased risk of disability (morbidity) or death (mortality). To achieve an optimal perinatal outcome, high risk factors must be recognized early so that appropriate and timely treatment can be implemented.

Nursing care for the family experiencing a high risk pregnancy focuses on the nurse's independent and collaborative roles. The independent role of the perinatal nurse is to diagnose and treat the expectant family's reactions or their concerns for potential risk of a high risk condition. This is founded on the American Nurses Association's definition of the unique role of the nurse (1980), that is, to diagnose and treat human responses of individuals, families, and groups to actual or potential health problems. The second and equally important role of the perinatal nurse is collaborative management of a high risk condition with other health team members. According to Carpenito (1997), the nurse's collaborative role is to monitor the high risk condition and implement physician-prescribed, as well as nurse-prescribed, interventions to minimize fetal and maternal complications.

PRENATAL ASSESSMENT

We have used the problem-solving process as the framework for patient care. To make appropriate nursing diagnoses, a comprehensive nursing data base must be collected. We chose Gordon's functional health patterns (1994) as the assessment tool, since they are relevant to all conceptual nursing models and provide a systematic method of data collection to determine an individual's or family's functioning response to a potential or actual threat to the optimal physical and emotional pregnancy outcome.

A prenatal assessment guide using the functional health patterns has been developed (Box 2-1). This tool can assist health care providers in their assessment of the expectant mother and family in the acute care setting or in home care. First, it provides a method of assessing prenatal physical and emotional risks to facilitate screening for a high risk complication. Second, it assesses the patient's and family's reactions if a high risk condition develops to facilitate formulation of nursing diagnoses. Third, to facilitate individualized care planning, it enhances assessment of the available supports and resources and the belief system of the family.

NURSING DIAGNOSES AND COLLABORATIVE PROBLEMS

After relating theoretic concepts of the high risk condition, gathering a comprehensive functional health pattern assessment of the patient's and her family's response to the high risk condition, and performing a complete physical assessment, an analysis of the data will define the nursing diagnoses and collaborative problems. The North American Nursing Diagnosis Association (NANDA)–approved nursing diagnoses are used in this book. As outlined by Carpenito (1997), the problem is stated in the form of a nursing diagnosis if the nurse can legally order the definitive interventions to prevent a complication or to achieve the patient-centered goals. The problem is stated in the form of a collaborative problem if the nurse monitors to detect onset or changes in the potential complication of the high risk condition and must collaborate with the physician as to the appropriate interventions or follow physician-prescribed treatment orders. The desired outcomes will then be nurse-centered goals to minimize or appropriately manage the risk.

HIGH RISK FACTORS

Factors that significantly influence the pregnancy's outcome may be divided into categories.

Text continued on p. 44

Box 2-1
Functional Health Pattern Assessment for High Risk Pregnancy

Health-perception/health management pattern

Individual assessment

Perceived or actual prenatal risks (ask questions in all the following areas)

Demographic risks: geographic location/socioeconomic status/educational attainment/marital status/age/racial-ethnic group/occupational hazards/blood type

Behavioral characteristics

When first sought prenatal care

Patterns of use and perception of effect on health of self and fetus of alcohol, tobacco, prescription and nonprescription drugs, illegal drugs, exposure to passive smoke, and sexual contact with an illegal drug user

Patterns of utilizing health screening such as physical, dental, and eye checkups, Pap smears, and immunizations (especially rubella)

Seat belt use

Breast self-examination pattern

Current general health (any of the following health problems?)

Anemia (severe)

Cardiac disease

Chronic hypertension

Chronic lung disease

Diabetes

Emotional problems

Metabolic diseases such as phenylketonuria (PKU)

Phlebitis

Renal disease

Seizure disorders

Sexually transmitted disease

Thyroid disease

Ulcers

Past medical history (describe your past health)

Childhood diseases

Emotional problems

Illnesses

Sexually transmitted diseases

Surgeries

Family medical history (any health problems in your family? If yes, what?)

Emotional problems

Genetic defects

Illnesses such as hypertension, diabetes, multiple birth, diethylstilbestrol (DES), or prematurity

Continued

Box 2-1
Functional Health Pattern Assessment for High Risk Pregnancy—cont'd

Environmental/chemical exposure (Since becoming pregnant, have you been exposed to any of the following factors or agents?)
Heavy metals
Organic solvents
Pollutants
Radiation/x-ray
Viral infections such as cytomegalovirus, rubella, or toxoplasmosis
Which prenatal health care resources have you utilized or do you plan to utilize, such as childbirth education classes, support groups, social services, and community agencies?
What are your expectations of the health care providers?
Do you wish to write a birth plan?
Do you desire to maintain control?
Family assessment
Who in the family determines such things as what the family eats, exercise pattern, or visits to the doctor?
What does your family do to stay healthy?
Community assessment
What, if anything, does the community do to help/hinder your attempts to be healthy?
What, if anything, does the community do to help/hinder you in raising children?
Cultural practice assessment
Beliefs about immunization: do you plan to immunize your child?
Beliefs about health care
How often do you or your family get routine checkups?
What is your belief about health care during pregnancy?
Nutritional-metabolic pattern
Individual assessment
What is a typical daily food and fluid intake/eating times/food likes and dislikes/dieting pattern/ways you like your meat cooked (rare)?
What is your understanding as to the needed dietary changes during (use the appropriate situation) normal pregnancy/high risk pregnancy/adolescent pregnancy/multiple gestation/lactation/postdelivery recovery?
Appetite?
Supplements used such as iron, vitamins, minerals?
Food restrictions, cravings, and pica?
What eating-related discomforts such as nausea or vomiting/leg cramps/heartburn/bleeding gums are you experiencing?
What is your nutritional status: height and weight/amount of weight gained or lost/condition of skin, teeth, hair, nails?

Box 2-1
Functional Health Pattern Assessment
for High Risk Pregnancy—cont'd

Family assessment
Which family member makes the nutrition-related decisions?
Is the cost of nutritional foods within the family's budget?
Community assessment
Are stores reasonably accessible to the expectant family?
Are any community resources such as WIC or food stamp program needed?
Is the water supply safe for the expectant mother or newborn?
Cultural practices assessment
Are there any cultural practices regarding foods or fluids that you or your
family value?

Elimination pattern
Individual assessment
Urinary elimination pattern: changes or problems perceived such as
frequency, odor, or burning pain on urination
Bowel elimination pattern: changes or problems perceived such as
flatulence, constipation, odor, or hemorrhoids
Remedies used
Family assessment
What is the family's use of laxatives?
If the family has an indoor cat, who changes the cat litter box?
Pest control/garbage disposal
Community assessment
What are the sanitation and disposal practices of the community?
Are there any hazardous waste disposal plants near the community?
What is the quality of air?
Cultural practices assessment
Are there any cultural practices in the area of elimination that you or your
family value?
When do you think a child should be toilet trained?

Activity-exercise pattern
Individual assessment
What is usual pattern of exercise, activity, use of leisure time, and
recreation?
Do you plan to change this pattern during pregnancy/high risk condition/
postdelivery recovery in any way? Be specific.
Are you experiencing any problems that interfere with the desired or
expected pattern of activity?
Since becoming pregnant, what has been your level of energy?
Have you been experiencing any discomforts such as backache, round
ligament pain, or varicosities?

Continued

Box 2-1

Functional Health Pattern Assessment for High Risk Pregnancy—cont'd

If a high risk condition develops and limited physical activity or bed rest becomes necessary, do you understand the reason for the treatment?

What are your bathing/dental hygienic practices?

Family assessment

What is the family's activity/leisure/recreational pattern?

Does the family have adequate transportation available?

Community assessment

What activities are available in the community for an expectant and a new family?

Cultural practices assessment

What activities/movements are prescribed during pregnancy or puerperium?

What activities/movements are forbidden during pregnancy or puerperium, such as bathing/type of water used?

Sleep-rest pattern

Individual assessment

What is your pattern of sleep, rest, and relaxation/problems with/remedies utilizing?

Which positions do you use to sleep?

Family assessment

What are the family's sleeping arrangements and plans for where the new baby will sleep?

When do you believe a child should start sleeping through the night?

Community assessment

Do any community activities interfere with the family's sleep?

Cultural practices assessment

How much sleep should the pregnant woman get?

In what position should one sleep?

Cognitive-perceptual pattern

Individual assessment

Do you find it easy or difficult to communicate with family members or health care providers?

Is there any information you would like to know about the following?

Reproduction

High risk condition at risk for

Screening methods to be ordered

Labor and delivery

Postdelivery recovery

Perception of the needs of the fetus and infant/proposed method to meet these needs

Box 2-1
Functional Health Pattern Assessment for High Risk Pregnancy—cont'd

Knowledge regarding infant care, prior experience/planned method of infant feeding

How do you learn best: teaching method/appropriate strategies/preferred method/level of education/language spoken/readiness and motivation?

Nature and location of pain/discomforts

Adequacy of sensory modes/prosthesis used

Family assessment

Family's decision-making process and pattern of communication: which family member decides whether to attend a childbirth education class?

Community assessment

Community resources needed and available such as a support group if a high risk condition develops or referral to facilitate teaching

Cultural practices assessment

What educational goals do you have for yourself, this child?

How should one respond to pain?

Self-perception/self-concept pattern

Individual assessment

How do you feel about yourself: general mood/body image/sense of worth/sense of control over life?

How do you feel about your life situation (use appropriate situation): health status/being pregnant/physical and emotional changes that you are experiencing/parenthood/pregnancy loss?

How would you describe your childhood?

Family assessment

What is your significant other's response to the present life situation (use the appropriate situation): the pregnancy/high risk condition/your physical and emotional changes/parenthood/pregnancy loss?

How would the father-to-be describe his childhood?

What is the general family's feeling?

What is the response of the other family members to the pregnancy, that is, siblings?

Community assessment

What are the housing conditions where you live?

What would you say is the overall feeling in your neighborhood?

Cultural practices assessment

Are there any cultural practices where you live that will influence parenting?

Role-relationship pattern

Individual assessment

Do you feel loved and secure in your family relationship?

What are your home responsibilities: child care, housework?

Continued

Box 2-1

Functional Health Pattern Assessment for High Risk Pregnancy—cont'd

What is your occupation: present/former?

Describe your work environment, commuting distance, hours at work, stress level, involvement in work activities such as lifting or standing, exposure to chemicals or infections.

What are your hobbies?

What is your perception of how pregnancy/a high risk condition will affect your responsibilities?

Anticipatory guidance: what would you do if you had to be hospitalized for a few days, or who will take care of your home/other children while you are in the hospital to have your baby?

Describe your greatest concern.

Family assessment

What is your family composition/living arrangements?

What are the responsibilities in the home/at work/in the community of each family member?

What is your and your significant other's perception of how parenthood will affect the future activities and plans of the family?

Community assessment

Referral services needed such as homemaker/child care/financial assistance

Cultural practices assessment

What is the family's beliefs about the role of the father during pregnancy, during labor, and in child care?

Sexuality/reproductive pattern

Individual assessment

Are your sexual relationships satisfying during this pregnancy?

Are you experiencing any sexuality problems?

How are you dealing with the modified or restricted sexual activity if indicated because of a high risk condition?

Menstrual history: length of menstrual cycles/length of period/last normal menstrual period/estimated date of delivery

Contraceptive history: method used/problems experienced/knowledge of alternative methods/plan for future contraception

Previous obstetric history

  Gravid/para (FPAL)/dates of previous pregnancies?

  History of spontaneous abortions/induced abortions/ectopic pregnancy/ abruptio placentae/placenta previa?

  History of low-birth-weight or large-for-gestational-age (LGA) infants?

  History of multiple birth?

  History of birth defects or intrauterine fetal death?

  History of preterm birth?

Box 2-1
Functional Health Pattern Assessment
for High Risk Pregnancy—cont'd

History of labor dystocia/operative delivery/breech delivery?

History of Rh or ABO incompatibility?

History of a high risk pregnancy complicated with gestational diabetes or preeclampsia?

History of postpartum depression?

Current obstetric status

When sought prenatal care?

Multiple gestation?

Fetal presentation?

Experiencing any bleeding?

Experiencing any complications?

Fundal height/quickening/gestational age when first heard FHR correlates with gestational age?

Diagnostic tests such as hemoglobin/urinalysis/blood sugar within normal limits?

Family assessment

What is the desired family size?

What is your significant other's sexuality response to pregnancy/sexual restrictions if necessary?

Community assessment

Community's patterns of reproduction: birth rates/teenage pregnancy rate/maternal and fetal mortality

Community resources: various prenatal care alternatives/family planning/abortion services/adoption services

Cultural practices assessment

Are there any beliefs about sexual practices during pregnancy that you practice?

Where should delivery take place?

What does the due date mean to you?

Coping/stress tolerance pattern

Individual assessment

Perceived life stressors

Is there anything in particular that is worrying you about yourself/significant other/your baby?

What do you think about childbirth/high risk condition/hospitalization?

Have you had or are you anticipating any other major life changes during this pregnancy?

How do you feel you are adjusting to the role of parent/life-style changes?

Have you ever been physically or emotionally abused by someone?

Have you ever been forced into participating in sexual activities?

Continued

Box 2-1
Functional Health Pattern Assessment
for High Risk Pregnancy—cont'd

Losses experienced
   Have you ever had an infant or a child who died?
   Have you had a recent death in your immediate family?
   Are you still grieving about the death?
Coping mechanisms utilized: what do you do when you are upset?
Perception of support system
   Who comforts you when you have a problem?
   Who is the person you talk with about your pregnancy?
   The baby's father is _____.
   Your mother is _____.
   What can the nurses do to provide you with more comfort and security?
Family assessment
Is there anything in particular that is worrying your significant other/family?
Community assessment
Does the community where you live cause you added stress?
Referral services needed: social worker/community health nurse/mental
   health nurse/mental health referral/support group
Cultural practices assessment
Are there any religious practices that are important to you?
Do you feel your faith in God is helpful to you? If so, how?
Is prayer important to you?

Demographic Characteristics

Geographic Location

Factors such as altitude, soil conditions, environmental exposures, and water contamination that are indigenous to certain regions of the United States should be considered.

Socioeconomic Status

Factors such as substandard living conditions, poor hygiene, inadequate nutritional status, limited income, and limited educational level are interrelated in adverse perinatal outcomes.

Educational Attainment

The risk of adverse prenatal outcome decreases as the length of education increases, probably related to the socioeconomic index, improved nutrition, and decreased substance use (Cogswell, Yip, 1995).

Marital Status

An unmarried mother or a mother from a broken marriage has twice the risk of an adverse perinatal outcome, which is usually related to a low birth weight and inadequate prenatal care (McIntosh and others, 1995).

Maternal Age

The ideal childbearing age is 20 to 34 years old, with a slightly increased adverse perinatal outcome for mothers younger than 20 years or older than 34 years (Cogswell, Yip, 1995).

Racial/Ethnic Origin

In different countries the ethnic group at risk will vary. In the United States, African-Americans are at increased risk (Centers for Disease Control and Prevention, 1995). According to the latest census statistics, overall maternal mortality was 5.7%. For African-American women, maternal mortality was 18.6% (Centers for Disease Control and Prevention, 1995). The reasons for the disparity in maternal mortality are unclear, but possible suppositions include lack of access to or use of early prenatal care and differences in pregnancy-related morbidity.

Occupational Hazards

A broad range of adverse perinatal risks are related to various occupational health hazards. Therefore the perinatal nurse has an important role in screening women as to various occupational hazards. Occupational hazards can be grouped into three categories (see Table 2-1 for potential hazards and possible effects). The risk to the growing fetus depends primarily on dose, timing of exposure, and maternal and fetal susceptibility (Mattison, 1992). The greatest risk for a congenital abnormality is during embryogenesis (the first 60 days). However, brain development can be affected significantly between 8 and 15 weeks of gestation and even up through the twenty-fifth week (Lidstrom, 1990). Exposure to occupational hazards later in the pregnancy most frequently restricts fetal growth. According to Bentur and Koren (1991), the most common hazardous occupational exposure encountered during pregnancy is lead. Persons most at risk for lead exposure are glass-staining artists and automotive and

TABLE 2-1 Occupational hazards and possible reproductive risk

Occupational hazards	Possible reproductive risk
Chemical hazards	
Lead	Spontaneous abortion, low-birth-weight infants, fetal death, impaired neurologic development, cognitive impairment (Bentur, Koren, 1991; Colie, 1996; Stapleton, 1996)
Passive smoking	Low birth weight (Rubin and others, 1986)
Pesticide	Decreased fertility, congenital anomalies (Keleher, 1991)
Organic solvents	Congenital defects (Bentur, Koren, 1991)
Physical hazards	
Severe fatigue caused by standing more than 3 hr or working long or double shifts	Prematurity, low birth weight (LBW) (Clapp, 1996; Colie, 1996)
Extreme heat (core temperature 38.9° C or more)	Spontaneous abortion; birth defects (Colie, 1996; Paul, 1993)
Noise	Decreased fertility, congenital anomalies, preterm labor, and small for gestational age (SGA) (Lidstrom, 1990)
Vibration	Decreased fertility, spontaneous abortion, preterm labor, and hyperemesis gravidarum (Lidstrom, 1990; Pelmear, 1990)
Radiation such as x-ray	Reduced fertility, congenital anomalies, and chromosome aberrations (Chamberlain, 1991; Keleher, 1991)
Biologic hazards	
Contact in crowded places/contact with a higher risk group such as school children and the sick	If the woman contracts an infectious disease, congenital anomalies and premature rupture of membranes (PROM) (Chamberlain, 1991)
Psychologic hazards	
Stress	Spontaneous abortion, prematurity, pregnancy-induced hypertension (PIH) (Keleher, 1991)

aircraft painters. Video display terminals do not appear to pose any reproductive risk (Bentur, Koren, 1991; Keleher, 1991; Lidstrom, 1990; Paul, 1993).

Behavioral Characteristics

Substance Abuse

Alcohol, tobacco, and illegal drug use is a significant risk factor for perinatal mortality. See Chapter 25 for specific factors.

Failure to Seek Prenatal Care

Failure to seek prenatal care is one of the most important factors influencing pregnancy outcome. It usually reflects a life-style less likely to promote health, especially in nutrition and exposure to fetal toxins such as alcohol, nicotine, and other drugs (Burks, 1992).

Nutritional Status

Inadequate nutritional intake and inadequate prenatal care are the two most significant factors influencing pregnancy outcome. A low prepregnancy weight and an inadequate pregnancy weight gain are important indicators of poor nutritional status. An inadequate pregnancy weight gain especially during the second trimester may negatively affect the maternal plasma value, reducing the transfer of nutrients to support appropriate growth (Abrams, Selvin, 1995).

Psychosocial Stressors

Extreme maternal stress and anxiety can negatively influence pregnancy outcome. They can affect the mother's health by compromising her immune state, increasing the risk of preterm labor, and decreasing fetal birth weight (Homer and others, 1990; Rothberg, Lits, 1991).

Abuse/Violence

Battering is a real problem, with the risk increasing during pregnancy (Campbell, 1995). Physical abuse during pregnancy increases the risk of preterm deliveries and low-birth-weight infants, possibly related to abdominal trauma and subsequent placental damage, infection from forced sex, or stress (Campbell, 1995). There is also an increased risk of child abuse once the baby is born (Campbell, 1994).

Medical Status

If the mother has a medical condition (see Unit IV) or is at high risk for developing a medical complication, the risk for an adverse perinatal outcome increases.

Obstetric Status

The obstetric variables that have the most significant effect are multiple gestation, malpresentations, and previous obstetric problems (Samueloff and others, 1989).

CONCLUSION

Meticulous, ongoing prenatal assessment is essential to achieve an optimal perinatal outcome. A thorough nursing assessment will focus the nurse toward (1) health-promoting activities that can prevent complications and (2) early recognition of developing complications while treatment is more effective.

BIBLIOGRAPHY

Abrams B, Selvin S: Maternal weight gain pattern and birth weight, *Obstet Gynecol* 86:163-169, 1995.

American Nurses Association: *The nursing practice act,* Kansas City, Mo, 1980, The Association.

Bentur Y, Koren G: The three most common occupational exposures reported by pregnant women: an update, *Am J Obstet Gynecol* 165:429-437, 1991.

Bernhardt J: Potential workplace hazards to reproductive health: information for primary prevention, *J Obstet Gynecol Neonatal Nurs* 19(1):53-62, 1990.

Burks M: Prenatal care, *Nurs Pract* 17(4):34, 1992.

Campbell J: Child abuse and wife abuse: the connections, *Md Med J* 43:165-166, 1994.

Campbell J: Addressing battering during pregnancy: reducing low birth weight and ongoing abuse, *Semin Perinatol* 19(4):301-306, 1995.

Carpenito L: *Nursing diagnosis: application to clinical practice,* ed 7, Philadelphia, 1997, Lippincott.

Centers for Disease Control and Prevention: Differences in maternal mortality among black and white women—United States, *MMWR Morbid Mortal Wkly Rep* 44(1):6-7, 1995.

Chamberlain G: Work in pregnancy, *Br Med J* 302:1070-1073, 1991.

Clapp J III: Pregnancy outcome: physical activities inside versus outside the workplace, *Semin Perinatol* 20(1):70-76, 1996.

Cogswell M, Yip R: The influence of fetal and maternal factors on the distribution of birth weight, *Semin Perinatol* 19(3):222-240, 1995.

Colie C: Preterm labor and delivery in working women, *Semin Perinatol* 17(1):37-44, 1993.

Colie C: Occupational hazards. In Queenan J, Hobbins J, editors: *Protocols for high-risk pregnancies,* ed 3, Mass, 1996, Blackwell Science.

Gordon M: *Nursing diagnosis: process and application,* ed 3, St Louis, 1994, Mosby.

Hein H, Burmeister L, Papke K: The relationship of unwed status to infant mortality, *Obstet Gynecol* 76:763-768, 1990.

Hogue C and others: Overview of the national infant mortality surveillance (NIMS): project design, methods, results, *Public Health Rep* 102:126, 1987.

Homer C, James S, Siegel E: Work-related psychosocial stress and risk of preterm, low birth weight delivery, *Am J Public Health* 80:173-177, 1990.

Keleher K: Occupational health: how work environments can affect reproductive capacity and outcome, *Nurse Pract* 16(1):23-34, 1991.

Keleher K: Primary care for women: environmental assessment of the home, community, and workplace, *J Nurse Midwifery* 40(2):88-96, 1995.

Kleinman J, Kessel S: Racial differences in low birth weight, *N Engl J Med* 317:749, 1987.

Lemasters G: Epidemiology methods to assess occupational exposures and pregnancy outcomes, *Semin Perinatol* 17(1):18-27, 1993.

Lidstrom I: Pregnant women in the workplace, *Semin Perinatol* 14(4): 329-333, 1990.

Mattison D: Minimizing toxic hazards to fetal health, *Contemp OB/GYN* 35(8):81-100, 1992.

McIntosh L, Roumayah N, Bottoms S: Perinatal outcome of broken marriage in the inner city, *Obstet Gynecol* 85(2):233-236, 1995.

Paul M: Physical agents in the workplace, *Semin Perinatol* 17(1):5-17, 1993.

Pelmear P: Low frequency noise and vibration: role of government in occupational disease, *Semin Perinatol* 14(4):322-328, 1990.

Rothberg A, Lits B: Psychosocial support for maternal stress during pregnancy: effect on birth weight, *Am J Obstet Gynecol* 165(2):403-407, 1991.

Rubin D and others: Effect of passive smoking on birth weight, *Lancet,* pp 415-417, Aug 23, 1986.

Samueloff A and others: Ranking risk factors for perinatal mortality, *Acta Obstet Gynecol Scand* 68(8):677-682, 1989.

Stapleton R: Silent hazard: lead poisoning in utero, *Childbirth Instructor Magazine* 6(3):12-14, 1996.

CHAPTER

3

Assessment of
Fetal Well-Being

Antepartum and intrapartum assessment of the fetus has gained momentum in the past 20 to 25 years. In the past it was assumed if the mother was well, the fetus was well. Several means of fetal surveillance are now available, and both patients (mother and fetus) can be assessed.

Sophisticated technology and biochemical analyses aid in the care of both patients. Nurses working in modern obstetric units must understand a myriad of technologic and laboratory data to effectively care for the mother and fetus. At the same time, family-centered concepts of care must be integrated in more creative ways.

FETAL HEART RATE MONITORING
Electronic Monitoring

Electronic fetal heart rate (FHR) monitoring provides a current and continuous observation of indirect, subjective information about fetal oxygenation. Continuous or intermittent FHR tracings provide a convenient and reasonably predictable means of assessing fetal well-being. Electronic FHR monitoring, although controversial, is suggested as a means of reducing perinatal morbidity and mortality.

The most recent U.S. health statistics, from 1990, indicate that overall infant mortality (deaths per 1000 through first year of life) is 9.1:1000 births, ranking the United States twenty-first among industrialized nations (Department of Health Services, 1992). Perinatal deaths (20 weeks of gestation through first 30 days after birth) are 13.8:1000, with morbidity estimated much higher (National Center for Health Statistics, 1991).

In the United States, continuous electronic fetal heart rate monitoring (EFM) has become routine in most hospital peri- natal/maternity centers. Perinatal mortality has improved in the past decade, and EFM is one explanation for the improve- ment. However, morbidity statistics have not improved and raise two main concerns regarding routine use of EFM (Freeman and others, 1991). The first concern involves the effects on the incidence of cerebral palsy (CP). The second concern in- volves the effects of routine continuous EFM on cesarean birth rates.

With improved neonatal care, especially for extremely prema- ture infants, the actual rate of CP has risen slightly in the past 25 years (Freeman and others, 1991). In fact, because of more surviving premature infants and their associated increased risk of birth asphyxia, CP rates are unlikely to improve (Creasy, Resnik, 1994; Freeman and others, 1991).

The most discussed risk of EFM is the rise of cesarean birth rates. In the United States the current cesarean birth rate is 21% to 25% (Creasy, Resnik, 1994; Freeman and others, 1991).

One study examined the cesarean birth rate in more than 7000 births at a large southwestern tertiary perinatal center in a different manner (Radin and others, 1993). Term primiparas, regardless of demographic data, physician practice, complications, inductions, regional anesthesia, or stage of labor when admitted, had an 18% cesarean birth rate. Those with multiple gestations, those with intrauterine fetal death, or those who were less than 35 weeks pregnant were not included in the study. The variables of assigned nurse (there is little to no opportunity for self-assignment) and phases of labor during care were examined. Three discrete groups of nurses were identified regardless of other variables. The low cesarean birth rate group had a cesarean birth rate lower than 5%. The middle group had an overall 18% cesarean birth rate. The high group had a cesarean birth rate as high as 35% to 49%. No significant differences existed in neonatal Apgar scores. This study suggests that some nurses may manage technologic data from EFM to provide expert nursing care and manage patients with epidurals differently, whereas other nurses may use the data solely to report fetal assessment data to the physician to alter medical management and use epidurals as an excuse to psychologically abandon patients who are not experiencing pain. This study warrants further investigation of specific differences in nursing care practices and effects on cesarean birth rates.

Intermittent Auscultation

When done at prescribed intervals and for 60 seconds, especially during and immediately after contractions, intermittent auscultation has been suggested to be equally valuable in predicting fetal outcomes (ACOG, 1995; Freeman and others, 1991). The value of EFM may, in fact, be that we now better understand what we hear. It therefore should not be discarded but, rather, should be used differently by nurses than by physicians for the management of intrapartum care. These studies also used a 1:1 ratio of nurse midwife to patient, with continuous bedside care.

With research findings supporting the use of both EFM and intermittent auscultation, it is apparent that perinatal nurses must understand the use of FHR monitoring. To do this, perinatal nurses must be fully acquainted with the following (Trepanier and others, 1996):

- Physiology and pathophysiology of fetal oxygenation
- Physiologic basis of FHR control
- Instrumentation and the application of external and internal fetal monitoring methods
- Baseline FHR, variability, patterns, periodic rate changes, dysrhythmias, and artifacts (describe effects of maternal contractions on FHR control)
- Nursing process related to EFM
- Skills and techniques for antepartum evaluation of fetal well-being through auscultation, EFM testing, and fetal movement counts
- Newer methods of fetal evaluation, such as biophysical profile and Doppler flow studies

Physiology and Pathophysiology of Fetal Oxygenation

Maternal Circulatory and Cardiovascular Adaptation

One of the most dramatic adaptations to pregnancy is the increase in maternal blood volume by 20% to 100% over prepregnant volume. Plasma increase plateaus around 32 to 34 weeks of gestation. Red blood cells increase in response to the plasma volume. Both volume and blood cell increases are in response to cell proliferation and growth of the uterus, placenta, and fetus.

Under physiologically nonstressful conditions, the vascular system in the maternal pelvic region remains widely dilated. In the presence of stressors, it is capable of marked constriction and reduction of uteroplacental blood supply. The most common and easily preventable stressor is mechanical obstruction of the maternal inferior vena cava and aorta by the gravid uterus when in a supine position. Activation of the maternal autonomic nervous system (ANS) in response to other hemodynamic changes may also trigger marked constriction of the pelvic vasculature, which is physiologically expendable to general maternal circulatory needs.

The usual state of the uterine vasculature is one of low resistance to blood flow. This occurs in part because of new vascularization of the uterus and in response to the systemic influence of estrogens, which increases overall vasodilation. It is estimated that uterine blood now increases from 50 ml/min in early pregnancy to 700 ml/min by term.

Because of vasodilation and increased volume, cardiac output (stroke volume × heart rate) is greater during pregnancy. The heart rate is generally 10 to 15 bpm faster than prepregnant rates, and stroke volume is increased, because of increased blood volume, by approximately 15%. The increase in cardiac output further facilitates uterine blood now during pregnancy.

Uteroplacental-Fetal Exchange

The placenta performs several major organ functions for the fetus. It acts as the following:

- Lung for respiratory functions of exchanging oxygen (O_2) and carbon dioxide (CO_2)
- Gastrointestinal tract for nutritive functions and exchange of waste products and electrolytes
- Skin for thermoregulation
- Kidney for renal functions of acid-base balance and electrolyte homeostasis
- Endocrine organ for production of hormones that promote placental perpetuation
- A barrier to maternal blood and bacteria

After implantation the placenta begins to form the chorionic tissues. By the fourteenth week the placenta is a discrete organ with independent functions and purpose. It is at this point that segments of the placenta, called *cotyledons,* form and connect by vascular channels to the umbilical cord. The surface of the placenta then thins to a membranous, single layer of cells. Maternal blood and fetal blood, although not mixing, are exposed to one another across this membrane. By this exposure, fetal respiration, acid-base and electrolyte homeostasis, nutrition, and excretion take place. The space in which these functions take place is the intervillous space, which contains maternal blood. The fetus therefore totally depends on its mother for most homeostatic mechanisms.

Transfer and exchange of molecules occur in the intervillous space. Molecules enter through the epithelial cells on the surface of the villi and move through the villous stroma and into the fetal capillary vessels within the villi. Molecules pass back and forth between maternal and fetal tissues. Exchange processes are accomplished by means of simple or selective diffusion.

Simple diffusion is a relatively uncomplicated process responsible for the rapid exchange of small molecules, such as O_2, CO_2, water, electrolytes, creatinine, and uric acid, across the placental membrane. Simple diffusion also allows such drugs as antibiotics, narcotics, barbiturates, and anesthetic agents, as well as other potentially harmful drugs, to cross quickly to the fetus. Simple diffusion depends totally on the adequacy of uterine blood flow and on the concentration gradient of the molecules.

Selective transfer is a complex process and therefore occurs more slowly than simple diffusion. It can occur against a concentration gradient by an energy-dependent process. Glucose, for instance, is transported in this manner from stores in the placenta.

Selective transfer can also be actively facilitated by specific enzyme systems. For example, amino acids and buffering substances are transferred using specific enzyme groups to facilitate the process. Selective transfer, by energy-dependent or enzyme-dependent processes, depends on the sufficiency of the placental surface area and placental thickness rather than on uterine blood flow.

Because simple diffusion is faster, taking only minutes, O_2, CO_2, and water can be transported and exchanged rapidly to correct fetal hypoxia if uterine and umbilical blood flow and maternal O_2 are sufficient. On the other hand, the more complex processes of selective transfer, which take hours, cannot correct an acid-base imbalance from hypoxia.

Fetal Capabilities for Withstanding Stressors

The fetus has certain remarkable capabilities that enable it to withstand stressors. Fetal stressors may be caused by physiologic maternal adaptation failures, disease, or mechanical or physiologic obstruction of maternal blood flow through the uterus and into the intravillous space. The fetus is equipped with a high concentration of hemoglobin in plasma (60% hematocrit). Each hemoglobin molecule, because of its unique shape, can be supersaturated with O_2. This is fortunate and necessary because by the time maternal O_2 is transferred to the fetus, the oxygen partial pressure (pO_2) is at best 35 to 40 mm Hg pressure. Compared with an adult pO_2 of 90 to 96 mm Hg pressure, the fetal pO_2 would be inadequate were it not for different fetal hemoglobin. The low fetal pO_2 causes the diffusion gradient to facilitate oxygen delivery from the mother to the fetus.

The fetal heart must have significant hypoxia before myocardial depression occurs. It is only after fetal myocardial depression that significant fetal central nervous system (CNS) hypoxia occurs. Protection from myocardial hypoxia is present in part because of the well-supplied and unimpeded blood supply from the coronary vessels. Impulses travel through the heart, originating at the sinoatrial (SA) node and traveling across the atrioventricular (AV) junction, down the bundle branches, and out the Purkinje fibers in the ventricles. When myocardial depression occurs from hypoxia, cardiac dysrhythmias may occur. The fetus can effectively compensate only by increasing FHR; it cannot increase output by changing the cardiac output.

Function of Amniotic Fluid Related to Evaluation of FHR

Amniotic fluid is produced primarily by maternal blood, although the fetus contributes to the volume through urinary excretion and diuresis. It has a number of functions. Amniotic fluid is a buoyant medium, allowing the umbilical cord to float and preventing entrapment between the wall of the uterus and the fetal body, especially during contractions. This function is imperfect but for the most part effective. The fluid medium, when filled with fetal meconium, also promotes stiffening and loss of flexibility of the cord with extended exposure to meconium.

Physiologic Basis of FHR Control

Central Nervous System Control

Regulation of the fetal heart rate originates in the fetal CNS. By the tenth week of fetal life, both the CNS and the cardiac systems are developed enough to begin and maintain the FHR.

Sympathetic. Initially the sympathetic portion of the rudimentary autonomic nervous system (ANS) is functionally active. The sympathetic branch is responsible for establishing and sustaining the FHR. The normal rate throughout fetal life ranges from 110 to 160 bpm for most babies, tending toward the upper range of 150 to 160 in early fetal life and the middle to lower ranges of 110 to 140 by term. The sympathetic branch of the ANS also serves as a reserve throughout intrauterine life, accelerating the FHR in response to various stimuli as needed for fetal circulation and supporting compensatory responses to physical insults.

Parasympathetic. As the fetus becomes more mature, early in fetal life, the parasympathetic branch of the ANS begins to influence the FHR. It serves as an opposing force against the steady beat sustained by the dominant sympathetic branch. This opposition exerts a differing strength of opposing force on each beat. Three effects of this opposing force are observed on the FHR (Freeman and others, 1991):

1. It gradually slows the intrinsic rate from early gestation through term.
2. It causes beat-to-beat differences in rate per minute of 2 to 3 bpm, referred to as *short-term variability (STV)*.
3. It results in three to six cyclic fluctuations per minute of 5 to 15 beats amplitude, referred to as *long-term variability (LTV)*.

Instrumentation and Application of Fetal Monitoring Methods

Although still indirect and somewhat subjective, EFM gives data slightly more objective than intermittent auscultation and infers information about current and ongoing fetal oxygenation. It does this by calculating and recording an average per minute FHR, indicating STV and LTV, and by providing a continuous graphic printout of rate patterns and periodic changes.

To fully appreciate patterns, it is helpful to have a continuous record for interpretation. Correct application of the monitor methods and an understanding of the operation of the monitor are helpful in obtaining accurate information. Fetal monitors are made by a variety of manufacturers and may have capabilities for external (indirect) monitoring only or for both external and internal (direct) monitoring of FHR and maternal contractions. Other features, such as fetal electrocardiogram (ECG) monitoring, twin monitoring, amnioinfusion, ambulatory monitoring, transmission of strips from one location to another, usually by telephone, central displays, and computer record storage, are also available from most manufacturers. See Fig. 3-1 for types of monitors.

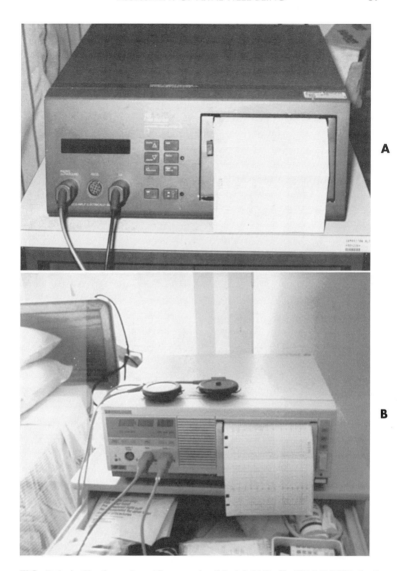

FIG. 3-1 A, Fetal monitor (Corometrics Model 115). **B,** HP M1350A fetal monitor from Hewlett-Packard Co. offers sophisticated monitoring capabilities, including dual-ultrasound twin monitoring, fetal movement profile (FMP), and tocodynamometer transducer.

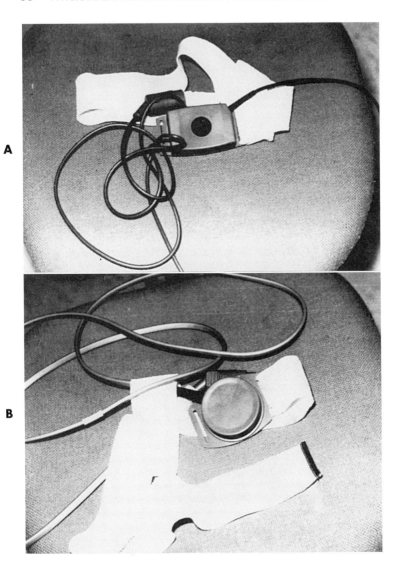

FIG. 3-2 A, Corometrics tocotransducer to be located over best-palpated area of uterus, usually near umbilicus near term. **B,** Corometrics ultrasound transducer to be located over fetal chest wall facing fetal heart.

External (Indirect) Monitoring

The external monitor parts are the tocotransducer (Fig. 3-2, *A*) for assessing contractions and the ultrasound transducer (Fig. 3-2, *B*) for assessing FHR. To place the transducers properly, it is important to ascertain by abdominal palpation how the baby is positioned.

Box 3-1
Advantages and Disadvantages of External Contraction Monitoring

Advantages
Noninvasive
Convenient
Provides continuous record of
  frequency and duration of
  contractions

Disadvantages
Cannot accurately measure
  strength
Loses some information at
  beginning and end of each
  contraction
Restricts patient movement or
  must be frequently adjusted
  with position change

Modified from Tucker SM: *Pocket guide to fetal monitoring and assessment,* ed 3, St Louis, 1996, Mosby.

External contraction monitoring. Near term, the tocotransducer should be placed over the fundus of the uterus, two to three fingers below the top and slightly off center from the umbilicus on the side where the fetal back is palpated. A good rule of thumb for placement of the tocotransducer for preterm contractions is to palpate the uterus for firmness and place the tocotransducer where this is best felt. The placement may be in any quadrant, including those lower than the umbilicus. There is a pressure-sensitive area on the underside of the tocotransducer that must respond to changes in the abdominal wall when the uterus contracts against it. The tocotransducer is secured in place with a belt and tightened only enough to keep it from slipping. The monitor then has an indicated dial or button to artificially set the reference for uterine resting tone, usually between 5 and 15 mm Hg on the graph paper. Box 3-1 presents the advantages and disadvantages of external contraction monitoring.

External FHR monitoring. The ultrasound transducer has sending and receiving crystals encased in a disk. If possible, it should be placed over the fetal chest wall for detection of the best signal. The signal is detected from the motion of the heart valves closing between the atria and ventricles.

The ultrasound transducer selects the complex of two sound waves from the motion of the two atrioventricular valve closures, or it selects the one sound wave that is timed within the logical sequence of events; and then it calculates the rate per minute.

Box 3-2

Advantages and Disadvantages of External FHR Monitoring

Advantages
Noninvasive
Does not require dilation or rupture of membranes
Convenient
Continuous recording of FHR
Can assess presence of cyclic fluctuations (LTV) and absence of both LTV and STV

Disadvantages
Cannot accurately assess presence of STV
Tracing quality affected by maternal position, obesity, and fetal movement

Modified from Tucker SM: *Pocket guide to fetal monitoring and assessment,* ed 3, St Louis, 1996, Mosby.
FHR, Fetal heart rate; *LTV,* long-term variability; *STV,* short-term variability.

Through a system of logic, it samples a set number of valve closures, compares the previous intervals, and decides which to count. The logic system tends to give the appearance of slightly greater rate differences than are truly present. This causes the appearance of "roughness" or a "jiggle" to the line (Freeman and others, 1991). If the rate differences are not logical compared with the previous calculated rates, blanks will appear in the tracing. Blanks also occur when the signal is lost from fetal movement or shift in maternal position. Box 3-2 presents the advantages and disadvantages of external FHR monitoring.

Internal (Direct) Monitoring

Internal monitoring uses different components: (1) an intrauterine pressure catheter (IUPC) (Fig. 3-3, *A*) and (2) a fetal spiral electrode (FSE) (Fig. 3-3, *B*).

Intrauterine pressure catheter. The IUPC may be inserted by qualified registered nurses (RNs) (NAACOG, 1991a). It is inserted before the spiral electrode, in an aseptic manner, into the uterine cavity.

The two types of IUPCs are a fluid-filled system and a solid catheter. The fluid-filled catheter must first be flushed with sterile water; a syringe is left attached to a three-way stopcock at the distal end. The catheter is a flexible, narrow-gauge tube with holes along a short distance and at the proximal end. It is partially enclosed in

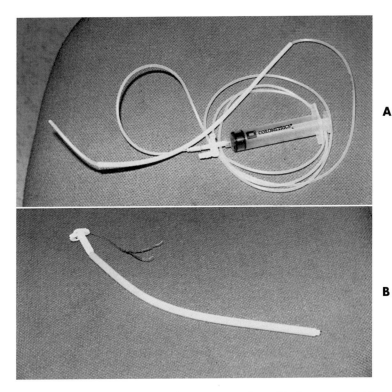

FIG. 3-3 A, Corometrics intrauterine pressure catheter. **B,** Corometrics fetal spiral electrode for attachment to leg plate.

a firmer plastic catheter introducer. The examiner's hand carefully lifts the presenting part and inserts the introducer with the catheter just through the dilated cervix. Then the fluid-filled catheter is carefully advanced to a specific marker visualized on the outside of the perineum. The introducer is drawn back toward the distal end, and the catheter remains behind. The catheter is then taped to the patient's abdomen or thigh. As the uterus contracts and relaxes, the intercavitary pressure is reflected against the fluid-filled catheter. The distal end is connected to a strain gauge and to the monitor. The three-way stopcock and transducer with dome allow the catheter to be referenced to the atmosphere by zeroing, flushing with additional fluid as necessary, and directing the reflected pressure from contractions to the strain gauge. Pressure of contractions is measured in millimeters of mercury (mm Hg).

Another type of IUPC is the closed or solid catheter with the transducer at or near the tip. Some are single-lumen catheters to measure pressure only, and others have a triple lumen to allow pressure monitoring, amnioinfusion, and sampling of the fluid. The solid catheters must be connected to the monitor by a cable and zeroed before placement into the uterine cavity. The triple-lumen catheter also allows the IUPC to be rezeroed after being disconnected and without replacing it with a new catheter. The single-lumen catheter does not allow this option.

Fetal spiral electrode. The FSE may also be placed by qualified RNs. It is attached to the presenting part of the fetus, avoiding such potentially dangerous areas as the fontanels, facial features, or genitalia if breech. The FSE has two color-coded wires attached to it. These are twisted together, and all are encased in an introducer. The examiner identifies the area of the presenting part and then inserts the introducer between the fingers and flush against the presenting part. The distal ends of the wires are rotated counter-clockwise and attached to the presenting part. A leg plate is strapped to the patient's thigh, and the leg plate cord is plugged into the FECG receiver on the monitor. The monitor in this way directly counts from the fetal R wave (the highest amplitude electrical impulse from the fetal heart). It does not need to respond to or disregard other fetal impulses but may count maternal R-R intervals if the fetus is dead. What is plotted on the graph paper is each rate from every R-R interval calculated as it would be for 1 minute. Thus the FSE can accurately assess beat-to-beat rate differences known as STV. Box 3-3 presents advantages and disadvantages of internal monitoring.

Baseline Fetal Heart Rate

The FHR is controlled by the fetal CNS, specifically the ANS. Because that portion of the fetal brain is developed first and is the most rudimentary, it requires a significant degree of hypoxia before FHR control evidences the effects. Observation of an entirely reassuring FHR and patterns predicts adequate CNS oxygenation. However, nonreassuring features are considerably more subjective and of less predictive value for fetal oxygenation. This is secondary to little being known about the degree or length of time of hypoxia (Freeman and others, 1991).

Each examination of a fetal monitor strip should follow the same systematic steps:

1. Evaluate patient history and status.
2. Evaluate contraction frequency, duration, and, if IUPC, intensity and resting tone.

Box 3-3
Advantages and Disadvantages of Internal Monitoring

Advantages

Contractions are measured accurately for:
- Strength
- Duration
- Frequency
- Resting tone

Can accurately assess presence of STV

Is more comfortable

Disadvantages

Requires ruptured membranes and dilation

If prolonged, ruptured membranes may carry a small increase in infection

Possible injury to uterine wall or fetus if forcefully introduced

Modified from Tucker SM: *Pocket guide to fetal monitoring and assessment,* ed 3, St Louis, 1996, Mosby.
STV, Short-term variability.

---

3. Determine the average baseline rate.
4. Describe LTV on external monitor and both LTV and STV on internal monitor.
5. Describe or, when possible, name patterns of periodic rate changes in response to documented stimuli.
6. Diagnose fetal response to stimuli, initiate independent nursing interventions, and collaborate with the physician for medical management.

Rate

Baseline FHR is the average rate lasting at least 10 consecutive minutes, observed as occurring between contractions and in the absence of other stimuli. If contractions are occurring quite close together, the usual place to observe is just before each contraction (Fig. 3-4) (Freeman and others, 1991). The baseline FHR is normally 110 to 160 bpm, although rates from 90 to 110 and from 160 to 180 may also be normal if all other features are reassuring and if that rate is appropriate for gestation, that is, faster in early pregnancy and slower in later pregnancy. Rates above the 160s for more than 10 minutes are termed *tachycardia,* and those below 110 for more than 10 minutes are termed *bradycardia.* Table 3-1 summarizes baseline FHR abnormalities.

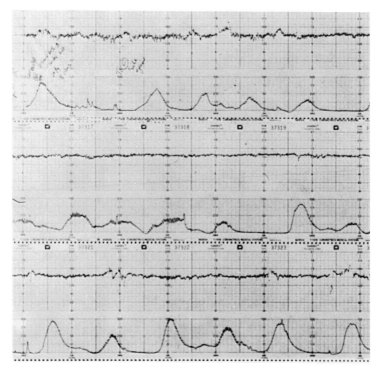

FIG. 3-4 Normal baseline fetal heart rate (FHR). Baseline FHR found between contractions, in absence of periodic changes, and observed in 10-minute segments *(panels 37317 through 37319 in center)* is 150 to 155. This is normal range.
Courtesy John P. Elliott, MD, Phoenix.

TABLE 3-1 Summary of baseline FHR abnormalities

Tachycardia (Fig. 3-5)

Description	Rate greater than 160 for at least 10 consecutive min
Etiology	Acute, short-term hypoxia
	Drugs given to mother such as beta-sympathomimetics (terbutaline, ritodrine)
	Recovery from stress
	Dysrhythmia
	Maternal fever
	Maternal hyperthyroid disease
Mechanism	Sympathetic response
Significance	Serious when greater than 180 bpm
Nursing interventions	Look for cause
	Turn patient to left side
	Hydrate to improve circulating volume
	O_2 at 8-10 L/min by tight face mask
	Reduce stressors (turn off oxytocin [Pitocin], treat maternal fever)

Bradycardia (Fig. 3-6)

Description	Rate less than 100 bpm for at least 10 consecutive min
Etiology	Chronic long-term hypoxia
	Drugs such as beta-blockers (propranolol [Inderal])
	Dysrhythmias
	Can be terminal event after severe stress
	Prolapsed cord
Mechanism	Parasympathetic response
Significance	Serious when less than 80 bpm or lasting more than 10 min
Nursing interventions	Turn side to side or to knee-chest position
	O_2 at 8-10 L/min by tight face mask
	Correct maternal hypotension
	Look for cause such as prolapsed cord
	Prepare for delivery by most expeditious means

Modified from Freeman R and others: *Fetal heart rate monitoring,* Baltimore, 1991, Williams & Wilkins.

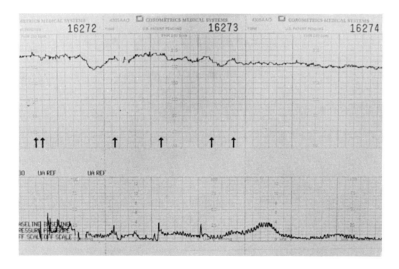

FIG. 3-5 Tachycardia. Baseline fetal heart rate (FHR) *between panels 16272 and 16274* is 180 to 200 bpm. Long-term variability (LTV) is present. *Arrows* are result of maternal use of remote marker to indicate fetal movement.

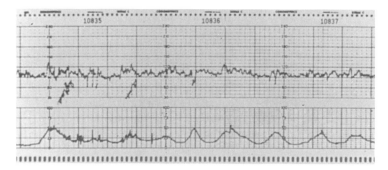

FIG. 3-6 Bradycardia. Baseline fetal heart rate (FHR) is 95 to 105 bpm. Long-term variability (LTV) is present.

Variability

Variability (Freeman and others, 1991) is described as long term (LTV) or short term (STV). It is always assessed in the baseline and therefore between contractions in the absence of other influences, such as accelerations, decelerations, or fetal movement, and for at least 10 minutes.

Long-term variability. LTV is defined as 3 to 6 cyclic fluctuations of 5 to 20 beats amplitude per minute. It is usually described as present, absent, increased, exaggerated, or decreased. The following definitions are useful in determining which descriptor to use (AWHONN, 1993; Freeman and others, 1991).

1. *Present:* 3 to 6 cycles per minute of 5 to 15 beats amplitude (Fig. 3-7, *B*)
2. *Decreased (minimal):* 2 or 3 cycles per minute of 3 to 5 beats amplitude
3. *Absent:* fewer than 3 cycles per minute of less than 3 beats amplitude (Fig. 3-7, *A*)
4. *Increased:* 3 to 6 cycles per minute of 15 to 25 beats amplitude (Fig. 3-7, *C*)
5. *Exaggerated (marked):* 3 to 6 cycles per minute greater than 25 beats amplitude

For purposes of documentation, a 3-, 4-, or 5-point scale may be used (NAACOG, 1990a; Schmidt, 1987). It is important for the scale and descriptive definitions to be agreed on within a clinical setting. It is relatively common to find increased or decreased LTV (Freeman and others, 1991).

Short-term variability. STV is defined as a rate that varies by 2 to 3 bpm when sampled by the monitor and is calculated every 20 to 30 milliseconds. It appears as either a "rough" line or a "jiggly" line (Freeman and others, 1991). It therefore is described as present when the line is rough and absent when the line is smooth (Table 3-2). When documenting observations pertaining to variability, the nurse should identify whether he or she is describing LTV or STV. With current technology in second- and third-generation monitors, it is possible to describe the presence of only LTV when using external monitoring. Presence of STV may be identified accurately only using the FSE. However, the absence of either STV or LTV may be accurately identified regardless of the use of external or internal monitoring.

When LTV is present on external monitoring, it can be safely assumed that STV is present in all but one rare periodic change, namely, sinusoidal (see Fig. 3-11, *A*). When LTV is not present but STV appears to be, causes such as fetal sleep, CNS depressants,

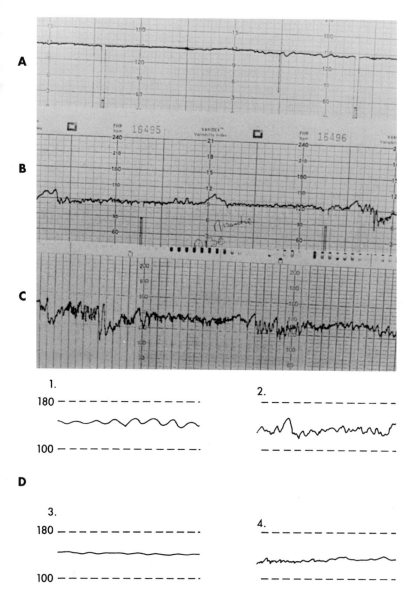

FIG. 3-7 A to C, Variability is depicted in each panel. All are traced from spiral electrode. **A,** Absent short-term variability (STV) and long-term variability (LTV). **B,** Present LTV and STV. **C,** Present STV and increased LTV. **D,** Components of fetal heart rate (FHR) variability for fetal electrocardiogram (FECG)–derived FHR. *1,* LTV without STV; *2,* LTV and STV present; *3,* LTV and STV absent; *4,* STV without LTV.

Modified from Freeman R and others: *Fetal heart rate monitoring,* Baltimore, 1991, Williams & Wilkins.

TABLE 3-2 Abnormalities of baseline variability*

Increased LTV (see Fig. 3-7, *C*)

Description	Persistent cyclic fluctuations, 3-6 times per min of 15-25 beats amplitude
Etiology	Recovery from previous insult
	Response to sudden stimuli
Mechanism	Increased interplay between sympathetic and parasympathetic branches of ANS
Significance	If episodic and less than 2-3 min in duration: benign
	If persistent, it is nonreassuring and should be treated
Nursing interventions	Look for cause and treat by repositioning laterally
	Start and/or increase IV
	Give O_2 at 8-10 L/min by mask

Exaggerated LTV (see Figs. 3-7, *C,* and 3-11, *B*)

Description	Persistent cyclic fluctuations 3-6 times per min of greater than 25 beats amplitude
Etiology	Sudden hypoxia often following nonreassuring variable decelerations (see Tables 3-3 and 3-5 and Fig. 3-11, *B*)
Mechanism	Loss of ANS control
Significance	Nonreassuring and if persistent may be pre-terminal
Nursing interventions	Same as for increased LTV and prepare for emergent delivery

Decreased LTV

Description	2-3 cyclic fluctuations per min of 3-5 beats amplitude
Etiology	Sleep, narcotic, barbiturate, or other CNS depressant; usually does not persist after 20-40 min or length of initial medication effect; early hypoxia
Mechanism	CNS depression during sleep or after medication
Significance	Usually benign
Nursing interventions	Continued observation
	Acoustic stimulation

*See Fig. 3-7.
LTV, Long-term variability; *ANS,* autonomic nervous system; *IV,* intravenous; *CNS,* central nervous system. *Continued*

TABLE 3-2 Abnormalities of baseline variability—cont'd	
Absent LTV or STV (see Figs. 3-7, *A* and *D-3*)	
Description	LTV: fewer than 2-3 cyclic fluctuations of less than 3 beats amplitude
Etiology	Severe degree of hypoxia
Mechanism	Loss of interplay between branches of ANS
Significance	Nonreassuring and indicative of fetal acidemia (pH <7.1)
Nursing interventions	Same as for increased LTV

STV, Short-term variability.

and hypoxia must be evaluated. Variability, both LTV and STV, is an important indicator of fetal oxygen reserve. Therefore if the absence of LTV or STV exceeds the usual 20 to 40 minutes for fetal sleep or reasonable time periods for maternal medication effects, decreased or absent fetal oxygen reserve may be the logical explanation. If LTV or STV is absent, intervention is demanded, and if either is present, intervention will do no harm. When absent, plans for an emergent delivery should be underway in the event that treatment is ineffective.

FHR Patterns and Periodic Rate Changes

FHR patterns or periodic rate changes express the mechanism of insult to the fetus. Knowing the mechanism facilitates appropriate nursing response and interventions. It also aids in predicting whether a change can be effected and how long it might take to accomplish. Periodic changes are also in response to some stimuli. When reassuring changes are observed, they are usually explained by fetal movement or a healthy response to contractions. The FHR can demonstrate patterns of acceleration or deceleration in response to most stimuli (Tables 3-3 to 3-5) (Freeman and others, 1991). Progressive FHR changes in response to gestation, oxygenation, and certain stimuli are shown in Fig. 3-8, p. 75.

Dysrhythmias and Artifact

Definition

A dysrhythmia occurs as a result of abnormalities in the automatic origination of impulses throughout the myocardium, a disruption of the normal impulse conduction pathway, or a combination of both.

TABLE 3-3 Summary of accelerations and decelerations

Reassuring rate changes

Uniform accelerations (Fig. 3-9, *A*)

Description	Uniform in shape
	Begins when contraction begins and ends when contraction ends
	Often mirrors intensity of contractions
Mechanism of insult	Sympathetic response to stimuli
Significance	Healthy CNS response
	Often associated with breech presentations
Nursing intervention	Totally benign so none needed

Nonuniform accelerations (Fig. 3-9, *B*)

Description	Nonuniform in shape
	Usually occur in response to fetal movement so vary in contraction cycle
Mechanism of insult	Sympathetic response to stimuli
Significance	Healthy CNS response; reassuring
Nursing intervention	None

Early decelerations (Fig. 3-10, *A*)

Description	Uniform in shape
	Frequently mirror contraction intensity
	Begin when contraction begins and end when contraction ends
	When noted, usually occurs between 4 and 7 cm dilation of cervix but can occur at any time
Mechanism of insult	Head compression
	Parasympathetic (vagal) reflex caused by pressure on fontanels against resisting cervix
Significance	Although not normal, since it does not occur in all fetuses, it is reassuring
Nursing interventions	Differentiate these from late decelerations
	No action necessary or helpful

Variable decelerations

Description	Variable in shape, often V or W shaped
	Variable in placement with contractions; may occur between or with contractions
	Heart rate falls abruptly and rises abruptly
Mechanism of insult	Cord compression
Significance	Reassuring if:
	Infrequent occurrence
	Low point is within normal heart rate range
	Lasts less than 45 sec
Nursing intervention	Change maternal position

Modified from Freeman R and others: *Fetal heart rate monitoring*, Baltimore, 1991, Williams & Wilkins; American College of Obstetricians and Gynecologists: *ACOG Tech Bull,* no. 207, 1995.

CNS, Central nervous system.

Continued

TABLE 3-3 Summary of accelerations and decelerations—cont'd

Nonreassuring rate changes

Variable decelerations (Fig. 3-10, *B*)

Significance	Nonreassuring if:
	Repetitive
	Falls below 90 bpm
	Lasts longer than 50 sec
	Followed by tachycardia
	Has slow return to baseline
	Has loss of variability between decelerations
Nursing interventions	Turn side to side or to knee-chest position
	Give O_2 at 8-10 L/min by tight face mask
	Improve circulating volume
	Expect expeditious delivery if ominous

Late decelerations (Fig. 3-10, *C*)

Description	Uniform in shape
	Sometimes reflect intensity of contractions
	Begin anywhere in contraction cycle, although common near peak
	End after contraction has ended with slow, sloping return to baseline
Mechanism of insult	Uteroplacental insufficiency leading to CNS hypoxia or myocardial depression
Significance	Always nonreassuring regardless of depth of deceleration or degree of variability
	Acute episodes usually demonstrate good variability and are more likely to be correctable
	Chronic episodes usually are accompanied by decreased or absent variability and are less likely to be correctable; usually associated with fetal acidosis
Nursing interventions	Turn patient to left side
	Administer O_2 at 8-10 L/min by tight face mask
	Infuse rapidly intravenous fluid
	Correct hypotension
	If oxytocin (Pitocin) used, turn it off
	Expect expeditious delivery if not corrected in 30 min

TABLE 3-4 Summary of nonreassuring or preterminal rate changes

Prolonged deceleration (Fig. 3-10, *D*)

Description	Abrupt deceleration lasting 2-10 min
	Usually falls below 90 bpm
Mechanism of insult	Prolonged cord compression
Significance	If lasts longer than 10 min, fetus may become acidemic, myocardial depression occurs; and is then a preterminal event
Nursing interventions	Notify physician or midwife of first occurrence
	Check for cord prolapse
	Turn patient side to side or to knee-chest position until change is effected
	Give O_2 at 8-10 L/min by tight face mask
	Correct maternal hypotension; increase intravenous fluids
	Continuous observation until delivery
	Be prepared for emergency delivery

Modified from Freeman R and others: *Fetal heart rate monitoring,* Baltimore, 1991, Williams & Wilkins.

TABLE 3-5 Preterminal rate changes

Sinusoidal (Fig. 3-11, *A*)

Description	Present LTV with absent STV
	Absence of all reassuring rate changes or patterns
	May have episodes of baseline rate that cannot be determined or appear to wander
Mechanism of insult	Derangement of CNS control of FHR secondary to increased arginine vasopressin
	When severe degree of hypoxia from fetal anemia is coupled with fetal hypovolemia, this unusual rate change occurs
Significance	Categorized as preterminal event that precedes fetal death if not immediately treated
	May only be treated successfully in utero by fetal intrauterine transfusion

Modified from Freeman R and others: *Fetal heart rate monitoring,* Baltimore, 1991, Williams & Wilkins.

LTV, Long-term variability; *STV,* short-term variability; *CNS,* central nervous system; *FHR,* fetal heart rate.   *Continued*

TABLE 3-5 Preterminal rate changes—cont'd

Sinusoidal—cont'd

Nursing interventions	Prepare for emergent delivery
	Prepare for intrauterine transfusion
	Position patient laterally
	Infuse IV fluids rapidly
	Administer O_2 at 6-10 L/min by mask
Saltatory (Fig. 3-11, *B*)	
Description	Exaggerated LTV with sharp increased variations of greater than 25 beats amplitude
Mechanism of insult	Loss of ANS control; when it occurs, frequently follows nonreassuring variable decelerations
Significance	Preterminal in most cases if not corrected immediately
Nursing interventions	Position patient laterally on hands and knees
	Infuse IV fluids rapidly
	Administer O_2 at 8-10 L/min by mask
	Prepare for expeditious delivery

ANS, Autonomic nervous system; *IV,* intravenous.

Dysrhythmias

Fetal dysrhythmias occur reasonably often, although significant fetal or neonatal morbidity is rare. Dysrhythmias can be recorded only with EFM using the internal (FSE) mode. On many monitors, the logic system is automatically disengaged when the FSE cable is plugged into the monitor. Most have a switch located in the paper holder or on the back of the monitor to override this or to engage it in certain situations (Freeman and others, 1991; NAACOG, 1990a).

Because the logic system is intended to be operational on the external (ultrasound) mode, dysrhythmias cannot be traced externally. The logic, or artifact rejection, system is intended to filter artifact when monitoring the heart rate externally. Because artifact is relatively common with the external Doppler method (ultrasound), without the artifact rejection (logic), the externally derived tracing would be virtually impossible to read (Freeman and others, 1991).

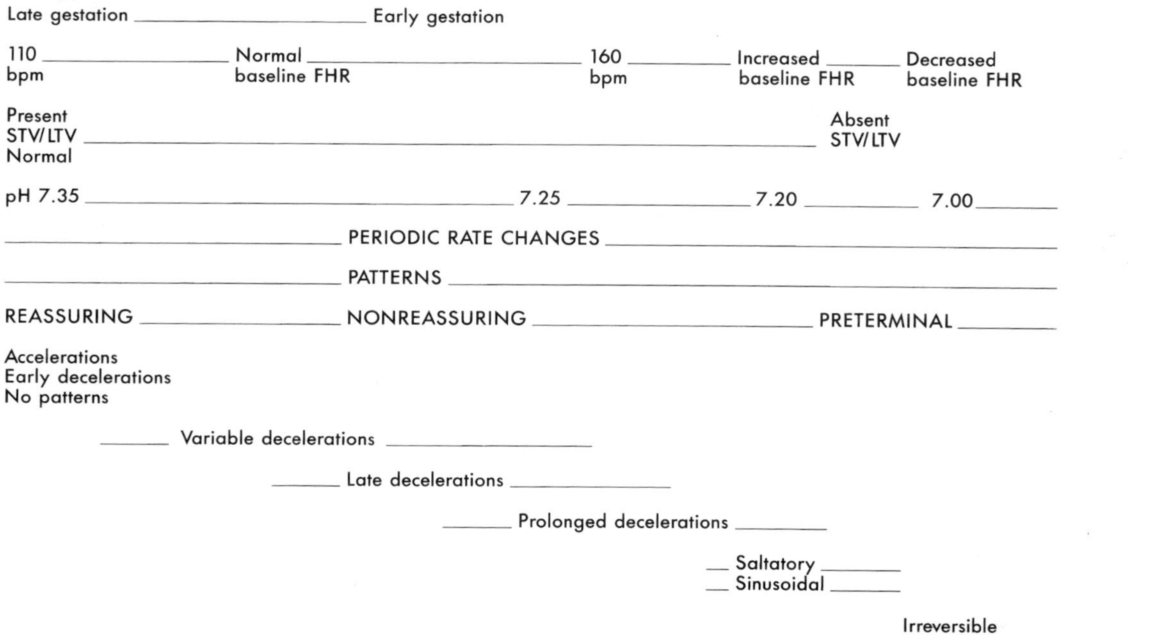

FIG. 3-8 Progressive fetal heart rate changes. *FHR*, Fetal heart rate; *STV*, short-term variability; *LTV*, long-term variability.

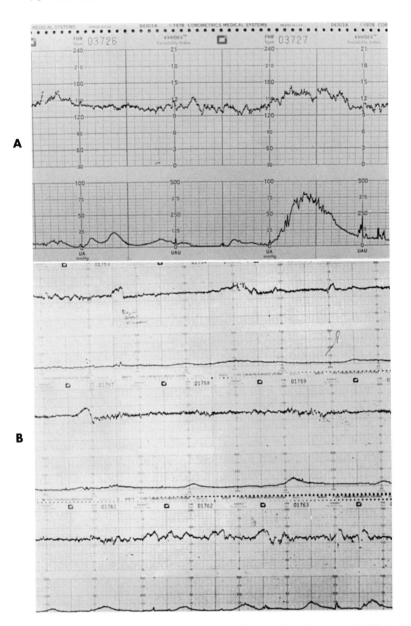

FIG. 3-9 A, Uniform acceleration is noted beginning in *panel 03727* in response to contraction beneath. **B,** Nonuniform accelerations can be seen between contractions. Baseline fetal heart rate (FHR) of 150 to 155 bpm with accelerations to 170 bpm.

B courtesy John P. Elliott, MD, Phoenix.

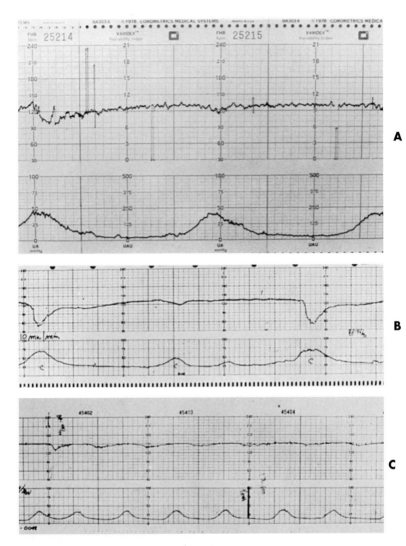

FIG. 3-10 A, Early decelerations. Baseline fetal heart rate (FHR) is 130 bpm. Gradual decelerations to 120 bpm are seen in *panel 25215.* The rate has returned to baseline FHR of 130 bpm by end of contraction. **B,** Severe nonreassuring variable decelerations. Note abrupt fall in heart rate from baseline of 130 bpm. Note also depth of deceleration to 55 to 60 bpm, sloping return to baseline, and absent variability. Those features make these severe decelerations, and prognosis for the fetal outcome is poor. **C,** Late decelerations. Baseline FHR is 150 bpm. Subtle decelerations are seen with each contraction beginning near or just after peak and not returning to baseline until 30 to 40 seconds after contraction has ended. Note poor to absent variability that accompanies baseline and is transmitted by external ultrasound.

Continued

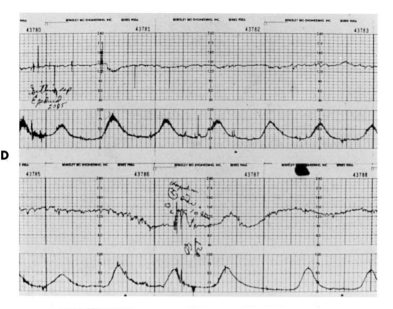

D,

FIG. 3-10, cont'd D, Prolonged deceleration in *panels 43786 and 43787.* This deceleration follows initiation of epidural anesthesia and frequently can be avoided with IV fluid preload. Note occurrence of late decelerations with good baseline variability following recovery period.
B to **D** courtesy John P. Elliott, MD, Phoenix.

Artifact

Conversely, with the artifact rejection (logic) system operational on internally derived EFM tracings, the true intervals from R wave to R wave would be rejected when varying from the preset, arbitrary normal values for the monitor. The arbitrarily defined limits are exceeded when dysrhythmias occur. Thus if left operational, the artifact rejection (logic) system will defeat the true intervals and a dysrhythmia will be missed or recorded as a deceleration or a baseline abnormality (Freeman and others, 1991).

Using the internal (FSE) mode, the logic system should be used only when artifact is suspected and dysrhythmia has been ruled out. To rule out dysrhythmia, troubleshooting the internal mode is necessary. The problem can be with the leg plate, the wires connecting to the leg plate, or the attachment to the fetal presenting part. The system can be tested by the following:

1. Plugging the leg plate into the back of the monitor and testing its function
2. Checking the connections of the wires to the leg plate
3. Replacing the FSE

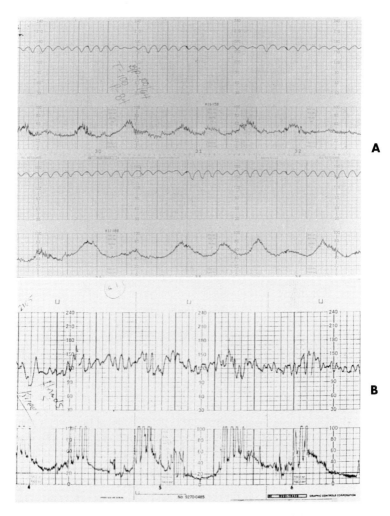

FIG. 3-11 A, Sinusoidal heart rate. Regular oscillations around baseline reflect present long-term variability (LTV) and absent short-term variability (STV). This unusual rate disturbance is preterminal occurrence. **B,** Saltatory heart rate. There are the usual 3 to 6 cycles per minute, but amplitudes are in excess of 25 beats.

If all parts appear to be functioning or attached properly and the auscultated heart rate sounds are regular, the problem must be artifact. Engaging the logic system will clean the tracing by filtering the artifact.

There are several ways to diagnose a dysrhythmia:

1. Listen to the rhythm; if irregular, it may be a dysrhythmia.

2. Analyze the internally derived tracing of the heart rate. A dysrhythmia appears as excursions above or below the line. These excursions are organized, straight, and purposeful. The baseline can generally be followed through the perpendicular excursions (Fig. 3-12 and Table 3-7).
3. Listen and calculate the heart rate with a fetoscope and a Doppler device. The fetoscope counts the sound of the ventricular contraction rate; the Doppler counts the reflected sound waves from the motion of the atrioventricular valves as they close. If the atria and ventricles have a rate and response difference, these will be detected by this method.
4. Connect the fetal monitor to an ECG module with high gain; the FSE will trace the fetal ECG, which can be analyzed like any other ECG tracing for rate and P, QRS, or T wave abnormalities.
5. Do an ultrasound evaluation of the fetal heart and rate. This is the most definitive method of dysrhythmia diagnosis.

The nurse is responsible, in analyzing the EFM tracing, for determining whether a dysrhythmia, an artifact, or normal rate and rhythm exist. It is important in determining interventions to recognize which dysrhythmia represents a benign rhythm or rate disturbance and which represents a significant abnormality. Table 3-6 describes and summarizes artifact versus dysrhythmia, and Table 3-7 describes and summarizes dysrhythmias and their significance.

Of all possible dysrhythmias, paroxysmal atrial tachycardia/supraventricular tachycardia (PAT/SVT) and congenital heart block are serious. PAT/SVT may be treated in utero, whereas heart block is not treatable. Medical management of PAT/SVT consists of pharmacologic fetal cardioversion. The pharmacologic agents used are usually digoxin and sometimes also quinidine, which potentiates the effects of digoxin. Digoxin may be administered to the fetus by the following methods (Freeman and others, 1991):

1. Administer oral digoxin to the mother in increasing doses until toxicity in the mother or cardioversion in the fetus occurs, whichever is first. Maternal heart rate should be appropriately assessed with a baseline ECG and then by apical radial counting. The mother should be monitored for other signs of toxicity and quinidine added as needed if dose must be decreased (Freeman and others, 1991).
2. Administer IV digoxin to the mother and monitor as just described.

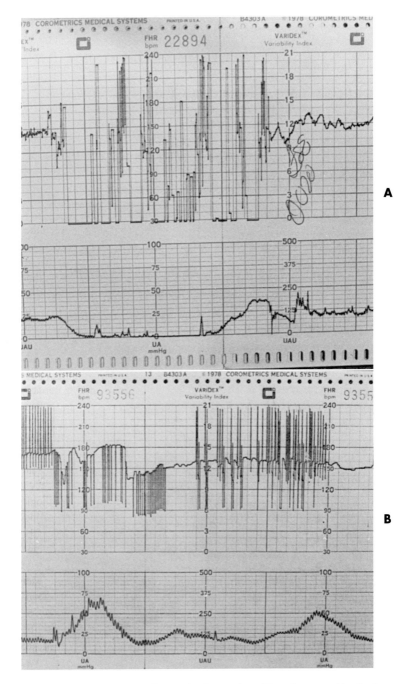

FIG. 3-12 A, Artifact. Note disorganized scattering of impulses traced by fetal scalp electrode. **B,** Dysrhythmia. Note organized distribution of impulses traced by fetal spiral electrode.

TABLE 3-6 Artifact versus dysrhythmia

Instrument	Artifact	Dysrhythmia
Auscultation device	Regular rate and rhythm	Abnormal rate or rhythm
FSE	Perpendicular excursions irregular and baseline completely obscured	Baseline can be read despite perpendicular excursions

FSE, Fetal spiral electrode.

3. Administer digoxin intraamniotically. The dose is calculated based on ultrasound estimation of fetal gram weight and amniotic fluid replacement per 24 hours. The fetus must not be affected by hydrops fetalis to such an extent that the fetus is unlikely to swallow the amniotic fluid.
4. Administer the digoxin directly to the fetus through a percutaneous fetal umbilical venous puncture.

ANTEPARTUM AND INTRAPARTUM FETAL SURVEILLANCE

The latest census statistics estimate that more than two thirds of fetal deaths occur in the antepartum period (Freeman and others, 1991). Certainly a means of surveillance that allows detection of that risk before damage occurs could greatly benefit those pregnancies. Antepartum monitoring provides a means of doing just that. When fetal compromise takes place, fetal activities are lost in reverse order of their development. FHR decelerations occur first, followed by loss of accelerations, then breathing movements, body movements, and muscle tone, and then death (Johnson and others, 1988). Decreased amniotic fluid can also indicate fetal compromise because decreased renal blood flow decreases fetal urinary output resulting in decreased amniotic fluid volume. Decreased amniotic fluid, on the other hand, can cause fetal compromise because of the increased risk of cord compression (ACOG, Technical Bulletin, 188, 1994).

The most common maternal conditions associated with fetal compromise are as follows:

1. Hypertensive disorders of pregnancy (PIH)
2. Chronic hypertension
3. Diabetes
4. Postterm pregnancy

TABLE 3-7 Dysrhythmias: appearances, audible features, and significance

Dysrhythmia	Appearance	Audible features	Significance
Premature atrial contractions (PACs)	Excursions above and below baseline	Compensatory pauses	Benign
Premature ventricular contractions (PVCs)	Same	Same	Usually benign unless superimposed on preterminal rate or wandering baseline
Paroxysmal atrial or continuous supraventricular tachycardia (PAT or SVT)	Rate too fast to trace	Rate above 240 bpm; irregular	Serious and treatable; can be converted while in utero Fetal hydrops (similar to adult congestive heart failure) may be fatal
Congenital heart block	Sudden drops by half	Fetoscope rate same as slowed rate Doppler rate twice the above = 2:1 block	May result in fetal death Associated with maternal connective tissue disease Newborn will need immediate placement of pacemaker
Sinoatrial arrest	In lowest point of variable deceleration, rectangular deflection appears	Absent audible impulse	Benign

5. Connective tissue disease
6. Renal disease
7. Hemolytic incompatibility
8. Multiple gestation
9. Placental abnormalities

The decision as to when to test is usually made based on viability (not before 26 to 28 weeks), severity of the condition, and when the condition is recognized. With the availability of regionalized centers and transportation capabilities, as well as long-distance telemetry, early detection of fetal compromise is possible and desirable for optimal treatment and outcome. The most frequently used tests to detect early fetal compromise are presented in Boxes 3-4 through 3-10, which may serve as useful guides for nursing policies and procedures (ACOG Technical Bulletin, 188, 1994).

NURSING PROCESS

NURSING DIAGNOSIS/COLLABORATIVE PROBLEM AND INTERVENTIONS

■ **POTENTIAL COMPLICATION: FETAL COMPROMISE** related to cord compression/stimulation or diminished uteroplacental blood flow. **_DESIRED OUTCOMES:_** Fetal compromise will be prevented or managed as manifested by an active fetus whose baseline is maintained between 110 and 160 bpm with normal LTV, STV, and reactivity and no decelerations. The biophysical profile will continue to be greater than 6 and the Doppler flow systolic/diastolic ratio less than 3.

Antepartum
  1. Auscultate FHR with fetoscope or Doptone for 60 seconds and record at appropriate intervals.
  2. In the presence of a high risk condition, be prepared to explain the reasons for testing and the procedure and to assist in antepartum surveillance using such tests as the nonstress test (NST), contraction stress test (CST), biophysical profile (BPP), or Doppler studies as ordered.
  3. Explain the significance of and the procedure for monitoring fetal movement at home on a daily basis. Teach the patient when to notify her health care provider.
  4. Explain the importance of follow-up care.
  5. Refer to social office for financial concerns if the family is without health benefits.

Text continued on p. 97

Box 3-4
Nonstress Test (NST)

Definition

A widely accepted method of evaluating fetal status by observing accelerations of the FHR following a stimulus such as fetal activity.

Procedure

1. Explain the testing procedure to the patient.
2. Have the patient empty her bladder and then position herself in a semi-Fowler's position. A wedge may be placed under her right hip to prevent supine hypotension if needed.
3. Place the ultrasound transducer and tocotransducer.
4. Document the date and time the test is started, make and model of monitor, the external modes used, patient's name, reason for test, and maternal vital signs.
5. Record maternal blood pressure every 10 to 15 minutes.
6. Run a 20-min FHR/contraction strip.
7. If at the end of the first 20 minutes a reactive criterion has not been met, stimulate the fetus acoustically and then wait an additional 20 minutes for criteria to be met.
8. At the end of the test, interpret the results and report to the physician or midwife.

Interpretation

1. *Reactive:* if there are at least two accelerations of peak amplitude of at least 15 bpm above the baseline lasting 15 or more seconds. Other reassuring features such as presence of variability and absence of nonreassuring periodic changes with any spontaneous contractions or fetal movement should also be described and expected for a test to read as reactive (Fig. 3-13).
2. *Nonreactive:* no accelerations or failure to meet above criteria (Fig. 3-14).

Management

1. A reactive NST should be repeated every 3 or 4 days for continued prediction of fetal well-being.
2. If the NST remains nonreactive after the second 20 minutes or if any nonreassuring periodic change is present, either a contraction stress test (CST) or another more definitive evaluation of the fetus such as ultrasound for a biophysical profile may be done.

Advantages

1. It is a noninvasive test requiring no initiation of contractions.
2. It is quick to perform.
3. There are no known side effects.
4. It has a low false-negative rate (1%) (Vintzileos and others, 1989).

Disadvantages

1. It is not as sensitive to fetal oxygen reserves as CST.
2. It has a high false-positive rate, greater than 75% (Vintzileos and others, 1989).

FHR, Fetal heart rate.

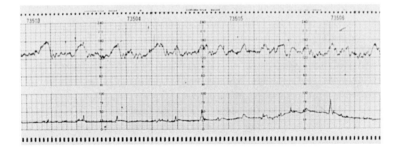

FIG. 3-13 Reactive nonstress test. Baseline fetal heart rate (FHR) of 130 to 140 bpm with numerous accelerations of greater than 15 beats lasting for more than 15 seconds. Small spikes in tocotransducer tracing are fetal activity.
Courtesy John P. Elliott, MD, Phoenix.

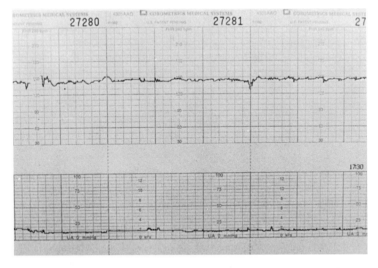

FIG. 3-14 Nonreactive nonstress test. Although there is apparent adequate beat-to-beat variability, no accelerations are seen that can be described as meeting criterion of 15 beats more than baseline for 15 seconds.

Box 3-5
Vibroacoustic Stimulation Test (VST)

Definition
A method of evaluating fetal status by observing accelerations of the FHR following a vibroacoustic stimulation.

Procedure
1. Explain the testing procedure to the patient and reasons for its use, and assure her it is not harmful to the fetus.
2. Have the patient empty her bladder and then position herself in a semi-Fowler's position. A wedge may be placed under her right hip to prevent supine hypotension if needed.
3. Place the ultrasound transducer and tocotransducer.
4. Document the date and time the test is started, make and model of monitor, the external modes used, patient's name, reason for test, and maternal vital signs.
5. Obtain a 5- to 15-minute FHR tracing to establish a baseline.
6. Record maternal blood pressure every 10 to 15 minutes.
7. If no fetal movements are observed, use an acoustic stimulation device by Corometrics or an electrolarynx to produce a vibratory sound stimulus.
8. Apply stimulus over fetal head for 1 second; wait 1 minute.
9. If no acceleration occurs after first stimulus, apply a second stimulus for 2 seconds; wait 1 minute.
10. If no acceleration occurs after second stimulus, apply for 3 seconds; wait 1 minute.
11. Repeat stimuli in same manner until two accelerations or 10 minutes have elapsed.

Interpretation
Reactive: two accelerations in 10 minutes. An acceleration should be characterized by a duration minimum of 15 seconds and a peak of at least 15 beats above the baseline.

Advantages
1. It decreases NST length (Gagnon, 1989).
2. It decreases the incidence of nonreactive NST (Gagnon, 1989).
3. In early labor this test correlates well with normal fetal pH (Sarno and others, 1990).
4. It reduces the need for fetal scalp pH during labor by as much as 50%.
5. There are no known risks if the above protocol is followed.

FHR, Fetal heart rate; *NST,* nonstress test.

Continued

Box 3-5
Vibroacoustic Stimulation Test (VST)—cont'd

Limitations
1. The influence of gestational age: for example, before 30 weeks of gestation, FHR response to vibroacoustic stimulation may be absent or less than 10 beats over baseline FHR.
2. The influence of prestimulation basal FHR: in the presence of fetal tachycardia, the FHR response can be absent in 50% of healthy fetuses after 30 weeks and therefore may be of limited value in predicting fetal outcome if absent.
3. The effect of labor and rupture of membranes may decrease fetal response to acoustic stimulation, especially during the active phase of labor and after rupture of membranes (Gagnon, 1989).
4. It is speculated that repeated use may cause fetal hearing damage (Sleutel, 1989).

Box 3-6
Fetal Movement Monitoring

Definition
The fetus reduces movement or stops moving in response to chronic hypoxia in an attempt to reduce oxygen consumption and conserve energy.
Procedure
1. Teach patient the significance of fetal movements.
2. Teach patient a fetal assessment method.
   Count fetal movements for a fixed period of time. Instruct the patient to lie down three times each day for 20 to 30 minutes and count the fetal movements felt (Rayburn, 1987).
   Record time taken to count a fixed number of fetal movements. Instruct the patient to start counting at 9 AM and stop counting for the day when 10 fetal movements have been noted. Then record the time taken (Baskett, Liston, 1989).
3. Demonstrate how to record movements on a daily fetal movement record.
Interpretation
Report decreased fetal movement compared to previous day's counts or fewer than four fetal movements in any 1 hour.
Management
If decreased fetal movement is reported, evaluate fetal status with an NST or a biophysical profile immediately and manage according to the results.

NST, Nonstress test.

Box 3-6
Fetal Movement Monitoring—cont'd

Gestational influences

Gestational age:	Fetal movements are constant after 24 weeks of gestation (Connors and others, 1988). There is *not* a decrease near to term.
Diurnal rhythm:	Normally fetal movement is increased in the late evening (Bocking, 1989).
Fetal behavior state:	There is no fetal movement during quiet sleep (20- to 40-min sleep cycles) (Baskett, Liston, 1989).
Drugs:	Depressant drugs such as barbiturates, narcotics, and alcohol can reduce fetal movement. In therapeutic doses, most drugs do not reduce fetal movement (Baskett, Liston, 1989).
Smoking:	Fetal movement may be temporarily reduced during smoking. Nicotine reduces fetal blood flow (Linblad and others, 1988).
Fetal malformation:	A fetus with a malformation is more likely to have reduced activity (Baskett, Liston, 1989).

Box 3-7
Contraction Stress Test (CST)

Definition

A commonly used fetal well-being test that determines how the fetus responds to relative hypoxia during a contraction. A compromised fetus, with a limited ability to compensate for mild hypoxia because of limited oxygen reserves, will demonstrate a consistent pattern of late decelerations during the test.

Procedure

1. Explain the testing procedure to the patient.
2. Have the patient empty her bladder and then position herself in a semi-Fowler's position. A wedge may be placed under her right hip to prevent supine hypotension if needed.
3. Place the ultrasound transducer and tocotransducer.

Continued

Box 3-7

Contraction Stress Test (CST)—cont'd

Procedure—cont'd
4. Document the date and time the test is started, make and model of monitor, the external modes used, patient's name, reason for test, and maternal vital signs.
5. Run a 20-min NST for baseline information regarding FHR and uterine contractions.
6. Stimulate contractions either by nipple stimulation of endogenous oxytocin or with intravenous oxytocin.
7. Observe for uterine hyperstimulation.
8. Assess maternal blood pressure every 10 to 15 minutes during the test and when the test is completed.
9. Interpret the test results and report findings to the physician or midwife.

Initiation of contractions with nipple stimulation
1. On one side begin nipple brushing. Continue until a contraction begins or for 10 minutes.
2. If no contraction in 10 minutes of brushing, change sides and continue for 10 minutes. If still not effective, brush both nipples simultaneously.
3. Continue nipple brushing on effective side or sides until a contraction occurs. Stop until contraction is over, and then begin again until three contractions occur in 10 minutes.

Stimulation of contractions with oxytocin
1. Start mainline intravenous normal saline.
2. Piggyback oxytocin diluted so that increments of 0.5 mU/min can be delivered.
3. Start at 0.5 mU/min; double amount every 15 to 20 minutes until 4 mU and then increase by 2 mU until three contractions occur in 10 minutes or maximum dose of 16 mU is reached.

Interpretation
1. *Negative* (Fig. 3-15): no decelerations noted on entire strip. LTV is present, and there is an absence of any nonreassuring changes.
2. *Equivocal:* a test may be equivocal for one of three reasons:
   a. *Suspicious:* less than 50% of the contractions on the entire strip have late decelerations. Variability is usually good (Fig. 3-16, *A*).
   b. *Hyperstimulation:* a contraction frequency greater than four in 10 minutes, less than 60 seconds between contractions, or a contraction lasting longer than 90 seconds with a late deceleration occurring (Fig. 3-16, *B*).
   c. *Unsatisfactory:* the quality of the tracing is too poor to accurately interpret FHR with contractions or the frequency of three contractions in 10 minutes cannot be obtained for an end point of the test (Fig. 3-16, *C*).

Box 3-7
Contraction Stress Test (CST)—cont'd

Interpretation—cont'd

3. *Positive* (Fig 3-17): 50% or more of the contractions on the strip have late decelerations associated with them even if the end point of three contractions in 10 minutes is not obtained. If associated with decreased variability, the prognosis is poor.

Management

1. A negative CST predicts continued fetal well-being for 7 days and need only be repeated weekly provided maternal well-being is the same (Freeman and others, 1991).
2. An equivocal CST should be repeated in 24 hours. If a test remains equivocal for 3 consecutive days, NSTs are usually used from then on instead of CSTs (Freeman and others, 1991).
3. A positive CST necessitates more vigorous management. If the variability is good and the fetus is mature by the proper dates and in a vertex position, a very carefully monitored induction can be attempted. If the fetus is immature, treating the maternal condition that might have precipitated the problem may be the treatment of choice to give the baby its best chance.
4. With a positive CST when variability is poor, delivery by an emergency cesarean is the only chance for optimal outcome for the baby regardless of maturity.
5. Regardless of test results, if variable decelerations are noted, an amniotic fluid index is recommended.

Advantages

1. It is more sensitive to fetal oxygen reserves than NST.
2. It has a low false-negative rate (2%) (Vintzileos and others, 1989).

Disadvantages

1. It is contraindicated in such high risk conditions as preterm labor and placenta previa.
2. It must be administered in a birthing setting.
3. It has a false-positive rate greater than 50% (Vintzileos and others, 1989).

NST, Nonstress test; *FHR,* fetal heart rate; *LTV,* long-term variability.

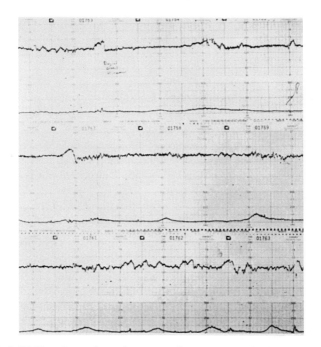

FIG. 3-15 Negative and reactive contraction stress test obtained with breast stimulation. No late decelerations are noted in any panel. Good apparent beat-to-beat variability is present, and fetal heart rate (FHR) accelerates periodically. Three contractions are present in 10 minutes *(panels 01761 through 01763).*   Courtesy John P. Elliott, MD, Phoenix.

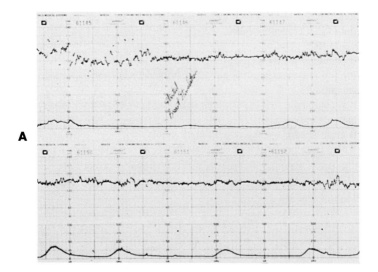

FIG. 3-16 A, Equivocal contraction stress test because of one late deceleration in panel 61145. Breast stimulation was started to further challenge placental function and determine if late deceleration would persist. Because remainder of test was negative for late decelerations and reactive, test was repeated the following day.   *Continued*

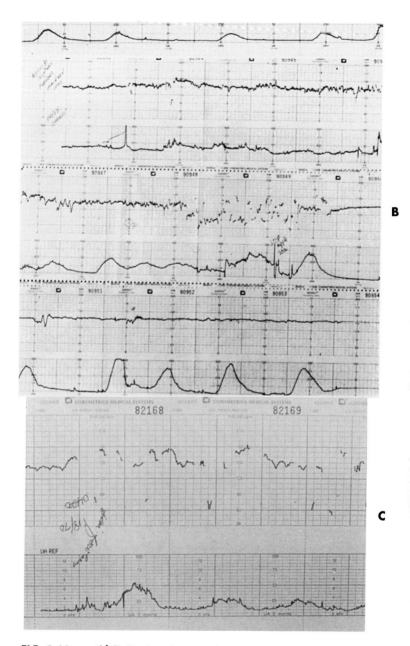

FIG. 3-16, cont'd B, Equivocal contraction stress test because of later and prolonged deceleration with excessive and hyperstimulated uterine activity in *panels 90948 and 90949.* Previous portion of strip had good apparent variability and reactivity, although remaining portion, during recovery, demonstrates poor variability. Tracing was continued until adequate recovery was evidenced. Then test was repeated the following day. **C,** Equivocal contraction stress test because tracing immediately following each contraction is unsatisfactory for accurate interpretation of fetal heart rate (FHR) response. **B** courtesy John P. Elliot, MD, Phoenix.

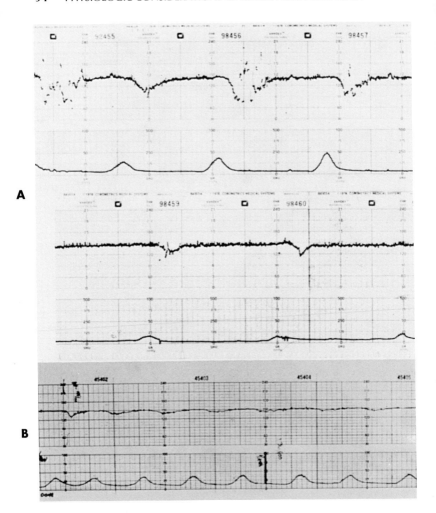

FIG. 3-17 A, Positive contraction stress test with adequate apparent beat-to-beat variability. Baseline fetal heart rate (FHR) is 140 to 150 bpm. Tracing was continued, and reactivity was also noted while decisions were made for delivery in postterm pregnancy. **B,** Positive nonreactive contraction stress test with poor to absent variability. Baby was delivered by emergent cesarean birth with Apgar scores below 6. Mother was stable with pregnancy-induced hypertension (PIH). **B** courtesy John P. Elliott, MD, Phoenix.

Box 3-8
Biophysical Profile (BPP)

Definition

Evaluation of fetal well-being through the use of various reflex activities that are CNS controlled and sensitive to hypoxia as well as the fetal environment that can affect fetal well-being (Manning and others, 1990).

Procedure

Scan the abdomen and assess fetal tone, movement, breathing, and amniotic fluid.

Interpretation

1. The biophysical activities that are the first to develop are the last to disappear when asphyxia occurs.

Fetal tone	Starts to function at 7.5 to 8.5 weeks of gestation
	Is abolished at a pH less than 7.1
Fetal movement	Starts to function at 9 weeks of gestation
	Is abolished when the pH is between 7.1 and 7.2
Fetal breathing	Starts to function at approximately 20 to 21 weeks of gestation
	Is abolished at a pH of 7.2
Reactive FHR	Starts to function at 26 to 28 weeks of gestation
	Is abolished at a pH of less than 7.19

2. Decreased amniotic fluid can be the result of chronic hypoxia or can cause hypoxia.
3. A grade III placenta represents an aged placenta that may function inadequately.

Scoring

1. 0 to 2 points each for fetal tone, movement, breathing, reactivity, and amniotic fluid volume.
2. An 8 to 10 BPP score is reassuring. The test need only be repeated weekly in a high risk pregnancy except in the diabetic or postterm pregnancy where it should be repeated twice weekly.
3. A 4 to 6 BPP score is nonreassuring. If fetal pulmonary maturity is assured and the cervix is favorable, deliver; otherwise, repeat in 24 hours. If score persists, deliver if fetal pulmonary maturity is certain. Otherwise, treat with steroids and deliver in 48 hours.
4. A 0 to 2 BPP score means immediate delivery.
5. Oligohydramnios constitutes an abnormal biophysical assessment regardless of the overall score (Manning and others, 1990).
6. Grade III placenta constitutes an abnormal biophysical assessment regardless of the overall score since it represents an aging placenta.

Continued

Box 3-8
Biophysical Profile (BPP)—cont'd

Advantages
1. It permits conservative therapy and prevents premature intervention.
2. There are fewer false-positive results than with NST or CST (Vintzileos and others, 1989).
3. The test can be completed in 20 minutes by a trained technician (Platt, 1989).
4. It is the most accurate test in being able to identify the compromised fetus (Vintzileos and others, 1989).

CNS, Central nervous system; *NST,* nonstress test; *CST,* contraction stress test.

Box 3-9
Amniotic Fluid Volume Index (AFI)

Definition
Evaluation of the quantity of amniotic fluid.
Procedure
Scan each of the four quadrants of the abdomen. Measure one pocket of fluid in each quadrant. The pockets are selected by areas that are free of fetal small parts. The centimeters of each measurement are added together.
Interpretation
1. 0 to 8 cm of amniotic fluid is abnormally low and indicates need for delivery.
2. 10 to 12 cm of amniotic fluid is normal (Rutherford and others, 1987).

Box 3-10
Doppler Flow Studies

Definition
Noninvasive method for studying intrauterine environment, specifically the uteroplacental blood flow in the umbilical arteries.
Procedure
1. The nurse should assist the patient to position herself in a supine position and place a wedge under her right side to facilitate adequate blood flow and reduce maternal positional side effects.
2. A pulsed Doppler device will be positioned over the fetus. The umbilical artery blood flow is distinguished from other blood flow by its characteristic waveform.

Box 3-10
Doppler Flow Studies—cont'd

Procedure—cont'd

3. The directed blood flow within the umbilical arteries is calculated using the difference between the systolic and the diastolic flow. Measurements are averaged from at least five waveforms.

Interpretation

1. Elevations of the systolic/diastolic (S/D) ratio above 3.0 are considered abnormal.
2. Elevations of the S/D ratio are seen in hypertensive disorders of pregnancy, fetal growth retardation, or other causes of uteroplacental insufficiency.

Intrapartum
Low risk patients

1. When the patient is admitted in labor, apply external EFM for 20 minutes. Then assess FHR by intermittent auscultation during and after contractions or by continuous fetal monitoring.
2. During latent phase of labor, assess and record FHR every 60 minutes (AWHONN, 1993).
3. During active labor, assess and record FHR every 30 minutes (AWHONN, 1993).
4. During second-stage labor, assess and record FHR every 15 minutes (American College of Obstetricians and Gynecologists, 1994; AWHONN, 1993).

High risk patients

1. When the woman is admitted in labor, apply external EFM for 20 minutes. Then assess FHR by intermittent auscultation during and after contractions or by continuous fetal monitoring.
2. During latent-phase labor, assess and record FHR pattern every 20 to 30 minutes (AWHONN, 1993).
3. During active-phase labor, assess and record FHR pattern every 15 minutes (AWHONN, 1993).
4. During second-stage labor, assess and record FHR pattern every 5 minutes (AWHONN, 1993).
5. FHR pattern assessment should include baseline heart rate, variability, and FHR changes over time.
6. On identification of a nonreassuring pattern, (a) reposition the patient laterally, turn from side to side, or have patient

get in a hands and knees or modified Trendelenburg position, depending on pattern and fetal response; (b) start and/or infuse intravenous fluids rapidly; (c) discontinue labor stimulant if being administered or, if not, obtain an order for 0.25 mg subcutaneous terbutaline; (d) administer oxygen at 8 to 10 L/min by mask; and (e) notify physician or midwife.

7. Assess maternal blood pressure, pulse, and respirations every 1 to 2 hours before the onset of active labor and every hour in active labor.

8. Assess maternal temperature every 1 to 4 hours depending on the stage of labor and status of membranes.

9. Monitor maternal contractions every 30 minutes and maintain a safe and effective labor pattern with maternal positioning (of choice and therapeutic), fluids, and comfort measures as appropriate. See Chapters 26 and 27.

10. Record fetal and maternal responses to nursing interventions. Notify physician or midwife of any adverse effects on fetal response (AWHONN, 1993).

BIBLIOGRAPHY

Electronic Fetal Monitoring

American Academy of Pediatrics/American College of Obstetricians and Gynecologists (ACOG): *Guidelines for perinatal care,* Washington, DC, 1993, The Academy.

American College of Obstetricians and Gynecologists: Antepartal fetal surveillance, *ACOG Tech Bull,* no. 188, 1994.

American College of Obstetricians and Gynecologists: *ACOG Tech Bull,* no. 209, 1995.

Association of Women's Health, Obstetric, and Neonatal Nurses (AWHONN): *1992 position statement. Fetal heart rate patterns: monitoring, interpretation, and management,* Washington, DC, 1992, The Association.

Association of Women's Health, Obstetric, and Neonatal Nurses (AWHONN): *Fetal heart rate monitoring principles and practices,* Washington, DC, 1993, The Association.

Bobak I, Jensen M: *Maternity care,* ed 4, St Louis, 1995, Mosby.

Carlton L: Basic intrapartum fetal monitoring. In Martin J, editor: *Intrapartum management modules: a perinatal education program,* Baltimore, 1990, Williams & Wilkins.

Creasy R, Resnik R, editors: *Maternal-fetal medicine: principles and practice,* ed 3, Philadelphia, 1994, Saunders.

Department of Health Services: *Arizona health status and vital statistics, 1990,* Phoenix, 1992, Public Health Service.

Ellison J and others: Electronic fetal heart rate monitoring, auscultation, and neonatal outcomes, *Am J Obstet Gynecol* 165(4):1281-1290, 1991.

Freeman R and others: *Fetal heart rate monitoring,* Baltimore, 1991, Williams & Wilkins.

Galvan B and others: Using amnioinfusion for the relief of repetitive variable decelerations during labor, *Clin Perinatol* 16(5):222-229, 1989.

National Center for Health Statistics: *Vital statistics of the United States: mortality,* Hyattsville, Md, 1991, Public Health Service.

Nurses Association of the American College of Obstetricians and Gynecologists (NAACOG): *NAACOG statement: nursing responsibilities in implementing fetal heart rate monitoring,* Washington, DC, 1988a, The Association.

Nurses Association of the American College of Obstetricians and Gynecologists (NAACOG): *Nurses' responsibilities in augmentation and induction of labor,* Washington, DC, 1988b, The Association.

Nurses Association of the American College of Obstetricians and Gynecologists (NAACOG): *Practice competencies and educational guidelines for nurse providers of intrapartum care,* Washington, DC, 1989, The Association.

Nurses Association of the American College of Obstetricians and Gynecologists (NAACOG): *Critical concepts in EFM video series,* Washington, DC, 1990a, The Association.

Nurses Association of the American College of Obstetricians and Gynecologists (NAACOG): *Nursing practice resource: fetal heart rate auscultation,* Washington, DC, 1990b, The Association.

Nurses Association of the American College of Obstetricians and Gynecologists (NAACOG): *Electronic fetal monitoring: nursing practice competencies and educational guidelines,* Washington, DC, 1991a, The Association.

Nurses Association of the American College of Obstetricians and Gynecologists (NAACOG): *Standards for the care of women and newborns,* Washington, DC, 1991b, The Association.

Parer J: Fetal heart rate. In Creasy R, Resnik R, editors: *Maternal-fetal medicine: principles and practice,* ed 3, Philadelphia, 1994, Saunders.

Radin T, Harmon J, Hanson D: Impact on cesarean birth rates, *Birth,* Mar/April 1993.

Schmidt J: Documenting EFM events, *Perinatal Press* 10(6):77-81, 1987.

Shiffrin B: *Exercises in fetal monitoring,* St Louis, 1990, Mosby.

Trepanier M and others: Evaluation of a fetal monitoring education program, *J Obstet Gynecol Neonatal Nurs* 25(2):137-144, 1996.

Tucker M, Hauth J: Intrapartum assessment of fetal well being, *Clin Obstet Gynecol* 33(3):515-525, 1990.

Tucker S: *Pocket guide to fetal monitoring and assessment,* ed 3, St Louis, 1996, Mosby.

Varney H: *Nurse midwifery,* Boston, 1987, Blackwell Scientific Publications.

Vintzileos A and others: A randomized trial of intrapartum electronic fetal heart rate monitoring versus intermittent auscultation, *Obstet Gynecol* 81(6):899-907, 1993.

Amniotic Fluid Volume Index

Rutherford S and others: The four quadrant assessment of amniotic fluid volume: an adjunct to antepartum fetal heart rate testing, *Obstet Gynecol* 70(3):353-355, 1987.

Biophysical Profile

Bocking A: Observations of biophysical activities in the normal fetus, *Clin Perinatol* 16(3):583-594, 1989.

Ferguson H: Biophysical profile scoring: the fetal Apgar, *Am J Nurs* 88(5):662-663, 1988.

Gaffney S and others: The biophysical profile for fetal surveillance, *MCN Am J Matern Child Nurs* 15(6):356-360, 1990.

Goldstein S: Embryonic ultrasonographic measurements: crown rump length revisited, *Am J Obstet Gynecol* 165(3):497-501, 1991.

Harding J and others: Correlation of amniotic fluid index and nonstress test in patients with preterm premature rupture of membranes, *Am J Obstet Gynecol* 165(4):1088-1094, 1991.

Iffath A and others: Variable decelerations in reactive nonstress tests with decreased amniotic fluid index predict fetal compromise, *Am J Obstet Gynecol* 165(4):1094-1096, 1991.

Johnson T, Besinger R, Thomas R: New clues to fetal behavior and well being, *Contemp OB/GYN* 31(5):108-123, 1988.

Manning F and others: Fetal assessment based on fetal biophysical profile scoring: experience in 12,620 referred high risk pregnancies, *Am J Obstet Gynecol* 162:918-927, 1990.

Platt L: Predicting fetal health with the biophysical profile, *Contemp OB/GYN* 33(2):105-119, 1989.

Sassoon D and others: The biophysical profile in labor, *Obstet Gynecol* 76:360-365, 1990.

Toohey J and others: Does amniotic fluid index affect the accuracy of estimated fetal weight in preterm premature rupture of membranes? *Am J Obstet Gynecol* 165(4):1060-1062, 1991.

Vintzileos A and others: Fetal biophysical profile scoring: current status, *Clin Perinatol* 16(3):661-669, 1989.

Doppler Flow Studies

Cundiff J and others: Umbilical artery Doppler flow studies during pregnancy, *Clin Perinatol* 19(6):475-488, 1990.

Trudinger B: Doppler ultrasound assessment of blood flow. In Creasy R, Resnik R, editors: *Maternal-fetal medicine: principles and practice,* ed 3, Philadelphia, 1994, Saunders.

Fetal Movement Monitoring

Ahn M and others: Antepartum fetal surveillance in the patient with decreased fetal movement, *Am J Obstet Gynecol* 157:860-864, 1987.

Baskett T: Gestational age and fetal biophysical assessment, *Am J Obstet Gynecol* 158(2):784-788, 1988.

Baskett T, Liston R: Fetal movement monitoring: clinical application, *Clin Perinatol* 16(3):613-625, 1989.

Bocking A: Observations of biophysical activities in the normal fetus, *Clin Perinatol* 16(3):583-593, 1989.

Connors G and others: Maternally perceived fetal activity from 24 weeks gestation to term in normal and at risk pregnancies, *Am J Obstet Gynecol* 158:294, 1988.

Davis L: Daily fetal movement counting: a valuable assessment tool, *J Nurse Midwifery* 32(1):11-17, 1987.

Freda M and others: Fetal movement counting: which method? *MCN Am J Matern Child Nurs* 18(6):314-321, 1993.

Gantes M and others: The daily use of fetal movement records in a clinical setting, *J Obstet Gynecol Neonatal Nurs* 15(5):390-393, 1986.

Linblad R and others: Effect of nicotine on human fetal blood flow, *Obstet Gynecol* 71:371, 1988.

Mikhail M and others: The effect of fetal movement counting on maternal attachments to the fetus, *Am J Obstet Gynecol* 165(4):988-990, 1991.

Rayburn W: Clinical implications of monitoring fetal activity, *Am J Obstet Gynecol* 148:823-827, 1987.

Reddy N and others: Fetal movement during labor, *Am J Obstet Gynecol* 165(4):1073-1077, 1991.

Nonstress and Contraction Stress Tests

American College of Obstetricians and Gynecologists (ACOG): Antepartum fetal surveillance, *ACOG Tech Bull* 107:1-4, 1987.

Baser I, Johnson T, Paine L: Coupling of fetal movement and fetal heart rate accelerations as indicators of fetal health, *Obstet Gynecol* 80(1):62-66, 1992.

Clark S: How a modified NST improves fetal surveillance, *Contemp OB/GYN* 35(3):45-48, 1990.

Dauphinee J: Antepartum testing: a challenge for nursing, *J Perinatal Neonatal Nurs* 1(1):29-49, 1987.

Freeman R and others: *Fetal heart rate monitoring,* Baltimore, 1991, Williams & Wilkins.

Harmon J, Barry M: Antenatal testing, mobile outpatient testing service, *J Obstet Gynecol Neonatal Nurs* 18(1):345-348, 1989.

Mayberry L, Intrurrisi-Levy M: Use of breast stimulation for contraction stress test, *J Obstet Gynecol Neonatal Nurs* 16(2):121-124, 1987.

Murray M: *Antepartal and intrapartal fetal monitoring,* Washington, DC, 1988, NAACOG Publication.

Murray M, Harmon J, Canfield S: Nipple stimulation contraction stress test for the high risk patient, *MCN Am J Matern Child Nurs* 11(5):331-333, 1986.

Vibroacoustic Stimulation

Auyeung R, Goldkrand J: Vibroacoustic stimulation and nursing intervention in the nonstress test, *J Obstet Gynecol Neonatal Nurs* 20(3): 232-237, 1991.

Clark S: Do we still need fetal scalp blood sampling? *Contemp OB/GYN* 33(3):75-85, 1989.

Gagnon R: Acoustic stimulation: effect on heart rate and other biophysical variables, *Clin Perinatol* 16(3):643-659, 1989.

Kisilevsky B, Kilpatrick K, Low J: Vibroacoustic induced fetal movement: two stimuli and the methods of scoring, *Obstet Gynecol* 81(2):174-179, 1994.

Paul R, Chez R: Fetal acoustic stimulation, *Contemp OB/GYN* 32(1):123-125, 1988.

Sarno A and others: Fetal acoustic stimulation in the early intrapartum period as a predictor of subsequent fetal condition, *Am J Obstet Gynecol* 162:762-767, 1990.

Slade D and others: Acoustic stimulation induced fetal response compared to traditional nonstress testing, *J Obstet Gynecol Neonatal Nurs* 20(2):160-165, 1991.

Sleutel M: An overview of vibroacoustic stimulation, *Obstet Gynecol Neonatal Nurs* 17(6):447-452, 1989.

Zimmer E and others: Vibroacoustic stimulation evokes human fetal micturition, *Obstet Gynecol* 81:178-180, 1993.

4

Technologic Advances

In the past 10 years major advances have been made in antepartum fetal surveillance, diagnosis, and medical therapies. These include the following:
- Prenatal genetic screening, such as chorionic villus sampling (CVS), amniocentesis, and serum alpha-fetoprotein
- Fetal percutaneous blood sampling
- Fetal therapies, such as transfusion, surgery, and selective reduction

PRENATAL GENETIC SCREENING

Three common methods of prenatal genetic screening are available. Amniocenteses have been used as a primary method of genetic screening for more than a decade. Maternal serum analysis for alpha-fetoprotein is a newer, less specific method of screening. Both amniocentesis and maternal serum alpha-fetoprotein (MSAFP) are done in the second trimester. When results pointed to a potential abnormality, an earlier method for genetic screening was needed. CVS can screen in the first trimester.

Purpose

Prenatal genetic screening is used to detect fetal congenital malformations and inherited disorders.

Indications

Several indications for prenatal genetic screening exist. They are as follows:

- Maternal age 35 years or older
- Abnormal genetic history of mother or father
- Previous child with genetic defect
- Maternal phenylketonuria (PKU) or congestive heart disease
- Maternal history of two or more miscarriages
- Either parent of Jewish descent at risk for Tay-Sachs disease
- Extreme parental anxiety or concern about potential for genetic abnormalities

CHORIONIC VILLUS SAMPLING
Definition

In chorionic villus sampling (CVS) a portion of the chorion is aspirated and analyzed for evidence of genetic, chromosomal, or biochemical abnormalities.

Routes

CVS is done by transabdominal aspiration (needle) or transcervical aspiration (catheter).

Risk

Fetal loss rate is less than 1% (Creasy, Resnik, 1994) but is greater than with amniocentesis. Both the transcervical and transabdominal approaches have been reported to carry a risk of limb anomalies and maternal bacteremia (Burton and others, 1992; Hsieh and others, 1995; Silverman and others, 1994).

Timing

Transabdominal needle aspiration is done in the first or second trimester. Transcervical catheter aspiration is done at 6 to 11 weeks of gestation.

Procedure for Abdominal Route

The woman drinks 300 to 400 ml of water before the procedure. With ultrasonographic guidance an 18-gauge spinal needle with stylet is inserted through the maternal abdominal wall and myometrium into the chorion. The stylet is withdrawn, and a 20-ml syringe is attached to an aspiration device. Chorionic villi are obtained by repeated (15 to 20) rapid aspirations of the syringe plunger to 20-ml negative pressure. Simultaneously, the needle tip is redirected several times within the placenta. The needle is withdrawn under continuous 20-ml negative pressure. The specimen is then transferred to a Petri dish for inspection under a microscope to judge quantity of tissue. After the specimen is transferred to a genetics laboratory, cells are harvested at 5 to 8 days (Elias and others, 1989).

Procedure for Transcervical Route

With ultrasound guidance, a speculum is placed in the vagina. The vagina is cleansed, and the cervix is secured with a tenaculum. A 20-mm catheter with a pliable stainless steel obturator is then passed through the cervix and into the chorion. The obturator is removed, and a 10-ml syringe is attached to the catheter. Chorionic villi are obtained by 2 to 5 ml of negative pressure applied at several sites on the chorion. The specimen is transferred to the genetics laboratory, where cells are harvested in 5 to 8 days (Hammer, Tufts, 1986).

Postprocedure Care

The fetal heart rate (FHR) is auscultated twice in 30 minutes. Unsensitized D-negative patients are given 300 µg of D immunoglobulin. A repeat ultrasound is scheduled to be performed at 16 weeks of gestation.

Comparison of Two Routes

The transabdominal route can decrease the risk of infection and spontaneous abortion (Elias and others, 1989). Also, it can be done after 12 weeks of gestation (Hogdall and others, 1988). Absolute contraindications for transcervical aspiration include the following:
- Vaginismus
- Vaginitis
- Inaccessible cervical canal

Relative contraindications include the following:
- Pronounced angle of uterine corpus on cervix
- Multiple pregnancy
- After 12 weeks of gestation (Brambati and others, 1987)

AMNIOCENTESIS
Definition

Amniocentesis is the transabdominal needle aspiration of 10 to 20 ml of amniotic fluid for laboratory analysis.

Timing

The previous standard for amniocentesis was 16 weeks. Now it may be done as early as 10 weeks of gestation. All sources report a loss rate less than loss with CVS (Creasy, Resnik, 1994).

Risks

Risks with amniocentesis include the following:
- Spontaneous abortion
- Trauma to the fetus or placenta
- Bleeding
- Preterm labor
- Infection
- Rh sensitization from fetal to maternal bleed

Preparation

The nurse explains the procedure to the patient. The patient is encouraged to void just before the procedure to avoid the risk of bladder puncture.

ALPHA-FETOPROTEIN SCREENING
Definition

Alpha-fetoprotein plus (AFP Plus) screening is useful in identifying pregnancies at risk for certain adverse outcomes and in detecting some types of fetal chromosomal abnormalities (McKeon, O'Reilly, 1990).

Timing

The optimal time for AFP screening is 16 to 18 weeks (American Academy of Pediatrics, Committee on Genetics, 1987).

Method

Maternal serum is routinely screened for the level of AFP. It is necessary to have accurate gestational dating.

Physiology

AFP is similar to serum albumin in chemical structure and is the major fetal serum protein (Burton, 1988). It is produced in the yolk sac for the first 6 weeks and then by the fetal liver and gastrointestinal tract (Myhre and others, 1989).

Although alpha-fetoprotein's biologic function is unknown, it may have an immunoregulatory role, protecting the fetus against maternal immunologic attack (Burton, 1988). It is normally present in amniotic fluid, presumably by way of fetal urinary excretion.

AFP reaches its peak amniotic fluid concentration between 10 and 14 weeks of gestation, decreasing steadily thereafter. It diffuses across the membranes and is detectable in maternal serum beginning at approximately 12 to 14 weeks of gestation. Triple screening is the usual method now used. The triple screen detects the alpha-fetoprotein (AFP), human chorionic gonadotropin (HCG), and unconjugated estriol (uEST). Combining all three chemical markers with the mother's age allows a detection rate of 50% to 77%, or two to three times the detection rate with maternal serum AFP alone. uEST is especially useful for women younger than 35 years. In addition to the trisomies, triple screening will detect 85% to 90% of open neural tube defects (MacDonald and others, 1993; Palomaki and others, 1992).

Conditions Associated With Elevated Levels

Elevated levels of AFP are found in the following:
- Neural tube defects
- Pilonidal cysts
- Esophageal or intestinal obstruction
- Liver necrosis
- Abdominal wall defects, such as omphalocele or gastroschisis
- Kidney disorders
- Low birth weight
- Oligohydramnios
- Multifetal gestation
- Decreased maternal weight
- Underestimated fetal gestational age

Conditions Associated With Low Levels

Low levels of AFP are found in the following:
- Chromosomal trisomies, such as Down syndrome
- Gestational trophoblastic disease
- Fetal death
- Increased maternal weight
- Overestimated fetal gestational age

Interpretation of Results

MSAFP levels are not diagnostic but, rather, serve as a screen for fetal risk factors. Elevated or low levels indicate a need to follow up with other diagnostic studies, such as ultrasound or amniocentesis, for assistance in making specific diagnoses. A normal MSAFP indicates there is a low risk for certain abnormalities but does not ensure a perfect, normal baby.

ALPHA-FETOPROTEIN-PLUS SCREENING
Definition

Alpha-fetoprotein-plus (AFP-Plus) screening is more accurate than AFP alone in detecting Down syndrome. This test is 60% to 70% accurate, whereas AFP alone is only 20% accurate. AFP is just as accurate as AFP-Plus in detecting open neural tube defects.

Timing

Timing for AFP-Plus screening is the same as for AFP screening.

Method

Three substances in the maternal serum are measured: alpha-fetoprotein (AFP), unconjugated estriol (uEST), and human chorionic gonadotropin (HCG). It is just as necessary, as in AFP screening, to have accurate gestational dating.

Physiology

Pregnancies affected with Down syndrome have lower serum levels of AFP and uEST and higher levels of HCG than unaffected pregnancies.

Interpretation of Results

AFP-Plus screening is 60% to 70% accurate in detecting Down syndrome and 85% accurate in detecting open neural tube defects. If the results are abnormal, additional screening is usually recommended. A normal result does not ensure a perfect, normal baby.

PERCUTANEOUS UMBILICAL BLOOD SAMPLING
Purpose

Percutaneous umbilical blood sampling is done to obtain fetal blood samples for rapid chromosomal analysis or to measure fetal hemoglobin (Baumann, McFarlin, 1994).

Timing

The sample may be drawn as early as amniocentesis but is generally done late in the second trimester when such diagnoses may change options and recommendations for medical management (Creasy, Resnik, 1994).

Method

With concurrent ultrasonographic visualization, a 23- or 25-gauge spinal needle is directed into the umbilical vein about 1 cm from the site of cord insertion into the placenta (Creasy, Resnik, 1994).

Postprocedure Care

External fetal monitoring is done for 1 to 2 hours after the procedure. Also, the nurse should instruct the mother in fetal movement counts and how to obtain results in 48 to 72 hours if the mother is discharged home.

FETAL INTRAUTERINE TRANSFUSION
Definition

Fetal intrauterine transfusion is a relatively new procedure that is now associated with increased success, new clinical applications, and more common use, but it is not a new concept. In the 1970s fetal intrauterine transfusions were being done experimentally and then only as a last resort in the most technologically sophisticated level III facilities. The procedure was first done by placing a parenteral catheter through the maternal abdominal wall and, by ultrasound guidance, placing it in proximity to the fetal diaphragmatic lymph system. The transfused blood was then indirectly absorbed through the lymphatics into the fetal circulation. The procedure was fraught with risks of maternal infection, fetal injury, and poor success. As a result, it was seldom used. At the time, ultrasound technology made placement difficult, and a safe procedure for fetal direct IV transfusion was improbable. Now, the direct route through percutaneous umbilical venous placement has changed and improved risks and success.

Purpose

Direct intrauterine fetal transfusion is indicated for the severely hydropic infant before 33 weeks of gestation in a D-negative sensitized pregnant woman. It is indicated also when percutaneously sampled umbilical venous blood demonstrates a significant lowering of fetal hemoglobin or hematocrit or if amniotic fluid samples indicate a rising bilirubin level and delta optical density (OD) increase.

Risks

Risks associated with intrauterine fetal transfusion surgery include the following:
- Maternal infection
- Overtransfusion
- Fetal vascular trauma
- Onset of preterm labor
- Fetal bradycardia

Method

Careful aseptic preparation of the maternal abdomen is necessary. The nurse should premedicate the mother with enough narcotic and tranquilizer to render the fetus quiet. The fetal vein is located using ultrasound. A 22-gauge long spinal needle is guided toward the vessel. Once the tip is placed correctly, blood, 20 to 50 ml/kg (depending on gestation), crossmatched to the mother and spun down tightly packed to a hematocrit greater than 70%, is then instilled slowly. Electronic fetal monitoring (EFM) is used for 1 to 2 hours after the procedure. The mother is instructed to continue fetal movement counts and other fetal testing (Creasy, Resnik, 1994).

FETAL INTRAUTERINE SURGERY*
Definition

Therapeutic advances in technology that led to fetal intrauterine surgical corrections evolved from interventions for D (Rh) sensitization and the effects on the fetus (Creasy, Resnik, 1994). Initially therapy was directed at disease acquired in utero. In the early 1980s, therapies for congenital disorders began to be attempted.

All forms of fetal surgery remain experimental, although some trends are becoming evident. These surgical procedures include the following:

1. Surgical correction of obstructive uropathies: the rationale for such therapy is to bypass the site of the obstruction and thereby prevent progressive renal damage.
2. Surgical correction of obstructive hydrocephalus: the rationale is to reduce ventricular size and expansion to minimize compression damage to the cerebral cortex.
3. In utero repair of fetal diaphragmatic hernia: presumably, repair of the hernia will provide release of compressive forces and restore normal lung development.

---

* Krummel and others, 1991; Longacker and others, 1991.

4. In utero plastic repair of such abnormalities as cleft palate and lip: theoretically, plastic repairs before birth would heal with less scarring.

Methods

The surgical corrections may be accomplished by ultrasound-guided percutaneous placement of catheter shunts or by hysterotomy with direct visualization and surgical repair. The type of congenital malformation as well as the skill and experimental training of the perinatologist will determine the exact method.

Risks

A number of problems arise when assessing the success and benefit of fetal intrauterine surgical corrections. Not the least of these are ethical dilemmas. Because of increased fetal and neonatal survival and the nature of accompanying disabilities, with surgical corrections of some disorders, more fetuses thus survive as infants with disabilities. Without fetal surgery many of these fetuses would not survive. Therefore it appears that increased survival will increase the societal problems of caring for infants with disabilities.

Some repairs corrected with intrauterine fetal surgery have better success than others. Infants with diaphragmatic hernia repair have the lowest survival rate. Those with repair of uropathologic conditions have the highest survival, although the best is with posterior urethral valve syndrome and the worst is with urethral atresia.

Hydrocephalic disorders are generally well screened for amount of adequate cerebral cortical tissue before attempting the repair. If other associated neurotube defects accompany hydrocephalus, the degree of handicap in surviving infants also varies (Creasy, Resnik, 1994; Krummel and others, 1991).

When hysterotomy is the chosen route for accomplishing the repair, there are other attendant problems. First, the incision into the uterus generally carries the risk of necessitating treatment of the uterine incision as similar to a classic cesarean. Second, as the procedure is being carried out, loss of amniotic fluid and interruption of the integrity of the amnion occur. The interruption of the integrity of the amnion is compensated for by using a stapling procedure of the amnion to the uterine wall as the incision is being made. Loss of amniotic fluid is restored by warmed normal saline as the cavity is closed. A third problem is keeping the fetus from having the head and upper respiratory system out of the fluid during the procedure and thus stimulating the switch from fetal cardiopulmonary circulation to neonatal circulation.

The limits on the number and type of fetal therapies for congenital disorders probably primarily result from the difference in the relative size of the fetus and the available technology and surgical instruments. It can be anticipated that those problems will be overcome as innovative and creative solutions are found to manage them.

The remaining serious problem society must wrestle with will continue to be the ethical dilemmas that arise more rapidly than our awareness of the long-term consequences of medical experimentation on the future (Holloway, 1990).

SELECTIVE REDUCTION
Definition

Selective reduction is a procedure to reduce the number of multiple embryos conceived usually by one of the fertility modalities. The concerns for nursing generally are related to the ethical dilemmas presented to the family and care providers. Because of their decision, parents are at high risk for complicated grief, potentially requiring referral for therapeutic psychologic support.

NURSING PROCESS

PREVENTION

The main functions of nursing care are to prevent uninformed decisions by parents, fetal compromise after intrauterine therapies, and unnecessary distress of the human spirit because of decisions for fetal testing or therapy.

Counselors and teachers are of prime importance. The ultimate goal is to empower families to make difficult decisions considering their ability to parent and the quality of life for their unborn child.

ASSESSMENT

Assessment of stressors, coping styles, and general knowledge and locus of control related to physical and emotional health assists in formulating nursing diagnoses. The nurse must articulate diagnoses and collaborative problems related to alterations in, risks to, complicating factors in, and strengths and deficiencies of individuals and the family as a unit.

NURSING DIAGNOSES/COLLABORATIVE PROBLEMS AND INTERVENTIONS

- **POTENTIAL COMPLICATIONS: FETAL INJURY** related to unexpected/unanticipated fetal outcome as a result of fetal therapy. *DESIRED OUTCOMES:* Parents will express an understanding of potential risks and benefits of fetal therapy. They will seek information about potential risks of fetal therapy and demonstrate tolerance for an unanticipated outcome. The nurse should do the following:
  1. Prepare for potential unexpected result.
  2. Establish a trusting relationship.
  3. Encourage and foster open communication with health providers.
  4. Coordinate a multidisciplinary conference with parents in attendance.
  5. Assist with preparations for extended family visitation while the patient is hospitalized.

- **RISK FOR KNOWLEDGE DEFICIT** related to unfamiliar tests, genetic screening, procedures, and environment. *DESIRED OUTCOMES:* Individuals will verbalize understanding of complicated and unfamiliar information and seek information about unexpected tests results or outcomes. The nurse should do the following:
  1. Encourage questions.
  2. Give anticipatory guidance.
  3. Be prepared to repeat information more than once.
  4. Provide more than one viewpoint or opinion.

- **RISK FOR INEFFECTIVE FAMILY COPING** related to unexpected outcome or test results, lack of knowledge, inadequate support system, or ineffective coping skills. *DESIRED OUTCOMES:* Individuals will discuss feelings, ask questions, and seek assistance. They will verbalize receptivity to explanations and demonstrate new, effective coping skills. The nurse should do the following:
  1. Assess for coping styles.
  2. Provide accurate information about fetal tests and therapy.
  3. Encourage and facilitate close family contact; eliminate separation.

- **DISTRESS OF THE HUMAN SPIRIT** related to fear for safety of the baby and difficulty with choosing care options from among alternatives that all conflict with values.

DESIRED OUTCOMES: Individual family members will verbalize distress and accept psychologic and spiritual support. Spiritual pain will be tolerated by the family without dysfunctional coping mechanisms. The nurse should do the following:

1. Refer to parents' spiritual or psychologic support person.
2. Communicate acceptance of expressed spiritual pain.
3. Encourage expression and exploration of feelings.
4. Assess parents' need for comforting spiritual rituals.
5. Support parents' decisions without expressing personal conflict and attitudes that may be in opposition to parents' attitudes.

CONCLUSION

The continued, rapid growth in technologic and innovative advances in fetal evaluation and therapies has exceeded considerations of physical, psychologic, and social consequences. It has become increasingly difficult for parents with a high risk pregnancy to obtain adequate information about expected benefits and negative consequences of fetal evaluation and therapies. The rapid growth also contributes to an inability to keep current with information needed to counsel and guide parents in making thoroughly informed decisions about fetal evaluation or therapy. Nurses have a professional responsibility to seek, be receptive to, and be intelligently critical of information that is on the cutting edge of the future.

BIBLIOGRAPHY

Amniocentesis

Creasy R, Resnik R, editors: *Maternal-fetal medicine: principles and practice,* ed 3, Philadelphia, 1994, Saunders.

Hanson F and others: Amniocentesis before 15 weeks gestation: outcome, risks, and technical problems, *Am J Obstet Gynecol* 156:1524-1531, 1987.

Chorionic Villi Sampling

Brambati L, Oldini A, Lanzani A: Transabdominal chorionic villus sampling: a free hand ultrasound-guided technique, *Am J Obstet Gynecol* 157:134-137, 1987.

Burton B, Schulz C, Burd L: Limb anomalies associated with chorionic villus sampling, *Obstet Gynecol* 79(5):726-730, 1992.

Copeland K and others: Integration of the transabdominal technique into an ongoing chorionic villus sampling program, *Am J Obstet Gynecol* 161:1289-1294, 1989.

Creasy R, Resnik R, editors: *Maternal-fetal medicine: principles and practice,* ed 3, Philadelphia, 1994, Saunders.

Elias S and others: Transabdominal chorionic villus sampling for first trimester prenatal diagnosis, *Am J Obstet Gynecol* 160:879-886, 1989.

Green J and others: Chorionic villus sampling: experience with an initial 940 cases, *Obstet Gynecol* 71:208, 1988.

Hammer R, Tufts M: Chorionic villi sampling for detecting fetal disorders, *MCN Am J Matern Child Nurs* 11(1):29-31, 1986.

Hogdall C and others: Transabdominal chorionic villus sampling in the second trimester, *Am J Obstet Gynecol* 158:345-349, 1988.

Hogge W, Schonberg S, Golbus M: Chorionic villus sampling: experience of the first 1000 cases, *Am J Obstet Gynecol* 154:1249-1252, 1986.

Hsieh FJ and others: Limb defects after CVS, *Obstet Gynecol* 85(1):84-88, 1995.

Jackson L: *CVS Newsletter,* no. 24, Feb 14, 1988.

McGovern M, Goldberg J, Desnick R: Acceptability of chorionic villus sampling for prenatal diagnosis, *Am J Obstet Gynecol* 155:25-29, 1986.

Rhoads C and others: The safety and efficiency of chorionic villus sampling for early prenatal diagnosis of cytogenic abnormalities, *N Engl J Med* 320:609-617, 1989.

Silverman N and others: Incidence of bacteremia associated with chorionic villus sampling, *Obstet Gynecol* 84(6):1021-1024, 1994.

Fetal Intrauterine Transfusion

Creasy R, Resnik R, editors: *Maternal-fetal medicine: principles and practice,* ed 3, Philadelphia, 1994, Saunders.

Seeds J, Bowes W: Ultrasound guided intrauterine transfusion in severe rhesus immunization, *Am J Obstet Gynecol* 154:1105, 1986.

Fetal Surgery

Birnholtz J, Frigoletto F: Antenatal treatment of fetal hydrocephalus, *N Engl J Med* 304:1021, 1981.

Clewell W, Meier P, Manchester D: Ventricularmegaly: evaluation and management, *Semin Perinatol* 9:98, 1985.

Creasy R, Resnik R, editors: *Maternal-fetal medicine: principles and practice,* ed 3, Philadelphia, 1994, Saunders.

Glick P, Harrison M: Correction of congenital hydronephrosis in utero. IV, *J Pediatr Surg* 19:649, 1984.

Harrison R, Bressack M, Chung A: Correction of congenital diaphragmatic hernia in utero, *Surgery* 88:260, 1980.

Holloway M: Fetal law: experimental surgery may feed ethical debates, *Sci Am* 263(3):46-48, 1990.

Krummel T and others: Characteristics of fetal repair, *Prog Clin Biol Res* 365:167-176, 1991.

Longacker M, Adzick N, Harrison M: Update on the status of fetal surgery, *Surg Ann* 23(2):53-68, 1991.

Stringer M, Librizzi R, Weiner S: Establishing a prenatal genetic diagnosis: the nurse's role, *MCN Am J Matern Child Nurs* 16:152-156, May/June 1991.

Maternal Alpha-fetoprotein

American Academy of Pediatrics, Committee on Genetics: Alpha fetoprotein screening, *Pediatrics* 80:444-445, 1987.

Bauman P, McFarlin B: Prenatal diagnosis, *J Nurse Midwifery* 39(2):35-57, 1994.

Burton B: Elevated maternal alpha fetoprotein (MSAFP): interpretation and follow-up, *Clin Obstet Gynecol* 31:293-304, 1988.

Creasy R, Resnik R, editors: *Maternal-fetal medicine: principles and practice,* ed 3, Philadelphia, 1994, Saunders.

Davis R and others: Decreased levels of amniotic fluid alpha fetoprotein associated with Down syndrome, *Am J Obstet Gynecol* 153:541-544, 1985.

Knight G, Palomaki G, Haddow J: Use of maternal serum alpha fetoprotein measurements to screen for Down syndrome, *Clin Obstet Gynecol* 31:306-327, 1988.

MacDonald M, Wagner R, Slotnick R: Sensitivity and specificity of screening Down's syndrome with AFP, HCG, UE3, and maternal age, *Obstet Gynecol,* Jan 1993.

McKeon V, O'Reilly M: Maternal serum alpha fetoprotein screening to detect fetal disorders, *IJCE,* 17-19, Feb 1990.

Myrhe C, Richards T, Johnson J: Maternal serum alpha fetoprotein screening: an assessment of fetal well being, *J Neonatal Nurs* 2:13-20, 1989.

Palomaki, Knight, Haddow: *Prenatal Diagn* 12:925-930, 1992.

Percutaneous Umbilical Blood Sampling

Creasy R, Resnik R, editors: *Maternal-fetal medicine: principles and practice,* ed 3, Philadelphia, 1994, Saunders.

II

Psychologic Implications of a High Risk Pregnancy

Nursing and the behavioral sciences point to the need to consider the high risk mother as a unique person who must cope with a complex group of psychologic and physiologic problems. In addition to undergoing the normal maturational process of childbearing, the high risk mother must cope with a great emotional burden and psychologic adjustment to a childbearing experience that may not culminate in a happy, healthy mother-infant dyad.

5

Psychologic Adaptations

To understand the emotional work and psychologic adjustments a high risk mother and her family must accomplish, certain concepts should be examined. Understanding concepts of attachment, the tasks of pregnancy, and the concept of adaptation in relation to crisis, anxiety, and frustration can be helpful when developing a plan of care for a high risk pregnant family.

ATTACHMENT

Attachment is a process influenced by many complex factors and is a permanent, interactional emotional bond that exists for life. Parent-infant attachment usually begins at the time the pregnancy is planned or during the pregnancy, even in many high risk pregnancies (Kemp, Page, 1987a; Klaus, Kennell, 1982).

Maternal

For the mother, attachment to the fetus is enhanced when she begins to feel the baby move, her body begins to change shape, and the uterus grows. Her focus is usually turned to the baby and its well-being, at which time she establishes a relationship with the fetus (Gay and others, 1988; Rubin, 1970). If the mother is afraid the fetus may die, this attachment may not take place because she is too fearful to establish a relationship. If family relationships are strained, it is more difficult for an expectant mother to form a positive attachment with her baby as well (Weingarten and others, 1990).

Clinicians have suggested that ultrasound examination of the fetus enhances attachment. However, research studies (Heidrich, Cranley, 1989; Lumley, 1990) have not shown that ultrasound examination significantly affects maternal attachment.

Paternal

For the father, attachment to the fetus differs from that for the mother. Most of his attachment centers on acceptance and support of the mother's changing physical and emotional state. When a threat to maternal or fetal health develops, the father may feel guilty for his inability to protect the mother and the fetus and ensure a safe passage for them (Wohlreich, 1987). This may affect his attachment.

Influencing Factors

Parent attachment to the fetus and newborn depends on the following factors:
1. Emotional maturity
2. Experience in being nurtured
3. Interpersonal relationships with significant others
4. Ability to cope with physiologic and psychologic stressors
5. Desire for pregnancy and self-concept of parenthood
6. Fears and fantasies during the pregnancy

There is a sensitive period, immediately after birth, when attachment is enhanced through the interactions of parents with their infant. These interactions are categorized into observable sensory levels (Rubin, 1984; Sherwen, 1987).

Tactile

When given the opportunity, most parents will make immediate tactile contact with their infant. The initial contact is exploratory and is made with the fingertips. Progression of tactile contact follows an orderly pattern but can vary in its length of time. After the fingertips, the palms of the hands are used to stroke and massage the baby. Then the baby is drawn into close contact with the mother and encompassed (Tulman, 1985).

Verbal

Some parents make early verbal contact by carrying on a continual stream of soft, high-pitched verbalization (Tomlinson, 1990). The context usually involves relating how the infant resembles other family members.

Visual

Early eye-to-eye contact is sought even when the infant is not being held. The parents usually try to position themselves so they and the infant are en face. If the infant does not open his or her eyes, they will implore him or her to do so.

Entrainment

The speech pattern of either parent has a powerful influence on the infant's activity. The infant very soon forms activity patterns in a reciprocal relationship that resembles a dance. The infant's response in this manner seems to lock the parent into repeating speech over and over.

Synchrony

The first act of synchrony occurs in the feeding process. The mother responds to the infant's sucking bursts and pauses for breath. Mothers learn to respond in the cycles of sucking and pausing at the appropriate points to stimulate or discourage sucking.

If the neonate is sick and the parents' interactions and caregiving opportunities are limited, attachment may lag behind. However, according to Klaus and Kennell (1984), these parents will become attached to their babies, but it might be delayed.

MATERNAL TASKS

A series of developmental tasks must be accomplished in pregnancy for the mothering, attachment behaviors to occur (Gay and others, 1988; Patterson and others, 1990; Rubin, 1975).

Pregnancy Acceptance

Pregnancy validation or acceptance usually takes place during the first trimester when the woman determines that she is pregnant and begins securing acceptance of the pregnancy from significant others. During this time, she is very concerned about herself and seeking "safe passage" for herself.

Establishing a Relationship With the Fetus

The pregnant woman begins to establish a relationship with the fetus when she can look beyond her concern about herself and focus on the fetus being part of her (fetal embodiment). This is when she becomes more dependent and wants to socialize with other pregnant women. As her relationship with her fetus grows, she begins to view the fetus as a separate individual from her (fetal distinction). The focus of safe passage at this time is for the fetus as well as for herself through prenatal care and making life-style changes.

Role Transition

Role transition involves preparing for the birth and early motherhood. Now she is seeking safe passage for herself and her baby during the delivery process.

PATERNAL TASKS

The expectant father's unconscious feelings and early memories of childhood play an important part in his emotional adjustment to the pregnancy. His involvement in the birth promotes and enhances nurturing behavior (Colman, Colman, 1971; Sherwen, 1987). The father's involvement and accomplishment of paternal tasks can be divided into three phases (Diamond, 1986; May, 1982).

Announcement Phase

The announcement phase is the period during the pregnancy when it is first recognized and the father informs others of the pregnancy. It varies in length from a few hours to a few weeks. It may be characterized by strong feelings of elation or shock, depending on the desire for the pregnancy. However, the father's response is usually mixed with pride, joy, concern, and conflict.

Moratorium Phase

The moratorium phase also varies in length but typically includes the twelfth to the twenty-fifth weeks. The pregnancy does not seem real to the father during this time and is characterized by emotional distancing. Distancing allows the man to work through any ambivalence about what he will give up because of the pregnancy, such as an exclusive relationship with the mother-to-be, privacy, a quiet home, and social freedom. He often spends more time at work because of his financial concerns. Marital tension and disrupted communication are common.

Focusing Phase

The focusing phase begins around the twenty-fifth to the thirtieth week and extends to the onset of labor. The expectant father focuses on his experience, begins to feel more in tune with the mother, and redefines his world in terms of his future father-hood role.

HIGH RISK STRESSORS
Situational and Maturational Stressors

Pregnancy itself is a situational stressor. The cognitive process of pregnancy is one of questioning and uncertainty (Affonso, Sheptak, 1989; Rubin, 1970). When a pregnancy becomes high risk and the expectant mother or her fetus is at risk for illness or death, the family is faced with a far greater situational stressor. At the same time the family is also faced with maturational stressors.

The development of a high risk condition may disrupt the accomplishment of maternal or paternal tasks, and added stressors may result. Fears for the mother's well-being can cause heightened ambivalence about the pregnancy. Previous pregnancy losses may be recalled and may complicate acceptance of the reality of a current pregnancy. If signs of bleeding or other ominous physical signs occur, it might be difficult to validate the pregnancy. Preparations for the baby may be halted. Prenatal education for self and partner also might not be an option offered to an ill or hospitalized mother. Unmet expectations for the pregnancy may be a source of frustration at a time when activities would otherwise be directed at preparation for parenthood.

Preparation for the birth process might be totally out of the parents' control if the mother's well-being is in question. Fears about procedures and care may take precedence over the usual plans. The growth rate of the mother's body may be a great concern. Choices for infant feeding, the birth process, or the coach's support might differ from what were desired.

When all or any of the developmental tasks are thwarted or interfered with, attachment can be slow in the neonatal period. If either the neonate or mother is ill immediately after delivery, early contact may not occur. When the neonate is premature or is connected to machinery, the parents might fear touching the infant. The appearance and behavior of the neonate can be so new to the parents that their visual inspection finds nothing to identify with. Finally, if the pregnancy was thought to be in jeopardy, efforts might have been devoted to "letting go" rather than "attaching to." If this is so, the parents must resolve these feelings before they can begin to attach. The depth of emotion surrounding the possible death of the baby can be so strong as to permanently interfere with attachment if feelings are not explored.

Hospitalization Stressors

Antepartal hospitalization can cause added stressors for the family of a high risk pregnancy. These stressors include separation from home, family, and other support persons, which can cause increased loneliness. Other stressors are feelings of added loss of control or powerlessness, changes in family circumstances causing stress on family functioning, and concern for the family members at home (Loos, Julius, 1989; Mercer and others, 1988). Dependency needs may not be fulfilled. Socialization with other pregnant women can be limited.

PSYCHOLOGIC RESPONSES

The family may react in a variety of ways to the diagnosis of a high risk pregnancy. It depends on what significance they place on the condition, their experience with coping skills, ability to effectively problem solve, and available situational supports (Aguilera, 1990).

Anxiety

Anxiety can arise when expectations are not met. In a high risk pregnancy, the expectation of a normal pregnancy culminating in delivery of a healthy baby is being threatened. The strength of the unmet needs and degree of awareness about them determine the extent of anxiety.

Threat to Self-esteem

If the expectant mother feels the diagnosis is a blow to her self-confidence, she may experience a sense of low self-esteem (Kemp, Page, 1987b). This may cause her to feel she has failed as a woman (loss of a perfect pregnancy) and as a mother (fear of loss of a perfect baby), lowering her confidence in her ability to be a mother.

Self-blaming

The parents may react by blaming themselves for real or imagined wrongdoing, or one may blame the other.

Frustration

Frustration occurs when obstacles prevent the achievement of a goal. The behavioral effects of frustration include anger, aggression, withdrawal, fixation, or finally even learning. Frustration occurs in a high risk pregnancy when goals such as a healthy pregnancy, having a perfect baby, or having the perfect birth experience have the obstacles of illness, separation, and rigid rules imposed on them.

Conflict

Conflict results when there are simultaneous, opposing goals of equal strength. If the desired pregnancy causes physical restrictions requiring financial strains or imposes difficulty in mothering tasks with other children, conflict can result. The choices offered to the mother might all be unappealing. If her goal is to have a vaginal delivery and a cesarean delivery is the only safe option for her, conflict will occur.

Crisis

A crisis occurs when a very important life goal is threatened and no immediate solution is apparent (Aguilera, 1990). The inability to function results, and a state of disequilibrium ensues.

HIGH RISK ADAPTATION

The ability to restore equilibrium depends on three balancing factors. First, an individual must have a realistic perception of the event. Second, there must be adequate support from significant others. Third, an individual must have developed adequate coping mechanisms in the past or the ability to problem solve (Aguilera, 1990).

To deal with the multiple crises a high risk pregnancy imposes, the mother and her family must call on past coping mechanisms and must learn new ones. The nurse should discuss with parents ways they have responded in the past and encourage the use of tactics that have worked before. Previous pregnancy loss should be discussed early in a current pregnancy to assess for coping strategies.

Information must be provided repeatedly about the disease or the condition the woman is facing and should be explained thoroughly to provide autonomy and choices where possible. Information will facilitate a realistic appraisal of the events and prepare the couple for potential future events. The mother should be accompanied by significant people, especially her partner, when information is given. Hospitalization should include flexible rules for the father's presence whenever he can be there, and separations should be minimized whenever possible.

When both the woman and her partner can be given choices in care, personal strategies for coping will be less limited and thus more effective. Skill in encouraging these coping mechanisms is necessary in a high risk obstetric setting because of the psychologic impact on the entire family. To maintain the unity of the family when the pregnancy is over, it is important to facilitate the sharing of events. Interventions in a crisis should be aimed at restructuring the present. They should suppress negative uses of energy and support positive efforts.

NURSING PROCESS

PREVENTION

A high risk pregnancy carries with it a threat not only to the physical well-being of the mother and fetus, but also to the emotional well-being of the entire family unit. Therefore serious consideration must be given to assisting all family members. The nurse must assess and assist the high risk family in the use of previously learned, effective coping styles and in the development of new coping skills. To do this, the focus of nursing care must be on identifying and exploring feelings of fear, anxiety, frustration, and the resolution of conflicts in needs. Maintaining the family as a unit as much as possible, especially the mother and her partner, is paramount. Except for situations when the mother's life may be in jeopardy, the father should be encouraged to spend normal family time with the hospitalized woman. Other children should be brought in for frequent supervised visits. Socialization needs and nesting preparations should be encouraged in creative and innovative ways.

ASSESSMENT

An initial and ongoing assessment to determine the individual's and family's functioning response to the actual threat to optimal physical and emotional pregnancy outcome is paramount. This is the basis for formulating appropriate nursing diagnoses and an individualized plan of care. This will eliminate making assumptions regarding how the expectant parents are feeling and how they are coping. A prenatal psychologic assessment guide, using the functional health patterns, has been developed (Box 5-1).

NURSING DIAGNOSES/COLLABORATIVE PROBLEMS AND INTERVENTIONS

- **FEAR** of threat to self-concept, health status, socioeconomic status, role functioning, interaction patterns, environment, and fetal or neonatal well-being.

Box 5-1

Psychologic Assessment for High Risk Pregnancy

Health-perception/health-management pattern

What choices in your birth plan have been limited, such as attendance at childbirth education classes, type of delivery, need for anesthesia, or other medical interventions, because of the development of a high risk condition?

Do you feel your control has been affected?

Nutritional/metabolic pattern

What dietary changes need to be made because of your high risk condition?

Why do you need to make these dietary changes?

Elimination pattern

What kinds of elimination changes, if any, have developed because of your high risk condition or treatment?

Activity/exercise pattern

What activity changes have been necessary because of your high risk condition?

Why do you need to make these activity changes?

What does bed rest or limited activity, if ordered, mean to you and your family?

Sleep/rest pattern

How do you feel after sleeping or resting at night?

Does this high risk condition affect your normal sleeping pattern? If so, how?

Cognitive/perceptual pattern

Explain your understanding of the high risk condition, proposed plan of treatment, and possible effects on self, fetus, and neonate?

Self-perception/self-concept pattern

What does this high risk condition mean to you and your family?

Are you or your family experiencing any guilt feelings?

Is anyone upset at you or blaming you for this high risk condition?

How do you feel it has affected your self-confidence, maternal role, and acceptance of the pregnancy?

Role/relationship pattern

What are the family stressors?

Who lives in the home?

How has this high risk condition affected your home, work, and other responsibilities?

How can the nurse help you and your family plan needed restructuring of roles and activities?

What are your financial concerns because of this high risk condition?

Box 5-1

Psychologic Assessment for High Risk Pregnancy–cont'd

Sexuality/reproductive pattern

How does the modified or restricted sexual activity affect you and your significant other?

Coping/stress tolerance pattern

What are you most worried or fearful about?

Identify stressors that are affecting you and your family because of this high risk condition.

How is this hospitalization affecting your life?

How supportive is the baby's father and your family and friends?

What coping techniques have been effective for you in the past?

What referral services would be helpful?

Value/belief pattern

Which values, if any, are being affected or threatened by this high risk condition?

DESIRED OUTCOME: The patient, her significant other, and siblings will be able to communicate and discuss their fears and concerns openly. The nurse should do the following:

1. Provide time for the patient and her family to express their concerns regarding the possible outcome for the baby and inconvenience to the mother and family during the treatment. Encourage them to vent any apprehension, uncertainty, fears, anger, and worry they may be experiencing. Talking about the event can help in identifying, analyzing, and understanding the events causing the fear. Beginning such discussion with a mother can be facilitated with statements such as "Many women in your situation feel. . . . "

2. Assess for increased wariness, poor eye contact, restlessness, trembling, insomnia, and tension.

3. Assess the family's expressed feelings of guilt, such as "What did we do to cause or contribute to this?"

4. Assess financial concerns such as medical bills, child care expenses, and traveling and lodging expenses for the out-of-town family.

5. Encourage the father to relieve his fear and anxiety in a positive way instead of keeping it to himself. Couples who

do not receive help together might otherwise increase each other's fear and anxiety.

6. Facilitate parents discussing their feelings with the other children in the family so the siblings can understand why their parents are upset. Allow the children to express any guilt they may be experiencing. If they wished that the fetus would "go away," provide reassurance that they did not cause the situation and that the parents still love them.

7. Encourage the expectant family to express feelings and concerns about the anticipated labor and delivery experience.

8. Explain the high risk condition, all treatment modalities, and reasons for each.

9. Define terms that health professionals use in talking to the family.

10. Clarify misconceptions. Explain causes of the condition and, if causes are unknown, any associations or lack of association with patient activities.

11. Keep patient informed of health status, results of tests, and fetal well-being.

12. Refer to a nurse specialist, counselor, social worker, or chaplain as appropriate and desired.

■ **RISK FOR SITUATIONAL LOW SELF-ESTEEM** related to perceived inability to accomplish pregnancy tasks satisfactorily, the "high tech" focus, or lack of support or acceptance of the unborn child from the baby's father.

DESIRED OUTCOMES: The patient will verbalize competency in coping with and accomplishing pregnancy tasks despite the altered situation. She will verbalize that her emotional needs are being appropriately met. The nurse should do the following:

1. Encourage verbalization of feelings by "active listening."

2. Provide emotional support as needed.

3. Assess and assist the patient in identifying strategies for accomplishing pregnancy acceptance, fetal embodiment, fetal distinction, and role transition.

4. Encourage participation in her care and decision making as much as possible. For example, allow self-administration of medications and encourage expectant parents' involvement in the treatment plan.

5. Support, encourage, and enhance information gathering for

childbirth preparation and acquisition of parenting skills. Special childbirth education classes designed to meet the unique needs of the high risk pregnant couple are clearly beneficial (Avery, Olson, 1987).

6. Alter the environment to meet the needs of the mother and the father for acquisition of parenting skills and parent/child interaction.
7. Allow the mother to choose her own foods within the restrictions, and allow foods to be brought from home if requested.
8. Develop flexible visiting policies for the high risk unit. Provide extra beds for fathers-to-be to feel welcome to spend the night. Encourage siblings-to-be to visit.
9. Make needed referrals, such as to social service and mental health specialists, if problems are identified.

■ **RISK FOR ALTERED FAMILY PROCESSES**   related to the treatment plan of limited activity, separation of the family members from each other, or ineffective adaptive behaviors in response to the high risk pregnancy.

DESIRED OUTCOME: Each member of the family will verbalize acceptance of the family's restructuring plan to meet the mother's roles and responsibilities. The nurse should do the following:

1. Assess the patient's responsibilities to determine difficulties she will face in implementing prescribed bed rest or limited activity.
2. Teach the patient and her significant others about the importance of bed rest or limited activity for her high risk condition.
3. Facilitate the family in problem solving difficulties in implementing maternal bed rest or limited activity.
4. Make needed referrals, such as to the social worker, if problems are identified that the family cannot work out.
5. Provide and encourage extended and private visiting time.
6. Involve appropriate family members in decisions.

■ **RISK FOR INEFFECTIVE INDIVIDUAL OR FAMILY COPING**   related to lack of previous coping strategies, separation during the pregnancy, change in usual communication patterns, anxiety, fear, frustration, or conflict arising from unacceptable alternatives.

DESIRED OUTCOMES: Family members will use previously developed coping skills, maintain effective communication patterns, meet basic family needs, and avoid dysfunctional coping strategies. The nurse should do the following:

1. Assess the expectant mother's family structure. How supportive are the family members? (Family relationships can have a positive or negative effect on the expectant mother's health [Ramsey and others, 1986].)
2. Assess the family's coping strategies and resources.
3. Problem solve with the family regarding past coping strategies that have proven effective for various family members.
4. Assess for change in communication patterns within the family.
5. Assess for inability to meet basic needs of family members.
6. Encourage each family member to verbalize about the complications.
7. Encourage and facilitate support-seeking activities such as socializing with other pregnant couples and attending specially designed childbirth preparation classes.
8. Refer to a perinatal clinical nurse specialist, a social worker, community support groups such as "High Risk Moms" (Beck, 1995; Snyder, 1988), and pastoral care as desired by the family.

- **DIVERSIONAL ACTIVITY DEFICIT** related to therapeutic treatment of limited activity.
  DESIRED OUTCOME: The patient will verbalize various activities she would like to do. The nurse should do the following:
    1. Assess patient's interest in various diversional activities within the activity limit.
    2. Provide crafts, reading, and puzzles that can be done in bed, or encourage patient to have these things brought in.
    3. Provide classes in preparation for childbirth by way of video, a hospital television, or group classes that can be attended while reclining.
    4. Refer to a diversional therapist or volunteer to provide reading materials, handicrafts, or other interesting things.

- **SLEEP PATTERN DISTURBANCE** related to worry, hospital disturbances, and change in the sleeping environment.
  DESIRED OUTCOME: The patient will have at least 8 hours of sleep at night and report that she feels rested in the morning. The nurse should do the following:
    1. Assess how the patient feels on waking.

2. Assess the patient's normal sleep time and pattern.
3. Assess for disturbing dreams.
4. Minimize interruptions at night if possible.
5. Adjust hospital routines, when possible, to match the patient's normal sleep pattern.
6. Encourage bed rest exercises.

■ **ALTERED SEXUALITY PATTERN** related to limitations imposed because of the treatment plan for the high risk condition.
   DESIRED OUTCOME: The patient and her significant other will discuss openly their sexual concerns and will verbalize mutual acceptance of the temporary limitations. The nurse should do the following:
   1. Assess understanding of the patient and her significant other of the need to modify or restrict sexual activity.
   2. Assess how each is affected by this sexual restriction.
   3. If the mother is hospitalized, allow some private time for the couple.
   4. Encourage closeness.

CONCLUSION

A high risk pregnancy imposes a myriad of psychologic stressors on individuals and the family unit. Supportive care that considers the needs of the family is a must. Without adequate support, families experiencing a high risk pregnancy are at high risk for permanent separation, divorce, substance abuse, and physically and emotionally abusive situations. With adequate support, family members can achieve a sense of accomplishment in the face of adversity and become emotionally closer to each other.

BIBLIOGRAPHY

Affonso D, Sheptak S: Maternal cognitive themes during pregnancy, *MCN Am J Matern Child Nurs* 18(2):147-166, 1989.

Aguilera D: *Crisis intervention: theory and methodology,* St Louis, 1990, Mosby.

Annie C, Groer M: Childbirth stress: an immunologic study, *J Obstet Gynecol Neonatal Nurs* 20(5):391-397, 1991.

Avery P, Olson I: Expanding the scope of childbirth education to meet the needs of hospitalized, high-risk clients, *J Obstet Gynecol Neonatal Nurs* 16(6):418-420, 1987.

Beck C: Perceptions of nurses' caring by mothers experiencing postpartum depression, *J Obstet Gynecol Neonatal Nurs* 24(3):814-821, 1995.

Colman A, Colman L: *Pregnancy: the psychological experience,* New York, 1971, Herder & Herder.

Diamond M: Becoming a father: a psychoanalytic perspective on the forgotten parent, *Psychoanal Rev* 73(4):41-64, 1986.

Gay J, Edgil A, Douglas A: Reva Rubin revisited, *J Obstet Gynecol Neonatal Nurs* 17(6):394-399, 1988.

Heidrich S, Cranley M: Effect of fetal movement, ultrasound scans, and amniocentesis on maternal-fetal attachment, *Nurs Res* 38(2):81-84, 1989.

Kemp V, Page C: Maternal prenatal attachment in normal and high-risk pregnancies, *J Obstet Gynecol Neonatal Nurs* 16(3):179-184, 1987a.

Kemp V, Page C: Maternal self-esteem and prenatal attachment in high-risk pregnancy, *Matern Child Nurs J* 16(3):195-206, 1987b.

Klaus M, Kennell J: *Parent infant bonding,* ed 2, St Louis, 1982, Mosby.

Klaus M, Kennell J: Bonding: another view, *Perinatology/Neonatology* 8(2):72-73, 1984.

Loos C, Julius L: The client's view of hospitalization during pregnancy, *J Obstet Gynecol Neonatal Nurs* 18(1):52-56, 1989.

Lumley J: Through a glass darkly: ultrasound and prenatal bonding, *Birth* 17(4):214-217, 1990.

May K: Three phases of father involvement in pregnancy, *Nurs Res* 31(6):337-342, 1982.

Mercer R and others: Effect of stress on family functioning during pregnancy, *Nurs Res* 37(5):268-275, 1988.

Patterson E, Freese M, Goldenberg R: Seeking safe passage: utilizing health care during pregnancy, *Image J Nurs Sch* 22(1):27-31, 1990.

Ramsey C, Abell T, Baker L: The relationship between family functioning, life events, family structure, and the outcome of pregnancy, *J Family Pract* 22(6):521-527, 1986.

Rubin R: Cognitive style in pregnancy, *Am J Nurs* 70(3):502-508, 1970.

Rubin R: Maternal tasks in pregnancy, *MCN Am J Matern Child Nurs* 4(3):143-153, 1975.

Rubin R: *Maternal identity and the maternal experience,* New York, 1984, Springer.

Sherwen L: Maternal role attainment. In Sherwen L, editor: *Psychosocial dimensions of the pregnant family,* New York, 1987, Springer.

Snyder D: Peer group support for high risk mothers, *MCN Am J Matern Child Nurs* 13(2):114-117, 1988.

Tomlinson P: Verbal behavior associated with indicators of maternal attachment with the neonate, *J Obstet Gynecol Neonatal Nurs* 19(1):76-77, 1990.

Tulman L: Mothers and unrelated persons' initial handling of newborn infants, *Nurs Res* 34(4):205, 1985.

Weingarten C and others: Married mothers' perceptions of their premature or term infants and the quality of their relationships with their husbands, *J Obstet Gynecol Neonatal Nurs* 19(1):64-73, 1990.

Wohlreich M: Psychiatric aspects of high-risk pregnancy, *Psychiatr Clin North Am* 10(1):53-68, 1987.

CHAPTER

6

Pregnancy Loss and Perinatal Grief

There is a growing awareness of the significance a fetal or newborn death has on parents. This parental crisis not only involves the actual death of the baby, but also shatters dreams and hopes for the future. Despite the fact that grief is a universal feeling at some time in life, the scientific study of the psychology of grief is only 54 years old, beginning with Lindemann's classic study of the survivors of the Cocoanut Grove fire in 1944. Although psychologic symptomatology associated with the death of a child, spouse, parent, or sibling has been widely accepted, only recently has the impact of pregnancy loss and infant death been acknowledged by society.

If one examines the incidence of miscarriage, including spontaneous events, induced abortions, and ectopic pregnancy, it is estimated that 15% to 20% of all pregnancies end very early in gestation. If stillbirth, newborn death, and sudden infant death syndrome in the first year of life are included, another 15% can be added to the estimation. Thus approximately one third of all pregnancies, by the end of the expected first year of life, do not culminate in the healthy, bouncing baby of societal dreams (Woods, Esposito, 1987).

Death is rarely predicted at any but the final stages of the life cycle. During gestation and shortly after birth, death seems a remote possibility. Uniformly recognized social rituals associated with death in later life are well known, whereas pregnancy loss has few accepted societal rituals. It is often said that fetal and neonatal deaths are celebrated only in the tears of the parents, yet the experience is a common occurrence among people during their childbearing years. It is an often repeated, poignant story told when women get together to describe their childbearing experiences or told in self-imposed control during a routine gynecologic or obstetric history. Usually many details of events surrounding pregnancy loss or infant death are told with great clarity and poignant remembrances.

It is imperative that health care professionals in the field of maternity and family care acknowledge and learn about helpful and comforting responses needed by families at the time of perinatal loss and assist in the acquisition of support in the following 1 to 2 years. To understand the dynamics of grief work and the mourning that takes place, it is necessary to do the following:

1. Explore the concepts of loss and grief.
2. Describe the different types of loss experienced at various stages of gestation and early newborn death.
3. Identify the feelings expressed by individual family members (mothers, fathers, and siblings), as well as other support people.
4. List strategies for care and follow-up that have been acknowledged by parents to be most helpful and comforting.
5. Describe the potential roles of various members of the health care team in providing support and comfort.
6. Discuss therapeutic communication skills relevant to grief support.

LOSS

Loss occurs when something or someone valued by a person is denied to him or her or taken away after acquisition. Although the definition appears relatively simple, the feelings surrounding the loss or losses are complex.

As pregnancy and infant loss become better understood and described, it is best not to compare losses at different times in gestation or the postnatal period but rather to identify those losses most significant to the individual. Some of the losses described by parents are as follows:

1. *Loss of a loved and valued person or relationship.* This loss includes adults, elderly persons, children, or infants.

2. *Loss of some aspect of self.* Loss of self may include self-worth, special qualities or position within society, providing "safe passage," attractiveness, body image, feeling special, or a visible or invisible body part.

3. *Developmental losses.* Developmental losses include such losses as parental status, social interaction with other parents, and sharing in firsts, such as holding one's infant for the first time, first birthday, first Christmas, and kindergarten.

4. *Loss of material or external objects.* Material objects may include nursery items, layette, toys, memorabilia such as photographs, baby book, handprints and footprints, and other tangible evidence of the baby's existence.

GRIEF
Terms

Three terms (grief, bereavement, and mourning) are commonly used, sometimes interchangeably. Definitions of these terms are helpful before discussion of the phases of psychologic work.

Grief is the total organismic response to and feelings about loss. Grieving is the process of assimilating the changes and meaning into a new sense or definition of reality (Woods, Esposito, 1987). *Bereavement* is the entire dynamic process precipitated by loss (Woods, Esposito, 1987). *Mourning* is the process through which integration and assimilation of the reality of loss are accomplished. Grieving and mourning are often used interchangeably. The four tasks of mourning (Worden, 1991) are as follows:

1. To accept the reality of the loss
2. To experience the pain of grief
3. To adjust to life without this baby
4. To withdraw emotional energy from grief for this baby and reinvest in other relationships

Phases

There are four interwoven phases of bereavement (Table 6-1) (Davidson, 1984). Phases, unlike stages, do not have sharp lines of demarcation. It is not possible to move from one phase into another without retaining a sense of those phases that came before or will come to be. Phases are dynamic, symbolically likened to interweaving a tapestry of life. Kubler-Ross (1969) contributed much to our understanding of a person facing his or her own death. Bowlby (1982) and more recently Peppers and Knapp (1985) have

TABLE 6-1   Phases of bereavement

Phases and times	Definition	Physical manifestations	Feelings	Psychologic characteristics
Phase 1: shock and numbness Highest peak at 1-2 wk and at 12 mo	Shock and numbness protect human spirit, although temporarily; these feelings allow a person time to sort through multitude of intense feelings surrounding event; this phase permits parents an opportunity to take one thing at a time and thus make initial events more manageable and controllable	Pain in various body parts, especially constriction of throat and heaviness in chest "Heavy" heart Empty arms or emptiness in abdomen Tears, weeping, screaming Dry mouth Sighing Loss of muscle power, uncontrolled trembling, startle response Sleep disturbance Loss of appetite	Disbelief Confusion Restlessness Feelings of unreality/ instability Regression/helplessness	Egocentric phenomena Preoccupation with thoughts of deceased Psychologic distancing of self; feeling as though looking at self from outside
Phase 2: searching and yearning Highest peak at 2 wk to 4 mo	During this phase, bereaved parents have enormous energy; they have a need to look for information and find answers; there are often	Crying Acting out feelings of anger Sleeplessness Change in eating habits	Separation anxiety Conflict Prolonged stress Sense of something sinister	Oversensitive Searching Disbelief/denial Anger/frustration Sense of presence/ phantom crying

	repeated descriptions of events leading up to and during time of death; awareness of reality of loss is beginning to be integrated into life			Dreaming/nightmares Fear Guilt/shame
Phase 3: disorganization and depression Highest peak at 4-6 mo	In this phase parents are struck by their keen sense of reality of their baby's death and the fact that nothing can be done to turn back time and change what has occurred; they have identified some of what they miss most and can never have with their child; depression is most predominant feature of this phase	Weakness Fatigue Need for a great deal of sleep Weakened immune system	Withdrawal/social isolation/loneliness Despair/depression Helplessness/powerlessness Sick/ailing	Hibernation/holding pattern Obsessional review Working at grieving, seeking to explain sense in experience Turning point/conscious decision to go forward with life or not Most dangerous time; three choices: move forward, status quo, or not survive

Continued

TABLE 6-1 Phases of bereavement—cont'd

Phases and times	Definition	Physical manifestations	Feelings	Psychologic characteristics
Phase 4: reorganization Highest peak begins at 1 yr and from then on	In this phase, parent has faced decision to survive and chosen survival and taken control of life; as healing of heart and mind begins, physical well-being also returns	Physical healing/immune restoration Increased energy Sleep restoration Appetite returns	Control Sense of restructured identity Responsible Can live with knowledge of baby's death	Forgiving of oneself and others Forgetting intense pain for longer periods of time Search for meaning and may reach out to help others experiencing similar loss Closing circle/having a place to go Has hope for future Lives for oneself and others Takes needed time to grieve Expects and prepares for anniversary reactions

laid the foundation for our understanding of parental grieving for the death of a wished for or expected child. Davidson (1984) has contributed to the understanding of the time involved in the progression of grief work or mourning. Finally, grieving parents provide the most important lessons in the tremendous effort involved in grief work.

Provided with time and support to grieve, parents may take 6 to 24 months to begin to feel renewed, reorganized, and generally okay. The time it takes does not depend on the length of the gestation. Rather, it depends more on the individual's strengths, coping strategies, and ability to seek and accept support and on other stressors in life at the time (Davidson, 1984; Rando, 1986; Woods, Esposito, 1987).

Types of Grief

Wheeler and Pike (1991) have described the following five distinct types of grief.

Anticipatory Grief

Anticipatory grief occurs when a perceived life-threatening diagnosis is given or the pregnancy is threatened. Anticipatory grief is somewhat different from conventional grief in the work that is done to adapt and the feelings expressed. Ambivalence is often described about hastening the end or the actual death so that the parent can "get on with life" versus doing "everything possible" to reverse the inevitable. With anticipatory grief work, the phases must be hastened to prepare for the inevitable; thus shock is less, and a sense of finality predominates.

Inhibited Grief

Inhibited grief is kept inward and private. Outward expressions of feelings are not acceptable to the individual. Commonly, there is an incongruence in feelings and expressions of them. Inhibited grief retards the ability to reach out for support and often leads to later manifestations of grief feelings and psychologic pain than would otherwise be expected.

Delayed Grief

When grief is delayed, decisions for care of the baby after death must be made by someone else. Preferably, the person designated will be most sensitive to the individual's desires and needs. However, in the case where grief is delayed because of the physical status of the mother, this often falls to the father. Caught in his own grief at the time, he may see it as his duty to protect the mother's feelings. It is generally best to refer assistance with necessary decisions to the family's spiritual advisor or close, reasonably objective friend.

Absent Grief

Absent grief may occur because of unresolved grief from a previous loss, because of death of one or more multiples with one or more survivors, or because of a concurrent mental disorder. Grief that is postponed or absent will in all likelihood assault the individual at a later, unexplained time.

Long-term Grief or Sorrow

Mourning persists in any one of the first three phases, and movement through or into another phase is seemingly impossible. When chronic sorrow is evidenced, life basically stops and simple activities are impossible. In a family, chronic grief on the part of one individual disables all members.

Complicated Grief

When progress in grief work halts and the parents have an emotional incapacity to continue the work of accomplishing the tasks, grief is complicated. Complicated grief requires referral to a professional psychologist or crisis intervention counselor. Signs of complicated grief, according to Wheeler and Pike (1991), include the following:

1. *Persistent thoughts of self-destruction.* The person focuses on self-destructive thoughts and develops a plan of self-destruction.
2. *Failure to provide for basic needs for survival.* Indications of this include social isolation; a weight gain or loss in excess of 24 pounds; increased or abusive use of alcohol, nicotine, or illegal drugs; sleep deprivation; an inability to care for basic needs of children in the home; or an inability to maintain or initiate basic activities of daily life.
3. *Persistent mourning or long-term depression.* This is characterized by being stuck in a phase of mourning for more than several months; no expression of grief after the loss; flat affect, with no demonstration of real feelings about anything; preoccupation with the image of the baby; expression of real guilt rather than only imagined guilt; or hostile reactions out of proportion to the situation.

4. *Abuse of controlling substances.* Use of such substances as alcohol or illegal drugs on a regular basis or verbalization of use to dull feelings indicates abuse.
5. *Occurrence or recurrence of mental illness.* This usually is seen as clinical depression or manic depression.
6. *Lack of balance in life.* This may be evidenced by workaholic activity, spending increasing time away from home, or religious fanaticism.
7. *Interpersonal relationship problems.* Relationship problems are manifested many times by blaming or hostile feelings.

EARLY PREGNANCY LOSS
Definition

Early pregnancy loss may occur through spontaneous events or elective, induced events. By definition, a *miscarriage* is a pregnancy loss that occurs before 20 weeks of gestation. In the United States, state laws often stipulate that, in addition, the weight is less than 350 g and signs of life are absent. *Abortion* is the medical term used for both spontaneous and elective, induced events occurring before 20 weeks of gestation (see Chapter 14).

Elective, induced abortions are generally done in the first or second trimester before 20 weeks. Those done in the first trimester are usually performed by dilation and curettage or evacuation, using either general anesthesia, regional anesthesia, or a paracervical block. First-trimester abortions are typically done for birth control reasons, although some may be done for maternal indications, such as uncontrolled seizure disorder, renal disease, or other underlying unstable medical condition. First-trimester abortions may be done also for fetal reasons, such as known teratogenic exposure.

Second-trimester abortions are most frequently done for maternal medical or fetal indications. Second-trimester abortions are generally induced with prostaglandin vaginal suppositories. The woman labors and delivers a fetus that may be born with signs of life. Some of the common fetal indications include diagnoses of abnormalities such as Down syndrome, Potter syndrome, neural tube defects, and other lethal and nonlethal fetal conditions. Maternal indications are less well defined, since many maternal contraindications for pregnancy are often worsened during labor and immediately postpartum regardless of gestation at the time of delivery. (See individual chapters on specific maternal medical complications and chapters about abortion and ectopic pregnancy.)

Feelings

Feelings Surrounding a First-trimester Spontaneous Abortion

In a first-trimester spontaneous abortion, a wide spectrum of feelings is expressed. These feelings vary from expressed relief to extreme sadness and despair.

Relief. The mother may express relief because she did not desire a pregnancy at this time. She may genuinely want this threat to herself and the embryo or fetus to end because she has been bleeding profusely off and on. Another reason may stem from her view of early pregnancy as the loss of a process, not the loss of a baby.

Sadness, grief, or despair. The mother may express sadness, grief, or despair if she has a high emotional investment in this pregnancy secondary to previous pregnancy loss or losses and has announced her pregnancy to family and friends. She may feel the need to "untell" and to acknowledge (1) her self-perception of "failure," (2) seeing the baby and heartbeat on a prior ultrasound, (3) spiritual beliefs and values surrounding life, (4) perfect planning for this pregnancy, or (5) incongruence of feelings between partners.

Neutral or unsure feelings. The mother may feel neutral or be unsure of her feelings secondary to validating the diagnosis of a positive pregnancy at the same time as miscarrying. She may have had no previous experience with loss of a loved person. This pregnancy may not have been planned (an "accident"). There may be a physical threat from excess bleeding, pain, and unfamiliarity with invasive procedures that obscures feelings at this time, or the woman may experience feelings of being alone or concerned for other family members, especially small children.

Feelings Surrounding a Second-trimester Spontaneous Abortion

It is important to understand that most women by 12 weeks have made some preparations for having a baby even if it is no more than seeking obstetric care (Swanson-Kauffman, 1986). Sometimes, at an early prenatal visit, an ultrasound is done and the woman can see the baby and its heartbeat. Validation of pregnancy and ultrasound confirmation of dates often change the perception of pregnancy from being only a process to a pregnancy that will result in a baby. When discussing the loss with a woman and being unsure of her feelings, it is best to start by referring to the "pregnancy" and listening for her use of either the "pregnancy" or "baby" when referring to the loss. The nurse's neutrality will encourage the expression of feelings without the encumbrance of "shoulds" and perceived expectations negatively influencing the woman.

Feelings Surrounding an Ectopic or Tubal Pregnancy

Ectopic or tubal pregnancy has some unique features surrounding the feelings. Pain may obscure initial feelings. Fear for one's own safety can cloud initial feelings. Body image disturbance may confuse feelings. Loss or potential loss of future fertility may complicate grief. Unfamiliar and invasive procedures may increase a sense of vulnerability.

Feelings Surrounding an Elective, Induced Abortion

Elective, induced abortion adds some dimensions to grief work. Some parents will have grief work complicated by strong feelings of guilt. This complication is particularly true for women who have referred to the "baby" in the first trimester and for women who have early second-trimester elective, induced abortions. Some of the feelings expressed describe having decided the time of death for the baby, choosing one's own or the family's convenience over a "helpless" baby, feeling pressured to do what someone else advised without seeking adequate information about alternatives, or believing that the baby suffered during the procedure.

Other feelings sometimes expressed are those centered on having extreme conflicts with beliefs and values and the need to do what was "right" for the family. Some women express surprise at feelings of guilt instead of sadness. Other feelings frequently expressed include feelings of abandonment by staff, physician, and even family and friends. The mother's feelings of guilt may lead to anger at those who cared for her or at those who encouraged and supported her in the decision. Although a certain amount of guilt and anger can be expected, getting stuck in these feelings or finding them totally unacceptable can adversely affect moving to another phase of bereavement. These feelings may necessitate referral for professional psychologic therapy.

Terminology

Terms used to identify the diagnosis should also be carefully chosen. Many women find the term *abortion* harsh and unkind when referring to spontaneous events. Some may feel insulted or misunderstood, believing that abortion refers only to an elective procedure. The term *miscarriage* is more neutral.

Some terms are too clinical and convey a lack of sincere feeling on the part of the caregiver. Products of conception are better referred to as "tissue" and the embryo or fetus as "baby." The term *habitual abortion,* which may be caused by an *incompetent cervix,* may also be offensive and prevent meaningful communication. Many women respond best to "consecutive" or "repeated" miscarriage caused by a "weakened" cervix.

Therapeutic Interventions

During and after early pregnancy loss, the following aspects are what parents say meant the most to them:

1. Support of a significant person during the experience
2. Seeing the tissue
3. Holding the baby
4. Saving mementos
5. Using symbolic mementos (When other mementos are not possible, symbolic mementos can be very important.)
6. Being allowed time to grieve
7. Being allowed choices (Allow time to make informed decisions about care of mother and baby.)
8. Sensitive caretakers (Assign caretakers who are educated and sensitive to feelings regarding early pregnancy loss.)
9. Being allowed options (Allow the option to bury or cremate the baby even though not required by state laws. If this method is chosen, most parents feel comforted when the baby's body is sent to the morgue rather than the pathology department.)

STILLBIRTH LOSS

The diagnosis of stillbirth causes grief at any gestational stage and regardless of personal situation. Stillbirth by definition is birth of a more than 19-week gestational baby without signs of life at the time of birth. Etiology of stillbirth varies from unexplained to severe maternal medical complications, such as diabetes, renal disease, cardiovascular disease, connective tissue disease/autoimmune disease, placental abruption, labor with a less than 24-week gestational fetus, malnutrition, maternal trauma, or postterm pregnancy beyond the estimated date of delivery by 2 or more weeks. Many unexplained stillbirths are attributed to possible cord accidents. Stillbirth related to the fetus is usually attributable to either extreme prematurity or congenital or genetic abnormalities incompatible with life.

In a stillbirth, often there has been little or no advance warning for the mother despite concurrent medical problems. Frequently the diagnosis is made immediately before the onset or induction of labor. On questioning, many women report decreased or absent fetal movement for several hours or a day or more before the stillbirth.

Feelings

At the time the diagnosis is made and the family is told, parents report a variety of feelings:

1. *Shock.* Parents may report feeling overwhelmed.
2. *Denial of reality.* They may wish the time could be reversed.
3. *Confusion.* They may be confused by medical information and anticipatory information aimed at assisting them with decisions that need to be made.
4. *Fear.* They may fear doing something very bad in a place where only good things should happen.
5. *Anger.* They may be angry with God or with their physicians and the staff.
6. *Guilt.* They may experience imagined guilt from inconsequential departures from perfect self-care, such as not taking prenatal vitamins regularly, not resting enough, or working during the pregnancy. They may experience real guilt about possible contributing factors such as substance abuse, including smoking and alcohol and crack cocaine usage.

Therapeutic Interventions

Some of the things parents remember as most helpful are summarized below:

1. *Being together.* Parents appreciated being together when the diagnosis was discussed with them.
2. *Simple explanations.* They appreciated being given simple explanations in nonclinical terms.
3. *Talked to directly.* They wanted to be talked to directly when confirmatory information is given, such as during the ultrasonic examination.
4. *Anticipatory guidance.* When anticipatory guidance is given, it should be done slowly and in small increments.
5. *Allowance to grieve.* Unrushed time to grieve should be provided.
6. *Mementos.* The ultrasound picture or tape as well as photographs after delivery should be offered to the parents.
7. *Being touched.* Parents were comforted by touch from each other and from the staff caring for them.

8. *Empathy from staff.* It was comforting to feel that the staff was grieving too or crying with them.

The time for labor and delivery does not usually need to be determined immediately except when the mother's physical well-being is in jeopardy. In fact, most parents can use additional time to begin to make plans for the labor and delivery experience, as well as the care of the infant after the delivery. Except when the mother is ill herself, she is usually able to participate in making better decisions for burial and services before the onset of labor fatigue.

During labor and immediately postpartum, what parents appreciate and remember is summarized according to Limbo and Wheeler (1986, 1995):

1. *Experience of closeness and being touched.* Parents appreciated being allowed to be close to each other and to family, important friends, and staff. Touch was especially appreciated.

2. *Being allowed to make independent decisions.* They appreciated the encouragement to make their own decisions about care with the support of educated and sensitive staff.

3. *Praise.* Liberal use of praise for a job well done during labor and delivery was therapeutic.

4. *Shielding from unnecessary questioning.* There is a need to be shielded from the necessity of telling their story or giving their health history to people not essential to the team.

5. *Continuity in care.* Allowing the same nurse to continue to care for the parents during her shift and preventing unnecessary moves from the labor room to delivery room to recovery room are helpful.

6. *Unlimited time with the infant after delivery.* Parents benefit from being encouraged and allowed to spend as much time as desired with the infant immediately following delivery. Then if the parents desire, they should be allowed additional opportunities to see the baby again. There are few rules or laws surrounding the seeing and holding of infants following death (Table 6-2).

7. *Being provided mementos.* Take many photographs and poses of the baby. Include poses with the baby clothed and unclothed, and include family member in the photographs. Collect as many mementos as possible. Mementos may include such things as the measuring tape, baby comb, blanket, clothing, footprints/handprints, blessing/baptismal certificate, the shell or other special receptacle used for

blessing water, other special memory certificates, and identification bracelets.

8. *Referral services.* Visits and supportive help from social service, support from hospital pastoral care or their own spiritual advisor, assistance with burial or cremation decisions, and follow-up from hospital staff involved in the care can be beneficial.

NEWBORN LOSS

Two unique features of grief are present when a death of a newborn occurs. First, parents experience anticipatory grief when a newborn is predicted to die. With that anticipatory grief comes ambivalence in expectations and hopes. On the one hand, parents want the baby to survive against all odds. On the other hand, parents want the baby not to suffer or go through extraordinary treatments. In addition, the grief work needed to prepare for the inevitable is greatly accelerated. Second, often tremendous differences exist in parents' reality and the reality of caregivers. Parents believe the baby ought to survive, whereas staff may know the baby cannot.

Parents' Feelings

Parents' feelings to be considered include the following:

1. Parents may feel abandoned, a loss of hope, and a sense of futility if given no choice as to delivery route or place.
2. Parents may fear high technology in the nursery.
3. There may be jealousy or anger at other parents whose babies are likely to survive.
4. Parents may wish that the baby would just die and get it all over with.
5. Parents may experience guilt about their wish for the baby to die and fear that their wish, if spoken aloud, may come true.
6. There may be guilt about minor or major departures from self-care during pregnancy.
7. There may be anger at each other if opinions differ about needed care for the baby, about decisions for removal of life support, or regarding parents' care of self or each other.
8. Guilt about having "bad genes" may be present.
9. Parents may feel helpless about their ability to care for their baby while he or she is so sick and dependent on technology. The parents may be detached from their idea of parental love for the baby.

T A B L E 6-2 Myths and truths related to parents seeing and holding their baby after death

Common myths	Truths
Body must be embalmed or refrigerated as soon as possible.	Some states do not require embalming for any body, and refrigeration can be postponed for up to 24 hr. However, because of the high percentage of water in a baby, the longer the baby is out of refrigeration, loss of moisture will hasten visual deterioration.
Parents cannot have the baby returned for additional visits related to risk of infection.	There is no risk of infection to parents, since the baby has not come into direct contact with any other body while being held in a morgue, if handled safely and properly.
A baby who looks macerated or clearly abnormal should not be viewed by the parents.	Studies have shown that parents who do not hold or see their infant after death regret it the most and often attribute that decision to the fact that staff either actively discouraged them from doing so or gave no encouragement (Woods, Esposito, 1987).
Once the parents have decided not to see or hold their stillborn baby, it would be cruel to suggest it later.	The first decision made by parents not to hold or see the baby is often made because of fear of the dead body and not knowing what to expect. It is a decision made when the feelings of shock and numbness take hold before the mind is ready to consider consequences and denial is in full force.

One visit with the parents is enough and should be limited in time.

The father or close family member knows best what each parent needs.

Once the autopsy is done, it is no longer possible for parents to view or hold the baby.

One visit with the parents is not enough for most parents. Visits are a part of searching and yearning and testing what is real.

Whenever possible each parent should be encouraged to make his or her own decisions about contact with the baby, making personal memories. Respect for the individuality of family members and the need to grieve in their own way are integral to mutual support.

Once the autopsy is done, hospital pathologists do not generally return anything to the body cavities nor do they suture their incisions. As a result, it is often more comforting to parents for the infant to be cosmetically acceptable before viewing. They need to be made aware of the alterations in the infant's appearance even after cosmetic treatment. Some parents will indeed still desire viewing. In that event, the nurse, social worker, or chaplain assisting in this should be adequately educated in the best way to support the parents. It is rarely recommended that the request be refused.

Issues and Concerns of Parents

Issues and concerns facing parents include the following:

1. Confusion regarding doing everything reasonable versus extraordinary resuscitation
2. How emotionally close to get to the baby
3. How often to visit
4. Concern that the baby will die in pain, cold, or alone

Therapeutic Interventions

Unified Plan

It is important for the health care team to create a unified plan, with parents' participation to whatever degree they are able and desire. This entails a combined approach between the obstetrician and pediatrician. Frequently the nurse and social worker become liaisons between the two physicians and the parents. Three important elements are needed for a successful unified approach: (1) a need for agreement among all parties; (2) a continuum of care; and (3) provision of information to the parents that presents both the pediatrician's view of the plan and the obstetrician's view. Communication of the plan should not catch parents in the middle of two opposing or conflicting plans.

Documentation of this plan should include the following:

- Plans for the birth and the anticipated outcome
- A brief summary of the clinical situation
- Description of the alternatives open for discussion with the parents
- Input from the parents
- Actual decisions made and parents' response

Helpful Strategies for Parents Experiencing a Newborn Death

- Parents are provided the opportunity to be close to each other and the baby.
- Parents know they can help with some care or comforting of the baby. For some mothers, it is important to pump breast milk, even if the baby never receives the milk.
- Parents know that when the baby dies, the baby was not alone, cold, or in pain. They trust and hope the nurse will take care of these things in their absence.
- Some parents want to hold the baby while it dies, whereas others prefer for someone else to do this. See Table 6-2 regarding myths and truths related to parents seeing and holding their baby after death.

- After death, parents participate in care, such as bathing, dressing, and holding after technologic equipment has been removed.
- Parents have been given advance information about the baby's chances for survival.
- Parents are informed and encouraged to participate in decisions about continuing or discontinuing life support as desired or not desired by them.
- The baby is kept alive long enough that parents can get to the hospital if absent when the baby's condition worsens.
- Parents have had the baby blessed or baptized before death.
- Parents have privacy at the time of death.
- Parents are being cared for by people educated in death and dying and who are sensitive to their needs.
- When called to come to the hospital after the baby has died or taken a turn for the worse, parents are met by the nurse, physician, or social worker as soon as possible.
- Parents have relatives or close friends included when desired.
- Parents take photographs of the baby before and after death.
- Parents collect all possible mementos, such as blanket, clothes, blood pressure cuff, comb, and remaining diapers.
- Parents make footprints and handprints.
- Parents assist with funeral arrangements and selection of a mortuary.
- Creative arrangements are made for letting the baby hear special music, breathe fresh air, and so on before death.
- A primary nurse cares for the mother before birth, and the primary nursery nurse attends the funeral.

Photographic Mementos

Perhaps the most important memento made or collected for the parents to treasure when a baby of any gestation dies is photographs of their infant. Some hints for creating good photographs follow:

- Take at least one roll of 12 photographs with a 35 mm, or similar quality, immediate-processing camera. The immediate photographs give parents something to keep and hold onto while awaiting processing of quality photographs. Generally, the clarity and color are more true with the latter.
- Take photographs of the baby clothed and unclothed whenever possible. Even a severely macerated baby usually has some acceptable unclothed pose.

- Take each photograph as a separate pose. For multiples, take one roll of each baby separately and one roll of all babies together.
- When taking pictures with infant on back, prop the nape of the neck with a small roll. This helps to keep the baby's mouth partially closed. It also poses the baby so that the features are fully visible (Fig. 6-1).
- Use different lighting, such as some with room light on, dimmed, and off.
- Remove technologic equipment and supplies from surrounding environment.
- Select background colors carefully. Pink rarely works well, whereas royal blue, purple, and lavender are excellent backgrounds.
- Use toys smaller and larger than baby and soft and fuzzy to create an environment with texture and size (Fig. 6-2).
- Include parents in some pictures, or include the nurse's arms or hands to communicate caring.

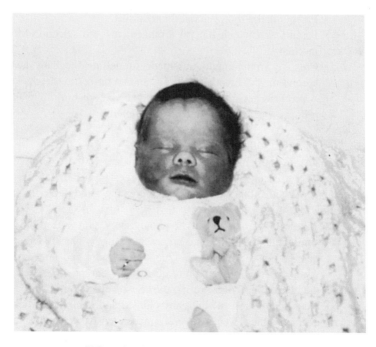

FIG. 6-1 Miranda: full-term, newborn death.

- Create a family portrait if desired. Include siblings when prepared for the experience.
- Very tiny babies, less than 20 weeks, often look best when a small-print blanket is used as a background (Fig. 6-3).
- Suggest inclusion of a religious medal or parents' wedding bands.
- Picture taking is a standard of care. It is not necessary or often advised to ask permission for photographs or to have a permit signed (Limbo, Wheeler, 1986). Parents risk saying no to something they later regret and cannot retrieve. Be aware, however, that some Native Americans may find photographs offensive to their spiritual beliefs and should be consulted first.

Other Keepsakes to Make or Collect
- Footprints and handprints can be made. Plaster of Paris can be used to make a mold in the shell used for the blessing, or a felt-tipped pen can be used to ink the foot or hand of a very premature baby who has no creases.
- Give a baby ring or other symbolic keepsake.
- Collect or write a special poem or message for this baby.
- Suggest the mother and father make a diary of their thoughts while their baby was alive.

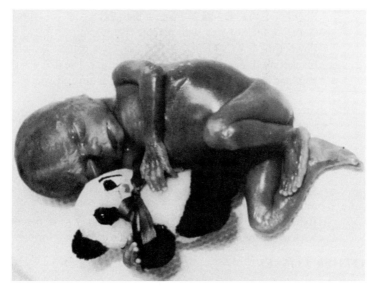

FIG. 6-2 Kimberly: 23 weeks of gestation, stillborn.

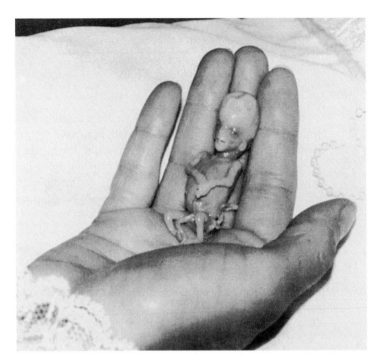

FIG. 6-3 Baby Weber: 12 weeks of gestation, miscarriage.

- Encourage the parents to make a baby book.
- Collect a lock of hair with parents' permission.
- Powder the baby's blanket before use. Give parents only the blanket used, even if soiled. Put blanket into a sealed plastic bag, and the powder scent will remain for several years.

Morgue or Pathology Preparation
- Use a soft wrap, without nap, next to the baby's skin.
- Position the baby's arms up alongside the head.
- Use soft rolls at either side of the baby's head and body and under the chin, if needed.
- Wrap outer cover snugly around the baby with head out. Use a third wrap to cover all of the baby.
- Babies going to the pathology departments whose parents wish to see them again should be put into saline, not formalin.

OTHER LOSSES

The unexpected nature of infant death and the relative lack of societal rituals make the loss of the wished-for baby especially sad.

Infant loss may also occur in ways other than death. Some such situations include the less than perfect baby with anomalies or early prematurity problems. It may occur through adoption. Feelings discussed in this chapter may not be solely limited to loss of a baby through death.

EFFECT OF GRIEF ON INDIVIDUAL FAMILY MEMBERS AND FRIENDS

Mother's Grief

A woman has a strong sense of both physical and emotional attachment to an unborn baby from the moment she begins to think of the concept of baby resulting from the process of pregnancy or when she first sees the baby on the ultrasound picture. Therefore the maternal task of fetal distinction may develop before fetal movement is felt. The woman may feel a distinct sense of failure when she has given birth to a baby who has died or will die. In addition, she may feel blamed by her partner. Women tend to find it easier to express feelings of sadness with tears and crying. As a result, it tends to be comparatively easier for them to reach out for understanding and empathy than it is for men.

Father's Grief

The father, on the other hand, often has less emotional attachment until the woman's body begins to take on a noticeably pregnant shape. Even then he does not have the almost constant physical reminder of the reality of baby and pregnancy. As a result, the father generally lags behind the mother in his accomplishment of the pregnancy tasks of validation, fetal distinction, and embodiment. It is only at the time of birth, when caretaking activities are assumed by both, that attachment feelings merge. Therefore when the baby is lost before term or born too premature for normal caretaking activities by the parents, the father's and mother's grieving is incongruent.

The father also experiences a learned role expectation of protector. This assumed and imposed role often prevents the father from expressing grief as sadness. Sometimes he is, in fact, more comfortable expressing it as anger at the situation, at those caring for the mother and baby, at the mother, and at himself for not protecting the family sufficiently.

Impact on Marital Stability

The father often feels forgotten because of his calm exterior and the frequent inquiries of family and friends as to the mother's well-being. At the same time, the mother feels misunderstood by him and alone in her grief, which she expected to have shared. If these troublesome feelings and misunderstandings are not discussed openly, tremendous resentment can result. When the mother becomes more preoccupied with her grief and the father feels more forgotten, the emotional distance between them widens. Absence of mutual support and sharing can be a significant contributor to complicated grief (Woods, Esposito, 1987).

Children's Grief

According to Wass and Corr (1984), childhood concepts of death occur in four stages.

Infancy

A baby has no real concept of death, although babies form internal images of people or things in their immediate environment.

Early Childhood

Children in early childhood are governed by their own experiences and believe that everything in their world is alive, even inanimate objects. They believe that wishes are made possible and events happen for personal reasons. Thus if they wished that a new baby would not enter their family, their wish might have come true. Children at this age also have difficulty comprehending things as final.

Late Childhood and Preadolescence

Death is understood as a final and permanent event. The child, however, feels it is an event that cannot happen to him or her. The child finds the process of dying and the dead body to be a source of curiosity and interest.

Mature Stage

Understanding death as an adult begins in adolescence. Death is finally understood to be irreversible and inevitable. By this stage, adolescents can develop abstract views toward death.

• • •

Siblings have varying degrees of attachment to an expected new baby in the family. When pregnancy loss occurs in a family, siblings may develop symptoms of depression, aggression, sleep disturbances, and anxiety. Children are vulnerable and very dependent on the adults in their world. When parents are perceived as withdrawn from the child because of grief over their loss, the other children feel threatened and unsafe.

It is advisable for parents to call on trusted extended family members or friends to be available to children, especially in the beginning. Siblings should be included in age-appropriate discussions and expressions of grief and sadness. Whereas it normally takes adults at least 1 to 2 years to work through their grief, a child may accomplish this in 3 to 6 months. This rapid progression may be distressing to parents. Parents with other children should receive education and assistance in providing support to their children.

Responses of Grandparents

Often grandparents of the baby who died find it very difficult to help their children, the parents. The inability to console and support is caused by their involvement in their own grief. Grandparents have grief for the death of their grandchild and are, at the same time, hurting from the pain their own child, the parent, must experience. These feelings may lead to an understandable although unhelpful overprotectiveness. Feeling this way may cause them to avoid the more desired approach of assisting the couple in making their own decisions. Instead, they make decisions for them and hasten the process, heedless of the parents' need to participate.

Later, grandparents may avoid future references to the baby and fail to acknowledge the grief in the misguided belief that it is kinder to their child, the parent. This chasm in expression of feelings leads to anger and loss of shared feelings at an important time. Therapeutic guidance and counseling of families during follow-up calls or visits should address this sensitive area of potential misunderstanding.

Responses of Friends

Friends and acquaintances may not know what to say or do to support the couple. This may cause them to avoid the parents or make insensitive or moralizing remarks.

Avoidance

Friends may avoid talking about the baby at all or avoid the parents. Usually they truly believe this is kinder. Occasionally, in ignorance, they believe that it is or should be finished business. Without similar experience of their own with loss, they are not self-educated in appropriate responses.

Insensitive or Moralizing Responses

Frequently used statements include the following:

- "At least you never knew the baby."
- "You can always have another."
- "You should get pregnant right away, and then you can put this behind you."
- "It was for the best. The baby would probably have been abnormal anyway."
- "God must have wanted a little angel in heaven."
- "If you had eaten better, stopped working, and so on, this wouldn't have happened to you."
- "I don't understand why you want to keep talking about the baby. If you'd get busy with . . . you'd feel better."
- "I understand just how you feel. My friend lost a baby from SIDS."

These responses are all well intended but tend to belittle the loss experienced by the parents. A simple "I'm sorry," "What can I do . . . to help?" or "I'm here for you, if you need to talk or tell me about it" can be very therapeutic. Self-disclosure of a personal loss that was truly similar also is appropriate and gives parents a sense of having a kindred spirit to share some of the troubled thoughts of being slightly crazy, falling apart, or not being able to make it because it hurts so much.

Supportive Responses

Remembering the baby on important anniversaries, calling the baby by name, and acknowledging the fact of the parents' parenthood also help to support the family. Expressed grief is healthy. Discussion of feelings helps the family get in touch with the reality of the experience and begin to move on to another phase of grief work. It also gives an underlying message of belief in the inner strength of the individual's ability to find solutions from within (Worden, 1991).

CULTURAL DIFFERENCES IN GRIEF

There is probably a biologic basis to grief. If this is true, grief is universal. Tears are thought to be the one common expression of grief and are believed to contain a chemical that has a cathartic effect when expressed. Another commonality is that the greater the personal crisis or stress, the greater the need to consider issues of personal space and touching expressions.

Although many similarities exist in the way various cultures deal with the death of a baby, it is important to become aware of some important distinctions. To work with different cultures effectively, the nurse must learn to be sensitive to what parents are saying they need and want when the family's cultural beliefs are unfamiliar. A broad understanding of generalities for that culture can be learned through study, but the unique needs of that family must be obtained through an assessment. Areas to consider are (1) What does death mean? (2) How are various family members expected to show their grief? and (3) What are the parents saying they need and want? Therefore the grief counselor should address predetermined cultural and ethnic needs, develop a cultural and ethnic sensitivity about grief issues, and provide caring to every person that reflects cultural sensitivity. It should be kept in mind that even members of the white American majority have intercultural differences.

Cultural differences of some populous groups in the United States are summarized in Box 6-1.

Box 6-1

Cultural Differences in Grieving

African-Americans
More than 50% are matriarchal households.
Extended family holds very special value.
Highest infant mortality (18.4/100 still births) in the United States (Giger, Davidhizar, 1991).
Illness beliefs
  Secondary to impaired social relationships
  Divine punishment
  Everything has an opposite, for example, birth—death
  Health is a gift from God
  Some continued reliance on folk medicine secondary to frequent humiliation in health care system

Hispanics
This group comprises Mexicans, Puerto Ricans, and Cubans.
Father makes decisions; mother directs home.
Children are essential; loss of a child is the loss of the future.
From caregivers, they want an understanding of the importance of family members' presence, the ability to speak Spanish, the need for touch, incorporation of home remedies, and folk beliefs.

Native Americans
Many tribal groups make it difficult to generalize their cultural values.
Their culture is in a state of flux.

Continued

Box 6-1
Cultural Differences in Grieving—cont'd

Native Americans—cont'd
Navajos are the largest subcultural group.
Most are agricultural.
The individual and nature, which are closely tied and interact, are highly valued.
Illness is the result of being out of harmony.
The infant is more susceptible to death while the fontanels are still open; the spirit leaves the child through the fontanels.
Taking photographs and naming the child steal the spirit; if the infant dies and the spirit is stolen, grieving must move the infant back to the spirit world, and it is therefore more difficult than if no photographs and no naming have taken place.
Healing and religion are inseparable; pregnant women often see both the medicine man and the doctor.
Eye contact is rude, but close proximity at a 45-degree angle is a must.
Chinese
There are good and bad deaths; yin and yang are belief in a balance of opposites.
Death ensures that the spirit will begin its next stage of existence in the best way.
The Chinese have a public sphere of self, which includes friends and acquaintances, and a private sphere where they only explore feelings and thoughts.
They will discuss perception of causes of death with family.
They believe in communication with the dead.
Southeast Asians
This group comprises Vietnamese, Cambodians, Laotians, and others.
Family is the basis for society; large families are valued.
Society is patriarchal.
They are proud of children, and their high value leads to deep mourning when death occurs.
They have a history of survival of recent horrible tragedies and loss.
They are often Buddhist and are warned against expression of strong emotion; if angry or distressed, they will respond with increased smiling.
Both agreement and respect are shown by smiling.

COUNSELING PRINCIPLES

According to Worden (1991), there are 10 principles of counseling to prevent complicated grief:

1. *Help the parents to actualize the loss.* This can be done by helping them tell their story by asking specific questions about the baby and their responses to the death.
2. *Interpret "normal" behavior.* To interpret behavior the health professional must have an understanding of what is normal. Then he or she can explain responses of family and friends.
3. *Allow for individual differences.* Each person's response to grief may differ.
4. *Provide time to grieve.* People need privacy and options offered. The health professional should use a nonjudgmental attitude in delivery of care and allow the grieving family time for decision making. An important question that requires a decision should be asked at least three times.
5. *Examine defenses and coping styles.*
6. *Assist the parents in living without the baby.*
7. *Facilitate emotional withdrawal from the baby.*
8. *Help the parents to identify and express feelings.* Parents should be helped to understand the importance of expressing anger, guilt, and sadness.
9. *Provide continuing support.* Continued support should be provided through follow-up telephone calls or visits after discharge, sending a sympathy card, and making a referral to self-help support groups.
10. *Identify complicated (pathologic) grief and refer.* The various family members' movement in phases of bereavement should be assessed, ineffective coping and defense mechanisms recognized, and appropriate referrals for therapy made when needed.

STRATEGIES OF CARING

It is important for caregivers to understand the nature of caring before offering support for healthy grieving. Swanson-Kauffman (1986) describes caring strategies as follows:

- *Knowing.* Knowing includes avoidance of assumptions, centers on the person being cared for, does thorough assessments, seeks clues, engages in the self, is able to recognize shock and keep in mind that parents might not hear you, and remembers the terror that is being felt.

- *Being with.* Being with means conveying availability, sharing feelings, not burdening, being there, keeping promises, slowing the system down if need be, and being with the parents after death through follow-up calls and sympathy notes.
- *Doing for.* Doing for encompasses comforting; anticipating; performing competently; and setting up a plan of help.
- *Enabling.* Enabling means to inform/explain, support/allow, focus, generate alternatives, and validate/give feedback by teaching and encouraging, providing time to make difficult decisions, and asking questions at least three times if a decision must be made.
- *Maintaining belief.* This can be done by manifesting belief in the individual, maintaining a hope-filled attitude about the individual's ability to cope, offering realistic optimism, and being willing "to go the distance" with the parents.
- *Respecting.* The nurse should respect the parent's knowledge of the person of the baby and their knowledge of what they need.

ROLES OF VARIOUS TEAM MEMBERS
Nurse

The nurse has several functions in providing support and comfort (Woods, Esposito, 1987):
- Communication with other hospital personnel and support services
- Consistency in responses
- Advocacy
- Support
- Continuity of care
- Assessment of each individual's needs
- Identification of pathologic responses
- Willingness to bend the rules
- Provision of privacy

Social Worker

The social worker is usually the advocate for the immediate and extended family. The social worker, as advocate, has several responsibilities (Woods, Esposito, 1987):
- Assesses family dynamics after the loss
- Responds to individual needs
- Interacts with the family after discharge
- Provides education about children's needs

- Counsels with extended family, such as the grandparents
- Makes needed referrals

Chaplain

The hospital chaplain is an important team member. It is generally best to involve him or her as early as possible. It is wise to let the chaplain explain his or her role. The major functions of the chaplain (Woods, Esposito, 1987) are as listed:

- Acts as a nonmedical friend and companion who has been educated in the skills of therapeutic listening
- Helps the family to define faith
- Allows the family to express negative feelings, especially anger
- Acknowledges parents' hopes and dreams
- Provides personalized approach to assisting with plans for memorial or funeral services as needed

Funeral Director

The funeral director is integral to assisting with the creation of a moment to acknowledge grief. The main role of the funeral director is to facilitate a special remembrance of the significance of this baby. According to Woods and Esposito (1987), the funeral director does this in the following manner:

- Provides choices
- Assists in selection of casket, vault, or urn
- May suggest a low-cost option for parents who have no funds (may include assuming the cost of honoraria, cemetery charges, newspaper notices, and flowers)
- Performs embalming procedures, dressing, and casketing
- Communicates with pathologists to preserve integrity of the body
- Guides parents as they dress, hold, and photograph their baby
- Comforts the extended family
- Provides visitation privacy if desired
- Assembles the family
- Conducts the service
- Offers a postfuneral reception
- Supplements extended support through education and referrals

Obstetrician, Primary Provider, or Practitioner

This physician has both inpatient and outpatient roles.

Inpatient Roles
- Discusses maternal and fetal conditions with parents
- Provides alternatives in medical plan from which parents have a right to choose
- Works with the grief support team, that is, nurse, social worker, chaplain
- Communicates important considerations to pathologist
- Plans with the pediatric or neonatal team when baby will or may be under his or her care

Outpatient Roles
- Provides 1-week follow-up postpartum care
- Discusses events and repeats explanations for events leading up to the delivery
- Assesses psychologic need for short-term or long-term counseling
- Makes psychologic referrals appropriate to parents' needs as couple or individuals
- Refrains from assuming the role of professional counselor when this would be inappropriate but also distinguishes between healthy grief and complicated grief

Pediatrician, Neonatologist, Primary Provider, or Practitioner

The physician and nursing team for the newborn should be involved in contributing to the plan and communicating with the family as soon as potential or probable problems are evident. Either the obstetrician or pediatrician should discuss autopsy or genetic study results with parents. This should be done at a scheduled conference and preferably in person (see Bibliography).

Geneticist

A geneticist should be involved when structural or genetic abnormalities are possible or obviously apparent. The geneticist provides information at the earliest possible time antecedent to the loss if possible. The two main functions of the geneticist are to provide information and to provide counseling relative to the genetic results.

Peer Support

Peer support may be nationally affiliated or locally affiliated with such sources as a church or voluntary agency. These groups may have several purposes:

- Education
- Professional facilitation
- Self-help support

Box 6-2 summarizes resources for dealing with perinatal loss.

NURSING PROCESS

PREVENTION

Nursing care is directed at care of the immediate family and prevention of the following:

1. Complicated grief
2. Ineffective coping
3. Individual reactive depression
4. Inability of the family system to meet the needs of various family members, carry out family functions, or maintain communications for mutual growth and maturation
5. Spiritual distress

NURSING DIAGNOSES/COLLABORATIVE PROBLEMS AND INTERVENTIONS

■ **RISK FOR DYSFUNCTIONAL GRIEVING** related to delay in expressing grief; chronic sorrow over previous losses; prevention of or lack of facilitation of normal grief expressions and bereavement work, especially on the part of health team members; the unexpected nature of infant death.

DESIRED OUTCOME: The individuals in the immediate family will express culturally appropriate, grief-related feelings within reasonable time frames for bereavement phases. The nurse should do the following:

1. Assess for expressions of normal grieving through the four phases of bereavement (see Table 6-1).
2. Encourage expression of feelings through the establishment of rapport. Bring up the subject and make references to the baby.
3. Facilitate an adequate amount of time to acquaint with and say good-bye to the baby or to acknowledge the pregnancy loss.
4. Slow down the system when time frames interfere with need for adequate time. Be a parent advocate.
5. Give simple explanations initially.
6. Answer only those questions that truly ask for answers. Understand that many times initial questions are a lament of emotional pain.

Box 6-2
Resources for Dealing With Perinatal Loss

Compassionate Friends: Infant Loss Support (602-641-1941)

This nondenominational self-help organization offers friendship and support to parents who have suffered the death of a child. Support and friendship are provided in the forms of monthly meetings, telephone friends, and resource material. Any bereaved parent can become a member by simply requesting assistance from the local chapter. There are no dues or membership fees.

Pregnancy and Infant Loss Center (PILC) 1421 E. Wayzata Blvd, Suite 40 Wayzata, MN 55391 (612-473-9372)

Founded in 1983 by a group of bereaved parents, this national organization works to promote an environment in which families can participate in healthy grieving, helps families find and use their own support networks, provides information and education to professionals, and serves as parent advocate after the death of a high risk neonate. PILC makes referrals to local support groups, publishes a quarterly newsletter, distributes literature on perinatal bereavement, and gives workshops and in-service programs.

Resolve Through Sharing La Crosse Lutheran Hospital 1910 South Ave La Crosse, WI 54601 (800-362-9567)

This comprehensive hospital-based perinatal bereavement program provides guidelines for professionals caring for families who have experienced miscarriage, ectopic pregnancy, stillbirth, or neonatal death. It aims to ensure consistent, sensitive care for grieving family members. Its activities include nationwide educational and certification programs for perinatal nurses and childbirth educators.

Source of Help in Airing and Resolving Experiences (SHARE) St. Elizabeth's Hospital 211 South 3rd St Belleville, IL 62222 (800-821-6819)

This organization aims to ensure support for parents from the time they anticipate a problem by helping them to express grief and related emotions. It maintains a national listing of relevant resources and helps parents to contact local support groups and other resources, such as fertility specialists and printed materials. SHARE publishes a bimonthly newsletter for caregivers and families and presents workshops throughout the United States and abroad.

7. Give anticipatory guidance for what is to come next in physical responses, responses of family and friends, and grief work.

8. Make memories and collect keepsakes that will provide comfort in the future.

9. Ensure follow-up support for healthy, functional adaptive grief work (refer to Box 6-2).

10. Refer to pastoral care if family desires.

11. Refer to social worker for assistance with funeral or other ritual memorial.

12. Refer to self-support group or psychotherapy as appropriate.

- **RISK FOR INEFFECTIVE INDIVIDUAL OR FAMILY COPING** related to situational crisis, pregnancy loss, or infant death; maturational crisis of parenthood; personal vulnerability; lack of information regarding reasons for the death or loss; problem-solving skills deficit; support system deficit; independence/dependence conflict; exhausted support capacity; role changes; developmental or situational crises; chronically unexpressed guilt, anxiety, or hostility; dissonant discrepancy of coping styles among members of the family, especially significant other; highly ambivalent family relationships.

  DESIRED OUTCOMES: The individuals of the family will demonstrate adequate coping skills and response to both the maturational/developmental crisis and the situational crisis of unexpected pregnancy loss or infant death. The individual members will provide role-appropriate support to each other. Grief work will progress at an expected rate throughout the phases of bereavement. The nurse should do the following:

  1. Evaluate normal family coping mechanisms and relationships among family members. Evaluate effectiveness of coping with the stress.

  2. Observe for signs of change, conflict, denial of role responsibilities, or inability to perform role responsibility as culturally appropriate.

  3. Assess family's support system.

  4. Screen for effective or ineffective management of adaptive tasks.

  5. Encourage both parents to experience the event together while supporting individual differences in expression of grief.

  6. Educate parents regarding individual responses.

7. Help parents to recognize signs of ineffective coping in siblings, for example, interpersonal problems at school or in the home, excessive quarreling, or regressive behaviors.
8. Provide information regarding cause or lack of cause of pregnancy loss or infant death.
9. Promote reliance on previously learned coping skills.
10. Refer to supportive therapy when reliance on maladaptive behaviors is diagnosis.

■ **RISK FOR HOPELESSNESS** related to perceived powerlessness resulting from long-term unresolved stress of life-style of helplessness.

DESIRED OUTCOMES: Parents will verbalize understanding and acceptance of individual needs for expression. Parents will allow and promote each family member's healthy expression of grief. Parents will accept treatment for maladaptive expressions of grief. Individuals will not abuse substances to mask feelings of grief. Depression will not last longer than 4 to 6 months in its severest form. The nurse should do the following:

1. Assess each grieving member of the family for persistent social withdrawal, immobilizing emotional pain resulting in incapacity to care for own basic needs, chronic low self-esteem, or signs of substance abuse.
2. Promote acceptance of outside support and assistance for the first 2 years.
3. Provide a resource of follow-up.
4. Refer for psychotherapy when powerlessness or hopelessness threatens the individual or family safety.

■ **RISK FOR SPIRITUAL DISTRESS (DISTRESS OF HUMAN SPIRIT)** related to questioning why God allowed this to happen and questioning their religious beliefs.

DESIRED OUTCOME: Each family member will verbalize acceptance of the situation. The nurse should do the following:

1. Assess the patient's and family's spiritual beliefs, needs, and practices.
2. Assess the patient's and family's faith; energize them by fostering whatever type of faith they wish to exhibit (Kennison, 1987).
3. Help to prevent considerable distress for parents who are of the Catholic, Eastern Orthodox, Episcopalian, or Lutheran religion by facilitating infant baptism before death. These

religions believe the unbaptized soul cannot go to heaven (Eich, 1987). If a priest or minister is not available, any nurse who believes in God can perform the baptism. Sprinkle water on the head or body while saying the words "I baptize you in the name of the Father, and of the Son, and of the Holy Spirit." For a stillborn, prefix the statement with "If this be valid."

4. Assess for persistent distress of the human spirit and anger at God.
5. Take note of expressions of inner conflict with meaning of life.
6. Encourage the various family members to express their beliefs, feelings of anger, and any perception of unfairness they are experiencing.
7. Listen and maintain a nonjudgmental attitude.
8. Refer to hospital chaplain, rabbi, or appropriate religious specialist.

- **RISK FOR ALTERED FAMILY PROCESSES** that are compromising, disabling, or result in breakup of the family unit related to disabling grief, maladaptive coping behaviors, or abusive disorders in dysfunctional family units.

  DESIRED OUTCOMES: Family members will care for, support, and provide for basic needs of individuals. Parents will do necessary parenting activities for the children. Parents will seek or accept therapy for ineffective coping, especially when substance abuse or neglect issues are identified. Parents will be into the fourth phase of bereavement by 2 to 3 years after the death of their baby and be reinvesting in a future together. The nurse should do the following:

  1. Assess for inability of family members to deal with death constructively, to meet basic needs of individual members, to accept and receive needed help, or to express and accept various family members' individualized expressions of feelings.
  2. Provide therapeutic listening and communication follow-up for a minimum of 3 to 12 months.
  3. Explain responses of others and incongruent grief of mothers and fathers.
  4. Follow the principles of counseling when making these follow-up contacts.
  5. Refer to appropriate therapy when the family unit is identified as dysfunctional.

CONCLUSION

The primary goals of the nurse in providing nursing care at the time of pregnancy loss or infant death are to maintain the integrity of the family unit and promote healthy, uncomplicated grief. This is best accomplished through compassionate, sensitive caring at the time of the event and through referring for appropriate follow-up during at least the first year after the loss.

BIBLIOGRAPHY

Bereavement

American College of Obstetrics and Gynecology (ACOG): Grief related to perinatal death, *ACOG Techn Bull,* no. 86, April 1985.

Appleton R, Gibson B, Hey E: The loss of a baby at birth: the role of the bereavement officer, *Br J Obstet Gynecol* 100:51-54, 1993.

Backer BA, Hannon NR, Russel NA: *Death and dying: understanding and care,* ed 2, Albany, NY, 1994, Delmar.

Bhattacharjee C: Improving the care of bereaved parents, *Nurs Standard* 4(22):18-20, 1990.

Black KD, Ecker M, Librizzi RJ: Prevention of recurrent fetal loss caused by antiphospholipid syndrome, *J Perinatol* 16:181-185, 1996.

Borg S, Lasker J: *When pregnancy fails: families coping with miscarriage, stillbirth and infant death,* New York, 1989, Bantam Books.

Bowlby J: *Attachment and loss,* vol I. *Attachment,* ed 2, New York, 1982, Basic Books.

Bridwell D: *The ache for a child,* Wheaton, Ill, 1994, Victor Books.

Brown Y: The crisis of pregnancy loss: a team approach to support, *Birth* 19(2):82-89, 1992.

Buckman R: *How to break bad news: a guide for health care professionals,* Baltimore, 1992, Johns Hopkins University Press.

Calabrese JR, Kling MA, Gold PW: Alterations in immunocompetence during stress, bereavement and depression: focus on neuroendocrine regulation, *Am J Psychiatry* 144(9):1123-1134, 1987.

Carr D, Knupp S: Grief and perinatal loss: a community hospital approach to support, *J Obstet Gynecol Neonatal Nurs* 14(2):130-139, 1985.

Cohen MD, editor: *The limits of miracles: poems about the loss of babies,* South Hadley, Mass, 1984, Bergin & Garvey Publications.

Conley BH: *Handling the holidays,* Elburn, Ill, 1993, Conley Outreach Publications.

Corr CA, Morgan JD, Wass H: *Statements on death, dying and bereavement,* London, Ontario, 1994, King's College.

Costello A, Gardner SL, Merenstein GB: State of the art: perinatal grief and loss, *J Perinatol* 8:361-370, 1988.

Davidson GW: *Understanding the death of the wished-for child,* Springfield, Ill, 1979, OGR Service Corp.

Davidson GW: *Understanding mourning,* Minneapolis, 1984, Augsburg Publishing House.

Davis DL: *Empty cradle, broken heart,* ed 2, Golden, Colo, 1996, Fulcrum Publishing.

Davis DL, Stewart M, Harmon RJ: Perinatal loss: providing emotional support for bereaved parents, *Birth* 15:242-246, 1988.

DeFrain J: Learning about grief from normal families: SIDS, stillbirth and miscarriage, *J Marital Family Ther* 17(3):215-232, 1991.

Ewy D, Ewy R: *Death of a dream: miscarriage, stillbirth, and newborn loss,* New York, 1984, Dutton.

Fretts RC and others: The changing pattern of fetal death, *Obstet Gynecol* 79(1):35-39, 1988.

Friedman R, Gradstein B: *Surviving pregnancy loss,* Boston, 1996, Little, Brown.

Galinsky E: *Between generations: the six stages of parenthood,* New York, 1987, Addison Wesley Publishing Co.

Graves S, Williams SL: *Holiday help: hope and healing for those who grieve,* Louisville, Ky, 1992, Accord.

Harrigan R and others: Perinatal grief: response to the loss of an infant, *Neonatal Network* 12(5):25-31, 1993.

Ilse S: *Empty arms: coping with miscarriage, stillbirth and infant death,* Maple Plain, Minn, 1990, Wintergreen Press.

Irwin M, Daniels M, Weiner H: Immune and neuroendocrine changes during bereavement, *Psych Clin North Am* 10(3):449-465, 1987.

Klaus MH, Kennel J: *Parent-infant bonding,* St Louis, 1982, Mosby.

Kohn I, Moffit PL: *A silent sorrow,* New York, 1992, Bantam Double-day Dell.

Kowalski K: Loss and bereavement: psychological, sociological, spiritual and ontological perspectives. In Simpson KR, Creehan PA, editors: *AWHONN's perinatal nursing,* Philadelphia, 1996, Lippincott-Raven.

Kübler-Ross E: *On death and dying,* New York, 1969, MacMillan.

Lasker JN, Toedter LJ: Acute versus chronic grief: the case of pregnancy loss, *Am J Orthopsychiatry* 61(4):510-522, 1991.

Lederman R: *Psychosocial adaption in pregnancy,* Englewood Cliffs, NJ, 1984, Prentice Hall.

Leon I: Psychoanalytic conceptualization of perinatal loss: a multidimensional model, *Am J Psychiatry* 149:1464-1472, 1992.

Leon IG: Understanding and coping with reproductive losses, *Women's Psychiatric Health* 3(1):1-3, 6-7, 1994.

Limbo R, Wheeler S: Coping with unexpected outcomes, *NAACOG Update Series* 5(3):1-8, 1986.

Limbo RK, Wheeler SR: *When a baby dies: a handbook for healing and helping,* La Crosse, Wis, 1995, Bereavement Services/RTS.

Lindemann E: Symptomatology and management of acute grief, *Am J Psychiatry* 101:141-148, 1944.

Locke SA: *Coping with loss: a guide for caregivers,* Springfield, Ill, 1994, Charles C Thomas.

Manning D: *Don't take my grief away from me,* San Francisco, 1984, Harper & Row for Insight Books.

Meier PR and others: Perinatal autopsy: its clinical value, *Obstet Gynecol* 67(3):349-351, 1986.

Nelson CW, Niederberger J: Patient satisfaction surveys: an opportunity for total quality management, *Hosp Health Services Administration* 35(3):409-427, 1990.

Oaks J, Ezell G: *Dying and death: coping, caring and understanding,* ed 2, Scottsdale, Ariz, 1993, Gorsuch Scaresbrich Publishing.

Peppers LG, Knapp R: *How to go on living after the death of a baby,* Atlanta, 1985, Peachtree Publishers.

Rando T: *Parental loss of a child,* Champaign, Ill, 1986, Research Press.

Rando T: *Treatment of complicated mourning,* Champaign, Ill, 1993, Research Press.

Rich L: *When pregnancy isn't perfect: a lay person's guide to complications in pregnancy,* New York, 1991, Penguin Books.

Rillstone P: Not all babies live, *Int J Childbirth Educ* 8(4):27-28, 1993.

Rubin R: Maternal tasks in pregnancy, *Matern Child Nurs J* 4:143-153, 1975.

Schwiebert P, Kirk P: *When hello means goodbye,* Portland, Ore, 1985, Perinatal Loss.

Shively P: *Reaching out: a guide for developing or enhancing a comprehensive bereavement program for hospitals, clinics, and other healthcare centers,* La Crosse, Wis, 1995, Bereavement Services/RTS.

Simonds W, Rothman BK: *Centuries of solace: expressions of maternal grief in popular literature,* Philadelphia, 1992, Temple University Press.

Swanson KM: Nursing as informed caring for the well-being of others, *Image J Nurs Sch* 25:352-357, 1993.

Swanson-Kauffman K: Caring in the instance of unexpected early pregnancy loss, *Top Clin Nurs* 2:37-46, 1986.

Swanson-Kauffman K: There should have been two: nursing care of parents experiencing the perinatal death of a twin, *J Perinat Neonat Nurs* 2(2):78-86, 1988.

Theut SK and others: Resolution of parental bereavement after perinatal loss, *J Am Acad Child Adolesc Psychiatry* 29(4):521-525, 1990.

VanderZalm JE: The perinatal death of a twin: Karla's story of attaching and detaching, *J Nurs Midwifery* 40:335-341, 1995.

Wallerstedt C, Higgins P: Perinatal circumstances that evoke differences in the grieving response, *J Perinat Educ* 3(2):35-40, 1994.

Wheeler S, Limbo RK, Gensch BK: Loss and grief. In Bobak IM, Jensen MD: *Maternity and gynecological care: the nurse and the family,* ed 5, St Louis, 1992, Mosby.

Witter DM, Tolle SW, Moseley JR: A bereavement program: good care, quality assurance, and risk management, *Hosp Health Services Administration* 35(2):263-275, 1990.

Care for Caregiver

Arlen SB: Good selfishness, *Bereavement Magazine,* pp 10-11, June 1990.

Borysenko J: *Minding the body, mending the mind,* New York, 1987, Bantam Books.

Callanan M, Kelly P: *Final gifts,* New York, 1992, Poseidon Press.

Cameron J: *The artist's way,* New York, 1992, GP Putnam's Sons.

Caring for the caregiver: coping with the death of a patient, *Bereavement Magazine,* pp 26-27, May 1990.

Carter R, Golant SK: *Helping yourself help others: a book for caregivers,* New York, 1994, Times Books.

Deits B: *Life after loss: a personal guide dealing with death, divorce, job change and relocation,* Tucson, 1988, Fisher Books.

Feldstein MA, Gemma PB: Oncology nurses and chronic compounded grief, *Cancer Nurs* 18:228-236, 1995.

Figley C, editor: *Compassion fatigue: secondary traumatic stress disorders from treating the traumatized,* New York, 1995, Brunner/Mazel.

Heinrich K, Killeen ME: The gentle art of nurturing yourself, *Am J Nurs* 93(10):41-44, 1993.

Katherine A: *Boundaries: where you end and I begin,* Park Ridge, Ill, 1991, Parkside Publishing Corp.

Klein A: *The healing power of humor,* Los Angeles, 1989, Jeremy P Tarcher.

Larson DG: *The helper's journey: working with people facing grief, loss and life-threatening illness,* Champaign, Ill, 1993, Research Press.

Osmont K: *More than surviving: caring for yourself while you grieve,* Omaha, Neb, 1990, Centering Corp.

Smith D: *The Tao of dying,* Washington, DC, 1994, Caring Press.

Springer LK: Caregiver characteristics as seen by patients, family, and caregivers, *The Forum,* pp 7-9, 1992.

Taigman M: Can empathy and compassion be taught? *J Emerg Medical Services,* pp 43-48, June 1996.

Travis JW, Callander MG: *Wellness for helping professionals,* Mill Valley, Calif, 1990, Wellness Associates.

Wolfelt AD: *Understanding grief: helping yourself heal,* Muncie, Ind, 1992, Accelerated Development.

Wolfelt AD: *Selfcare for the bereavement caregiver: the codependent syndrome,* Fort Collins, Colo, 1992, Companion Press (training video tape [3 hours]).

Children and Grief

American Academy of Pediatrics Committee on Psychosocial Aspects of Child and Family Health: The pediatrician and childhood bereavement, *Pediatrics* 10(3):516-518, 1992.

Arnold JH, Gemma PB: *A child dies: a portrait of family grief,* Philadelphia, 1994, Charles Press.

Baker JE, Sedney MA, Gross E: Psychological tasks for bereaved children, *Am J Orthopsychiatry* 62(1):105-116, 1992.

Bowden V: Children's literature: the death experience, *Pediatr Nurs* 19:17-21, 1993.

Cohn J: *Molly's rosebush,* Morton Grove, Ill, 1994, Whitman & Co.

Dodge N: *Thumpy's story,* Springfield, Ill, 1983, Prairie Lark Press.

Goldman L: *Life and loss: a guide to help grieving children,* Bristol, Pa, 1994, Accelerated Development.

Grollman E: *Talking about death: a dialogue between parent and child,* Boston, 1990, Beacon Press.

Haasl B, Marnocha J: *Bereavement support group program for children,* Muncie, Ind, 1990, Accelerated Development.

Heiney SP: Sibling grief: a case report, *Arch Psychiatr Nurs* 5(3):121-127, 1991.

Johnson PP, Williams DR: *Morgan's baby sister,* San Jose, Calif, 1993, Resource Publications.

Kubler-Ross E: *On children and death,* New York, 1983, MacMillan.

O'Toole D: *Aarvy aardvark finds hope: a read-aloud story for people of all ages about loving and losing, friendship and hope,* Burnsville, NC, 1988, Rainbow Connection.

Overbeck B, Overbeck J: *Helping children cope with grief,* Dallas, 1992, TLC Group.

Ragourzeos B: *A grieving student in the classroom: guidelines and suggestions for school personnel and classroom teachers of grades 1-12,* Lancaster, Pa, Hospice of Lancaster County.

Resler R: *Remembering you: a book for children and teenagers who experience the loss of a brother or sister,* Cleveland, 1996, Rainbow Babies' and Children's Hospital.

Sanders C: *How to survive the loss of a child,* Rocklin, Calif, 1992, Prima Publishing.

Schaefer D, Lyons C: *How do we tell the children?* New York, 1993, Newmarket Press.

Schonfeld DJ: Talking with children about death, *J Pediatr Health Care* 7:269-274, 1993.

Silverman PR, Worden JW: Children's reactions in the early months after the death of a parent, *Am J Orthopsychiatry* 62(1):93-104, 1992.

Van-Si L, Powers L: *Helping children heal from loss: a keepsake book of special memories,* Portland, Ore, 1994, Portland State University.

Wass H, Corr C: *Helping children cope with death: guidelines and resources,* Washington, DC, 1984, Hemisphere.

Wolfelt AD: *Healing the bereaved child,* Fort Collins, Colo, 1995, Companion Press.

Clergy/Spiritual Issues

Carpentino LJ: Spiritual distress. In *Nursing diagnosis: application to clinical practice,* Philadelphia, 1993, Lippincott.

Coleman GD: Baptizing dying infants not always required, *Health Progress,* pp 46-66, Oct 1986.

Corrine L and others: The unheard voices of women: spiritual interventions in maternal-child health, *Matern Child Nurs* 17:141-145, 1992.

Cox G, Fundis R: *Spiritual, ethical and pastoral aspects of death and bereavement,* Amityville, NY, 1993, Baywood.

DiMeo E: Rx for spiritual distress, *RN,* pp 22-24, March 1991.

Doka KJ, Morgan JD, editors: *Death and spirituality,* Amityville, NY, 1993, Baywood.

Eich W: When is emergency baptism appropriate? *Am J Nurs* 87(12): 1680-1681, 1987.

Feinstein D, Mayo PE: *Mortal acts: eighteen empowering rituals for confronting death,* San Francisco, 1993, Harper.

Fickling KF: Stillborn studies: ministering to bereaved parents, *J Pastoral Care* 47:217-227, 1993.

Fish S, Shelly J: *Spiritual care: the nurse's role,* ed 3, Downer's Grove, Ill, 1988, Intervarsity Press.

Haase JE and others: Simultaneous concept analysis of spiritual perspective, hope acceptance and self-transcendence, *Image J Nurs Sch,* 24(2):141-147, 1992.

Kennison M: Faith: an untapped health resource, *J Psychosoc Nurs* 25(10):28-30, 1987.

Meyer C: *Surviving death,* Mystic, Conn, 1991, Twenty-Third Publications.

Parrott C: *Parent's grief: help and understanding after the death of a baby,* Redmond, Wash, 1992, Medic Publishing Co.

Rybarik F: Ask the experts: what are the roles of pastoral caregivers and funeral directors in dealing with perinatal loss? *AWHONN Voice* 3(8):8, 1995.

Thearle MJ and others: Church attendance, religious affiliation and parental responses to sudden infant death, neonatal death and stillbirth, *Omega* 31(1):51-58, 1995.

VandeCreek L: Patient and family perceptions of hospital chaplains, *Hosp Health Services Administration* 36:455-467, 1991.

Wolfelt AD: *Death and grief: a guide for clergy,* Muncie, Ind, 1988, Accelerated Development.

Communication

Black RB: Women's voices after pregnancy loss: couple's patterns of communication and support, *Soc Work Health Care* 16(2):19-36, 1991.

Burley-Allen M: *Listening: the forgotten skill,* ed 2, New York, 1995, Wiley & Sons.

Crowther ME: Communication following a stillbirth or neonatal death: room for improvement, *Br J Obstet Gynecol* 102:952-956, 1995.

Davis H, Hallowfield L, editors: *Counseling and communication in health care,* New York, 1991, Wiley.

Gerken KM: What (and what not) to say after pregnancy loss, *Bereavement Magazine,* pp 24-25, July/Aug 1993.

Nance T: Intercultural communication: finding common ground, *J Obstet Gynecol Neonat Nurs* 24:249-255, 1995.

Range LM, Walston AS, Pollard PM: Helpful and unhelpful comments after suicide, homicide, accident or natural death, *Omega* 25(1):25-31, 1992.

Rybarik F: Ask the experts: what communication skills are most helpful with families grieving a perinatal loss? *AWHONN Voice* 4(6), 1996.

Tannen D: *You just don't understand: women and men in conversation,* New York, 1990, Morrow.

What does a good listener do? Career Track Tapes, MS 20-13, Boulder, Colo.

Cultural Issues

Beeman PB: Cultural concepts in clinical care, *J Obstet Gynecol Neonatal Nurs* 24:327-369, 1995.

Counts DR, Counts DA: *Coping with the final tragedy: cultural variation in dying and grieving,* Amityville, NY, 1993, Baywood.

DeSpelder L, Strickland A: *The last dance: encountering death and dying,* Palo Alto, Calif, 1992, Mayfield Publishing Co.

Geissler EM: *Pocket guide to cultural assessment,* St Louis, 1994, Mosby.

Giger J, Davidhizar R: *Transcultural nursing,* ed 2, St Louis, 1995, Mosby.

Henry-Jenkins W: The Muslim way of death, *Bereavement Magazine,* pp 33-34, Jan 1993.

Hutchinson MK, Baqi-Aziz M: Nursing care of the childbearing Muslim family, *J Obstet Gynecol Neonatal Nurs* 23:767-771, 1994.

Irish DP, Lundquist KF, Nelsen VJ, editors: *Ethnic variations in dying, death and grief: diversity in universality,* Washington, DC, 1993, Taylor & Francis.

Layne LL: Motherhood lost: cultural dimensions of miscarriage and stillbirth in America, *Women Health* 16(3/4):69-97, 1990.

Mehta L, Verna IC: Helping parents to face perinatal loss, *Indian J Pediatr* 57(5):607-609, 1990.

Randall E: *Strategies for working with culturally diverse communities and clients,* Washington, DC, 1994, Association for Care of Children's Health.

Stroebe W, Stroebe MS: Is grief universal? Cultural variations in emotional reaction to loss. In Rulton R, Bendiksen R, editors: *Death and identity,* ed 3, Philadelphia, 1994, Charles Press.

York CR, Stichler J: Cultural grief expressions following infant death, *Dimens Crit Care Nurs* 4(2):120-127, 1985.

Depression

Agency for Health Care Policy and Research: *Depression in primary care: detection, diagnosis and treatment,* Silver Spring, Md, 1993, AHCPR Publications Clearinghouse.

American Psychiatric Association: *Diagnostic and statistical manual of mental disorders,* ed 4, Washington, DC, 1994, The Association.

Bowlby J: *Attachment and loss,* vol II, ed 2, New York, 1982, Basic Books.

Horowitz JA and others: Postpartum depression: issues in clinical assessment, *J Perinatol* 15:268-278, 1995.

Leahy JM: A comparison of depression in women bereaved of a spouse, child, or parent, *Omega* 26:207-217, 1993.

Neugebauer R and others: Depressive symptoms in women in the six months after miscarriage, *Am J Obstet Gynecol* 166:104-109, 1992.

Ectopic Pregnancy

Breault CM: Ectopic pregnancy is also a perinatal loss, *J Emerg Nurs* 15(3):217, 1989.

Grainger DA, Seifer DB: Laparoscopic management of ectopic pregnancy, *Curr Opin Obstet Gynecol* 7:277-282, 1995.

Maiolatesi CR, Peddicord K: Methotrexate for nonsurgical treatment of ectopic pregnancy: nursing implications, *J Obstet Gynecol Neonatal Nurs* 25:206-208, 1996.

Powell MP, Spellman JR: Medical management of the patient with an ectopic pregnancy, *J Perinatal Neonatal Nurs* 9(4):31-43, 1996.

Rolnick S and others: Decrease in the rate of ruptured ectopic pregnancies: a successful team approach, *HMO Pract* 8:105-109, 1994.

Ethics

Cox G, Fundis R: *Spiritual, ethical and pastoral aspects of death and bereavement,* Amityville, NY, 1993, Baywood.

McFadden EA: Moral development and reproductive health decisions, *J Obstet Gynecol Neonatal Nurs* 25:507-512, 1996.

Miya PA and others: Ethical perceptions of parents and nurses in NICU: the case of Baby Michael, *J Obstet Gynecol Neonatal Nurs* 24:125-130, 1995.

Monagle JF, Thomasma DC: *Medical ethics: policies, protocols, guidelines and programs,* Gaithersburg, Md, 1992, Aspen.

Family Relationships/Gender Issues

DeFrain J: Learning about grief from normal families: SIDS, stillbirth and miscarriage, *J Marital Family Ther* 17(3):215-232, 1991.

Doerr MW: *For better or worse—for couples whose child has died,* Omaha, Neb, 1992, Centering Corp.

Gilbert KR: Interactive grief and coping in the marital dyad, *Death Studies* 13:605-626, 1989.

Gilbert KR: "We've had the same loss, why don't we have the same grief?" Loss and differential grief in families, *Death Studies* 20:269-283, 1996.

Goldbach KR and others: The effects of gestational age and gender on grief after pregnancy loss, *Am J Orthopsychiatry* 61(3):461-467, 1991.

Kissane DW, Bloch S: Family grief, *Br J Psychiatry* 164:728-740, 1994.

Lang A, Gottlieb LN, Amsel R: Predictors of husbands' and wives' grief reactions following infant death: the role of marital intimacy, *Death Studies* 20:33-57, 1996.

Lister MK, Lovell SM: Healing together: helping couples cope with miscarriage, stillbirth or early infant loss, *Bereavement Magazine,* pp 12-13, Oct 1990.

Rosof BD: *The worst loss: how families heal from the death of a child,* New York, 1994, Holt.

Wallerstedt C, Higgins P: Facilitating perinatal grieving between the mother and the father, *J Obstet Gynecol Neonatal Nurs* 25:389-394, 1996.

Wheeler S, Pike M: *Seasons of a woman's grief.* Presentation at the National NAACOG Convention, Orlando, June 1991.

Follow-up

Ewton DS: A perinatal loss follow-up guide for primary care, *Nurse Pract* 18(12):30-36, 1993.

Piper WF, McCallum M, Azim HFA: *Adaptation to loss through short-term group psychotherapy,* New York, 1993, Guilford Publications.

Worden JW: *Grief counseling and grief therapy,* ed 2, New York, 1991, Springer.

Funerals

Lamb JM, editor: *Bittersweet . . . hello goodbye: a resource in planning farewell rituals when a baby dies,* St Charles, Mo, 1989, SHARE.

Manning D: *A minister speaks about funerals,* Springfield, Ill, 1992, Human Services Press.

Morgan E: *Dealing creatively with death: a manual of death education and simple burial,* ed 13, Bayside, NY, 1993, Zinn Communications.

Silverman PR, Worden JW: Children's understanding of funeral ritual, *Omega* 25(4):319-331, 1992.

Wolfelt A: *Interpersonal skills training: a handbook for funeral home staffs,* Muncie, Ind, 1990, Accelerated Development.

Interventions/Supportive Care

Brost L, Kenney JW: Pregnancy after perinatal loss: parental reactions and nursing interventions, *J Obstet Gynecol Neonatal Nurs* 21:457-463, 1992.

Calhoun LK: Parents' perceptions of nursing support following neonatal loss, *J Perinatal Neonatal Nurs* 8(2):57-66, 1994.

Catlin AJ: Emotional support for early pregnancy loss: how you can do it, *Matern Child Health Educ Resources* 7(2):1-3, 1992.

Conrad BH: *When a child dies: ways you can help a bereaved parent,* Santa Barbara, Calif, 1995, Fithian Press.

Courtney SE, Thomas N, Predmore BK: Reverse transport of the deceased neonate—an aid to mourning, *Am J Perinatol* 2(3):217-222, 1985.

Limbo RK, Wheeler SR: *When a baby dies: a handbook for healing and helping,* La Crosse, Wis, 1995, Bereavement Services/RTS.

Maloni JA and others: Transforming prenatal care: reflections on the past and present with implications for the future, *J Obstet Gynecol Neonatal Nurs* 25:17-23, 1996.

Neumann M, Hudson PO: Solution-oriented therapy techniques for women's health nurses, *J Obstet Gynecol Neonatal Nurs* 23:16-20, 1994.

Rybarik F: Coping with perinatal loss: the role of a perinatal bereavement team, *Adv Nurs Pract* 2(12):21-22, 32, 1994.

Scott MS, Grzbowski M, Webb S: Perceptions and practices of registered nurses regarding pastoral care and the spiritual needs of hospital patients, *J Pastoral Care* 48:171-179, 1994.

Sexton PR, Stephen SB: Postpartum mothers' perceptions of nursing interventions for perinatal grief, *Neonatal Network* 9(5):47-51, 1991.

Thearle MJ, Gregory H: Evolution of bereavement counseling in sudden infant death syndrome, neonatal death and stillbirth, *J Pediatr Children's Health* 23:204-209, 1992.

Welch ID: Miscarriage, stillbirth or newborn death: starting a healthy grieving process, *Neonatal Network* 9(8):53-57, 1991.

Wolfelt AD: *Growth-oriented grief counseling: therapeutic interventions for caregivers,* Muncie, Ind, 1992, Accelerated Development.

Men/Fathers

Hughes CB, Page-Lieberman J: Fathers experiencing a perinatal loss, *Death Studies* 13(6):537-556, 1989.

Merrill SE: *Miscarriage and the fathers: the need for an availability of social support,* unpublished master's thesis, Eau Claire, Wis, 1986, University of Wisconsin–Eau Claire School of Nursing.

Nelson JD, editor: *The rocking horse is lonely: and other stories of fathers' grief,* Wayzata, Minn, 1994, Pregnancy and Infant Loss Center.

Page-Lieberman J, Hughes CB: How fathers perceive perinatal death, *Matern Child Nurs* 15:320-323, 1994.

Staudacher C: *Men & grief,* Oakland, Calif, 1991, New Harbinger Publications.

Wheat R: *Miscarriage: a man's book,* Omaha, Neb, 1995, Centering Corp.

Wolfelt AD: Gender roles and grief: why men's grief is naturally complicated, *Thanatos,* pp 20-25, Fall 1990.

Young-Mason J: Baby Susan, *Clin Nurs Specialist* 6(2):104, 1992.

Miscarriage

Allen M, Marks S: *Miscarriage: women sharing from the heart,* New York, 1993, John Wiley & Sons.

Flagler S, Nicoll L: A framework for the psychological aspects of pregnancy, *NAACOG'S Clin Issues Perinatal Women's Health Nurs* 1(3):267-278, 1990.

Friedman R, Gradstein B: Miscarriage—an unrecognized loss. In *Surviving pregnancy loss,* Boston, 1992, Little, Brown.

Frost M, Condon J: The psychological sequels of miscarriage: a critical review of the literature, *Aust NZ J Psychol* 301:54-62, 1996.

Harris BG, Sandelowski M, Holditch-Davis D: Infertility . . . and new interpretations of pregnancy loss, *Matern Child Nurs* 16:217-220, 1991.

Hutti MH: Parents' perceptions of the miscarriage experience, *Death Studies* 16:401-415, 1992.

Ramsden CA: Miscarriage counseling: an accident and emergency perspective, *Emerg Nurs* 3(2):68-73, 1995.

Reed KS: The effects of gestational age and pregnancy planning status on obstetrical nurses' perceptions of giving emotional care to women experiencing miscarriage, *Image J Nurs Sch* 24(2):107-110, 1992.

Roberts H: Managing miscarriage: the management of the emotional sequelae of miscarriage in training practices in the west of Scotland, *Fam Practitioner* 8(2):117-120, 1991.

Winslow S: Miscarriage, the unrecognized tragedy, *Bereavement Magazine,* p 25, March/April 1991.

Zaccardi R, Abbott J, Kosiol-McLain J: Loss and grief reactions after spontaneous miscarriage in the emergency department, *Ann Emerg Med* 22:799-804, 1993.

Newborn Death/Neonatal Intensive Care Unit

Davis DL: *Loving and letting go,* Omaha, Neb, 1993, Centering Corp.

Downey V and others: Dying babies and associated stress in NICU nurses, *Neonatal Network* 14(1):41-45, 1995.

Frey D: "Does anyone here think this baby can live?" *New York Times Sunday Magazine,* pp 22-31, 36, 44, 47, July 9, 1995.

Gustaitis R, Young EWD: *A time to be born, a time to die: conflicts and ethics in an intensive care nursery,* Reading, Mass, 1986, Gustaitis and EWD Young.

Miya PA and others: Ethical perceptions of parents and nurses in NICU: the case of Baby Michael, *J Obstet Gynecol Neonatal Nurs* 24:125-130: 1995.

Swanson K: Providing care in the NICU: sometimes an act of love, *Adv Nurs Sci* 13(1):60-73, 1990.

Todd A: *Journey of the heart,* Nashville, Tenn, 1995, Medical Center North.

Photography

Brown CE, Kozich P: Reconstructing reality: reserving memories through the creation of impressions, *Int J Childbirth Educ* 9(1):38-40, 1994.

For K: *Tips for picture taking,* Beech Grove, Ind, 1991, St Francis Hospital Center.

Griesbach S: A medical photographer's role on a perinatal bereavement team, *J Biological Photography* 56(4):149-153, 1988.

Johnson J, Johnson SM: *A most important picture: a tender manual for taking pictures of stillborn babies and infants who die,* Omaha, Neb, 1985, Centering Corp.

Lamb JM Sr: Baby pictures questionnaire, part II. Quotes from parents, *SHARE Newsletter* 11(4), July/Aug 1987.

McGhie J: Portraiture of the stillborn . . . should we or should we not? *J Audiovisual Media Med* 12:9-10, 1989.

Primeau MR, Recht CK: Professional bereavement photographs: one aspect of a perinatal bereavement program, *J Obstet Gynecol Neonatal Nurs* 23:22-25, 1994.

Ruby J: Portraying the dead, *Omega* 19(1):1-20, 1988-1989.

Schweibert P: *When hello means goodbye,* Portland, Ore, 1985, Perinatal Loss.

Wright J: What's wrong with this picture? *Am Baby,* pp 32-34, Feb 1991.

Physician Articles

American Academy of Pediatrics Committee on Psychosocial Aspects of Child and Family Health: The pediatrician and childhood bereavement, *Pediatrics* 89(3):516-518, 1992.

Buckman R: *How to break bad news: a guide for health care professionals,* Baltimore, 1992, Johns Hopkins University Press.

Chez RA, Davidson G: Helping patients and doctors cope with perinatal death, *Obstet Gynecol* 85(6):1059-1061, 1995.

Curry CJ: Pregnancy loss, stillbirth and neonatal death: a guide for the pediatrician, *Pediatr Clin North Am* 39(1):157-192, 1992.

Forrest GC, Standish E, Baum JD: Support after perinatal death: a study of support and counseling after perinatal bereavement, *Br Med J* 285(20):1475-1479, 1982.

Freeman RR, Poland RL, editors: *Guidelines for perinatal care,* ed 3, New York, 1990, American Academy of Pediatrics and American College of Obstetrics and Gynecology in conjunction with March of Dimes.

Lake MF, Knuppel RA, Angel JL: The rationale for supportive care after perinatal death, *J Perinatol* 7(2):35-89, 1992.

Leash RM: *Death notification: a mutual guide to the process,* Hinesburg, Vt, 1994, Upper Access.

Lemmer CM: Parental perceptions of caring following perinatal bereavement, *West J Nurs Res* 13(4):475-493, 1991.

Leon IG: Perinatal loss: a critique of current hospital practices, *General Pediatrics* 31:366-374, 1992.

Newman L, Williams J: The family physician's role following a neonatal death, *J Family Practice* 29(5):521-525, 1989.

Schmidt TA, Tolle SW: Emergency physicians' responses to families following patient death, *Ann Emerg Med* 19(2):125-128, 1990.

Statham H, Dimavicius J: Commentary: how do you give the bad news to parents? *Birth* 19(2):103-104, 1992.

Wiseman B: Death of a child: a bereaved doctor's perspective, *Bereavement Magazine,* May/June 1994.

Woods J, Esposito J: *Pregnancy loss: medical therapeutics and practical considerations,* Baltimore, 1987, Williams & Wilkins.

Prenatal Diagnosis and Decision Making

Blasco PM, Blasco PA: Prenatal diagnosis: current procedures and implications for early interventionists working with families, *Infants Young Children* 7(2):33-42, 1994.

Dallaire L and others: Parental reaction and adaptability to the prenatal diagnosis of fetal defect or genetic disease leading to pregnancy interruption, *Prenatal Diagn* 15:249-259, 1995.

Delp KJ, Minnick MA: *Support group manual: a training manual for conducting support programs for parents who have interrupted pregnancies secondary to fetal anomalies,* St John's, Minn, 1995, Pineapple Press.

Green JM: Obstetricians' views on prenatal diagnosis and termination of pregnancy: 1980 compared with 1993, *Br J Obstet Gynecol* 102:228-232, 1995.

Isle S: *Precious lives, painful choices,* Maple Plain, Minn, 1993, Wintergreen Press.

Kilker A, Burke BM: Grieving the wanted child: ramifications of abortion after prenatal diagnosis of abnormality, *Health Care Women International* 14:513-526, 1993.

Lyon W: *A mother's dilemma,* St John's, Minn, 1992, Pineapple Press.

Minnick M, editor: *Yesterday, I dreamed of dreams . . . ,* St John's, Minn, 1991, Pineapple Press.

Seller M and others: Grief and midtrimester fetal loss, *Prenatal Diagn* 13:341-348, 1993.

Zeanah CH and others: Do women grieve after terminating pregnancies because of fetal anomalies? A controlled investigation, *Obstet Gynecol* 82:270-275, 1993.

Research

Carter SL: Themes of grief, *Nurs Res* 38(6):354-358, 1989.

Cleiren M: *Bereavement and adaptation,* Washington, DC, 1992, Hemisphere.

DeVries B, Dalla Lana R, Falk V: Parental bereavement over the life course: a theoretical intersection and empirical review, *Omega* 29:47-69, 1994.

Discher TA, Haggerty PA: *The bereavement needs of family members in a hospital setting.* Poster session presented at RTS Bereavement Conference, Naperville, Ill, Oct 1995.

Gilbert KR: Interactive grief and coping in the marital dyad, *Death Studies* 13:605-626, 1989.

Goldbach KR and others: The effects of gestational age and gender on grief after pregnancy loss, *Am J Orthopsychiatry* 61(3):461-467, 1991.

Harper MB, Wisian NB: Care of bereaved parents: a study in patient satisfaction, *J Reprod Med* 39:80-86, 1994.

Janssen H and others: Controlled prospective study on the mental health of women following pregnancy loss, *Am J Psychiatry* 153:226-230, 1996.

Lasker JN, Toedter LJ: Satisfaction with hospital care and interventions after pregnancy loss, *Death Studies* 18(1):41-64, 1994.

Lemmer CM: Parental perceptions of caring following perinatal bereavement, *West J Nurs Res* 15:199-215, 1993.

Moos NL: An integrative model of grief, *Death Studies* 19:337-364, 1995.

Ponzetti JJ: Bereaved families: a comparison of parents' and grandparents' reactions to the death of a child, *Omega* 25(1):63-71, 1992.

Schaefer C, Quesenberry CP, Wi S: Mortality following conjugal bereavement and the effects of a shared environment, *Am J Epidemiol* 141:1142-1152, 1995.

Solari-Twadell PA and others: The pinwheel model of bereavement, *Image J Nurs Sch* 27:323-326, 1995.

Swanson K: Empirical development of a middle range theory of caring, *Nurs Res* 40(3):161-166, 1991.

Theut SK and others: Resolution of parental bereavement after a perinatal loss, *J Am Acad Child Adolesc Psychiatry* 29(4):521-525, 1990.

Standards/Guidelines

Association of Women's Health, Obstetric, and Neonatal Nurses (AWHONN): *AWHONN standards for the nursing care of women and newborns,* ed 4, Washington, DC, 1991, The Association.

Association of Women's Health, Obstetric, and Neonatal Nurses (AWHONN): *Competencies and program guidelines for nurse providers of perinatal education,* Washington, DC, 1993, The Association.

Association of Women's Health, Obstetric, and Neonatal Nurses (AWHONN): *Didactic content and clinical skills verification for professional nurse providers of perinatal home care,* Washington, DC, 1994, The Association.

Freeman RK, Poland RL, editors: *Guidelines for perinatal care,* ed 3, Washington, DC, 1992, American Academy of Pediatrics and American College of Obstetricians and Gynecologists in conjunction with the March of Dimes.

Gracey KM and others: Certification: hospital versus national standards, *J Nurs Staff Development* 12:93-97, 1996.

Joint Commission on Accreditation of Healthcare Organizations: Patient rights and organizational ethics. In *1995 Accreditation manual for hospitals,* vol 2, no. 1, Oakbrook Terrace, Ill, 1994, The Commission.

Stillbirth

Dalla Grana W: Stillbirth: the silent birth cry, *Bereavement Magazine,* pp 24-26, 1993.

DeFrain J.: *Stillborn: the invisible death,* Lexington, Mass, 1986, Heath and Co.

Mitchell S: Stillbirth—a patient's perspective, *Practitioner* 232:1368-1371, 1988.

Reid J: *Lifeline: a journal for parents grieving miscarriage, stillbirth or early infant death,* St John's, Minn, 1994, Pineapple Press.

Subsequent Pregnancy

Bourne S, Lewis E: Delayed psychological effects of perinatal deaths: the next pregnancy and the next generation, *Br Med J* 289(6438):147-148, 1984.

Bourne S, Lewis E: Pregnancy after stillbirth or neonatal death, *Lancet* II(8393):31-33, 1984.

Brost L, Kenney JW: Pregnancy after perinatal loss: parental reactions and nursing intervention, *J Obstet Gynecol Neonatal Nurs* 21:457-463, 1992.

Parker L, O'Leary J: Impact of prior prenatal loss upon subsequent pregnancy: the function of the childbirth class, *Int J Childbirth Education,* pp 7-9, August 1989.

Schwiebert PL, Kirk P: *Still to be born,* Portland, Ore, 1986, Perinatal Loss.

Stumpf V: The promise of tomorrow: subsequent pregnancy after prenatal loss, *Int J Childbirth Education* 9(1):29-30, 1994.

Theut S and others: Pregnancy subsequent to perinatal loss: parental anxiety and depression, *J Am Acad Child Adolesc Psychiatry* 27(3):289-292, 1988.

Support Groups

Braun L, Coplon J, Sonnenschein P: *Helping parents in groups: a leader's handbook,* Boston, 1984, Resource Communications.

Guillory BA, Riggin OZ: Developing a nursing staff support group model, *Clin Nurs Specialist* 5(3):170-173, 1991.

Holm MA: Strategies for developing a family support group, *Focus on Critical Care—AACN* 18(6):444-459, 1991.

Humm A: *How to organize a self-help group,* New York, 1979 (order from National Self-Help Clearinghouse).

Kellet J: Facilitating support groups: a pilot study, *Nurs Standard* 6(23):34-36, 1992.

Limbo R, Wheeler S: *A parent support group guide,* La Crosse, Wis, 1994, Bereavement Services/RTS.

Nugent K and others: A practice model for a parent support group, *Pediatric Nursing,* 18(1):11-16, 1992.

Overbeck B, Overbeck J: *Starting/running support groups,* Dallas, 1992, TLC Group (Publications for Transition, Loss and Change).

Rootes LE, Aanes DL: A conceptual framework for understanding self-help groups, *Hosp Community Psychiatry* 43(4):379-381, 1992.

Ryan PF, Cote-Arsenault D, Sugarman LL: Facilitating care after perinatal loss: a comprehensive checklist, *J Obstet Gynecol Neonatal Nurs* 205(5):385-389, 1991.

Wheeler S, Limbo R: Bereavement support . . . get it going and keep it growing, *The Director,* pp 34-41, Jan 1991.

III

Ethical Dilemmas and Legal Considerations in Perinatal Nursing

As technologic advances have occurred, new methods of maternal and fetal diagnoses and medical therapies have emerged. Nurses are confronted daily with unexpected ethical dilemmas for which they may be unprepared. The first chapter in this unit provides a basis for understanding the elements of ethical decision making and lists some possible clinical examples in perinatal nursing care. The rapid expansion of available technology in perinatal medical management and nursing care has also had an impact on the increase in litigation when unexpected outcomes occur. Legal considerations have become a common concern for the perinatal team. The second chapter in this unit discusses professional liability, related legal terminology, risks, and litigation processes and lists examples of common clinical concerns.

CHAPTER

7

Ethical Decision Making

Perinatal nurses are confronted daily with ethical dilemmas. This chapter examines the nature of values clarification, introduces a framework for ethics, provides a model for ethical decision making, outlines the individual nurse's responsibility for participation and involvement, and lists relevant clinical perinatal examples that commonly confront the perinatal nurse.

VALUES CLARIFICATION

Educators, psychologists, anthropologists, sociologists, and theologians have influenced the definition of values. They consider values to be attitudes, beliefs, and moral judgments that are chosen freely and thoughtfully and are prized and acted on (Uustal, 1985).

Process of Valuing

The process of valuing has three aspects: choosing, prizing, and acting.

Choosing

Choosing involves the cognitive component of valuing. Logical, critical, creative thinking and moral judgment development are included. Important elements of choosing include the following:

- Chosen freely
- Chosen from available alternatives
- Chosen after considering the consequences of each alternative
- Complements other values previously internalized

Prizing

Prizing involves the affective component. This feeling component of valuing includes the following aspects:
- An awareness of one's position on the matter
- The expression of one's value
- Experiencing positive self-esteem as a result of the expression of the value
- Communication and sending of clear messages about the value
- Empathetic listening
- Pride and happiness with the choice

Acting

Acting involves the behavioral component and results in the following (Uustal, 1985):
- Personal, professional, and academic competence
- Resolution of conflict
- Willingness to affirm the choice publicly
- Making the choice part of personal behavior
- Consistent repetition of the choice

MORAL JUDGMENT DEVELOPMENT

Moral judgment development theory complements valuing. Kohlberg in 1981 contributed to the study of moral development by expanding on the work of Piaget and describing six stages of moral development (Uustal, 1985).

Stages

Preconventional Level

The child at the preconventional level is responsive to cultural rules and labels of good and bad, right and wrong. These labels are considered by the child in the context of punishment, reward, or exchange of favors. This level is divided into two stages.

Stage 1. Stage 1 is the stage of punishment and obedience. Avoidance of punishment and deference to power are ends in themselves. The physical consequences of an action determine if it is good or bad. For example, the reason for doing right is to avoid punishment from those with more power.

Stage 2. Stage 2 is the stage of instrumental purpose and exchange. Right action is that which pragmatically satisfies one's own needs and occasionally the needs of others. Right is following the rules because it is in the immediate interest. Right is also what is fair, equal, a deal, or an agreement. Reciprocity is given for the actual reward rather than out of loyalty or gratitude.

Conventional Level

At the conventional level of moral judgment development, the person considers the expectations of others and conformity as valuable in their own right, regardless of the immediate consequences. There is an attitude not only of conformity, but also of active maintenance, support, and justification of the order. Stages 3 and 4 are at this level.

Stage 3. Stage 3 is the stage of mutual interpersonal expectations, relationships, and conformity. Good behavior is that which pleases and helps others and is approved by them. Conformity to stereotypes is common. Behavior is frequently judged by intention, as in meaning well. Right behavior is being nice and living up to what is expected.

Stage 4. Stage 4 is the stage of social system and conscience maintenance. Right action is doing one's duty in a group, showing respect for authority, and upholding the prescribed social order for its own sake. Orientation is toward authority, fixed rules, and maintenance of the social order.

Postconventional Level

The postconventional level is also called the *autonomous* or *principled level.* The individual attempts to define moral values and principles that have validity and application apart from the authority of society and the individual's identity with societal groups. There are two stages at this level.

Stage 5. Stage 5 is the stage of a priori rights and social contract or utility. This stage has utilitarian overtones. Right action is defined in terms of standards that have been agreed on by society in terms of individual rights. Right action is described as upholding basic rights, values, and legal contracts of society even when they conflict with concrete rules and laws of the group.

Awareness of relativism of personal values and opinions exists, with an emphasis on reaching consensus. Right action is also a matter of personal values aside from what is constitutionally agreed on. There is an emphasis on the legal point of view, with the possibility of changing law in terms of rational consideration of societal utility.

Stage 6. Stage 6 is the stage of universal ethical principles. Right action is defined by a decision of conscience in accord with self-chosen ethical principles. Specific laws usually rest on these principles. When, however, laws violate these principles, acts must be in accord with principles rather than law. Principles are abstract, ethical, and universal, such as the principles of justice, reciprocity, equality, and respect for human dignity.

Qualities

In addition to the six stages of moral development, Kohlberg in 1981 described six qualities of the stages of moral development (Uustal, 1985):

1. The development of morality proceeds in an invariant sequence as the individual matures and as the environment offers the necessary stimulation and opportunities to learn.
2. Subjects cannot comprehend moral reasoning at a level more than one stage beyond their development.
3. Subjects are cognitively attracted to reasoning one level above their own predominant level.
4. Movement through stages is effected when cognitive disequilibrium is created by conflicting values.
5. Although the time it takes to move through the stages varies, the sequence is always the same.
6. Movement to higher stages of moral development is advantageous for the individual and society.

FRAMEWORK FOR ETHICS

Definitions

Ethics

Ethics is the study of values in human conduct or the study of right conduct. It is a branch of philosophy that attempts to state and evaluate principles by which ethical dilemmas may be resolved. It is not a science with right or wrong answers but rather strives to provide a systematic, critical, rational, defensible, intellectual approach to determining what is best in a situation with conflicting values. The result will ultimately be unfavorable and pit one or more ethical principles against another.

Metaethics

Metaethics is the part of ethics that focuses on the extent to which ethical judgments are reasonable or justifiable.

Normative Ethics

Normative ethics is the part of ethics that raises questions about what is right or ought to be done in a situation that calls for an ethical decision.

Ethical Principles

Several basic principles help to identify values, morals, beliefs, and attitudes and to clarify ethical dilemmas (Table 7-1).

Ethical principles comprise the sixth stage of Kohlberg's 1981

TABLE 7-1 Definitions of ethical principles

Ethical principle	Definition
Beneficence	Duty to do good
Nonmaleficence	Duty to do no harm
Veracity	Duty to tell the truth
Justice	Equitable distribution of risks and benefits
Fidelity	Duty to keep one's promise or word
Reparation	Duty to make up for a wrong
Gratitude	Duty to make up for a good
Autonomy	Being one's own person without constraints by another's action or psychologic and physical limitations
Informed consent	Contains four elements: Disclosure of information Comprehension Voluntary agreement Competency to make decision
Confidentiality	Holding information entrusted in context of special relationships as private
Utility	Greatest good or least harm for the greatest number
Universality	Same principle must hold for everyone, regardless of time, place, or persons involved
Generality	Must not refer to specific people or situations
Finality	May override demands of law and custom
Publicity	Principles must be known and recognized by all
Ordering	Ethical principles must be prioritized even though they may be conflicting

moral development (Uustal, 1985). The characteristics of ethical principles are as follows:

1. They suggest direction or propose certain behaviors.
2. They serve as guides to organizing and understanding ethically relevant information in an ethical dilemma.
3. They propose how to resolve competing claims.
4. They are the reasons justifying moral actions.
5. They are universal in nature. They are not absolute and do have exceptions.
6. They are neither rules (means) nor values (ends).
7. They are unchangeable and discovered by humans rather than invented.

MODEL FOR ETHICAL DECISION MAKING
Characteristics of Ethical Dilemmas

We live in an era where technologies develop faster than we can consider consequences. Changes affect clinical practice before guidelines for use are developed and before the social and ethical impact can be considered. Recent advances in reproductive technologies and endocrinology, genetics, neonatal and maternal-fetal medical care, and fetal therapies have created numerous ethical dilemmas for the recipient of care and the caregiver. These dilemmas and the resultant decisions have a considerable impact on society.

The characteristics of an ethical dilemma are as follows (Nosek, 1988; Uustal, 1985):

1. The choice is between equally undesirable alternatives.
2. Real choices exist between possible courses of action.
3. The people involved place a significantly different value judgment on possible actions or the consequences.
4. Data alone will not help to resolve the dilemma.
5. "Answers" to the dilemma come from a number of different disciplines, such as psychology, sociology, and theology.
6. Actions taken in an ethical dilemma will result in unfavorable outcomes or constitute a breach of one's duty to another individual.
7. The choices made in an ethical dilemma have far-reaching effects on our perception of human beings and our definition of personhood, our relationships, and people and society as a whole.
8. Any ethical decision involves the allocation and expenditure of resources that are finite.

9. Ethical dilemmas are not solvable but rather resolvable.
10. There is no right or wrong when dealing with two equally unfavorable actions.

Theories in Ethics

Two classic schools of thought—teleology and deontology—dominate ethical theory.

Teleology

According to the theory of teleology the rightness or wrongness of an action is determined by the consequences, not by whether it is inherently right or wrong. This approach to decision making is goal or outcome based. It is also called *utilitarianism* or *consequentialism.*

Deontology

The theory of deontology holds that the inherent characteristics of the decision can be judged independent of its outcome or consequences. Duty-based or rights-based approaches are examples of deontologic thoughts.

Relativism

A pure application of either theory may not be useful. A third dimension of ethical theory was described by Neibuhr in 1963 (Uustal, 1985). It adds the notion of relativism or pragmatism and describes individual responsibility. The application of paradigm cases, anecdotal experiences, and ethical principles to clinical problems exemplifies relativism.

The root principles of ethical theory are beneficence, justice, and autonomy (see Table 7-1). Decision making is always colored by the individual's values, attitudes, knowledge, desires, cultural mores, experiences, and background (Archer-Drusté, 1988).

Steps in Decision Making

The steps in ethical decision making are described in Box 7-1.

Nursing Responsibility

The concepts central to nurses' responsibility in participation in ethical decision making are caring, coordination, and advocacy (Archer-Drusté, 1988). These are based on the unique relationship between the nurse and patient. Clinical ethics, existing aside from medical ethics, incorporates the ethical problems the nurse encounters in the independent and collaborative domains of

---

Box 7-1
Steps in Ethical Decision Making

1. Identify the problem:
   a. Who are the people involved?
   b. How are they interrelated?
   c. What is involved?
2. Identify the values, issues, or ethical dilemmas, and make a concise statement of the problem and conflicts in values.
3. State your values and ethical position related to the case.
4. Generate alternatives for resolving the dilemma or dilemmas.
5. Examine and categorize the alternatives:
   a. List alternatives.
   b. Identify those consistent and those inconsistent with your own values and ethics.
6. Predict the possible consequences for those acceptable alternatives:
   a. Identify physical, psychologic, social, spiritual, and short- and long-range consequences.
   b. Identify those consequences consistent with your values and ethics.
7. Prioritize acceptable alternatives.
8. Develop a plan of action.
9. Implement the plan.
10. Evaluate the action taken.

---

practice. Nursing is owned by society and as such is an essential part of society with a responsibility to the whole.

Caring

Caring, described by Swanson-Kaufman (1986; Swanson, 1993) and outlined in Chapter 6, provides the first mandate for nurses' participation in and assumption of ethical practice. The second mandate is derived from the social contract and the American Nurses Association (ANA) code for nurses (Box 7-2). The third mandate for participation in ethical decision making is the pivotal position of nursing within the health care organization. Professional nursing practice is ethical nursing practice (Archer-Drusté, 1988).

PATIENT SELF-DETERMINATION ACT

A federal law, The Patient Self-Determination Act, went into effect in December of 1991 for all health care facilities receiving federal monies. This act requires that all patients be informed of their rights to make decisions concerning their health care.

Box 7-2

American Nurses Association Code of Ethics

The nurse provides services with respect for human dignity and the uniqueness of the client unrestricted by considerations of social or economic status, personal attributes, or the nature of health problems.

The nurse safeguards the client's right to privacy by judiciously protecting information of a confidential nature.

The nurse acts to safeguard the client and the public when health care and safety are affected by the incompetent, unethical, or illegal practice of any person.

The nurse assumes responsibility and accountability for individual nursing judgments and actions.

The nurse maintains competence in nursing.

The nurse exercises informed judgment and uses individual competence and qualifications as criteria in seeking consultation, accepting responsibilities, and delegating nursing activities to others.

The nurse participates in activities that contribute to the ongoing development of the profession's body of knowledge.

The nurse participates in the profession's efforts to implement and improve standards of nursing.

The nurse participates in the profession's efforts to establish and maintain conditions of employment conducive to high-quality nursing care.

The nurse participates in the profession's effort to protect the public from misinformation and misrepresentation and to maintain the integrity of nursing.

The nurse collaborates with members of the health professions and other citizens in promoting community and national efforts to meet the health needs of the public

From American Nurses Assocation: *Code for nurses with interpretive statements,* Kansas City, Mo, 1985, The Association.

ADVANCE DIRECTIVE

An advance directive, also known as a *living will* or a *durable power of attorney,* recognizes the patient's right to control decisions relating to acceptance or refusal of aspects of his or her own medical care. When the patient has decision-making capacity, that control can be exercised by formulating an advance directive.

If the patient loses decision-making capacity, a durable power of attorney can appoint another person to make those decisions. A living will can direct the physician to provide, withhold, or withdraw life-sustaining care.

Box 7-3
Clinical Examples of Perinatal Ethical Dilemmas

Voluntary pregnancy termination
Selective reduction in multiple gestation
Previable termination of pregnancy for maternal reasons
Harvesting of fetal organs or tissue
In vitro fertilization and decisions for remaining fertilized ova
Allocation of resources in pregnancies complicated by substance abuse and
    other antisocial behaviors
Allocation of resources in pregnancy care during previable period
Fetal surgery
Maternal serum alpha-fetoprotein (MSAFP), amniocentesis, chorionic
    villus sampling (CVS) diagnosis, routine ultrasonography
Routine use of electronic fetal monitoring (EFM) for cesarean delivery
    indication in cases of previous cesarean delivery
Equal access to prenatal care
Health care rights
Maternal rights versus fetal rights
Extraordinary medical treatment for pregnancy complications
Court-ordered cesarean section

Lindgren S: *J Obstet Gynecol Neonatal Nurs* 25:653-656, 1996; Pryde P and others:
Obstet Gynecol 80:52-56, 1992.

In the case of a pregnant woman, however, the advance directive does not allow her to make decisions in advance that may affect fetal survival or quality of life. For example, if a pregnant woman is involved in a motor vehicle crash and sustains a head injury that permanently affects her cardiorespiratory center, she may be kept on life-sustaining care despite instructions in her living will to the contrary. If sustaining her on life support can successfully maintain the pregnancy, which shows no evidence of fetal compromise, her living will requesting no life support will be disregarded. In such situations it has been determined that postponement of maternal death does less harm to her when balanced against the fetal right to survive.

CLINICAL EXAMPLES OF ETHICAL DILEMMAS

Some clinical examples of ethical dilemmas that perinatal nurses face are listed in Box 7-3.

CONCLUSION

The list of perinatal ethical decisions is much longer than that given in Box 7-3. Some dilemmas are everyday issues. Others are likely to be encountered infrequently and then only in select tertiary perinatal centers. However, it is impossible to work in perinatal nursing and not become involved in ethical dilemmas or participate in ethical decision making. The nurse must not only examine issues in light of what she or he is willing to participate in, but also facilitate an environment where colleagues and patients can participate in ethical decisions. The nurse functions as educator, support person, counselor, administrator, researcher, and care provider. Nurses spend more time with patients than any other health care team members do. As a result, nurses must take an active and assertive role in the development of ethical guidelines for areas of perinatal practice.

BIBLIOGRAPHY

American College of Obstetricians and Gynecologists (ACOG): Ethical decision-making in obstetrics and gynecology, *ACOG Techn Bull* 136:1-7, Nov 1989.

American Nurses Association Committee On Ethics: *Ethical dilemmas confronting nurses,* Kansas City, Mo, 1985, The Association.

Archer-Drusté H: Clinical ethics: a mandate for nursing, *J Perinatal Neonatal Nurs* 1(3):49-56, 1988.

Aumann G: New chances, new choices: problems with perinatal technology, *J Perinatal Neonatal Nurs* 1(3):1-10, 1988.

Bushy A, Rauh R, Matt B: Ethical principles: application to an obstetric case, *J Obstet Gynecol Neonatal Nurs* 18(3):207-212, 1989.

Cerase P: Ethical dilemmas in the resuscitation of the very low birth rate infant, *J Perinatal Neonatal Nurs* 1(3):69-76, 1988.

Creighton H: *Law every nurse should know,* Philadelphia, 1986, Saunders.

Erlen J: Anencephalic infants as sources of organs: issues and implications for nurses, *J Obstet Gynecol Neonatal Nurs* 19(3):249-253, 1990.

Francis G: Ethical considerations in contemporary reproductive technologies, *J Perinatal Neonatal Nurs* 1(3):37-49, 1988.

Herz E: Infertility and bioethical issues of the new reproductive technologies, *Psychiatr Clin North Am* 12(1):117-131, 1989.

Jones S: Decision making in clinical genetics, *J Perinatal Neonatal Nurs* 1(3):11-24, 1988.

Lindgren S: Maternal fetal conflict: court ordered cesarean section, *J Obstet Gynecol Neonatal Nurs* 25:653-656, 1996.

Martin B, Curtis J: *Ethics in nursing,* ed 2, New York, 1986, Oxford University Press.

Minogue J, Reedy N: Companioning parents in perinatal decision making, *J Perinatal Neonatal Nurs* 1(3):25-35, 1988.

Nosek J: Ethics, *J Perinatal Neonatal Nurs* 1(3):1-87, 1988.

Nurses Association of the American College of Obstetricians and Gynecologists (NAACOG): *NAACOG practice guide: ethical decision making in OGN nursing,* Washington, DC, 1988, The Association.

Pryde P and others: Determinants of parental decision making to abort or continue after nonaneryoloid ultrasound detected fetal abnormalities, *Obstet Gynecol* 80:52-56, 1992.

Swanson KM: Nursing as informed caring for the well-being of others, *Image J Nurs Sch* 25:352-357, 1993.

Swanson-Kaufman K: Caring in the instance of unexpected pregnancy loss, *Top Clin Nurs* 8(2):37-46, 1986.

Uustal D: *Values and ethics in nursing: from theory to practice,* East Greenwich, RI, 1985, Educational Resources in Nursing and Wholistic Health.

CHAPTER

8

Legal Issues and Risk Management

Professional liability is a concept that explains a system of accountability. This system is expected to compensate for losses and deter negligent or substandard practices by the professional. Unfortunately, the professional liability system does a poor job of both compensation and deterence.

The system does not focus so much on poor performance and incompetence as it does on unexpected outcomes. Litigation in health care fields has increased sharply in the past 15 years, both in number of lawsuits and in the amount of awards.

Approximately 80% of all lawsuits in American history have occurred in the past 20 years (NAACOG, 1987). More than 75% of obstetricians and gynecologists are sued, and more than one third of them are sued more than three times. More than half the cost of insurance premiums and the award amounts comes from transaction costs to pay attorney fees and court costs (Cohn, 1987; Creighton, 1986; NAACOG, 1987).

MALPRACTICE INSURANCE

Nurses are more frequently being included among the separately named parties in a lawsuit. As a result, more nurses carry their own malpractice insurance. For specialty nursing practice, such as perinatal care, the insurance premiums are purchased at a greater expense than for other less litigious nursing specialties. Nurses in the specialty of perinatal care find themselves in a difficult position as part of the team, and therefore they are often not acting independently to reduce personal risk. Some issues to examine before deciding to carry a personal insurance policy (Creighton, 1986) include the following:

- Is the frequency of exposure high in the setting where the nurse practices? High exposure may occur where there are high risk patients more than 25% of the time.
- Do the policies and procedures represent a safe standard of care?
- Is the practice of the nurse sometimes outside a hospital setting in independent practice or always as an employee where liability insurance includes nurse practice? A physician's malpractice insurance does not cover the practice of office nurses. Examples of practice outside the hospital setting include teaching childbirth preparation classes, giving frequent telephone advice, doing outreach education, or doing contract care.
- Is the nurse working in a setting where physician response is not timely or where physicians are overworked?
- Is staff/patient ratio commonly less than standard?
- Are continuing education programs encouraged, and are they supported?

REASONS PARENTS SUE

Part of the cause of increased frequency and severity of perinatal litigation is unrealistic and inflated patient expectations of the health care system to correct all ills and the overconfidence of the health care professional.

Reasons parents sue vary. Some common reasons (Angelini, Gibes, 1987) are as follows:

- Injured or dead infant
- Urging of family and friends, who believe that if fault can be found, parents will feel better or that justice has been done
- Monetary concerns related to expense of continued care for an injured infant
- Anger, a need to blame, and belief that the provider is at fault
- Complicated grief
- Surprise that anything could go wrong, unrealistic expectations, or inadequate information before giving consent for care

- Belief that litigation will be profitable
- Poor communication with health care providers

When parents sue for their damaged child, the award sought is generally for the expenses involved in the continued and future care of that child. A small amount of the award may be for the emotional damages the parents have suffered; this must be proved separately from the child's damages. When parents sue because of a dead child, the award is almost solely for the emotional damages suffered from loss of the relationship and for any impairment in other relationships.

LITIGATION RISK

There are three common sources for risk of litigation:
1. Failure to keep current
2. Inadequate supervision, management, or administration of services
3. Communication inadequacies, errors, or inaccuracies

Failure to Keep Current

Ways to keep current include the following:
1. Exercising professional responsibility by attending continuing education programs consistently
2. Participating in a detailed orientation program when employed in new settings
3. Maintaining familiarity with relevant policies and procedures
4. Being aware of sources and relevant guidelines for standards of care
5. Keeping abreast of current relevant legal issues and decisions

Inadequate Supervision

The following aspects will help to prevent inadequate supervision:
1. The immediate supervising nurse who is present (head nurse, charge nurse, team leader, designee, or other similar title) is required to respond to all issues of supervision of the nurse at the bedside. This includes responding to issues related to who was informed of any difficulties or immediate identification of problems.
2. Nurses must know the chain of command when a problem is identified, especially when there is conflict in needed response to patient care issues.

3. Consultation with other staff members more experienced or expert may help.
4. Problematic staffing patterns or ratios must be identified. Such issues as adequate nurse/patient ratios for numbers and acuity, staff shift rotation or on call, and staff orientation, experience, and qualifications for assignment must be considered and responded to by the supervisor.

Inadequate Communication

Patient/Family and Nurse

Some areas of patient and nurse communication risks are described below.

Patient education and childbirth preparation. There may be risks associated with misinformation, incomplete information, or no information.

Telephone advice. Generally, it is best to view a telephone call requesting advice as a call for assistance to the patient in focusing on the key elements of the complaint and empowering her in self-advocacy with her concerns.

Amount of information. Caution should be exercised in giving too little information or vague responses, giving too much information or more than requested, giving misinformation or conflicting information, or withholding information.

Nurse to Physician

When there is disagreement between the nurse and physician, the nurse should do the following:

1. Settle it privately.
2. Get agreement before documenting.
3. Use "I" messages rather than "you" messages. For example, "I am concerned that this problem is not being evaluated" or "I need a physician to see this strip and evaluate the patient."
4. Follow the chain of command when differences cannot be immediately resolved.
5. Document the situation (just the facts), but not in the patient record.

Verbal Orders

There are increased risks with verbal orders because of translation and transmission. Also, some risk exists with telephone orders because the physician relies entirely on relayed information to diagnose the problem. This increases potential errors in treatment decisions. It is the nurse's responsibility to acknowledge that the physician's response seems to be in error.

Refusal or Inability to Comply

When the nurse clearly believes that to follow the physician's orders, to fail to obtain orders, or to fail to convince a physician of the necessity to see the patient will result in harm to the patient, the nurse has an obligation to assertively follow through with chain of command and alternative notification of medical team members.

EFFECT OF INCREASED LITIGATION ON HEALTH CARE

Cost and practice in health care are affected by the following risks and the failure to reduce them:

1. Increased cost of health care premiums
2. Increased cost of health care
3. Increased cost of malpractice/liability insurance
4. Decreased access to prenatal care as physicians limit their practice
5. Decreased quality of care as access is limited, especially for the medically indigent for whom risk is often the greatest

Rather than deterence of incompetent or substandard care, increased litigation has led to defensive medical practice with more costly and frequently questionably indicated testing. In addition, the personal, trusting relationship with providers has been less trusting, with referrals to specialists who do not have a long-term care relationship with the patient. Fragmented care with increased referrals may actually result in less continuity and thus increased risk for negligence (Angelini, Gibes, 1987; Cohn, 1987; Creighton, 1986; NAACOG, 1987).

SYSTEMS OF LAW

The four systems of law in the United States are martial, military, criminal, and civil law.

Martial Law

Martial law is invoked only in times of social emergency. An example of a social emergency is a national disaster. Civil rights can be selectively suspended.

Military Law

Military law operates in the military services and supersedes laws of states or other countries.

Criminal Law

Criminal law is the system for the state to prosecute criminal behavior. It is subject to a court of appeals and is based on precedent. Intent is an important element of proof, as well as proof of the criminal act itself. The defendant is considered innocent until proven guilty by the state as plaintiff.

Civil Law

Civil law serves for noncriminal behavior and seeks to recover compensation for proven damages. It is guided by torts, which put some of the burden of proof on the defendant. There are four elements to be proven and defended: duty, breach of duty, proximate cause, and damages (Angelini, Gibes, 1987; Creighton, 1986).

Duty

Duty is that special relationship, recognized by law, that establishes a duty by the health care professional to render a reasonable degree of care expected by a professional with the same or similar experience in the same or a similar situation.

Breach of Duty

Breach of duty is a failure to meet the minimum standard of care as defined by standard-setting bodies.

Proximate Cause

Proximate cause is an act or omission that, unbroken by any intervening cause, produces an injury. In a medical malpractice case, failure to adhere to the minimum standard of care must be the proximate cause of the injury.

Damages

Damages are the sum of money a court or jury awards as compensation. The law recognizes certain often imprecise and inconsistent categories of damages (Angelini, Gibes, 1987; Creighton, 1986):

1. General damages: typically intangible damages such as pain and suffering, disfigurement, and interference with ordinary enjoyment of life
2. Special damages: out-of-pocket expenses for medical expenses, lost wages, and rehabilitation
3. Punitive exemplary damages: damages awarded the plaintiff for intentional acts or gross negligence and used to punish the defendant or act as a deterrent to others

Table 8-1 defines common terms used during the litigation process and with which nurses are generally unfamiliar.

LITIGATION SEQUENCE

Once parents decide to sue, the following sequence of events occurs:

1. Parents seek the services of a lawyer. They explain their view of the situation and events. During that conference, the parents name physicians, one or more hospitals, and nurses involved. They may bring medical records from current providers with documentation of existing problems.
2. The attorney reviews the information, files the complaint, and requests records. The defense attorneys are notified.
3. The attorney notifies the court of intent to bring suit and states the elements of the complaint.
4. During this period, called *discovery,* a list of all possible parties to be deposed is reviewed.
5. The defense attorney or attorneys for each of the listed parties also begin discovery.
6. Potential experts for physicians and the hospital as well as the nursing care are contacted to begin reviewing records.
7. Some depositions are taken. The plaintiff's attorney takes the depositions of the physician or physicians and the most closely involved nurses. The defense attorneys are present.
8. The defense attorney or attorneys take depositions of the parents. The plaintiff's attorney is present.
9. Experts are named with the court after their agreement is obtained. Some attorneys give the experts the affidavit, which is a legal document stating in general terms what the expert is prepared to stipulate as expert opinion. This statement usually involves their position regarding their opinion of whether the standards of care were met.
10. Depositions are taken from experts and from other persons listed in the medical records.
11. Some states have a system for screening cases before deciding to settle or go to court.
12. The attorneys for both sides begin to make offers and counteroffers for settlement out of court.
13. If no settlement can be reached, a court date is filed by the plaintiff's attorney.
14. All filings of complaints, experts named, and court dates have deadlines to meet within the statute of limitations.

15. The attorneys orchestrate the timetable for presentation of witnesses and experts. The plaintiff has the first and last word in presentation of the case.
16. Subpoenas are issued to the witnesses. Experts are paid by the attorneys with whom they are working. The defense attorney recovers those costs from the insurance companies for the physicians, the hospital, or the nurse or nurses.

NURSE'S DEPOSITION
Players

Persons involved in the nurse's deposition are the hospital's attorney, plaintiff's attorney, physician's attorney, various paralegals and nursing consultants, a court recorder, and the witness.

Process

Swearing In

The court recorder swears in the witness by having the witness state name and current address and then swear or promise to tell the truth.

Introductory Questioning

The plaintiff's attorney begins with general questions such as name, marital status, current and past employment, and schooling. These questions are designed to put the nurse at ease, gain his or her trust, and evaluate body language when telling the truth for comparison when later answers may be about sensitive issues and might be untruthful.

Questioning Regarding the Case

The rest of the questions are related to the care given by that nurse to the mother. These questions usually are designed to nail down the facts from the witness or the opinions of the expert. They vary in style and associated pitfalls.

Helpful Guidelines

1. *Answering yes or no questions:* if the plaintiff's attorney asks for a yes or no response, and the question does not lend itself to either, the best answer is "I don't understand the question" or "I don't know." It is not wise to rephrase the question or answer yes or no and then try to explain the conditions. Sometimes the questions will be fired in rapid succession with a string of yeses or nos. The tendency is to answer all the same when, if one stopped to think, one

TABLE 8-1 Definitions of commonly used legal terms

Term	Definition
Accreditation	Official authorization providing credentials for maintaining standards and ensuring quality of care
Case law	Legal principles derived from judicial decisions; differs from statutory law
Complaint	Legal document that is initial pleading on part of plaintiff in a civil lawsuit; purpose is to give defendant notice of alleged facts constituting cause of action
Court trial	Trial without jury
Credentialing	System based on accepted standard criteria for determining competence and capabilities of a professional to provide consistent quality care and to minimize risks
Defendant	Individual or individuals who are named in suit by plaintiff; medical malpractice or professional negligence cases usually include multiple defendants, such as hospital, physician or physicians, and potentially individual nurse or nurses if insured separate from hospital
Deposition	A discovery procedure whereby each party may question the other party or any person who may be a possible witness
Evidence	Facts presented at trial through witnesses, records, documents, and concrete objects for purpose of proving or defending a case, such as standard of care testimony in medical malpractice case or opinion, which is testimony of expert witness based on special training or background, rather than on personal knowledge of facts at issue
Expert opinion	Testimony of person who has specialized knowledge, training, skill, and experience in area relevant to resolution of the legal dispute
Foreseeability	Requirement that case be judged on facts as they were known at the time of the occurrence, not in retrospect, with hindsight, or with knowledge gained since that time

Incident report	Term for report of situation that is not consistent with entire operation of hospital or routine care of patient; more appropriately termed *occurrence* or *situation report*; usually privileged, protected from discovery unless described in patient record
Malpractice/negligence	Legal cause of action involving failure to exercise degree of diligence and care that a reasonable and ordinarily prudent person would exercise in same specialty acting under similar circumstances
Plaintiff	Individual initiating lawsuit; in case of injured minor, parents or state brings suit
Professional negligence	In medical terms, malpractice is failure to exercise that degree of care, as it is used by reasonably careful health care professionals in same or similar situation or like qualifications; failure to meet this acceptable standard of care must be direct cause of injury
Respondent superior	Legal principle that makes employer liable for civil wrongs committed by employees within course and scope of their employment
Risk management	Systems approach to prevention of malpractice claims; involves identification of system problems, analysis, and treatment of risks before a suit is brought, as well as identification of patients who may sue
Standards of care	Norms of behavior and action defined by a particular profession and described and applied by professional and accrediting organizations
Statutory law	Law enacted by legislature
Statute of limitations	Time period in which plaintiff may file lawsuit; varies from state to state and is extended in most states for birth injury for discovery to take place after school age has been reached; then time is specified for complaint to be filed after discovery

From Creighton H: *Law every nurse should know*, Philadelphia, 1986, Saunders; NAACOG: *Professional liability series*, Washington, DC, 1987, The Association.

answer might vary. The best strategy is to stop, rephrase the question silently, and then answer thoughtfully.

2. *Answering long, difficult, complex questions:* do not answer the question in a long form. State that the question is confusing. If asked to explain the confusion, ask for the question to be separated into smaller parts; do not rephrase it.

3. *Response when hospital's attorney objects to question:* if the hospital's attorney objects to a question, there is no judge to arbitrate. You must have a response. Consider the objection to be a clue to reconsider carefully the response. The two common problems may be that the question is phrased to force you to contradict yourself or that the question is asking for an opinion that is not in your purview. The two best answers are "I don't know (understand)" and "the question is confusing."

4. *Always answer truthfully:* even when the answer is perceived by you as less than helpful to the defense, a truthful answer is always best.

5. *Always look directly at the plaintiff's attorney.*

6. *Dress professionally and comfortably:* position your body to occupy all of your allotted space with glasses, tissues, small purse, or a glass of water to mark boundaries. Do not curl into a small space in the chair; occupy it. Avoid caffeinated beverages before or during the deposition.

7. *Never argue:* do not argue with the attorney if he or she mistakenly rephrases your responses; state that you did not understand your response to have been as repeated.

8. *Simply answer the question being asked:* never explain unless specifically requested to do so.

9. *Preparation before deposition:* study the scientific principles underlying the situation. Study the applicable standards and policies and procedures in force at the time of the incident.

THE TRIAL
Players

The same players as for the deposition plus the judge and jury are present. There may be some onlookers, including the parents and hospital staff if approved by both attorneys.

Process

1. Opening statements are read by all attorneys.
2. The plaintiff presents his or her case first; then the defense presents. The plaintiff has some rebuttal time.

3. The judge may sustain or overrule attorneys' objections. If the objection is overruled, you answer; if it is sustained, you do not.

4. Look at the attorney when he or she questions you, and look at the jury when you answer.

The trial can be very threatening to self-esteem. A suit may require giving information to the state board of nursing, and there may be requirements for continuing education or assertiveness training with a limitation on your practice. The experience can be viewed as an opportunity for professional growth. Support groups or individual therapy is available through many employee assistance programs. Be aware of vulnerability in concurrent practice. Avoid discussing the case with any other involved staff members for your protection and theirs.

PREVENTION

Nurses have both professional and personal responsibilities for prevention of litigation and for assistance in reduction of awards. Those responsibilities include the following:

1. Knowledge of the sources of standards as well as specific standards of care: Table 8-2 describes relevant sources.

2. Participation in formulating and writing nursing policies and procedures: Box 8-1 describes elements of policies and procedures that should be considered.

3. Knowledge and application of components of risk management and quality assurance in clinical practice: Box 8-2 describes components of risk management and quality assurance.

4. Documentation of clinical practice that is complete, is concise, is accurate, and reflects communication among health team members and with patients and family: Box 8-3 describes guidelines for documentation.

5. Awareness of potential risks in clinical practice: Box 8-4 lists some clinical examples of common issues.

CONCLUSION

Prospective risk management is currently our only solution to a litigious society. With high expectations for the outcome of any pregnancy being the norm for human nature and the forces promoting increased numbers of and amounts of awards in birth injury cases, it is little wonder that health care costs have soared and access to prenatal care is at an all-time crisis.

Text continued on p. 215

TABLE 8-2 Sources of standards

Organizations	Description
Joint Commission on the Accreditation of Healthcare Organizations (JCAHO)	Joint commission accreditation is voluntary and a paid-for service. It scrutinizes specialty services and requests proof of quality assurance, staff education, policies and procedures, staff ratios, and documentation of the nursing process to name a few.
American Nurses Association (ANA)	The American Nurses Association provides statements of standards of maternal child care and the Code for Nurses, 1976. It thus provides guidelines for minimum care standards in the specialty area of maternal child nursing.
Association of Women's Health, Obstetric, and Neonatal Nurses (AWHONN, formerly NAACOG)	The Association of Women's Health, Obstetric, and Neonatal Nurses promotes excellence in nursing practice to improve the health of women and newborns. The Association publishes standards of practice and education. For more information, contact AWHONN, 700 14th St. NW, Suite 600, Washington, DC, 20005-2019. Telephone: 800-673-8499.
Community standards	Community standards are superseded by a national standard. However, a like-level designation is compared to similar-level designations. Where designation has not been requested by state accreditations such as through health department or perinatal association, the facility remains undesignated. It is compared to the level I (primary care) facilities in that state.

Box 8-1
Policy and Procedure Writing

Practice statements
Write policies so that a wide range of acceptable practice is possible and
flexibility is allowed.
When restrictions or limitations for acceptable practice are necessary, they
should be specified.
Policy statements
Specific care to be rendered
Staff
    Patterns of staffing
    Educational preparation
    Special credentialing/certification/validation
New orientation and continuing education
Equipment
    Care, repair, and testing
    Cleaning and storage
Environment where care can or cannot be provided
Suggested organization of policy and procedure
Institution name
Department
Title
Dates of origination, review, and revision
Approval signature/committee
Date of approval
Purpose/patient desired outcomes
Policy statement
Equipment
Procedure
Additional information
Cross index
References

Box 8-2
Components of Risk Management and Quality Assurance

Policy revision
Writing new or reviewing/revising existing policies and procedures
Updating references to meet current standards of care
Educating and providing in-service education for staff about new or revised policies and procedures
Monitoring quality assurance
Document a quality assurance program with provision for monitoring patient outcomes, process outcomes if patient outcomes do not meet established levels, and operational/administrative outcomes
Risk management plan for problematic perinatal clinical risks
Electronic and auscultative monitoring of fetal heart rate (FHR)
Oxytocin administration and safe use of labor stimulants
Nursing response to obstetric emergencies such as:
   Fetal stress/nonreassuring response to labor or antepartum events
   Maternal hemorrhage
   Eclamptic seizures
   Hypertensive emergencies
   Precipitous delivery
   Hypoglycemia
Cardiac and respiratory emergencies
Parenting skills
Breast feeding
Perinatal grief support
Documentation
Quality assurance indicators
Monitoring results
Correction plan and implementation

From NAACOG: *Professional liability series,* Washington, DC, 1987, The Association; NAACOG: *OGN nursing practice resonance quality assurance,* Washington, DC, 1990, The Association.

Box 8-3
Guidelines for Documentation

Documentation on fetal monitor strip
Identifying patient information

Dates, times, and strip sequence information

Monitoring mode, equipment used, adjustments, and calibrations

Maternal status: vital signs, activity/position changes, vaginal examinations, status of membranes

Medications: route, dosage, time of analgesics/anesthesia, oxytocin (Pitocin), tocolytics

Cervical assessment

Interventions/treatments: position changes, oxygen, oxytocin, hydration

Delivery information: time and type of delivery

Infant information: gender, Apgar scores, weight, newborn findings, cord pH

Documentation on maternal record
Time electronic fetal monitor (EFM) was applied and mode of monitoring

Patient status/activity

Fetal heart rate (FHR)
  Baseline FHR
  Presence or absence of short-term variability
  Description of long-term variability
  Description of reassuring or nonreassuring information by naming the identified patterns according to established criteria

Uterine activity
  Presence, frequency, and duration
  Intensity and resting tone if intrauterine pressure catheter (IUPC)

Assessment
  Vital signs
  Cervical assessments

Interventions, including patient response and time of physician notification

Antepartum and postpartum patient education, verbalization/demonstration of understanding

Referrals

Terms to be avoided*
Uteroplacental insufficiency (UPI)

Hypoxia

Fetal distress

"Decreased" variability

From Creighton H: *Law every nurse should know,* Philadelphia, 1986, Saunders; MMA advisory: *Electronic heart monitoring documentation,* Sept 1987; NAACOG: *Professional liability series,* Washington, DC, 1987, The Association; Schmidt J: Documenting EFM events, *Perinatal Press* 10(8):79-81, 1987.
*These terms have not been given consistently accepted definitions.

Continued

Box 8-3
Guidelines for Documentation—cont'd

Storage
Safe and confidential storage must be provided by the hospital to last for at least the statute of limitations; fetal monitor strips are the fetal record and should be stored with the maternal record

Purpose of documentation
Provides record of patient assessment and assists with planning care
Evaluates patient condition and ongoing response to treatment
Allows assessment of developing patterns in patient condition
Provides a history for future admissions
Provides communication among health care professionals contributing to patient care and documents that communication
Explains diagnosis and course of illness management and treatment
Assists in utilization review for appropriate use of hospital and resources
Provides data in continuing education and research
Provides information for Joint Commission on the Accreditation of Healthcare Organizations (JACHO)
Provides information for billing and reimbursement
May constitute a legal document
Identifies and provides necessary information for incident management

Box 8-4
Clinical Examples of Common Issues

- Electronic fetal heart rate monitoring: continuous versus intermittent
- Nurse's responsibilities in induction/augmentation
- Nurse's response to obstetric, cardiac, or respiratory emergencies
- Patient education for self-care antepartum and postpartum
- Birth plans
- Childbirth education and patient expectations
- Genetic or teratogenic advice
- Preterm labor response to need for treatment
- Precipitous delivery
- Nursing care impact on cesarean birth rate
- Maternal stabilization and transport; regionalized care
- Standards for three levels of perinatal care

Nurses are increasingly exposed to the risk of being named as one of the parties to a birth injury case. It is important to realize that being found liable does not necessarily mean one is incompetent or likely to be punished by loss of employment or licensure. Becoming educated in terminology and the litigation process will facilitate maintenance of self-esteem in a difficult and threatening experience. Nurses have an evolving role as expert witnesses as well. Until recently, physicians most often gave expert testimony about the nurse's duty and standard of care. As nurses become better educated about the process and their responsibilities as professionals and as citizens, it is appropriate for them to give expert testimony in malpractice cases involving specific nurses or the hospital's quality of nursing care.

BIBLIOGRAPHY

Angelini D, Gibes R: The malpractice crisis: trends in risk management and liability, *J Perinatal Neonatal Nurs* 1(2):1-83, 1987.

Chez B and others: Interpretations of nonstress tests by obstetric nurses, *J Obstet Gynecol Neonatal Nurs* 19(3):227-232, 1990.

Cohn S: Trends in perinatal nursing professional liability, *J Perinatal Neonatal Nurs* 1(2):19-29, 1987.

Creighton H: *Law every nurse should know,* Philadelphia, 1986, Saunders.

Divoll M: The role of the perinatal and neonatal nurse in risk management, *J Perinatal Neonatal Nurs* 1(2):29-39, 1987.

Johnson L: Preparing for a deposition, *Nurs 90* 20(7):44-47, 1990.

MMI advisory: *Electronic heart monitoring documentation,* Sept 1987.

Nosek J: Expanded role liability in perinatal nursing, *J Perinatal Neonatal Nurs* 1(2):39-48, 1987.

Nurses Association of the American College of Obstetricians and Gynecologists (NAACOG): *Professional liability series,* Washington, DC, 1987, The Association.

Nurses Association of the American College of Obstetricians and Gynecologists (NAACOG): *OGN nursing practice resource: quality assurance,* Washington, DC, 1990, The Association.

Nurses Association of the American College of Obstetricians and Gynecologists (NAACOG): *Standards for the nursing care of women and newborns,* ed 4, Washington, DC, 1991, The Association.

O'Neil S: Deposition do's and don'ts, *Contemp OB/GYN* 33(special issue):76-86, 1989.

Regan M: Documentation for the defense, *J Perinatal Neonatal Nurs* 1(2):49-60, 1987.

Robbins D: Incident report analysis: the experience of one large labor and delivery unit, *J Perinatal Neonatal Nurs* 1(2):9-18, 1987.

Schmidt J: Documenting EFM events, *Perinatal Press* 10(8):79-81, 1987.

UNIT

IV

Health Disorders Complicating Pregnancy

Various health disorders can complicate pregnancy. In the past, major medical disorders precluded pregnancy achievement either because maternal well-being could not be guaranteed or because the fetal effects were devastating. Now, with more sophisticated medical management of maternal conditions and with high technology for fetal surveillance, outcomes for both the mother and the neonate have improved. Common health disorders complicating pregnancy that are discussed in this unit are diabetes, cardiac disease, renal disease, and connective tissue disease.

CHAPTER

9

Diabetes

Diabetes is a disease characterized by the inability to produce or use sufficient endogenous insulin to metabolize glucose properly. This inability to metabolize glucose leads to altered metabolism. Pregnancy is a diabetogenic state. Metabolism of glucose, fats, and proteins is altered, and antiinsulin forces are present. This may affect the already altered metabolism.

There are four types of diabetes according to the National Diabetes Data Group Classification (The Expert Committee on the Diagnosis and Classification of Diabetes Mellitus, 1997) (Table 9-1). Types 1 and 2 diabetes are pregestational in that the woman has either one before becoming pregnant. In type 1 diabetes mellitus, there is insulin deficiency related to islet cell loss. In type 2 diabetes mellitus, there is insulin resistance because receptor sites at the tissue level are not responsive to insulin. Therefore it takes more insulin to first shut off the release of glucose from the liver. Second, it takes higher levels of insulin to open the receptors and facilitate muscle glucose uptake. The pancreas is overworked to meet the increased demand of extra insulin, and hyperglycemia develops. Gestational diabetes mellitus (GDM) is defined as carbohydrate intolerance that is first recognized during pregnancy (ADA, 1997a). Impaired glucose tolerance (IGT) is defined as impaired glucose but not severe enough to be diagnosed as type 1 or 2 or GDM. In pregnancy, diabetes is classified also according

TABLE 9-1 National Institutes of Health classification of diabetes

Classification	Previous names	Definition
Type 1	Juvenile-onset diabetes Brittle diabetes IDDM (insulin-dependent diabetes mellitus)	Insulin-deficient diabetes Pancreatic beta cells in islets of Langerhans virtually do not produce insulin Ketone prone
Type 2	Adult-onset diabetes NIDDM (non-insulin-dependent diabetes mellitus)	Insulin-resistant diabetes Pancreatic beta cells in islets of Langerhans produce normal or increased amounts of insulin Increased tissue resistance to insulin because of ineffective cell receptors
GDM (gestational diabetes mellitus)	Gestational diabetes	Carbohydrate intolerance that develops during pregnancy, regardless of severity At least two abnormal values on a 3-hr oral glucose tolerance test (100-g glucose)
IGT (impaired glucose tolerance) and IFG (impaired fasting glucose)	Prediabetes Secondary diabetes	Intermediate stage between normoglycemia and diabetes IGT—2-hr postprandial $\geq$140 mg/dl but <200 mg/dl IFG—fasting plasma glucose $\geq$110 mg/dl but <120 mg/dl

to the age at which it was diagnosed, the length of time the disease has been present, and the degree of vascular changes that have occurred. This classification was helpful in the past to provide prognostic indicators for neonatal outcome (Table 9-2). Recent research indicates that the degree of metabolic control and the presence or absence of long-term complications better delineate maternal and fetal risk (Greene, 1993; Miller, 1994; Willhoite and others, 1993).

INCIDENCE

Diabetes in pregnancy has long been recognized as a serious problem for both the mother and fetus. Before the availability of insulin in the 1920s, women with diabetes rarely became pregnant. Those who did become pregnant rarely carried a fetus to viability. Diabetes occurs now in approximately 2% to 3% of the pregnant population (Gabbe, 1996). Gestational diabetes will develop in another 12% of pregnancies (Bung, Artal, 1996). Maternal survival is 99.5%. Fetal survival is approximately that of the general population, 95% to 97%, if glucose is adequately controlled before and during the pregnancy.

ETIOLOGY

The etiology of diabetes is inherent in pancreatic inability to produce sufficient insulin to transport glucose into the cells. Insulin deficiency may result from pancreatic beta-cell damage, inactivation of insulin by antibodies, or increased insulin requirements. Type 1 diabetes is a chronic autoimmune disorder of the pancreatic islet cells that develops in individuals who carry a genetic marker that has been identified on chromosome 6 (Cunningham and others, 1997; Foster, 1994). Viral-induced, immune-stimulated antibodies against the beta cells form. This autoimmune response causes gradual destruction of the pancreatic beta cells. Persons with type 2 diabetes do not carry a genetic marker but, rather, have a genetic susceptibility. This type of diabetes is characterized by insulin resistance and pancreatic islet cell dysfunction. When insulin resistance occurs, there is increased insulin secretion but ineffective insulin postreceptor binding (Lesser, Carpenter, 1994). Thus glucose uptake by cells is decreased and hyperglycemia results. In 80% to 85% of patients with type 2 diabetes, obesity, especially of the abdominal region, causes their insulin resistance.

NORMAL PHYSIOLOGY

Pregnancy is a diabetogenic state characterized by mild fasting hypoglycemia, postprandial hyperglycemia, and hyperinsulin-

TABLE 9-2 Guide to classification of perinatal diabetes: revised White's classification

Class	Description	Vascular disease	Treatment
A_1	Gestational diabetes characterized by abnormal glucose tolerance test (GTT) without other symptoms; fasting glucose normal	None	Diet control
A_2	Gestational diabetes characterized by abnormal glucose tolerance test (GTT); fasting glucose elevated	None	Diet and insulin required to control
B	Diabetes onset at age 20 yr or older or diabetes is of less than 10-yr duration	None	Diet and insulin
C	Diabetes onset between ages 10 and 19 yr or duration of 10-19 yr	None	Diet and insulin
D	Diabetes onset at less than 10 yr of age or duration of more than 20 yr	Benign retinopathy	Diet and insulin
E	Diabetes onset at any age	Pelvic vascular disease	Diet and insulin
F	Diabetes onset at any age	Nephropathy	Diet and insulin
R	Diabetes onset at any age	Proliferative retinopathy	Diet and insulin
RF	Diabetes onset at any age	Nephropathy and retinopathy	Diet and insulin
H	Diabetes onset at any age	Atherosclerotic heart disease	Diet and insulin
T	Diabetes onset at any age	After renal transplant	Diet and insulin

Data from American College of Obstetricians and Gynecologists: *Management of diabetes mellitus in pregnancy*, ACOG Technical Bulletin No. 92, Washington, DC, 1986, ACOG Resource Center.

emia. These changes occur to ensure a continuous supply of glucose to the fetus. There is marked individual variation in the renal threshold for glucose.

Hyperinsulinemia: Increased Insulin Production

Estrogen and progesterone stimulate pancreatic beta-cell hyperplasia. As insulin secretion is increased, peripheral glucose utilization is enhanced, leading to a decreased fasting blood glucose level in the first trimester. During the second and third trimesters, rising placental hormones increase insulin resistance; decreased hepatic glycogen stores and an increased hepatic production of glucose cause elevated postprandial blood sugar levels. This increased glucose presence further stimulates pancreatic islet cell hypertrophy, increasing insulin levels.

Increased Tissue Resistance to Insulin

During the second and third trimesters, pregnancy hormones (estrogen, progesterone, human placental lactogen hormone, and cortisol) antagonize insulin's effectiveness because of postreceptor cellular changes and stimulates hepatic glucose production. Also, the placental enzyme *insulinase* accelerates degradation of insulin. The net effect is decreased insulin effectiveness causing reduced peripheral uptake of glucose, which facilitates glucose available to the fetus for accelerated fetal growth (Lesser, Carpenter, 1994).

PATHOPHYSIOLOGY
Pregestational Diabetes

In theory, the cause of faulty metabolism in the diabetic person is one or more of the following:
- Production of defective insulin
- Overproduction of insulin antagonist
- Increased tissue resistance to insulin
- Inadequate amount of insulin production
- Inappropriate timing of insulin release

When insulin is not available or effective in transporting glucose into the cell, glucose remains in the bloodstream in abnormal quantities. Because of cellular starvation, the body begins breakdown of fats (ketogenesis) and proteins (gluconeogenesis) for energy. Table 9-3 describes the manifestations and consequences of insulin lack.

If hyperglycemia is allowed to become severe, ketoacidosis can develop. The resultant diuresis causes loss of water and electrolytes, hyperosmolarity, and volume depletion. This in turn causes

TABLE 9-3 Manifestations and consequences of insulin lack

	Adaptation to cellular starvation	Urinary and blood alterations	Metabolic acidosis, water and electrolyte imbalance	Vascular effects
Insulin lack	Decreased glucose utilization and storage	Hyperglycemia, glycosuria	Cellular dehydration, osmotic diuresis	Peripheral circulatory failure leading to decreased blood pressure, coma, and death
	Increased metabolism of fatty acids	Increased ketogenesis leading to increased ketonemia, increased ketonuria, and increased glyconeogenesis, in turn leading to aminoacidemia, nitrogen in urine	Ketoacidosis, metabolic acidosis	
	Increased breakdown of amino acids		Catabolism leading to sodium and potassium loss	
	Signs and symptoms of insulin lack (hyperglycemia)			
Manifestations of hyperglycemia	Period of increased appetite, unusual thirst, loss of weight and strength and stamina, leg cramps or muscle fatigue, nausea and vomiting	Glycosuria, polyuria, ketonuria, ketonemia, aminoacidemia, hyperglycemia, pruritus	Kussmaul respiration, increased nausea and vomiting, listlessness, dehydration, altered blood chemistries, increased hemoglobin	

TABLE 9-4   Long-standing vascular effects

Consequences	Manifestations
Microvascular	
Neuropathy	Decreased perception of pain
Nephropathy	Proteinuria, oliguria, renal failure
Retinopathy	Visual changes that can lead to blindness
Macrovascular	
Atherosclerotic heart changes	Cardiovascular disease, coronary artery disease
Atherosclerotic vascular changes	Poor healing and gangrene

a release of stress hormones, impairs insulin action, and contributes to insulin deficiency.

When lack of insulin becomes a long-term or recurrent event, there are long-standing vascular effects (Table 9-4).

When glucose is low in relation to the amount of insulin, a diabetic person experiences different physiologic responses, manifested by hypoglycemia. Table 9-5 describes manifestations and consequences of an abundance of insulin in relation to glucose. During pregnancy, hypoglycemia is characterized by rapid onset. It can result from several causes:

- Too much insulin might have been prescribed or taken inadvertently, or the dose might be more than needed because of altered activity at the time.
- Delays in mealtimes can cause the onset of insulin action to occur in the absence of adequate glucose.
- *Hypoglycemia can be caused by skipping meals or failure to eat all that is prescribed.
- *Placental failure leading to decreased levels of the insulin antagonists can increase the effectiveness of available insulin, leading to hypoglycemia. This is a warning sign in the third trimester and precedes intrauterine death.
- Hypoglycemia can also be exaggerated in early control of hyperglycemia. This is called the *Somogyi effect.* A high blood sugar level rapidly brought down to normal ranges can cause an excessive blood sugar response, and wide variations from low to high blood sugar levels can result. Somogyi effects can

*Most common causes.

TABLE 9-5 Manifestations and consequences of relative abundance of insulin

	Adaptation to decreased glucose	Urinary and blood alterations	Metabolic acidosis, water and electrolyte imbalance	Vascular effects
Insulin abundance	Increased release and depletion of glycogen stores from liver	Hypoglycemia	Cellular death	Peripheral vascular circulatory collapse and decreased glucose to brain and other organ cells, coma, and death
	Increased metabolism of fatty acids	Increased ketogenesis leading to increased ketonemia, increased ketonuria	Ketoacidosis Metabolic acidosis	
	Increased breakdown of amino acids	Increased glyconeogenesis leading to aminoacidemia, nitrogen in urine	Catabolism leading to sodium and potassium loss	
Behavioral and physiologic manifestations of hypoglycemia	Increased appetite, sweating, lethargy, irritability, palpitations, weakness, headache, loss of consciousness	Ketonuria, ketonemia, aminoacidemia, hypoglycemia	Rapid onset of coma, altered blood chemistries, brain death	

also be seen when inadequate treatment of a hypoglycemic episode has taken place. It is extremely important that hypoglycemia be treated with a measured amount of complex carbohydrate and protein. Thus the body does not rapidly utilize the glucose and then drop blood sugars even lower than the previous levels, because no other source of glucose is being gradually formed and released from fats and proteins.

Woman With Gestational Diabetes

Gestational diabetes is defined as carbohydrate intolerance of variable severity with onset or first recognition during pregnancy (Metzger, The Organizing Committee, 1991). The pancreatic beta-cell functions are impaired in response to the increased stimulation and induced insulin resistance. It is a disorder typically of late gestation. Hyperglycemia during the first trimester usually means type 2 diabetes mellitus (ADA, 1997d).

SIGNS AND SYMPTOMS
Gestational Diabetes

Signs of gestational diabetes in a previous pregnancy are as follows:
- Prior delivery of an infant weighing more than 9 pounds
- Previous stillbirth or an infant with congenital defects
- History of polyhydramnios
- History of recurrent monilial vaginitis

Signs of gestational diabetes in the current pregnancy are as follows:
- Glycosuria on two successive office visits
- Recurrent monilial vaginitis
- Macrosomia of the fetus on ultrasound
- Polyhydramnios

Pregestational Diabetes

In the woman with pregestational diabetes, diabetic symptoms vary by trimester. Table 9-6 outlines the trimester manifestations and consequences.

Ketoacidosis

Signs and symptoms of ketoacidosis in the pregnant woman include the following:
1. Hyperventilation
2. Mental lethargy

TABLE 9-6 Trimester manifestations and consequences of diabetes

	Insulin requirements	Blood glucose alterations	Complicating factors
First trimester	Reduced, related to inhibition of anterior pituitary hormones Developing embryo is glucose drain Decreased maternal caloric intake Increased insulin production	Frequent low blood glucose levels leading to increased numbers of hypoglycemia episodes, increased incidence of starvation, ketosis, and ketonemia	Loss of appetite, nausea, or vomiting common in any early pregnancy Recovery from an acidemic state is more difficult because of insulin antagonists
Second trimester	Increase related to placental hormones (cortisol, insulinase) and their antiinsulin properties	Hyperglycemia leading to ketonemia, aminoacidemia	Exaggerated ketone response to caloric restriction Decreased renal threshold from increased blood flow makes urine sugar levels meaningless Body produces lactose or milk sugar, which further increases urinary sugar
Third trimester	Marked increase related to increased placental hormones but level off after 36 weeks of gestation	Hyperglycemia leading to ketonemia, acidemia	Same
Labor	Decrease related to workload of labor and increased metabolism	Hypoglycemia, acidemia from starvation ketosis	Usually kept NPO pending cesarean delivery
Postpartum	Decrease markedly related to loss of placental hormones	Hypoglycemia	Lactation lowers insulin; can initially complicate as supply is established and scheduled

3. Dehydration
4. Hypotension unless complicated by pregnancy-induced hypertension (PIH)
5. Abdominal pain and nausea and vomiting
6. Fruity odor to the breath
7. Blood glucose levels in excess of 300 mg/dl

MATERNAL EFFECTS

In general, the diabetic state in the mother does not deteriorate because of the pregnancy itself. In fact, most women, regardless of their classification during pregnancy, are in better control than when not pregnant. Despite the antagonistic forces of hormones, control is often better because of the close observation of blood sugar levels by the patient and health care team.

A diabetic pregnancy is more vulnerable to certain complications. The diabetic woman who develops hyperemesis gravidarum is at risk for severe metabolic disturbances. In addition to the obvious risks of dehydration and electrolyte imbalance that are always encountered with hyperemesis, starvation ketosis becomes a very real threat to the mother and the developing fetus. Hospitalization with appropriate intravenous therapy for fluids and calories is essential to prevent complications.

A pregnancy complicated by diabetes is at significant risk for the complications outlined below. However, the risk is directly related to glucose control initiated before conception and continued throughout the pregnancy (Evans and others, 1995; Miller, 1994).

Spontaneous Abortion

Diabetes mellitus has been reported to increase the risk of miscarriage related to inadequate glycemic control during the embryonic phase (first 7 weeks of gestation) indicated by an elevated Hb A_{1c} (Evans and others, 1995; Hollingsworth, 1992).

Preeclampsia

The pregnant woman with diabetes has two times the normal risk of preeclampsia (Garner, 1995). This is particularly true when there is already evidence of renal and vascular compromise. Hypertension and the resultant vasospasm can be the final blows to an already marginally effective placenta.

Preterm Labor

The woman with diabetes is at greater risk of developing preterm labor if she has increased uterine volume, has a hypertensive disorder, develops a kidney or urinary tract infection, or has vascular compromise (Neiger, Kendrick, 1994). Magnesium sulfate is the drug of choice in the treatment of preterm labor in the diabetic patient (Reece and others, 1991). Because intravenous beta-sympathomimetic tocolytic agents can cause significant deterioration of maternal glucose control, they should be used only with great caution (ACOG, 1994).

Polyhydramnios

Polyhydramnios is also more frequently encountered in the pregnant diabetic woman. Approximately 18% of all diabetic women during pregnancy develop polyhydramnios. Although the mechanism for this is not fully understood, fetal hyperglycemia is thought to result in increased fetal diuresis. The significance of polyhydramnios varies with sources. There may be a threat of premature rupture of the membranes because of uterine overdistention, and polyhydramnios is known to be associated with an increased incidence of fetal anomalies. In severe polyhydramnios, repeated therapeutic amniocenteses can be performed to relieve the pressure. Amniocentesis, when repeated, places the mother at increased risk of rupture of the membranes and infection associated with the procedure.

Infection

The pregnant diabetic woman is at significant risk for development of an infection involving almost any organ system. Approximately 80% of all diabetic women during pregnancy develop at least one infection as compared with 26% of nondiabetic women (Stamler and others, 1990). These infections can occur during the antepartum or postpartum period. Vaginitis, especially monilial, occurs very frequently. This is related primarily to the altered pH of the vaginal canal common to all pregnancies. Because of the increased incidence of vaginitis, which makes a prime medium for bacterial growth, the pregnant diabetic woman has an increased risk of pyelonephritis and urinary tract infections. These infections can be dangerous to the woman's health and increase the likelihood of preterm labor. Insulin-dependent diabetic women are five times more likely to develop postpartum endometritis or a wound infection (Miller, 1994).

Cesarean or Instrumental Birth and Induction

The pregnant woman with diabetes is more likely to deliver by the cesarean route because of concurrent complications, fetal distress, fetal macrosomia, and induction failures before term.

FETAL AND NEONATAL EFFECTS

The effects of diabetes on the fetus are directly related to the degree of strict glycemic control achieved before conception (Evans and others, 1995). The effects depend somewhat on the presence of maternal vascular complications. If the mother has class D or more advanced disease, vascular deficits can affect the sufficiency of the placenta. Placental insufficiency can also cause varying degrees of nutritional or hypoxic damage to the fetus. It is manifested by intrauterine growth restriction (IUGR) and oligohydramnios.

Hypoglycemia

Hypoglycemia normally has a minimal effect on the fetus if the mother is treated appropriately. The embryo draws its glucose from stores in the lining of the uterus, and the fetus draws from stores in the placenta. Glucose is transferred across the placental membrane by selective transfer. The immediate effects of maternal hypoglycemia on the fetus therefore are minimized over time. However, severe episodes of maternal hypoglycemia that result in ketosis have been shown to cause abnormal postnatal neurologic development (Moore, 1994).

Hyperglycemia

Hyperglycemia can have numerous deleterious and sometimes fatal effects.

Congenital Defects

Congenital defects occur four times more often in diabetic women (ACOG, 1994). Chronic hyperglycemia in the mother contributes to decreased synthesis of deoxyribonucleic acid (DNA) and ribonucleic acid (RNA) and is thought to be a reason for an increased incidence of congenital anomalies. Faulty carbohydrate, protein, and fat metabolism also occurs in the embryo and adversely affects organ development. Common fetal anomalies found in infants of diabetic mothers include skeletal and central nervous system defects such as neural tube defects, congenital cardiac anomalies, gastrointestinal malformations, and congenital renal anomalies. Congenital anomalies are directly related to diabetic control in the 3-month period before conception and during the first 2 months of pregnancy as indicated by glycosylated hemoglobin levels greater than 10% (ACOG, 1994).

Macrosomia

Elevated maternal glucose results in elevated fetal glucose. This stimulates fetal pancreatic production of insulin, which causes fetal hyperinsulinemia. Hyperinsulinemia increases growth and fat deposition, which are referred to as macrosomia. This is seen especially in classes A to C diabetes. These large-for-gestational-age (LGA) infants are at greater risk for birth trauma, particularly shoulder dystocia, brachial plexus injuries, facial nerve injuries, and asphyxia.

Intrauterine Growth Restriction

IUGR is less frequent than macrosomia, occurring in conjunction with placental insufficiency resulting from maternal diabetic vascular disease. This is seen especially in women with class D or higher diabetes and with existing vascular disease before their pregnancy.

Intrauterine Fetal Death

There is an increased risk of unexplained as well as explicable stillbirths. When placental insufficiency occurs as the result of vascular complications or an abruption, there is a clear reason for stillbirth. However, stillbirth occurs at times without obvious placental insufficiency as indicated by decreased fetal growth and oligohydramnios being present. These infants are usually LGA with polyhydramnios. It appears that severe prolonged hyperglycemia interferes in the transport of oxygen and carbon dioxide, leading to decreased fetal pH and increased pCO_2, lactate, and erythropoietin incompatible with life (Garner, 1995).

Delayed Lung Maturity

Various studies have suggested that diabetes causes a delay in fetal lung maturity (Piper, Langer, 1993). Elevated blood glucose appears to interfere with the production of phosphatidyl glycerol. Therefore a mature fetal surfactant may not be present until 38 to 39 weeks of gestation (Piper, Langer, 1993).

Neonatal Hypoglycemia

The fetus is programed to produce high quantities of insulin, and the neonate does not turn this off immediately. At birth the supply of increased glucose is suddenly cut off, but increased production of insulin continues, resulting in neonatal hypoglycemic episodes.

Neonatal Hyperbilirubinemia

Because of possible long-term stress, the compensatory mechanism of increased production of red blood cells is stimulated. After delivery the increased red blood cell breakdown frequently overworks the young hepatic system, resulting in hyperbilirubinemia.

Neonatal Polycythemia

Polycythemia is the result of decreased oxygenation stimulating the fetal kidneys to release glycoprotein hormone. This hormone stimulates the production of erythrocytes as a compensatory mechanism to increase the oxygen-carrying capacity of the blood. Therefore, in the presence of uteroplacental insufficiency, the newborn may have polycythemia.

Learning Disabilities

Fetal brain cell damage and decreased brain growth result from prolonged exposure to hyperglycemia This will increase the incidence of learning disabilities, lower intelligence quotient (IQ), and motor impairment (Cousins and others, 1991).

Childhood Obesity and Type 2 Diabetes Later in Life

Children exposed to hyperglycemia as a fetus have a greater risk of developing childhood obesity and type II diabetes later in life because they may have suffered islet cell injury (Doshier, 1995).

Ketoacidosis

Diabetic ketoacidosis can be life threatening to the mother and the fetus. Fetal mortality is approximately 20% if ketoacidosis develops (Cunningham and others, 1997). The cause of diabetic ketoacidosis is insufficient insulin to move glucose into cells, leading to hyperglycemia. The liver tries to compensate by increasing its production of glucose, only to further raise blood glucose levels. The body then starts to break down fat for energy, which results in ketone release. When the woman's buffering system is unable to compensate, metabolic acidosis develops. The excessive glucose and ketone bodies result in osmotic diuresis with subsequent fluid and electrolyte loss, volume depletion, and cellular dehydration. Acidosis leads to decreased uterine blood flow and thereby reduces fetal oxygenation.

DIAGNOSTIC TESTING

Gestational Diabetes Screening

Glucola Screen

According to a position statement of the American Diabetes Association, *all* patients except low-risk women should be screened for gestational diabetes between 24 and 28 weeks of gestation. The low-risk group includes women who are younger than 25 years and of normal body weight, have a negative family history (no first-degree relative) of diabetes, and are not a member of a high-risk ethnic/racial group, such as African American, Asian, Hispanic, or Native American (The Expert Committee on the Diagnosis and Classification of Diabetes Mellitus, 1997).

Any pregnant woman whose history indicates that she is at high risk for developing gestational diabetes should be screened at her first prenatal visit as well as the prenatal visit between 24 and 28 weeks of gestation (York and others, 1990). The health care provider may elect to run another glucose screen between 32 and 34 weeks of gestation. High risk factors include the following (Dooley and others, 1993; Dornhorst and others, 1992):

- Positive family history in parents or siblings
- Previous unexplained stillbirth
- Prior traumatic delivery
- Prior infant with a birth weight of 9 pounds or more
- Prior fetal anomalies
- Poor reproductive history, especially recurrent spontaneous abortions
- Obesity
- Hypertensive disorder
- Recurrent monilial vaginitis
- Polyhydramnios without demonstrated fetal anomalies
- Glycosuria on two consecutive office visits
- Of Native American, Hispanic-American, Asian-American, African-American, or Pacific Islander ethnic descent

A glucola screening is performed by giving 50 g of a cola beverage and 1 hour later testing the blood sugar. Boyd and others (1995) found 18 jelly beans to be an acceptable alternative to the glucola. A blood sugar level of 140 mg/dl or greater should be followed up with a 3-hour glucose tolerance test to confirm gestational diabetes. Adjustment of this threshold has been proposed according to race (African-Americans, 130 mg/dl; Fillipinos, 145 mg/dl; Asians, 150 mg/dl) (Nahum, Huffaker, 1993).

Three-hour Glucose Tolerance Test

For 3 days before the glucose tolerance test (GTT), 50 mg of complex carbohydrate should be eaten each day. Instruct the woman to abstain from eating, drinking, and smoking for 8 hours before the test. Have the patient rest for approximately 30 minutes before the test. Begin the test by drawing a fasting blood sugar sample. Start the timer and have the patient drink 100 g of glucose solution within 5 minutes. Subsequent blood samples are drawn at

TABLE 9-7   Normal serum values of 3-hour glucose tolerance test in pregnancy

Time of measurement	Blood glucose (mg/dl)
Fasting	<105
1 hr	<190
2 hr	<165
3 hr	<145

Data from The Expert Committee on the Diagnosis and Classification of Diabetes Mellitus: Report of the Expert Committee on the Diagnosis and Classification of Diabetes Mellitus, *Diabetes Care* 20(7):1183-1197, 1997.

1, 2, and 3 hours. During the test the patient should rest and abstain from smoking. Gestational diabetes is diagnosed if two or more plasma glucose blood values are elevated or exceed the values listed in Table 9-7 (ACOG, 1994; ADA, 1997a). A single abnormal value indicates impaired glucose tolerance. These women have been found to be at increased risk for fetal macrosomia (Evans and others, 1995). The GTT is repeated at 32 to 34 weeks in patients with one abnormal value.

Detection of Maternal Complications

Women who have already been diagnosed as diabetic, either during a previous pregnancy or in the absence of pregnancy, usually will be classified as previously described (see Table 9-2). If insulin dependent, the woman should be screened for renal, retinal, and cardiac involvement. Some commonly ordered tests are blood urea nitrogen (BUN) and serum creatinine, 24-hour urine collection for creatinine clearance and total protein, electrocardiogram, ophthalmology examination for retinopathy, and urine culture.

Glycosylated Hemoglobin

Hemoglobin A is a normal minor hemoglobin that has a glucose link. Glucose attaches to this hemoglobin during its normal 120-day life span. The amount depends on the glucose in the bloodstream. Glycosylated hemoglobin (Hb A_{1c}) is a blood test to determine the level of hemoglobin A that has become "sugar coated." Therefore the test reflects adequacy of glucose control for the previous 4 to 6 weeks. Hb A_{1c} levels above 7 indicate elevated glucose during the past 4 to 6 weeks and are associated with an increased incidence of congenital anomalies. Therefore this test is used to screen diabetic women before conception or at the initial prenatal visit. Some endocrinologists will continue to screen for adequacy of control every 2 to 3 months throughout the pregnancy.

USUAL MEDICAL MANAGEMENT AND PROTOCOLS FOR NURSE PRACTITIONERS
Preconception Management

Preconception planning is the key to a successful pregnancy, decreasing risks for the woman with pregestational diabetes. Refer to Box 9-1 for a nurse practitioner preconception assessment.

Antepartum Management

The goals of management of the pregnant woman with diabetes according to the ADA (1995) are as follows:

- Maintain fasting glucose levels between 60 and 90 mg/dl
- Maintain glucose levels before lunch, dinner, and bedtime snack between 60 and 105 mg/dl
- Keep 1- and 2-hour postprandial glucose levels between 100 and 120 mg/dl
- Keep the 2 AM to 4 AM blood glucose between 60 and 120 mg/dl
- Achieve a normal Hb A_{1c} concentration (below 6.1%)
- Prevent episodes of hypoglycemia
- Prevent diabetic ketoacidosis

Home monitoring and control consist of the following six facets in the insulin-dependent diabetic patient. Hospitalization may become necessary if euglycemia cannot be maintained with home monitoring and outpatient surveillance.

Glucose Monitoring

Self-monitoring of blood glucose (SMBG) should be done two to ten times per day depending on difficulty of control. The blood glucose samples are taken before meals and snacks, 1 to 2 hours after meals, at bedtime, and between 2 and 4 AM. Glucose monitoring should begin before conception. If this is not possible, it should begin as soon as pregnancy is suspected or determined. This can be done by using chemical test strips that are read by a portable blood glucose reflectance meter readily available to rent or buy. The results should be keep in a log book and brought to each prenatal visit.

Urine Testing
Ketones. Urine testing for ketones should be done three times per week during pregnancy on the first void of the day. If the patient

Box 9-1

Nurse Practitioner Preconception Assessment for Women With Diabetes

Health perception functional health pattern
History
  Type of diabetes
  Complications if present
  Current diabetes regimen
  Determine glucose control
    Home glucose monitoring record
    History of recent severe ketoacidosis or hypoglycemic episodes
  History of recent infections, particularly skin, foot, dental, or genito-urinary
  Other medications being taken
  Patterns of use and perception of effect on health of tobacco, alcohol, street drugs
  Patterns of using health screening such as physical, dental, and eye checkups, Pap smears, and immunization (especially rubella)
Physical examination
  General
    Age
    Weight
    Height
  Vital signs
    Blood pressure to rule out hypertension
    Pulse
    Respiration
    Temperature
  Skin
    Inspect for any rashes or lesions
    Inspect injection sites
    Inspect hands and feet for lesions, calluses
    Refer to podiatry services as indicated
  Eyes
    Examine to rule out retinopathy
    Referral to ophthalmologist for a dilated eye examination if had diabetes for 5 or more years
  Oral examination
    Evaluate oral and dental health
    Emphasize importance of twice yearly dental checkups with cleaning
  Neck
    Thyroid evaluation to rule out hypothyroidism

Box 9-1

Nurse Practitioner Preconception Assessment for Women With Diabetes—cont'd

Heart
   Rule out cardiovascular disease
Abdomen
   Rule out abnormal pulsation, organomegaly especially of the liver
Genital
   Pelvic examination and Pap smear to rule out vaginal infection
Extremities
   Test reflexes
   Check pulses
   Inspect hands and feet for lesions, calluses
   Refer to podiatry services as indicated
Neurologic
   Sensory system intact for light touch and pinprick in lower extremities
Laboratory evaluation
  Blood glucose level
  Hb A_{1c}
  Complete blood count (CBC), electrolytes, metabolic profile
  Fasting lipid profile: total cholesterol, low-density lipoprotein (LDL), high-density lipoprotein (HDL), triglyceride
  Thyroid panel: thyroxine (T_4), thyroid-stimulating hormone (TSH), antimicrosomal antibodies if indicated
  Rubella titer to check for immune status
  Microalbumin
  Urinalysis and culture
  24-hour urine for creatinine clearance and total protein to rule out nephropathy
  Electrocardiogram (ECG)
  Diabetes for more than 10 years or signs or symptoms of cardiac disease present, do a treadmill test
Instruct regarding habits to promote health
  If smoker, facilitate stopping if at all willing
  Attain or maintain ideal weight
Nutritional functional health pattern
Obtain a detailed dietary history
Determine eating patterns
Determine ideal body weight for height and body frame (100 pounds for first 5 feet of height + 5 pounds for each inch over 5 feet; + 10% for large frame or − 10% for small frame)
Determine daily caloric requirements
Determine amount of folic acid in the diet; current recommendation to decrease neural tube defect is 400 μg; supplement if low

Continued

Box 9-1

Nurse Practitioner Preconception Assessment for Women With Diabetes—cont'd

Elimination functional health pattern
Check urine sample for protein and ketones
Pattern of urination and bowel movements
Sleep/rest functional health pattern
Pattern of rest and sleep
Level of fatigue
Activity functional health pattern
Evaluate amount and type of exercise
Teach need for regular, repeatable level of daily activity
Teach benefits of regular exercise
Cognitive functional health pattern
Teach risks of pregnancy and importance of maintaining tight glucose control
Assess knowledge of the disease to determine learning needs
    Disease process
    Effects of pregnancy on disease process
    Dietary changes
    Insulin administration
    Exercise plan
    Glucose monitoring
    Signs of hypoglycemia
    Treatment for hypoglycemia
    Urine testing for ketones
Self-perception functional health pattern
Assess feelings about the disease
Assess feelings about managing a pregnancy complicated with diabetes
Role/relationship functional health pattern
Assess how pregnancy and the management of diabetes will affect responsibilities; assess ability to interrupt occupation and accommodations for job absences
Economic considerations and insurance coverage
Assess commitment of woman and her family
Sexuality functional health pattern
Assess if experiencing any sexuality problems
Menstrual history
Contraceptive history; emphasize a planned pregnancy
Previous obstetric history: preeclampsia, preterm labor, polyhydramnios, cesarean birth
Fetal and neonatal history: congenital anomalies, macrosomia, birth injury, neonatal metabolic abnormalities
Coping functional health pattern
Level of stress
Family and social support in the event pregnancy complications require lost time from job or bed rest

becomes ill or if blood glucose levels are elevated, it should be done daily. In pregnancy, ketonuria is caused by such dietary insufficiencies as low carbohydrate intake, low calorie intake, or skipped meals or snacks, as well as when ketoacidosis is present. Ketonemia during pregnancy has been associated with decreased intelligence in the offspring (Rizzo and others, 1991).

Sugar. Because of the lowered renal threshold for glucose, glucosuria is not used as a means of determining management.

Insulin Management

Types of insulin. The usual type of insulin used for the pregnant diabetic woman is a biosynthetic human insulin (Humulin), which is made by genetically programing *Escherichia coli* bacteria that produce insulin. Adverse reactions to insulin, which include hypersensitivity or allergic skin reactions, lipodystrophy, and tissue resistance, rarely occur with biosynthetic human insulin as compared with the animal-based insulins (Heppard, Garite, 1996). Human insulins also have a more rapid onset and shorter duration of activity (ADA, 1997b). A new, rapid-acting insulin called Humalog (Lispro) is now on the market. The advantages are that Humalog (Lispro) works faster (within 15 minutes) and has a shorter duration (lasting only 3 hours). Therefore Humalog (Lispro) matches the body's insulin needs at mealtime. In contrast, the onset of Regular Humulin is slower, taking 30 minutes or longer, and Regular Humulin has a longer duration time of 5 to 8 hours, which lasts past the mealtime.

Insulin classifications. The current classifications of insulin today are rapid-acting Humalog (Lispro), short-acting regular (Humulin R), intermediate-acting neutral protamine Hagedorn (NPH; Humulin N), and Lente (Humulin L) or long-acting Ultralente. Both rapid- and intermediate-acting insulins are used during pregnancy. See Table 9-8 for onset, peak, and duration of insulins. Refer to Box 9-2 for differences to be considered when using Humalog (Lispro).

Insulin dosage. The patient's 24-hour insulin dosage is usually calculated according to trimester. For women with gestational diabetes or class B diabetes who had been controlled with oral agents, the 24-hour insulin dosage is usually calculated according to the patient's present weight and weeks of gestation. Refer to Table 9-9 for one method to calculate the variable 24-hour insulin dosage during the three trimesters. Refer to Table 9-10 for common causes and treatment of early-morning hyperglycemia. Individualized modifications of insulin need depend on various factors. If the patient is thin, her need will be less than normal. However, if

TABLE 9-8 Insulin comparison chart for human insulins

Type	Preparation	Appearance	Onset	Peak (hr)	Duration (hr)
Rapid-acting Humalog	Lispro	Clear solution	15 min	1½	3
Short-acting Humulin	Regular insulin	Clear solution	0.5 hr	3-4	8
Intermediate-acting Humulin	NPH	Cloudy suspension	2-4 hr	4-12	12-24
	Lente	Cloudy suspension	2-6 hr	6-15	14-24

NPH, Neutral protamine Hagedorn (insulin).

Box 9-2
Nurse Practitioner Hints for Humalog (Lispro) Insulin Dosing

- Insulin regimen is a morning long-acting insulin, an evening long-acting insulin, and Humalog (Lispro) before each meal and to lower highs.
- Teach patient to eat as soon as she takes her injection of Humalog (Lispro) unless lowering a high blood glucose.
- High glycemic index foods such as bread, rice, potatoes, and sucrose products are covered much better with Humalog (Lispro), but with slow glycemic foods it may cause hypoglycemia because of its fast action.
- Hypoglycemia within 3 hours of an injection is probably related to Humalog (Lispro) and needs to be treated with a fast-acting carbohydrate. Hypoglycemia 3 hours after an injection of Humalog is probably related to the long-acting insulin and can be treated with the Rule of 15:15 g of carbohydrate and wait 15 minutes; then retest.
- Premeal hyperglycemia can be treated by increasing the premeal Humalog (Lispro) dose and waiting a time period dependent on the glucose level to eat the meal. Postmeal hyperglycemia indicates a need for increasing the Humalog dose. The immediate postmeal hyperglycemia can be treated with an extra one-time injection. To determine the amount of Humalog (Lispro) to give, the Rule of 1500 should be modified to an 1800 Rule. 1800 Rule: Total of insulin units per day ÷ 1800 = Amount of mg/dl the blood glucose will drop with each unit of Humalog (Lispro).

Data from Walsh J, Roberts R: *Diabetes Interview*, pp 20-21, Nov/Dec 1996.

she is extremely overweight, her need will be increased from the norm. For pregestational diabetic women already on insulin, the insulin dosage will be evaluated and adjusted based on current control and weeks of gestation. Early in pregnancy, insulin requirements may decrease slightly. As pregnancy advances, the insulin requirements will gradually increase until approximately 36 weeks of gestation. After 36 weeks of gestation, insulin requirements usually level off or slightly decrease. A rapid decrease may indicate placental compromise.

The 24-hour insulin requirement is normally divided into two to four injections each day to be given 20 to 30 minutes before a meal if Humulin is used or just before the meal if Humalog (Lispro) is used. For a *two-dose regimen,* the morning dose is usually two thirds of the woman's 24-hour dose, of which one third is regular insulin and two thirds is NPH. Her predinner dose is the remaining one third of her 24-hour dose, of which one half is

TABLE 9-9 Calculation pattern for insulin during pregnancy

Trimester	Insulin dosage
First trimester	0.6 U/kg body weight
Second trimester	0.7 U/kg body weight
Third trimester	0.8 U/kg body weight

Data from Heppard M, Garite T: *Acute obstetrics: a practical guide,* ed 2, St Louis, 1996, Mosby.

U/kg, Units per kilogram.

regular insulin and one half is NPH. This regimen may be used for the gestational diabetic woman, but it is not usually effective in pregnancy for the woman with type 1 DM or type 2 DM in maintaining euglycemia.

For a *three-dose regimen,* the morning dose is usually NPH with or without regular insulin, regular insulin before dinner, and NPH at bedtime.

For a *four-dose regimen,* regular is to be given before each meal and NPH before the bedtime snack.

A *fourth method* is an insulin dosage based on premeal blood glucose levels and grams of carbohydrate in the meal to be eaten. A basal dose of approximately 50% of the day's total insulin requirement is given as a long-acting insulin, such as Ultralente insulin, in the morning and evening. The morning dose is one third of the long-acting dose, and the predinner dose is two thirds of the long-acting dose. The patient then gives herself a short-acting insulin before each meal based on the number of carbohydrate grams in the planned meal and her premeal blood glucose level. The equation used is 1.5 units of regular insulin per 10 carbohydrate grams at breakfast and 1 unit of regular insulin per 10 carbohydrate grams at lunch and dinner. No additional insulin is given if the blood glucose is in the normal range (70 to 100 mg/dl). If the blood glucose is less than 70 mg/dl, the dose is decreased by 2 units of regular insulin. If the blood sugar is between 100 and 140 mg/dl, 2 extra units of regular insulin is given, and if the blood sugar is greater than 140 mg/dl, 4 extra units of regular insulin is given (ADA, 1995).

When using the two–, three–, or four–insulin dose regimen and blood sugar levels are in the hyperglycemic range, it might be necessary to give additional doses of regular insulin to maintain adequate control. These additional regular insulin doses may be given routinely with the intermediate insulin for the effect on

TABLE 9-10 Early-morning hyperglycemia

Causes	Definition	2-4 AM Blood sugar	Treatment
Somogyi effect	Nocturnal hypoglycemia causes a surge of counterregulatory hormones that increase the morning blood glucose	Low	Decrease evening NPH or increase kilocalories of bedtime snack or Change the evening NPH from predinner to prebedtime snack
Dawn phenomenon	Exaggerated growth hormone effect between 5 and 8 AM in conjunction with the waking process	Normal	Change the evening NPH from predinner to prebedtime snack Cautious use of early-morning regular insulin (3-6 AM)
Waning insulin	Inadequate insulin coverage relative to evening caloric intake	Elevated	Increase evening NPH dose Change evening NPH dose from predinner to prebedtime snack

NPH, Neutral protamine Hagedorn (insulin).

lunchtime and bedtime snack blood sugar levels. They may also be given alone in response to high blood sugar levels occurring episodically. Usual insulin changes recommended on an outpatient basis are described in Table 9-11. The Rule of 1500 is another way to determine how much additional insulin is needed to control the hyperglycemic state. The rule is 1500 divided by the daily insulin dosage the patient is taking. This equals the amount the glucose level will drop with 1 unit of regular insulin. A second formula that is used (blood sugar minus 200 divided by 10) equals number of regular units needed. Refer to Box 9-3 for helpful hints in Humulin insulin dosing for the nurse practitioner.

Insulin pump. The usual means of administering insulin at home is through multiple subcutaneous injections. However, a device for continuous infusion is used in certain circumstances. It is recommended only if the woman cannot achieve adequate control with multiple-dose injections because of the risk of nocturnal hypoglycemia with the use of the pump during pregnancy. The open-loop system infuses insulin at a basal rate and, before meals, delivers a bolus of insulin. The basal rate is generally 2.5 to 5 mU/kg/hr. Some open-loop systems require resetting after each bolus dose; others do this automatically. These systems are small and portable, usually worn around the waist with a belt.

Diet Management

Diet is the cornerstone of therapy in the management of diabetes. The *1994 Nutrition Guidelines* for the diabetic diet have made the diet far less restrictive and encourage individualization (Diabetes Education Society, 1995). Consideration must be given to pre-pregnancy weight, general health status, dietary habits, activity level, and insulin therapy. Folic acid supplements of 400 μg/day are recommended before conception and throughout the first trimester to decrease the risk of neural tube defects.

Caloric needs. Caloric intake should be increased during pregnancy by approximately 300 calories daily and modified to provide at least a 25-pound weight gain plus additional nutrients for mother and fetus. Daily caloric intake for a pregnant woman whose preconception body weight was ideal for her height and body frame is calculated as 30 to 35 calories/kg of body weight per day. If the woman was underweight before conception, her daily caloric intake is calculated as 35 to 40 calories/kg of body weight. When the pregnant woman was over her ideal weight starting pregnancy, her daily caloric intake is calculated as 25 calories/kg or as low as 12 to 15 calories/kg if she is extremely obese (greater than 150%

TABLE 9-11 Changes with split-dose insulin

Time	Blood sugar level (mg/dl)	Action
Fasting blood sugar	<60	Call physician for adjustment
	60-120	No change in 4 PM dose
	120-150	Increase evening NPH insulin by 2 U, and check fasting blood sugar next day
	150-210	Increase evening NPH insulin by 4 U, and check fasting blood sugar next day
	>210	Call physician for adjustment
Lunch blood sugar	<60	Call physician for adjustment
	60-120	No change in morning regular insulin
	120-150	Increase morning regular insulin by 2 U
	200-240	Increase morning regular insulin by 6 U
	>240	Call physician for adjustment
Dinner (PM) blood sugar	<60	Call physician for adjustment
	60-120	No change in morning dose
	120-150	Increase morning NPH insulin by 2 U, and check 4 PM blood sugar next day
	200-240	Increase morning NPH insulin by 6 U, and check 4 PM blood sugar next day
	>240	Call physician for adjustment
Bedtime snack blood sugar	<60	Call physician for adjustment
	60-120	No change in evening regular insulin
	120-150	Increase evening regular insulin by 2 U
	200-240	Increase evening regular insulin by 6 U
	>240	Call physician for adjustment

Private practice protocols of Drs. D. O'Keeffe and J. Elliott, perinatologists, Phoenix, 1991.

NPH, Neutral protamine Hagedorn (insulin); *U*, unit.

Box 9-3
Helpful Hints in Humulin Insulin Dosing for the Nurse Practitioner

- Fix the fasting blood sugar first because the fasting affects control for the remainder of the day.
- If blood glucose is high as indicated by the premeal blood sugar level, give insulin 45 minutes before the meal.
- Midmorning snack decreases late-morning hypoglycemia when using NPH or Lente insulin.
- As regular insulin dosages increase, their peaks of action are delayed.

NPH, Neutral protamine Hagedorn (insulin).

---

of ideal body weight) (Committee on Dietary Allowances, Food and Nutrition Board, 1990).

Nutrient balance. The ratio of nutrients for the pregestational diabetic woman should follow the Dietary Guidelines for Americans, which is 50% to 60% carbohydrates, 12% to 20% protein, and 20% to 30% fat (ACOG, 1994; ADA, 1997c). Less than 10% of the daily calories should be from saturated fat. Simple carbohydrate foods that are devoid of nutrients should be limited because of the postprandial hyperglycemic risk during pregnancy. Protein foods and foods high in soluble dietary fiber are recommended, since they slow gastric emptying and reduce intestinal glucose absorption. Because of a greater difficulty in controlling the postprandial blood glucose levels and frequently higher fasting blood glucose in gestational diabetic women, the current recommendations for these patients are to lower carbohydrates to 40% to 50%, increase fat to 30% to 40%, and increase protein to 20% to 25%. Within these parameters, complex carbohydrates, monounsaturated and polyunsaturated fats, and foods high in soluble fiber are encouraged.

Meal/snack pattern. The pattern of meals and snacks can be individualized, but the calorie intake should be divided throughout the day. A diet composed of three meals and three or four snacks daily decreases both postprandial hyperglycemia and between-meal hypoglycemia. To decrease nocturnal hypoglycemia, a bedtime snack of 25 g of carbohydrate and some protein is recommended for all persons with diabetes.

Individualized diet plan. First, the patient's individual calorie needs, nutrient balance, and meal/snack pattern are determined. Then a registered dietitian figures the number of different exchanges for each meal and snack (Table 9-12 summarizes the exchange plan) or figures the number of different servings in each food group of the food guide pyramid.

Exercise Recommendations

Exercise is an important component in establishing and maintaining glucose control; improved insulin sensitivity is evident after 4 weeks of exercise (Cunningham and others, 1997). Appropriate exercises are those that use the upper-body muscles and place minimal stress on the trunk region (Metzger, The Organizing Committee, 1991). When the lower body muscles are spared excessive weight bearing, there is less shunting of blood away from the placenta. If the pregnancy is also complicated with hypertension or vascular disease, a regular exercise program may be contraindicated (Miller, 1994).

Antepartum Fetal Surveillance

Antepartum monitoring is essential to early and periodic evaluation of fetal condition and to aid in timing the delivery to coincide with optimal outcome.

Ultrasound. Ultrasound examinations are usually done at intervals throughout the pregnancy. They are done to assist in accurately predicting gestational age and for reassurance about fetal organ development They also give information about fetal growth rate, quality of activity, volume of amniotic fluid, and a biophysical profile evaluation.

Fetal movement. Fetal movement counts are a valuable component of fetal surveillance. They should be used for daily surveillance of fetal well-being from 24 weeks of gestation until delivery. There are several methods that can be used (see Chapter 3).

Fetal echocardiogram. If the initial Hb A_{1c} was elevated, a fetal echocardiogram may be considered between 20 and 22 weeks of gestation to rule out a cardiac anomaly (Shields and others, 1993).

Biophysical profile. Biophysical profiles are the primary means of surveillance of fetal well-being and uteroplacental adequacy. For classes A_2, B, C, and D diabetes, the biophysical profile is started at or near week 32 and is done weekly until delivery. For more advanced disease indicated by proteinuria, IUGR, or

TABLE 9-12 Exchange plan summary

Food exchange groups	Nutrients provided	Calories per serving	Serving sizes
Starch (bread, cereals, grains, starchy vegetables)	15 g carbohydrate 3 g protein 3 g fiber	80	½ C cereal, grain, or pasta 1 slice of bread
Fruits	15 g carbohydrate 3 g fiber	60	½ C fresh fruit ½ C fruit juice ½ C dried fruit
Vegetables	5 g carbohydrate 2 g protein 2-3 g fiber	25	½ C cooked vegetables ½ C vegetable juice 1 C raw vegetables
Other carbohydrates: snack foods and sweet desserts	15 g carbohydrate Protein varies Fat varies	Varies	2 small cookies ½ C ice cream
Milk Skim/very-low-fat	12 g carbohydrate 8 g protein Trace grams of fat	90	1 C skim milk 8 oz plain nonfat yogurt
Low-fat	12 g carbohydrate 8 g protein 5 g fat	120	1 C 2% milk 8 oz plain low-fat yogurt

Whole	12 g carbohydrate 8 g protein 8 g fat	150	1 C whole milk 8 oz whole plain yogurt
Meat and substitutes			
Very lean	7 g protein 0-1 g fat	35	1 oz chicken: white meat, no skin ¼ C nonfat cottage cheese 2 egg whites
Lean	7 g protein 3 g fat	55	¼ C 4.5% fat cottage cheese 1 oz lean pork or beef 1 oz chicken: white meat with skin
Medium-fat	7 g protein 5 g fat	75	1 egg 4 oz tofu 1 oz roast beef, pork, or lamb
High-fat	7 g protein 8 g fat	100	1 oz processed sandwich meats 1 oz American, cheddar, or Swiss cheese
Fat	5 g fat	45	2 tbs peanut butter Variable

Developed from information in The American Diabetes Association, American Dietetic Association: *Exchange lists to meal planning*, Chicago, 1995, The Associations.

hypertension, it is started by week 26 to 28. For class A diabetes it should be started by week 40 (Heppard, Garite, 1996).

Contraction stress test. The contraction stress test (CST) may be the primary means of fetal surveillance when biophysical profiles are not readily available.

Nonstress test. Because the nonstress test (NST) is not as sensitive as the CST, the NST may be done between weekly CSTs so that testing is performed every 3 to 4 days (Heppard, Garite, 1996). In some centers it is used in place of CSTs. If so, it should be done twice each week instead of weekly.

Doppler umbilical artery velocimetry. Doppler umbilical artery velocimetry may be used early to detect IUGR. If the mother has vascular insufficiency, risk is increased for placental vascular disease. In these cases Doppler studies may be done.

Amniocentesis. The usual use of amniocentesis is to ascertain the lecithin/sphingomyelin (L/S) ratio and the presence of phosphatidyl glycerol (PG). An L/S ratio of 2.0 or greater when PG is present is sufficient to expect that surfactant levels are high enough in the fetus to prevent the development of respiratory distress syndrome (RDS). The amniocentesis is generally done after week 38 of gestation.

Management of Ketoacidosis

Diabetic ketoacidosis occurs when the fasting blood sugar rises to more than 250 mg/dl. The most common presenting symptoms are nausea and vomiting. Diagnostic indicators are moderate to large amount of urine ketones, plasma bicarbonate less than 15 mg/dl, serum acetone positive at a 1 : 2 dilution, and/or arterial pH less than 7.3. The treatment protocol for ketoacidosis is summarized in Table 9-13.

Intrapartum Management

The well-controlled diabetic woman with no complications does not have to deliver before term if the fetus is not macrosomic and the biophysical profile is reassuring. Early delivery may be necessary if the woman has not been in good glucose control, the woman has a history of a previous stillbirth, the woman has developed complications such as a hypertensive disorder of pregnancy or vasculopathy, fetal estimated weight is large for gestation, or there is an indication of fetal compromise (Moore, 1994). Then an induction or cesarean birth may be scheduled. Because of the danger of fetal compromise, it is not recommended to wait for spontaneous labor after 40 weeks of

TABLE 9-13 Protocol for treatment of perinatal ketoacidosis

Goal of treatment	Type of treatment	Treatment protocol
Hydrate	Fluids	1 L NS over first hr Then 200-500 ml/hr until 75% fluid deficit corrected
Reduce blood glucose levels	Insulin	IV bolus with 10-20 U of regular insulin; may repeat in 1 hr if glucose fails to drop by 10% Give 5-10 U of regular insulin per hr IV for 24 hr (50 U regular Humulin insulin in 500 ml of NS to run at 100-150 ml/hr) Perform capillary glucose testing q 2 hr
Clear ketones	Glucose	When serum glucose <250 mg/dl, decrease insulin infusion and change IV to: 5% dextrose and ½ NS (D$_5$ ½ NS) if Na$^+$ >145 mEq/L or 5% dextrose and NS (D$_5$NS) if Na$^+$ <145 mEq/L (piggyback at approximately 100 ml/hr to administer 5-10 g glucose per hr) Once serum glucose <150 mg/dl, feed patient appropriate dietary intake
Restore electrolyte balance	Potassium	Following the initial liter of fluid and urine output at least 30 ml/hr, administer K$^+$ as follows: K$^+$ >6 mEq = No added K$^+$ K$^+$ 5-6 mEq = 10 mEq K$^+$ added K$^+$ 4-5 mEq = 20 mEq K$^+$ added

Continued

Developed from information in Moore T. In Creasy R, Resnik R, editors: *Maternal-fetal medicine: principles and practice*, ed 3, Philadelphia, 1994, Saunders; Chauhan S and others: *J Perinatol* 16(3):173-175, 1996.

NS, Normal saline solution; *Na$^+$,* sodium; *IV,* intravenous; *K$^+$,* potassium.

TABLE 9-13 Protocol for treatment of perinatal ketoacidosis—cont'd

Goal of treatment	Type of treatment	Treatment protocol
		K^+ 3-4 mEq = 30 mEq K^+ added
		K^+ <3 mEq = 40 mEq K^+ added
		When K^+ is low on admission, add K^+ immediately to IV infusion; if patient remains oliguric, reduce rate
	Bicarbonate	If pH <7.0 give 44-89 mEq q 2 hr until pH >7.0
		If pH >7.0, do not give bicarbonate
Supportive	General measures	If comatose, place nasogastric tube and urinary catheter
		Oxygen by mask at 8-10 L/min
		Anticipate need for invasive hemodynamic monitoring
		Rule out infection and administer antibiotic treatment if needed
		Treat precipitating cause such as urinary tract infections, noncompliance with insulin administration, or dietary indiscretion
Evaluation of treatment plan	Monitoring	Level of maternal consciousness
		Assess for signs of cerebral edema
		Deteriorating mental status
		Sluggish pupillary light reflex
		Headache
		Urine for culture and sensitivity
		Hourly urinary output
		Continuous FHR monitoring; prepare for delivery if nonreassuring tracing persists after initial stabilization
		Maternal VS

Assess for signs of pulmonary edema
  Dyspnea
  Tachypnea
  Tachycardia
  Wheezing
  Productive or nonproductive cough
Assess for hypovolemia
  Urine output <30 ml/hr
  Hypotension
  Tachycardia
Perform capillary glucose testing q 1-2 hr
Continuous ECG monitoring for:
  ST-segment depression
  Inverted T waves
  Appearance of U waves following T wave
Obtain serum Na^+ K^+, HCO_3^-, Ca^{++}, Cl^-, venous pH levels every 2-4 hr as
  ordered until DKA has cleared

FHR, Fetal heart rate; *VS*, vital signs; *ECG*, electrocardiogram; HCO_3^-, sodium bicarbonate; Ca^{++}, calcium; Cl^-, chloride; *DKA*, diabetic ketoacidosis.

gestation. During an induction or spontaneous labor, intermittent subcutaneous insulin or a continuous insulin infusion will be required.

Insulin Infusion

If a continuous insulin infusion is needed, 25 U of regular insulin is added to 250 mg of normal saline (NS) (ACOG, 1994). Piggyback insulin infusion to mainline IV of NS, lactated Ringer's solution (LR), or D_5LR. The intravenous rate and supplemental regular insulin will vary based on every 1- to 2-hour blood glucose values. Refer to the section on Potential Complication: Hypoglycemia, Intrapartum later in this chapter.

Intermittent Subcutaneous Insulin

If intermittent subcutaneous injections are used, one third to one half of the patient's prepregnancy dosage of insulin may be given the morning of the induction. A long-acting insulin most likely will not be used because of the drop in insulin requirement after delivery (Cunningham and others, 1997). A continuous 5% glucose infusion is started at approximately 100 ml/hr. Supplemental regular insulin will be given based on glucose values obtained every 1 to 2 hours to maintain glucose between 70 and 90 mg/dl.

Cesarean Birth

In the event a cesarean birth is planned, fetal lung maturity should be predetermined. The cesarean is then scheduled for early morning. The woman should drink nothing after midnight and hold her evening and morning dosages of insulin. Her capillary glucose level should be checked before and immediately following the delivery. Glucose will be administered intravenously.

Postpartum Management

At delivery there is an abrupt loss of the antagonistic placental hormones and suppression of the anterior pituitary growth hormone. Therefore there is a significant decrease in insulin need during the immediate postpartum period. For the type 2 diabetic woman, the insulin dose is typically minimal for 1 to 3 days. The type 1 diabetic woman may require small doses determined by the blood glucose levels. By the third or fourth postpartum day, insulin requirements will usually increase to about two thirds of the prepregnancy dosage.

Frequent blood glucose monitoring may be necessary for the

first 48 hours to determine the individual patient's need. Women who were not insulin dependent before pregnancy most likely will not need insulin. See Table 9-14 for a summary of the new oral hypoglycemic agents. During the early postpartum period, the importance of ongoing glycemic control even when not pregnant should be stressed. The Diabetes Control and Complication Trial from 1983 to 1993 showed that keeping blood glucose levels within normal limits reduced the risk of diabetic complications such as retinopathy by 76%, nephropathy by 50%, neuropathy by 60%, and cardiac problems by 35%.

To continue normal blood glucose levels after delivery, ongoing self-monitoring of blood glucose (SMBG), comprehensive meal planning, and regular exercise along with possible oral hypoglycemic agents and/or insulin regimen are required. According to one of the ADA's position statements (1997c), the required diet is an individualized dietary prescription based on the Dietary Guidelines for Americans. Usually 10% to 20% of the kilocalories are from protein unless nephropathy is present, and the remaining 80% to 90% of kilocalories are distributed between dietary fat and carbohydrates. The percentage of calories from fat depends on maintaining glucose control, lipid levels, and weight goals. If the woman is obese, weight loss is a priority and dietary fat should be limited to less than 30% of the total calories with less than 10% saturated fat. If low-density lipoprotein cholesterol is elevated, fat should be less than 30% of the total calories with saturated fat restricted to less than 7% of total calories and dietary cholesterol less than 200 mg/day. However, if triglycerides and very-low-density lipoprotein cholesterol are elevated, a moderate increase in monounsaturated fat intake (up to 20% of total calories), with less than 10% of calories each from saturated and polyunsaturated fats, along with exercise and weight loss may be beneficial.

All women following a pregnancy complicated with gestational diabetes should understand the need for ongoing, long-term follow-up. Women who have had gestational diabetes mellitus (GDM) have more than a 50% risk of developing type 2 diabetes mellitus within the next 20 years (Kjos, 1994; O'Sullivan, 1991). This has been shown to decrease to a risk of 25% if the woman maintains a normal weight and exercises regularly (ADA, 1995). Refer to the Nursing Diagnosis of altered health maintenance: postpartum section of this chapter for appropriate postpartum teaching.

TABLE 9-14 Oral hypoglycemic agents

Drug	Method of action	Dosages	Side effects	Contraindications
Second-generation sulfo-nylureas Glyburide (Micronase; DiaBeta)	Sensitize pancreas to secrete first-phase insulin appropriately and thus normalize postprandial blood glucose Increase the number of insulin receptors Improve the postreceptor defect	1.25-20 mg in 1 or 2 doses Does not cause hypo-glycemia	Skin rash Headaches Occasionally N/V Hypoglycemia	Pregnancy Surgery Allergic to sulfa drugs
Glipizide Glucotrol Glucotrol XL	Decrease hepatic glu-cose production and thus decrease fasting hyperglycemia	2.5-40 mg in 1-3 doses 5-20 mg in 1 dose		

Biguanides: metformin (Glucophage)	Lowers blood glucose only if elevated and thus does not cause hypoglycemia	Phase in:
		Week 1
		  AM: 500 mg
		  PM: 500 mg
		Week 2
			Nausea
			Diarrhea
			Abdominal pain
			Metallic taste
			Megaloblastic anemia
				Pregnancy
				Lactation
				Liver disease
				Kidney disease
				Lactic acidosis
				Cardiopulmonary insufficiency
				History of alcoholism
				Binge drinking

Drug	Action	Dosage	Side Effects	Contraindications
	Decreases hepatic glucose production and thus decreases fasting hyperglycemia Increases glucose utilization by muscle cells Does not stimulate insulin secretion and thus rests the pancreas Improves lipid profile by ↓ total cholesterol; ↓ LDLs; ↓ triglycerides; ↑ HDLs	AM: 1000 mg PM: 500 mg Week 3 AM: 1000 mg PM: 1000 mg Take with meals to decrease side effects Maximum dose 2500 mg May be used in combination with sulfonylureas		Binge drinking
Acarbose (Precose)	Decreases appetite Delays digestion of carbohydrates and thus smaller rise in blood sugar Does not increase insulin production Does not cause hypoglycemia alone; but can occur in combination therapy	Take with first bite of meal Weeks 1 and 2: 25 mg qd Weeks 3 and 4: 25 mg bid Weeks 5-12: 25 mg tid Maintenance dosage: 50-100 mg tid May be used in combination with sulfonylureas	GI symptoms Flatulence Diarrhea Abdominal pain Elevated AST/ALT Hypoglycemia if in combination therapy If hypoglycemia develops, cannot treat with food	Pregnancy Lactation Hypersensitivity to the drug Intestinal malabsorption syndrome Inflammatory bowel disease Intestinal obstruction Hepatic disease or cirrhosis Moderate or severe renal disease

LDLs, Low-density lipoproteins; HDLs, high-density lipoproteins; N/V, nausea/vomiting.

NURSING PROCESS

PREVENTION

The two major goals of care for pregnant women with diabetes are to promote a healthy, normally developed newborn and to prevent complications of diabetes from adversely affecting the pregnant woman. Counseling before conception should be aimed at planning a pregnancy rather than simply allowing it to occur. Euglycemia should be attained and maintained for a minimum of 3 months before conception to reduce the risks of birth defects and congenital abnormalities to no more than the general population. Education in diet, glucose monitoring, and insulin adjustments is necessary for the woman to self-manage diabetes during pregnancy. Education and referrals should be aimed at promoting as much independence as the woman is willing and cognitively able to assume.

NURSING DIAGNOSES/COLLABORATIVE PROBLEMS AND INTERVENTIONS

- **ALTERED HEALTH MAINTENANCE** related to insufficient knowledge of diabetes and pregnancy.

  DESIRED OUTCOMES: The patient will verbalize understanding of the disease diabetes; how it affects pregnancy; the importance of maintaining fasting blood glucose levels between 60 and 90 mg/dl, premeal blood glucose levels between 60 and 105 mg/dl, 1-hour postprandial blood glucose levels less than 140 mg/dl, 2-hour postprandial blood glucose levels less than 120 mg/dl, and Hb A_{1c} less than 7%; and the interaction of diet, daily activity or exercise, and insulin. The patient and at least one member of her family will be able to correctly return demonstrate blood glucose monitoring, insulin administration, and urine testing.

  INTERVENTIONS
  Antepartum
  1. Emphasize the importance of weekly or biweekly prenatal visits or as often as indicated.
  2. Stress the importance of continually maintaining the blood glucose between 60 and 120 mg/dl during pregnancy to prevent adverse outcomes for mother and baby.
  3. Assess the patient's and her family's knowledge of the disease process and treatment, including the relationship among diet, exercise, insulin, illness, and stress.
  4. Determine the patient's and her family's understanding of the effects of diabetes on pregnancy and the effects of pregnancy on diabetes.

Glucose monitoring

1. Explain or review the importance of self-monitoring of blood glucose (SMBG) using a reflectance meter and enzyme strips. Demonstrate the procedure, and observe a return demonstration.

2. Educate to check blood glucose two to ten times daily as indicated. For types 1 and 2 diabetes the ideal frequency for SMBG testing is once before each meal, 1 hour after each meal, at bedtime, and in the middle of the night (ADA, 1995). However, an eight-test-per-day regimen is difficult to maintain, and the most common preferred standard is at least fasting, prelunch, predinner, at bedtime daily, and a 2-hour postprandial test weekly (Diabetes Control and Complication Trial Research Group, 1993).

3. Teach the patient and family to evaluate the blood glucose values according to the normal ranges for pregnancy and to notify the physician if the glucose values are outside the normal range. Normal glucose values during pregnancy are (a) before breakfast, 60 to 90 mg/dl; (b) before lunch, before dinner, and at bedtime snack, 60 to 105 mg/dl; and (c) 1 hour after meals, 120 mg/dl or less. To lessen stress, reinforce that the fetus will not usually be affected until the blood sugar level rises over 140 mg/dl, but a rising trend needs to be reversed immediately (Moore, 1994; Reece, Homko, 1993).

4. Explain the reasons oral hypoglycemia medication is not used during pregnancy. That is, oral agents cross the placenta and stimulate increased fetal secretion of insulin. This can promote complications such as macrosomia and neonatal hypoglycemia (Hollingsworth, 1992).

Insulin administration

1. Define the physiologic effect, dosage, and adverse reactions of insulin.

2. Explain that intermediate- and long-acting insulins are in a suspension and require mixing by gently rolling the vial between the palms of the hands.

3. Explain the importance of insulin being injected 30 minutes before mealtime unless Humalog (Lispro) is being used, which is injected within 15 minutes of the meal.

4. Demonstrate and request a return demonstration of correct injection technique using a systematic rotation pattern. A line drawing of the human body with an illustrated method of recording each injection is shown in Figs. 9-1 and 9-2. Each injection should be given 1 inch from the last injection. The

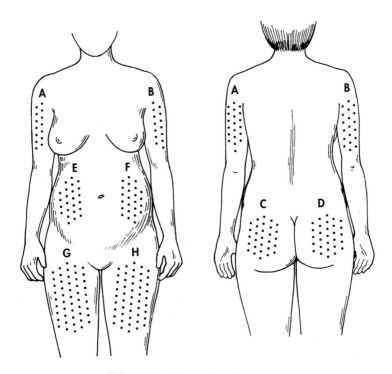

FIG. 9-1 Insulin rotation of sites.

angle of the needle should be 90 degrees to ensure deep subcutaneous administration unless the patient is very thin, in which case the 45-degree angle may be used to prevent an intramuscular injection.

5. Emphasize that the rate of insulin absorption depends on such variables as massage of the injection site, smoking, and choice of injection sites. Massage increases insulin absorption by increasing blood flow to the area. Smoking decreases insulin absorption. Absorption is fastest from the abdomen, followed by the arms, buttocks, and last the thighs (ADA, 1997b; Moore, 1994).

6. Advise the patient to record the expiration date on the insulin bottle after opening. To ensure continued sterility, bottles should be discarded after 3 months of use. All insulin in current use should be stored at room temperature, protected from direct sunlight and extreme temperature, to facilitate adequate absorption and utilization.

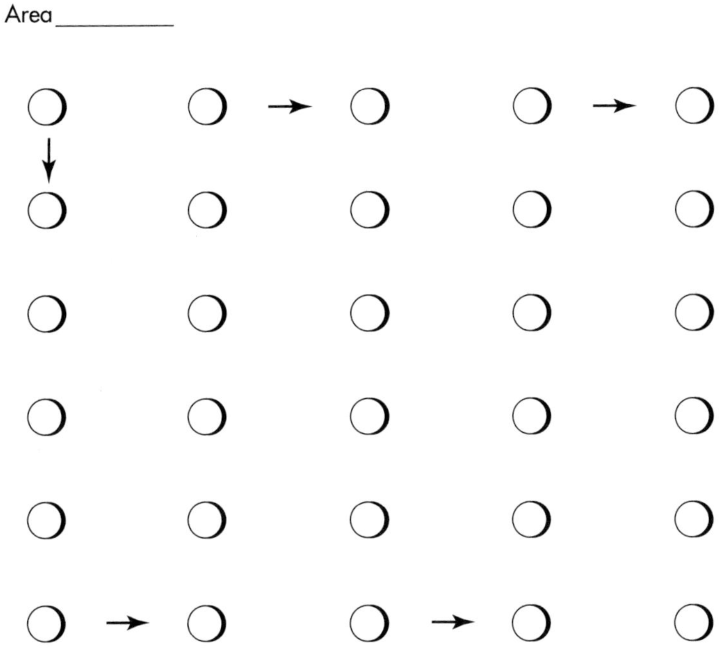

Area_____

FIG. 9-2 Charting insulin rotation.

Exercise
1. If the patient does not have any signs of hypertension or vascular damage, encourage a moderate consistent exercise program that lowers blood glucose by enhancing glucose uptake by the skeletal muscles. A long-term exercise program can reduce the cardiovascular risk of diabetes by increasing high-density lipoproteins (HDL) and lowering cholesterol (Winn, Reece, 1989).
2. Teach the patient to exercise for 20 to 30 minutes at 50% VO_2 maximum as long as the fetus has been active and blood glucose is within normal limits (Bung, Artal, 1996).
3. Teach the patient to use upper body muscles, putting little mechanical stress on the trunk and limiting an excessive weight-bearing load to the lower extremities.
4. Teach the patient to palpate the uterus for contractions during the exercise and stop if any occur.

Diet
See the nursing diagnosis on altered nutrition.

Urine testing

Explain or review urine testing for ketones, which should be done at least three times per week during pregnancy on the first void of the day. If the patient becomes ill or if blood glucose levels are elevated, it should be done daily.

General

1. Recommend keeping a diary of blood glucose results, insulin dosage, diet, exercise, any reactions, and general feelings of well-being.
2. Give a contact telephone number that is available on a 24-hour basis.
3. Advise of the importance of carrying a diabetic identification card and wearing a Medic-Alert bracelet or necklace.

Postpartum

1. Advise the gestational diabetic woman of her increased risk (50%) of developing type 2 diabetes mellitus (Kjos, 1994; O'Sullivan, 1991). Advise of the importance of the screening program for early detection of development of diabetes. This includes a 75-g, 2-hour oral glucose tolerance test at the 6-week postpartum checkup and a random or fasting blood glucose annually. Refer to Box 9-4 for protocol for postpartum testing.
2. Educate as to the relationship between maintaining an optimum weight and the decreased risk of later development. If the woman is or becomes obese, the risk of diabetes increases to 70% (Chamberlain, 1991). If the woman is obese, especially with increased abdominal fat, a weight loss of 5 to 10 pounds will make a difference in the amount of insulin the pancreas must produce. For example, an active thin person's pancreas may produce only 35 to 40 U/day as compared with a person who is overweight, whose pancreas may be required to produce 150 U/day to clear the same amount of glucose. Encourage the woman to follow a nutritional diet and exercise regularly to decrease risk.
3. Assess the woman's knowledge of approved contraception. The barrier methods of contraception are very safe for the diabetic woman. Oral contraceptives have been reported to alter carbohydrate metabolism by causing insulin resistance. Therefore in the past the diabetic woman has been encouraged to avoid oral contraception. Recent research has indicated that the current low-progestin and low-estrogen preparations have minimal effect on carbohydrate metabo-

Box 9-4

Nurse Practitioner Protocol for Postpartum Testing Following GDM

1. Perform a 75-g glucose tolerance test at the first postpartum checkup between 6 and 8 weeks after delivery or shortly after the woman stops breast feeding.
2. Test preparation: instruct the patient to eat an additional 150 g of complex carbohydrates (example: 12 additional slices of bread each day) for 3 days before the test.
3. Instruct to abstain from eating, drinking (except water), or smoking for 8 hours before the test.
4. Have patient rest in office for 30 minutes just before the test.
5. Draw a fasting plasma glucose level.
6. Administer 75 g of oral glucose drink.
7. Draw plasma glucose at 2 hours.
8. Interpret and reclassify GDM following pregnancy according to new criteria for the diagnosis of diabetes mellitus (The Expert Committee on the Diagnosis and Classification of Diabetes Mellitus, 1997).

   Normal—medical diagnosis: previous abnormality of glucose tolerance

Fasting plasma glucose	<110 mg/dl
2-Hour postprandial	<140 mg/dl

   Impaired glucose tolerance

Fasting plasma glucose	110-125 mg/dl
2-Hour postprandial	140-199 mg/dl

   Type 2 DM

Fasting plasma glucose	≥126 mg/dl
2-Hour postprandial	>200 mg/dl
Random plasma glucose	≥200 mg/dl with symptoms (polyuria, polydipsia, and unexplained weight loss)

9. Annual well-woman examination should include a fasting blood glucose following a 3-hour fast. If 110 or greater, further testing is needed.

GDM, Gestational diabetes mellitus.

lism. These include triphasic oral contraceptives, low-dose combined oral contraceptives, and the progestin-only pills. According to *Contraceptive Technology 1994-1996,* the diabetic woman may use oral contraceptives provided she does not have a personal or family history of vascular disease, does not smoke, and has a normal blood pressure (Hatcher and others, 1994). Even though no adverse effects have been noted on levels of total cholesterol, low-density lipoprotein, high-density lipoprotein, or triglycerides, ACOG (1994) is recommending a yearly lipid profile when oral contraceptives are prescribed. The intrauterine device is not ideal because of the increased risk of pelvic inflammatory disease and should be used with caution only for the multiparous diabetic woman.

4. Encourage breast feeding. Breast feeding decreases fasting and postprandial blood glucose levels and increases high-density lipoprotein cholesterol levels (Kjos and others, 1993). Therefore, during breast feeding, the insulin requirement is usually considerably less. The woman's dietary needs will increase the usually 500 to 800 calories. According to Lawrence (1994), the 24-hour kilocalorie need is 35 kcal/kg/day based on preconception weight. Teach the patient to expect fluctuations in her glucose levels during weaning and to continue close glucose monitoring. Reassure the mother that insulin does not cross into breast milk. However, elevated glucose levels will be present in the breast milk if her blood glucose is high. Monitor for mastitis and nipple infections because of their increased risk. Sore nipples that do not respond to the usual nonspecific treatment should be treated with nystatin ointment to the nipples and nystatin suspension for the infant as well.

- **RISK FOR NUTRITIONAL DEFICIT OR EXCESS** related to ineffective glucose uptake within cells and cellular dehydration related to increased vascular osmotic pressure. This is caused by the glucose concentration or excessive intake, lack of knowledge as to the appropriate diet, or ineffective handling of difficult situations.

  DESIRED OUTCOMES: Euglycemia will be reestablished or maintained. The patient will gain appropriate weight according to her prepregnancy status while avoiding excessive weight gain. The patient will follow her prescribed individualized meal plan.

INTERVENTIONS
Pregestational diabetes
1. During the first trimester, assess for the presence of nausea and vomiting.
2. Assess caloric intake and dietary pattern using the 24-hour recall.
3. Educate regarding the importance of healthy food choices within the individualized dietary prescription: total caloric intake of 300 calories more than nonpregnancy requirements; 10% to 20% low-fat protein, less than 10% polyunsaturated fat, and the remaining 60% to 70% monounsaturated fats and carbohydrates.
4. Explain the importance of seldom choosing concentrated sweets. They are usually empty calories and provide little if any other nutrients and may contain high saturated fat. However, when eaten, they should be part of the total carbohydrate intake, not extras.
5. Educate on how to use the American Diabetes Association exchange lists to facilitate meal-planning variety or the food guide pyramid. Teach the importance of eating a healthy diet to facilitate ongoing normal blood glucose levels. If the woman is having problems with blood glucose swings, carbohydrate counting is an alternative plan.
6. If the woman is insulin dependent, review importance of regularity of meals and snacks.
7. Educate as to the importance of folate, 400 μg/day, to decrease the risk of a neural tube defect.
8. Educate regarding the importance of soluble fiber such as legumes, fruits, and oat bran in slowing the absorption of glucose, which allows for a more gradual influx of glucose into the blood.
9. Explain the significance of notifying the physician if dietary intake is altered.
10. Refer to a registered dietitian or nutritionist for development of an individualized dietary plan.
11. Discuss problems associated with strict adherence to the prescribed diet, and assist patient to identify problems and solutions.
12. Provide patient with materials such as the American Diabetes Association's series on "Diabetes Day-by-Day."
Gestational Diabetes
1. Teach the importance of preventing fasting and postprandial hyperglycemia.

2. Teach dietary factors that affect the glycemic index of foods (the percent rise in blood glucose after ingesting a food compared to glucose). Such factors are processing, preparation, ripeness, storage, fiber, presence of other foods, and digestibility of the starch component.

3. Educate to avoid sugars and concentrated sweets because these foods are high in calories and low in nutrients and have a higher glycemic index.

4. Educate to avoid highly processed foods because these foods have a higher glycemic index.

5. Educate to eat smaller, more frequent meals (about every 3 hours) to decrease the risk of postprandial hyperglycemia, preprandial starvation ketosis, and nausea and heartburn discomforts of pregnancy.

6. Educate to eat a very small breakfast (10% to 15% of the day's calories), low in carbohydrates (less than 10%), because fasting blood glucose is likely to be high. Therefore avoid highly processed cereals, milk, fruit, and fruit juices for breakfast.

7. Educate to choose high-fiber foods such as whole grain breads, fresh and frozen vegetables, legumes, and fresh fruit because they have a lower glycemic index, except for breakfast.

8. Educate to choose low-fat protein foods because they lower the glycemic index of the meal (American Diabetes Association, American Dietetic Association, 1995).

- **POTENTIAL COMPLICATION: HYPOGLYCEMIA** related to first-trimester pregnancy problems, being newly placed on exogenous insulin, or failure or inability to eat prescribed diet.

    DESIRED OUTCOMES: Hypoglycemia will be prevented or managed appropriately as indicated by blood glucose levels between 60 and 120 mg/dl, and the patient will be asymptomatic. The patient will verbalize understanding of the influence of early pregnancy and insulin on rapid onset of hypoglycemia.

    INTERVENTIONS

    Antepartum

    1. Assess for signs and symptoms of hypoglycemic reactions by inquiring about and evaluating the patient's self-recorded log.

    2. Assess patient's knowledge about signs and symptoms of hypoglycemia, change in the suddenness of onset of reactions, and knowledge of self-treatment.

3. Evaluate knowledge and willingness of family members in assisting with self-monitoring and management.
4. Teach or review the signs and symptoms of hypoglycemia, such as circumoral numbness, hunger, sweating, irritability, tremulousness, a feeling of fatigue, tachycardia, or headache.
5. Instruct regarding the importance of obtaining a glucagon kit, and instruct family in glucagon administration.
6. Teach treatment for mild hypoglycemia. If hypoglycemia occurs within 30 minutes before mealtime, the patient should eat the meal immediately. If hypoglycemia occurs between meals, the patient should apply the 15:15 rule. The patient should take 15 g of carbohydrate (sugar), wait 15 minutes, and then recheck blood sugar; if it is greater than 70 mg, the patient should eat; if it is less than 70, the 15:15 rule should be repeated. Fifteen grams of fast carbohydrate can be obtained from products designed to treat low blood sugar, 1 C of low-fat milk, ½ C of orange juice, ½ C of regular soda, or five or six hard candies. After the blood sugar is above 70 mg, the patient should stabilize with food. She should eat if it is time for a meal or snack; if not, she should have some additional food such as low-fat cheese and crackers, half of a turkey sandwich, low-fat milk, or peanut butter crackers (Diabetes Education Society, 1995).
7. Teach the patient that if severe hypoglycemia is manifested with confusion or unconsciousness, a family member or knowledgeable person should administer 0.5 mg of glucagon subcutaneously and obtain emergency medical assistance.

Intrapartum

Intermittent subcutaneous insulin method
1. Assess blood glucose every hour or as appropriate.
2. Test for urinary ketones every 4 hours.
3. Be prepared to give one third to one half of the patient's pregnancy dosage of insulin in the morning.
4. Start a continuous infusion as ordered based on glucose levels.
5. Administer regular insulin in 2 to 5 U per dose to maintain the blood sugar between 70 and 90 mg/dl.

Insulin infusion method
1. Withhold usual AM insulin dosage and breakfast. Give nothing by mouth except ice chips.
2. Obtain baseline blood glucose and every 1 to 2 hours.
3. Start continuous intravenous infusion of NS or LR at 125

ml/hr unless urine ketones are present or blood glucose is less than 70 mg/dl. Then use 5% dextrose at a rate of 2.5 mg/kg/min (ADA, 1995).

4. Set up insulin solution by diluting 25 U of regular insulin in 250 ml of NS and flush line with 25 ml. Piggyback insulin infusion to mainline intravenous line at connection closest to insertion site.

5. Use an infusion pump and adjust rate based on blood glucose levels (ACOG, 1994):

Blood glucose (mg/dl)	Insulin dosage (U/hr)
<100	0
100-140	1.0
141-180	1.5
181-220	2.0
>220	2.5

The intravenous rate and supplemental regular insulin are adjusted according to the every 1- to 2-hour blood glucose values.

Postpartum
1. Evaluate maternal blood sugar levels immediately following vaginal or cesarean birth and frequently thereafter for the first 48 hours if insulin dependent during pregnancy.
2. Be prepared to administer insulin as indicated by blood glucose levels.

■ **POTENTIAL COMPLICATION: HYPERGLYCEMIA** related to the influence of pregnancy hormones, precipitated by an infection, or related to failure to follow diet.

DESIRED OUTCOMES: Hyperglycemia will be prevented or managed appropriately as indicated by blood glucose levels between 60 and 120 mg/dl. The patient and her family will verbalize understanding of signs and symptoms, effects on the mother and especially on the fetus, and importance of strictly adhering to schedule of prescribed diet and insulin.

INTERVENTIONS
1. Examine dietary intake for adherence.
2. Assess for signs of an infection.
3. Treat based on cause by changing only one facet of management at a time.
4. Observe closely for signs of hyperglycemia if the patient receives a corticosteroid to induce fetal lung maturity.

- **POTENTIAL COMPLICATION: KETOACIDOSIS** related to hyperglycemia.

  DESIRED OUTCOMES: Signs and symptoms of ketoacidosis will be minimized and managed and complications prevented as manifested by a normal fetal heart rate (FHR) pattern, normal fetal activity, and restoration of the blood glucose and electrolyte balance to normal within 24 hours.

  INTERVENTIONS

  1. Monitor for signs of diabetic ketoacidosis such as presence of ketonuria, altered level of consciousness, Kussmaul breathing, and acetone breath.
  2. Monitor FHR after 22 weeks continuously by electronic fetal monitor (EFM) during treatment of ketoacidosis.
  3. Evaluate fetal well-being with ultrasound, biophysical profile, or contraction stress test at the time maternal acidosis develops and for the remainder of pregnancy at appropriate intervals.
  4. Stabilize and prepare patient for maternal transport to tertiary facility.
  5. Be prepared as ordered to implement treatment protocols outlined in Table 9-13.

- **FEAR** related to lack of predictable outcome for self and her fetus as well as self-management requirements.

  DESIRED OUTCOME: The patient and family members will verbalize their fears and seek information to identify solutions to problems in self-management.

  INTERVENTIONS

  1. Encourage and facilitate a trusting relationship for the woman and her partner to discuss and name their fears related to pregnancy and diabetes.
  2. Determine the family's support system.
  3. Dispel anxiety regarding unrealistic fears and assist with identifying solutions to obstacles to self-management. (Lower anxiety regarding self-management increases compliance [York and others, 1990].)
  4. Encourage family members' participation and presence, especially when woman is hospitalized.
  5. Strive to normalize those aspects of pregnancy care that can be normalized.
  6. Refer to a diabetic support group or a high risk pregnancy support group.

- **FAMILY COPING: POTENTIAL FOR GROWTH** related to stressors that include time management problems, financial strain, or previous poor coping styles for disease management.

  DESIRED OUTCOMES: Family members and the patient will identify stressors and solutions that can be instituted before potential complications occur or are irreversible. The patient and family members will verbalize commitment to making pregnancy outcome positive for mother and baby. The patient will report self-monitoring problems promptly and early.

  INTERVENTIONS
  1. Discuss and anticipate potential problems at the earliest possible time in the pregnancy.
  2. Problem solve ways to decrease stress that will facilitate glucose stability.
  3. Encourage family members' participation in formulation of a plan.
  4. Establish a trusting relationship with the pregnant woman by expressing empathetic understanding of time and financial commitment.
  5. Make appropriate referrals for financial assistance such as American Diabetic Association and social service agencies.
  6. Assist with and facilitate development of a plan that meets the demands of the family values and beliefs where possible.

- **RISK FOR INFECTION,** especially monilial, incisional, and urinary tract infections, related to increased susceptibility secondary to the disease process such as hyperglycemia and poor circulation.

  DESIRED OUTCOMES: The signs and symptoms of an infection will be minimized and managed as measured by no burning on urination, no vaginal itching, normothermia, negative cultures, and the white blood cell count between 4500 and 10,000/mm^3.

  INTERVENTIONS
  1. Teach the patient how to recognize signs of an infection.
  2. Explain the significance of notifying the physician promptly of the first signs of an infection or any illness. Emphasize signs of a urinary tract infection or vaginal infection.
  3. Be prepared to obtain a urine culture and sensitivity periodically throughout the pregnancy to screen for asymptomatic bacteriuria.
  4. Explain the relationship between an infection and a possible increased insulin need.
  5. Assess incisional healing (episiotomy or abdominal incision) after birth.

■ **RISK FOR FETAL INJURY** related to the increased risk of congenital malformation if the mother's blood glucose is abnormal during the embryonic phase of development. If the mother has class A, B, or C diabetes, the fetus is at increased risk for birth injury because of possible macrosomia. If the mother has class D or above diabetes, there is an increased risk of IUGR or stillbirth because of vascular changes within the placenta.

DESIRED OUTCOMES: The fetus will remain active and maintain an appropriate growth for gestational age. The fetus will be free of any congenital defect.

INTERVENTIONS

Antepartum

1. Be prepared to assess patient's glucose control before conception or on the first prenatal visit with an Hb A_{1c} test and then every trimester. Begin folic acid supplementation before conception to reduce risk of fetal neural tube defects.

2. Be prepared to obtain a serum alpha-fetoprotein (AFP) sample between 6 and 8 weeks of gestation.

3. Assess fundal height measurements, and report any deviation of 3 cm or more from weeks of gestation.

4. Explain rationale and procedure for weekly biophysical profiles, contraction stress tests, and/or nonstress tests, starting at 32 weeks or as early as 26 to 28 weeks if patient is manifesting signs of hypertension or IUGR.

5. Teach mother to keep a daily fetal monitoring chart after 24 weeks of gestation.

6. Explain procedure and rationale for amniocentesis to determine fetal lung maturity with L/S ratio and phosphatidyl glycerol for elective delivery before 39 weeks.

7. Review the importance of ultrasound studies for gestational dating, assess fetal growth, and rule out fetal anomalies. Fetal echocardiography may be indicated at 20 weeks.

8. Prepare the patient and her family for the possible need of early delivery if signs of uteroplacental insufficiency (UPI) develop.

Intrapartum

1. Evaluate electronic fetal monitor for reassuring or nonreassuring baseline FHR, variability, and patterns that develop in response to labor.

2. Evaluate labor progress and ultrasound results for potential problems with dystocia, arrest of descent, or failure to progress (see Chapters 26 and 27).

- **POTENTIAL NEONATAL COMPLICATIONS: HYPOGLYCEMIA, HYPOCALCEMIA, AND HYPERBILIRUBINEMIA**

- **POTENTIAL COMPLICATION: END-STAGE RENAL DISEASE** related to diabetic sequelae. See Chapter 11.

- **POTENTIAL COMPLICATION: HYPERTENSIVE DISORDERS OF PREGNANCY.** See Chapter 20.

CONCLUSION

The ultimate goal of nursing care for a pregnant woman with diabetes is to minimize the effects of risks and complications. This is accomplished by educating the woman and her family in recognition of early signs and symptoms of management failures and in identifying and solving management issues that they are capable of solving and by promoting a relationship that encourages mutual work among the patient, her family, and members of the health care team. The outcome of the pregnancy should be a mother without additional diabetic complications, a healthy newborn, and a family who is ready and able to integrate the new baby into their family. An added side benefit of educating the pregnant woman who is already insulin dependent is that she will commonly learn useful skills that will aid in her self-management of diabetes for the remainder of her life.

BIBLIOGRAPHY

American College of Obstetricians and Gynecologists (ACOG): Diabetes and pregnancy, *ACOG Techn Bull,* no. 200, Dec 1994.

American Diabetes Association (ADA): *Medical management of pregnancy complicated by diabetes,* ed 2, Alexandria, Va, 1995, The Association.

American Diabetes Association (ADA): Position statement: gestational diabetes mellitus, *Diabetes Care* 29(suppl 1):S44-S45, 1997a.

American Diabetes Association (ADA): Position statement: insulin administration, *Diabetes Care* 20(suppl 1):S46-S49, 1997b.

American Diabetes Association (ADA): Position statement: nutrition recommendations and principles for people with diabetes mellitus, *Diabetes Care* 20(suppl 1):S14-S17, 1997c.

American Diabetes Association (ADA): Position statement: screening for diabetes, *Diabetes Care* 20(suppl 1):S22-S23, 1997d.

American Diabetes Association and The American Dietetic Association: *Exchange lists for meal planning,* Alexandria, Va, 1995, The Association.

Avery M, Rossi M: Gestational diabetes, *J Nurse Midwifery* 39(2 suppl):9s-19s, 1994.

Boyd K, Ross E, Sherman S: Jelly beans as an alternative to a cola beverage containing fifty grams of glucose, *Am J Obstet Gynecol* 173:1889-1892, 1995.

Bung P, Artal R: Gestational diabetes and exercise: a survey, *Semin Perinatol* 20(4):328-333, 1996.

Chamberlain G: ABC of antenatal care: medical problems in pregnancy, *Br Med J* 302(6787):1262-1266, 1991.

Chauhan S and others: Diabetic ketoacidosis complicating pregnancy, *J Perinatol* 16(3):173-175, 1996.

Committee on Dietary Allowances, Food and Nutrition Board: *Recommended dietary allowances,* ed 9, Washington, DC, 1990, National Academy of Sciences.

Cousins L and others: Screening recommendations for gestational diabetes mellitus, *Am J Obstet Gynecol* 165:493-496, 1991.

Coustan D: Screening and diagnosis of gestational diabetes, *Semin Perinatol* 18(5):407-413, 1994.

Coustan D: Gestational diabetes. In Queenan J, Hobbins J, editors: *Protocols for high-risk pregnancies,* ed 3, Cambridge, England, 1996, Blackwell Science.

Cunningham F and others: *Williams obstetrics,* ed 20, Stamford, Conn, 1997, Appleton & Lange.

Damm P and others: Predictive factors for the development of diabetes in women with previous gestational diabetes mellitus, *Am J Obstet Gynecol* 167:607-616, 1992.

Diabetes Control and Complications Trial Research Group: The effect of intensive treatment of diabetes on the development and progresson of long-term complications in insulin-dependent diabetes mellitus, *N Engl J Med* 329:977, 1993.

Diabetes Control and Complications Trial Research Group: Pregnancy outcomes in the Diabetes Control and Complications Trial, *Am J Obstet Gynecol* 174:1343-1353, 1996.

Diabetes Education Society: *Lifeskills teaching guides,* Denver, 1995, The Society.

Dooley S, Metzger B, Cho N: Gestational diabetes mellitus: influences of race on disease prevalence and perinatal outcome in a U.S. population, *Obstet Gynecol* 81:517-522, 1993.

Dornhorst A and others: High prevalence of gestational diabetes in women from ethnic minority groups, *Diabet Med* 9:820-835, 1992.

Doshier S: What happens to the offspring of diabetic pregnancies? *MCN Am J Matern Child Nurs* 20(1):25-28, 1995.

Evans A, deVeciana M, Benbarka M: Endocrine disorders. In Niswander K, Evans A: *Manual of obstetrics,* ed 5, Boston, 1995, Little, Brown.

Foster D: Diabetes mellitus. In Isselbacker K and others, editors: *Harrison's principles of internal medicine,* ed 13, New York, 1994, McGraw-Hill.

Gabbe S: Diabetes mellitus. In Queenan J, Hobbins J, editors: *Protocols for high-risk pregnancies,* ed 3, Cambridge, England, 1996, Blackwell Scientific.

Garner P: Type I diabetes mellitus and pregnancy, *Lancet* 346:157, 1995.

Goer H: Gestational diabetes, *Childbirth Educator* 5(5):8-10, 35-38, 1995.

Greene M: Prevention and diagnosis of congenital anomalies in diabetic pregnancies, *Clin Perinatol* 20:533-547, 1993.

Hare J: Diabetic complications of diabetic pregnancies, *Semin Perinatol* 18(5):451-458, 1994.

Hatcher R and others: *Contraceptive technology 1994-1996,* ed 16, New York, 1994, Irvington Publishers.

Heppard M, Garite T: *Acute obstetrics: a practical guide,* ed 2, St Louis, 1996, Mosby.

Hollingsworth D: Pregnancy, diabetes and birth: a management guide, ed 2, Baltimore, 1992, Williams & Wilkins.

Kaufmann R and others: Gestational diabetes diagnostic criteria: long-term maternal follow up, *Am J Obstet Gynecol* 172:621-625, 1995.

Kjos S: Maternal implications of gestational diabetes, *Semin Perinatol* 18(5):470-474, 1994.

Kjos S and others: The effect of lactation on glucose and lipid metabolism in women with recent gestational diabetes, *Obstet Gynecol* 82: 451-455, 1993.

Lagrew D and others: Antepartum fetal surveillance in patients with diabetes: when to start? *Am J Obstet Gynecol* 168:1820-1826, 1993.

Lawrence R: *Breastfeeding: a guide for the medical profession,* ed 4, St Louis, 1994, Mosby.

Lesser K, Carpenter M: Metabolic changes associated with normal pregnancy and pregnancy complicated by diabetes mellitus, *Semin Perinatol* 18(5):399-406, 1994.

Metzger B, The Organizing Committee: Proceedings of the Third International Workshop-Conference on Gestational Diabetes Mellitus, *Diabetes* 40(suppl 2):197-202, 1991.

Miller E: Metabolic management of diabetes in pregnancy, *Semin Perinatol* 18(5):414-431, 1994.

Moore T: Diabetes in pregnancy. In Creasy R, Resnik R, editors: *Maternal-fetal medicine: principles and practice,* ed 3, Philadelphia, 1994, Saunders.

Nahum G, Huffaker B: Racial differences in oral glucose screening test results: establishing race-specific criteria for abnormality in pregnancy, *Obstet Gynecol* 81:517-522, 1993.

Neiger R, Kendrick J: Obstetric management of diabetes in pregnancy, *Semin Perinatol* 18(5):432-450, 1994.

O'Sullivan J: Diabetes mellitus after GDM, *Diabetes* 40(suppl 2):131-135, 1991.

Piacquadio K, Hollingsworth D, Murphy H: Effects of in-utero exposure to oral hypoglycemic drugs, *Lancet* 338:866, 1991.

Piper J, Langer O: Does maternal diabetes delay fetal pulmonary maturity? *Am J Obstet Gynecol* 168:783-786, 1993.

Reece E, Homko C: Diabetes-related complications of pregnancy, *J Natl Med Assoc* 85:537, 1993.

Reece E, Homko C, Hagay Z: When the pregnancy is complicated by diabetes, *Contemp OB/GYN* 40(1):43-61, 1995.

Reece E and others: Assessment of carbohydrate tolerance in pregnancy, *Obstet Gynecol Surv* 46(1):1-14, 1991.

Rizzo T and others: Correlations between antepartum maternal metabolism and intelligence of offspring, *N Engl J Med* 325:911-916, 1991.

Ryan E, Enns L: Role of gestational hormones in the induction of insulin resistance, *J Clin Endocrinol Metab* 67:341-347, 1988.

Salvesen D and others: Fetal plasma erythropoietin in pregnancies complicated by maternal diabetes mellitus, *Am J Obstet Gynecol* 168:88, 1993.

Shields L and others: The prognostic value of hemoglobin A1c in predicting fetal heart disease in diabetic pregnancies, *Obstet Gynecol* 81:954-957, 1993.

Stamler E and others: High infectious morbidity in pregnant women with insulin-dependent diabetes: an understated complication, *Am J Obstet Gynecol* 163:1217-1221, 1990.

The Expert Committee on the Diagnosis and Classification of Diabetes Mellitus: Report of the Expert Committee on the Diagnosis and Classification of Diabetes Mellitus, *Diabetes Care* 20(7):1183-1197, 1997.

Walsh J, Roberts R: Switching to Humalog? Try these helpful hints, *Diabetes Interview,* pp 20-21, Nov/Dec 1996.

Willhoite M and others: The impact of preconception counseling on pregnancy outcomes: the experience of the Maine Diabetes in Pregnancy Program, *Diabetes Care* 16:450-455, 1993.

Winn H, Reece E: Integrating management of diabetic pregnancies, *Contemp OB/GYN* 33(1):91-102, 1989.

York R and others: Diabetes mellitus in pregnancy: clinical review, *J Perinatol* 10(3):285-293, 1990.

CHAPTER

10

Cardiac Disease

Pregnancy complicated with cardiac disease can be potentially dangerous to maternal well-being. The understanding of normal and abnormal cardiovascular physiology in pregnancy can aid enormously in anticipation of problems and prevention of complications.

INCIDENCE

The incidence of cardiac disease in the pregnant population ranges between 0.5% and 2%. Rheumatic fever, once responsible for 88% of cardiac disease cases in pregnancy, is now on the decline, responsible for only about 50% of cardiac disease cases in pregnancy. Congenital disease now plays a more prominent role. Mitral valve disease is still the most frequently seen valve defect in pregnant women. However, because of better childhood management of congenital heart disease, pregnancy outcomes are generally positive. Other cardiac diseases are rarely seen in pregnancy (Ueland, 1994).

ETIOLOGY

Cardiac disease in pregnancy takes a variety of forms and varies in functional severity. Some of the specific forms are as follows:
1. Rheumatic fever
2. Valve deformities (Kendrick, 1991; Rokey and others, 1994)

3. Congenital heart disease (Shime and others, 1987)
4. Developmental abnormalities
5. Congestive cardiomyopathies (Schmidt and others, 1989)
6. Cardiac dysrhythmias

NORMAL PHYSIOLOGY

Antepartum

Cardiac Output

In the antepartum period, cardiac output (the amount of blood pumped by the left ventricle into the aorta) rises significantly as early as the first trimester of pregnancy. It continues to rise and reaches a plateau between 28 and 34 weeks. It rises in response to the plasma volume increase, hormonal influences, and autonomic nervous system influences. This increase in cardiac output can cause patients to report signs and symptoms that mimic to some degree those of cardiac disease (Ueland, 1994), including the following:

- Dyspnea
- Orthopnea
- Dyspnea with exertion
- Edema
- Fatigability
- Infrequent palpitations

Blood Volume

Blood volume increases by plasma volume expansion and red blood cell multiplication. The mean plasma volume increase is 45% over the prepregnant volume, and red cell multiplication is in proportion to volume expansion if nutritional requirements are met. In early pregnancy the increased volume with each heart stroke increases cardiac output. As pregnancy continues, the heart rate increases to offset increased stroke volume. Increased volume maintains a dilated systemic vasculature.

Hormonal Influences

Hormonal influences affect resistance to blood flow and contractility of the myocardium. Increased estrogen leads to systemic vasodilation. Vasodilation increases cardiac output because of lowered peripheral resistance. Prolactin increases myocardial contractility (Capeless, Clapp, 1989).

Autonomic Nervous System

During pregnancy, autonomic nervous system (ANS) influences on blood flow become more prominent. In the nonpregnant state, when the ANS is blocked, there is little effect on blood pressure. However, in pregnancy, when the ANS is activated or blocked, dramatic changes in the maternal blood pressure can result. The cardiovascular system is hyperfilled from increased blood volume and hyperdynamic because of the predominance of the ANS (see Chapter 1).

Venous Pressure

Increased venous pressure, especially in the lower extremities, occurs in pregnancy. This can lead to a normal finding of an accentuated jugular pulse.

Heart

A slightly enlarged heart sometimes occurs in pregnancy because of the upward and leftward displacement of the heart anatomically. Benign dysrhythmias can occur, presumably because of the normal influences on myocardial contractility.

Inferior Vena Cava

When the weight of the gravid uterus lies against the inferior vena cava, partial or total occlusion reduces return volume to the heart and subsequent output.

Intrapartum

Hemodynamic responses to labor are also important; labor can be a critical period in the care of a pregnant woman with cardiac disease. Uterine contractions normally increase cardiac output and stroke volume because of increased intravascular volume, which leads to an increase in the workload of the heart. The workload can be relieved by positioning laterally and by pain relief, especially with caudal or epidural anesthesia (Forster, Joyce, 1989).

Postpartum

In the immediate postpartum period, there is a high risk for fluid volume overload caused by remobilization of fluid into vascular compartments. It is important to be cautious with intravenous fluids and with oxytocin administration after birth, both of which may further complicate the risk.

PATHOPHYSIOLOGY

To understand the pathophysiology of cardiac disease in pregnancy, one must understand what functional lesion is present. It is also necessary to understand various terms describing cardiac function (Dennison, 1990).

Stroke Volume

Stroke volume is the amount of blood ejected with each contraction of the left ventricle. It is affected by four interrelated factors:
1. Diastolic filling pressure (preload)
2. Distensibility of the ventricle
3. Myocardial contractility
4. Aortic pressure, which is the amount of pressure the ventricle must overcome to push blood into the aorta (afterload)

Contractility

There is a direct relationship between diastolic volume and the amount of blood pumped during systole. The greater the diastolic filling pressure, the more the fibers of the left ventricle stretch during diastole and the harder they contract during systole, increasing stroke volume and cardiac output. However, if the muscle fibers are stretched beyond a certain point, there is a loss of distensibility. This loss decreases the force of contractions and therefore decreases cardiac output.

Preload

Preload is the force responsible for stretching the ventricular muscles. It is also called *diastolic filling pressure.* If the preload is low, the ventricular muscle will not stretch enough for effective contractility. This leads to decreased stroke volume. If preload is too high, the muscle fibers will be overstretched. This also results in decreased contractility, leading in turn to decreased stroke volume.

Afterload

Afterload is the amount of pressure resistance in the aorta to the emptying of the left ventricle. It is the volume in the ventricles at the end of diastole and is also called *systemic vascular resistance.* Systemic vascular resistance (or afterload) is measured by taking blood pressure readings. The higher the afterload, the greater the force required by the left ventricle to overcome aortic pressure with systolic pressure to force the aortic valve to open. A high after-load decreases stroke volume and cardiac output if the pressure cannot be effectively overcome (Dennison, 1990; Ueland, 1994). Right heart failure may result from a high afterload that persists.

SIGNS AND SYMPTOMS

With cardiac disease in pregnancy, the actual lesion is responsible for the specific symptoms. Basically, cardiac disease causes problems with preload or afterload (Dennison, 1990; Ueland, 1994). Listed below are the usual signs that the cardiac condition is deteriorating in a patient with preexisting cardiac disease:

1. Dyspnea severe enough to limit usual activity
2. Progressive orthopnea
3. Paroxysmal nocturnal dyspnea
4. Syncope during or immediately following exertion
5. Chest pain associated with activity

In addition, a pregnancy with preexisting cardiac disease can increase predisposition to thromboembolic changes, palpitations, and fluid retention. These complications sometimes require prophylactic treatment or increases in dosage of current drug therapy. Other conditions of the cardiovascular system, such as chronic hypertension, can also rapidly deteriorate. Patients with chronic hypertension may develop cardiac functional compromise during pregnancy because of the increased volume expansion (see Chapter 20).

Symptoms of cardiac disease in general are classified by the functional incapacity. The classification does not change in pregnancy although symptoms may worsen. The classifications of cardiac disease (Creasy, Resnik, 1994) are as follows:

Class I: asymptomatic at all degrees of activity; uncompromised

Class II: symptomatic with increased activity; slightly compromised

Class III: symptomatic with ordinary activity; markedly compromised

Class IV: symptomatic at rest; incapacitated

These are prognostic indicators of maternal and fetal complications (Clark, 1991). Box 10-1 outlines the three maternal risk subgroups (Clark, 1991).

MATERNAL EFFECTS

Sudden, severe pulmonary edema occurs if afterload is high. If pulmonary hypertension is present in cardiac lesions such as mitral

---

Box 10-1
Maternal Cardiac Disease Risk Groups

Group I (mortality 1%)
Corrected tetralogy of Fallot
Pulmonic/tricuspid disease
Mitral stenosis (classes I, II)
Patent ductus
Ventricular septal defect
Atrial septal defect
Porcine valve
Group II (mortality 5%-15%)
Mitral stenosis with atrial
    fibrillation
Artificial heart valves
Mitral stenosis (classes III, IV)
Uncorrected tetralogy
Aortic coarctation (uncomplicated)
Aortic stenosis

Group III (mortality 25%-50%)
Aortic coarctation (complicated)
Myocardial infarction
Marfan's syndrome
True cardiomyopathy
Pulmonary hypertension

---

stenosis or tetralogy of Fallot, right cardiac failure occurs with a resultant increase in preload and decreased stroke volume.

Quite independent of hemodynamic changes, systemic emboli can occur. Patients with atrial fibrillation or mitral valve problems causing atrial fibrillation are particularly susceptible to embolic episodes if not treated adequately with anticoagulants.

Cyanotic heart disease generally does not decrease the pregnant woman's ability to oxygenate herself unless there is pulmonary hypertension. In atrial or ventricular septal defects, pulmonary hypertension may progress and reverse existing shunts. If this occurs, maternal mortality is 50% (Clark, 1991; Ueland, 1994).

A dissecting aneurysm, either with coarctation of the aorta or in Marfan's syndrome, is associated with a 50% maternal mortality. A dissecting aneurysm can develop suddenly as the pregnancy advances and fluid volume increases.

FETAL AND NEONATAL EFFECTS

Fetal effects are the result of decreased systemic circulation or decreased oxygenation. If maternal circulation is compromised because of cardiac functional incapacities, uterine blood flow may be reduced severely. In early pregnancy this can result in spontaneous abortion. If the uterine blood flow reduction occurs with advancing pregnancy, the fetus can experience effects of deprivation ranging from growth retardation to central nervous system hypoxia. Preterm delivery may be necessary if maternal life is threatened, and the resultant neonatal morbidity associated with prematurity is high.

If maternal oxygenation is impaired, as in cyanotic heart disease or in acute pulmonary edema, fetal oxygenation is also impaired. Depending on the severity and length of time of decreased oxygenation, fetal central nervous system hypoxia can result in degrees of mental retardation, fetal distress, or even fetal death (Brar and others, 1988; Garite, 1988).

If either parent has a congenital cardiac defect, the fetus has an increased risk for having a congenital cardiac defect. This could be devastating to the neonate already compromised by hypoxia or prematurity.

DIAGNOSTIC TESTING

Diagnosis of cardiac disease is made by the presentation of symptoms. Definition of the cardiac lesion, if unknown, is usually made by a cardiologist. An electrocardiogram (ECG), echocardiogram, series of laboratory tests including cardiac enzymes and electrolytes, and a chest x-ray film are the usual means, during pregnancy, for definition of the lesion or assessment of current status. When the pregnant woman is given anticoagulant therapy, coagulation studies are done. If the woman is taking digitalis, therapeutic blood levels are ascertained.

USUAL MEDICAL MANAGEMENT AND PROTOCOLS FOR NURSE PRACTITIONERS
General Management

Usual medical management is accomplished with the obstetrician and cardiologist working as a team, involving the pregnant cardiac patient in the management of her care. Cardiac medications are usually adjusted to be compatible with pregnancy, and dosages are adjusted when symptoms first present or worsen.

Early ultrasound of the fetus helps in accurate dating. Later, near 28 weeks, ultrasound can be used serially to document continued fetal growth and well-being. Fetal heart rate monitoring or biophysical profiles may be started by 24 weeks.

Bed rest, or at least restricted activity, is necessary for women with class III heart disease throughout the last trimester. If symptoms present in women with class I or ll heart disease, limitations may be necessary for maternal comfort and well-being and also for adequate fetal oxygenation. The time of presentation of symptoms of cardiac decompensation is usually when maternal fluid volume expansion is greatest. This occurs during the pregnancy near 28 weeks or in the postpartum period as the then unneeded volume is remobilized.

When cardiac disease is caused by rheumatic fever, prophylactic antibiotic therapy should be instituted during labor and continued into the postpartum period. Penicillin is the antibiotic usually used.

Throughout pregnancy and labor, care is aimed at reduction of cardiac workload, especially from the effects of tachycardia. During labor, pain relief is provided by regional anesthesia. Assistance with the delivery through the use of forceps in the second stage is often necessary. Vaginal delivery is preferred, if possible, because there are fewer hemodynamic disturbances. Sometime after 36 weeks of gestation, a plan for labor induction is made after amniocentesis shows lung maturity. In addition to other monitoring, an invasive line for hemodynamic monitoring of the mother will be necessary during labor and during the unstable postpartum period. Central venous pressure and pulmonary wedge pressure readings aid in management of preload and afterload pressures. Careful titration of fluid volume can aid in preventing pulmonary edema and cardiac overload. Oxygen at 5 to 6 L/min may be needed if cyanotic cardiac disease is present. When decompensation of the cardiac disease occurs, placing the mother's life in jeopardy, termination of the pregnancy might be necessary. This can occur before fetal viability or can result in extreme prematurity of the neonate. Consideration is first given to the safety of the mother (Gonik, 1994).

The number of cardiac transplants for young people in the chronic end stage of disease, including congenital heart disease and primary pulmonary hypertension, has increased in the past 20 years. Young females have reached childbearing years, are experiencing a good quality of life, and are thus occasionally embarking on planned pregnancies. Immune suppression is an important concept with such pregnant women because these drugs are given lifelong. The drugs are usually a combination of prednisone with either cyclosporine or azathioprine. Cyclosporine crosses the placenta, and therefore the newborn may experience immunosuppressive effects during the first week of life. In addition, cyclosporine crosses into breast milk, and therefore it is not advisable for the mother to breast-feed (Jordan, Pugh, 1996). Long-term immunosuppression poses other problems for the mother and fetus, predisposing both to infection. During the antenatal period, the pregnant woman must be closely monitored for rejection of the heart transplant and myocardial biopsies should be scheduled every 1 to 4 weeks (Fleschler, Sala, 1995; Jordan, Pugh, 1996).

Issues in the intrapartum period include planning ahead for the route of delivery, hemodynamic monitoring, analgesia-anesthesia options, and antibiotic prophylaxis. Those issues are best addressed with the team, including representatives from perinatology, neonatology, cardiology, and anesthesiology (Jordan, Pugh, 1996; Kennedy, 1995).

Drug Therapy

Drug therapy depends on the cardiac lesion. Consideration should be given to maternal benefits and fetal risks. Common drugs used in cardiac disease and pregnancy are heparin, furosemide (Lasix), digitalis, beta-blockers such as propranolol (Inderal), antidysrhythmics such as quinidine, or disopyramide phosphate (Norpace). Drugs from newer classifications may be continued from the prepregnant state if stabilization of the mother has been difficult when she is taking the drugs just mentioned.

Heparin

Heparin is the only anticoagulant recommended during pregnancy. Warfarin crosses the placenta and may have teratogenic effects and cause bleeding in the fetus. Heparin, however, has no such problems associated with its use. Ideally, the pregnant woman receiving anticoagulation therapy should be given heparin before pregnancy or as soon as possible. Prophylactic doses range from 5000 to 7500 U twice daily, 12 hours apart.

Furosemide

Furosemide (Lasix) is a commonly used diuretic. Dosage can vary from 40 to 80 mg one or two times daily. Intravenous dosage is usually ordered by the single dose and is also 40 to 80 mg, depending on the severity of fluid overload. Thiazides are rarely used because of the severe potassium deficiency that can result. Diuretics will reduce amniotic fluid volume and cross the placenta to the fetus and therefore may cause vitamin K deficiency in the fetus.

Digitalis

Digitalis is a glycoside commonly used in cardiac disease because it increases contractility and decreases heart rate. Although it does cross the placental barrier, it does not affect fetal cardiac function. However, this can decrease maternal concentrations and require dosage adjustment. In addition, it must be kept in mind that, just as myocardial contractility is increased, so can uterine contractility be affected, leading to preterm labor (Few, 1987).

Tocolytics

The drugs ritodrine and terbutaline are contraindicated in the treatment of preterm labor for the woman with cardiac disease. Beta-sympathomimetics increase cardiac rate and workload and increase the potential for pulmonary edema. Magnesium sulfate decreases calcium levels and has a direct effect on myocardial contractility. If magnesium sulfate is used to treat preterm labor, magnesium and calcium levels must be monitored frequently, because magnesium may upset the delicate balance of cardiac electrolytes, cause vasodilation, and lead to decreased blood pressure and therefore decreased cardiac output.

Propranolol

Propranolol (Inderal) may be used to treat hypertension because of the decreased pulsating effect on the aorta, or it may be used as an antidysrhythmic. It can increase uterine tone and lead to preterm labor. Propranolol decreases cardiac output and therefore can reduce uterine blood flow. Other antidysrhythmics used during pregnancy include quinidine and disopyramide phosphate. Most antidysrhythmics have not been well studied for their fetal effects (Creasy, Resnik, 1994).

Quinidine

Quinidine is used as an antidysrhythmic because it depresses myocardial excitability, conductive velocity, and contractility. It has never been studied in animals for effects on the fetus. Therefore, as with most antidysrhythmics, it is given when the benefits outweigh the risks. Because quinidine has been used for many years, as with most of the older drugs, experience with it in pregnancy is more common than with newer antidysrhythmic drugs.

Disopyramide Phosphate

Disopyramide phosphate (Norpace) is an antidysrhythmic drug with effects similar to those of quinidine. However, it is chemically unrelated to any other antidysrhythmics. It decreases the sinus node recovery period and lengthens the response time in the atrium. It has no effect on alpha- or beta-adrenergic receptors but has been reported to cause increased uterine contractility. Its use in pregnancy has been studied in animals, and no fetal anomalies have been found.

NURSING PROCESS

PREVENTION

Nursing measures must be directed toward prevention of complications. Nutrition should be adequate in iron and folic acid to prevent anemia, which would increase cardiac workload. Sodium restriction may be necessary, but intake should not fall below 2.5 g/day during pregnancy. It is important to differentiate symptoms associated with blood volume increased in normal pregnancies from early signs of volume overload in the pregnant cardiac patient.

Plans should be made early in the pregnancy for restriction of activities and possible prolonged bed rest. Relief from emotional stress can be facilitated if family care can be prearranged. During the pregnancy, attention must be directed at reducing and eliminating anxiety. The patient's anxiety regarding her own well-being, fetal well-being, and her family's care in her absence is likely to increase cardiac work load. Sedation provides only a partial solution. Realistic information about risks and benefits for mother and fetus will facilitate adequate coping and reduce anxiety over uncertainties.

When pregnancy termination must occur for the mother's safety and well-being, consideration of her future childbearing is very important. Contraceptive means may be limited. Permanent surgical intervention is often not a safe procedure for a woman with class III or IV cardiac disease. Birth control pills also are often contraindicated because of thromboembolic potential. For the sexually active couple, consistent use of the diaphragm, condoms, or foam might be a problem. Careful counseling in the area of contraception must include a realistic examination of the hazards of subsequent pregnancy to the health of the woman. Her sexual partner should be included in the counseling.

NURSING DIAGNOSES/COLLABORATIVE PROBLEMS AND INTERVENTIONS

GENERAL CARE

- **RISK FOR ALTERED HEALTH MAINTENANCE** related to cardiac limitations and knowledge deficit.

  DESIRED OUTCOMES: The patient will verbalize understanding of how pregnancy will affect her heart condition and the plan of management to prevent cardiac decompensation complications. The patient will administer drugs as ordered and verbalize understanding of side effects and beneficial effects. The woman and her family will verbalize understanding of needs for modification of activities and frequent follow-up.

  INTERVENTIONS

  Cardiac decompensation prevention

  1. When taking the initial history, determine which drugs the patient is taking. (The nurse should be aware of specific drugs commonly used in cardiac disease that are contraindicated in pregnancy and note the dosage, which may need to be changed. Women are usually very aware of potential fetal harm from any drug therapy and often have numerous questions that the nurse should be prepared to answer.)

  2. At each prenatal visit, assess blood pressure, apical/radial pulses, lung sounds, weight gain, edema, Homan sign, and chest pain.

  3. Report any signs of dysrhythmia such as palpitations, irregular heart rate, apical/radial differences, and progressive edema.

  4. Report any signs of pulmonary edema such as rales, abnormal heart sounds, a cough, and dyspnea.

  5. Report signs of thromboembolism such as pain, redness, tenderness, or swelling in the extremities or chest pain.

  6. Emphasize the importance of more frequent prenatal visits. During the first half of pregnancy, the patient is usually seen every 2 weeks. During the last half of pregnancy, she is usually seen weekly.

  7. Determine the patient's and her family's understanding of the effects of her heart disease on pregnancy and the effects of pregnancy on her heart disease.

  8. Assess for factors that increase stress.

  9. Emphasize the importance of observation for and immediate reporting of any signs of cardiac decompensation or

congestive heart failure. Such signs are generalized edema, distention of neck veins, dyspnea, pulmonary rales, frequent moist cough, or heart palpitations.

10. Instruct the patient as to the importance of daily weight. A sudden weight gain indicates fluid retention.

11. Provide the patient with information on the importance of avoiding constipation and the need to strain during a bowel movement.

12. Teach the importance of limiting activity (depending on the classification of heart disease). Patients with classes I and II need 10 hours of sleep every night and ½ hour of rest after meals in a semi-Fowler position. Patients with classes III and IV usually need bed rest for most of each day.

13. Refer to home health care or nurse specialists as indicated.

14. Refer to a high risk pregnancy support group.

Infection prevention

1. Instruct as to the importance of reporting any signs of infection immediately.

2. Be prepared to administer prophylactic antibiotics as ordered to prevent bacterial endocarditis.

Nutritional needs

1. Assess nutritional intake using a 24-hour recall. Pay particular attention to protein, iron, and folic acid intake.

2. Provide the patient and the family members who will be assisting with shopping and food preparation with information on the importance of a well-balanced diet. This will lessen the stress on the heart and decrease the risk of edema. (Protein deficiency and sodium excess can contribute to fluid retention. Inadequate iron can cause an increased workload on the heart. Decreased fiber can increase the risk of constipation.)

3. If the patient is taking a diuretic, she should be instructed to reduce dietary intake of sodium. Foods high in potassium, such as bananas, citrus fruits, and whole grains, should be included in her diet to prevent potassium deficiency, particularly when diuretics are part of the pharmacologic management.

4. Refer to a registered dietitian for nutritional advice and modifications to meet both the requirements of cardiac complications and pregnancy requirements.

5. Refer to social services for assistance with food supplementary programs.

Anticoagulation therapy

1. In the event anticoagulants become necessary, if injections are subcutaneous, be prepared to teach or reinforce heparin administration as follows (Wooldridge, Jackson, 1988):
   a. The sites should be rotated in the fatty tissue of the thighs, hips, and abdomen.
   b. The area should be cleansed in a circular motion with alcohol and then iced for 1 minute with an ice cube to reduce bruising.
   c. The injection should be given in one motion without aspiration. A syringe with a short, 25-gauge needle should be used.
   d. The area should not be rubbed after the injection.
   e. A return demonstration of the technique can be provided with normal saline.
   f. At least three correctly executed injections should be demonstrated by the woman and also by one family member.
   g. Instruct to take the medication at the same time each day.
   h. Instruct the woman to report side effects, such as bleeding gums, nosebleeds, and easy bruising or excessive tissue trauma, at injection sites.
2. Heparin can also be infused continuously subcutaneously by a pump designed for home use. Home care nursing care should be involved.

Early detection of preterm labor

1. Educate regarding recognition of signs and symptoms of preterm labor because most of the cardiac medications used in pregnancy are reported to increase uterine contractility.
2. Teach the benefits of bed rest in reducing uterine irritability and improving uterine blood flow.
3. Provide instructions as to what a contraction feels like, warning signs of preterm labor, and the importance of reporting immediately any of these signs.

Birth plan

1. Discuss with the couple their birth plan.
2. Explain any alterations such as epidural, episiotomy, and outlet forceps to decrease the workload on the heart.

Postpartum

1. Assess blood pressure, apical/radial pulses, lung sounds, weight loss, and Homan sign as condition indicates. (The first hours after delivery can be critical for maternal safety

because of the remobilization of the large blood volume of pregnancy.)

2. Assess for presence of edema and chest pain.
3. Provide relief from discomfort to reduce cardiac workload.
4. Discuss with the patient and her family their plans on discharge. Help at home will be necessary for several weeks until the patient can gradually resume her previous activities.
5. Lactation is not contraindicated since cardiac output is not compromised by lactation. The patient's medications should be evaluated for safety during lactation (Lawrence, 1989). Teach the patient to conserve energy during breast-feeding by obtaining a resting position and allowing others to burp the baby if possible. Emphasize the importance of adequate nutrition.
6. Provide counseling to the patient and her sexual partner in the area of contraception to include a realistic examination of the hazards of a subsequent pregnancy to the health of the mother. Assess knowledge of birth control methods, efficacy, and proper use. Oral contraceptives are often contraindicated because of thromboembolic potential (Hatcher and others, 1990).

- **RISK FOR IMPAIRED FETAL GAS EXCHANGE** related to specific cardiac lesion, diminished blood flow to the uterus, and decreased maternal cardiac output.

  DESIRED OUTCOMES: The fetus will remain active, and its heart rate will be maintained at a baseline between 110 and 160 with normal variability, normal reactivity, and no decelerations. The biophysical profile will continue to be greater than 6, and a nonstress test (NST) will be reactive.

  INTERVENTIONS
  1. Monitor fetal heart rate (FHR) as indicated (depending on mother's condition).
  2. Teach mother to keep a daily fetal movement chart after 24 weeks of gestation.
  3. Explain rationale and procedure for fetal surveillance studies as ordered, such as biophysical profiles or NST.
  4. When using the electronic fetal monitor (EFM), evaluate FHR for tachycardia, bradycardia, late or variable decelerations, and loss of long- or short-term variability.
  5. During labor, encourage the mother to lie on her side with oxygen by face mask.

CRITICAL CARE

- **POTENTIAL COMPLICATIONS: DYSRHYTHMIAS, CONGESTIVE HEART FAILURE (CHF), THROMBOEMBOLISM, PULMONARY EDEMA, ELECTROLYTE AND FLUID IMBALANCE, HYPERTENSION, DISSEMINATED INTRAVASCULAR COAGULATION (DIC), AND SUPERIMPOSED PREGNANCY COMPLICATIONS** related to increased circulating volume, increased workload during labor, and postpartum remobilization of fluid superimposed on an already compromised cardiac state.

  DESIRED OUTCOME: The complications will be minimized or managed as indicated by a normal sinus rhythm without S_3 or S_4 heart sounds; no signs of CHF; normal pulmonary artery pressure (PAP), pulmonary arterial wedge pressure (PAWP), and central venous pressure (CVP); absence of chest pain, frothy or bloody sputum, and pain or redness in lower extremity vascular beds; clear lung fields; and normal fluid balance and serum electrolytes.

  INTERVENTIONS

  1. If any fluid complications develop, be prepared to assist with insertion of invasive monitoring lines and transport when stabilized to a level III perinatal center if not already in one of these centers.
  2. Begin ECG monitoring of mother.
  3. Set up equipment for insertion of invasive lines.
  4. As the line is being inserted, the ECG monitor should be observed for dysrhythmias, especially premature ventricular contractions. Observe waveforms for changes indicating specific passage through the right atrium (low-amplitude waves), right ventricle (tall-amplitude waves), and pulmonary wedge (smaller, lower pressures with diastolic and systolic waves).
  5. Following insertion, continuous ECG monitoring for the cardiac rate is usual.
  6. Obtain CVP, PAP, and pulmonary capillary wedge pressure (PCWP) waveform readings every 1 to 4 hours as appropriate to degree of stabilization. (Table 10-1 outlines normal readings for each and the significance of low or high readings.)
  7. Report S_3 and S_4 heart sounds; increased PAP, PAWP, or CVP; or any dysrhythmias observed.
  8. Monitor vital signs every 1 to 4 hours as indicated, including maternal temperature.
  9. Assess lung fields every 1 to 4 hours, and report all abnormalities.

TABLE 10-1 Hemodynamic pressure readings

	Normal pregnancy	Low	High
CVP (measures right ventricular end-diastolic pressure when tricuspid valve is open and therefore right atrium and ventricle are common chambers)	1-10 mm Hg	Reflects inadequate circulatory volume from: Hemorrhage Third spacing Extreme vasodilation	Reflects: Increased preload High pulmonary resistance such as pulmonary embolus Poor cardiac contractility
Systolic PAP (reflects pressure in pulmonary artery when right ventricle is contracting and pulmonic valve is open)	15-25 mm Hg	Reflects a decreased venous return to heart from: Hemorrhage Third spacing Extreme vasodilation	Reflects: Increased blood volume Pulmonary arteriole constriction in response to increased pCO_2 and decreased pO_2 Increased with pulmonary disease such as embolus or edema
Diastolic PAP (reflects left heart when pulmonary valve is closed and left valves are open)	8-10 mm Hg		
PCWP (reflects only pressure from left side of heart)	3-10 mm Hg	Results from: A low circulating volume Extreme vasodilation	Reflects: Increased preload Poor contractility Increased afterload Increased pCO_2

CVP, Central venous pressure; *PAP*, pulmonary artery pressure; *PCWP*, pulmonary capillary wedge pressure.

10. Insert Foley catheter, and monitor intake and output hourly. (Urinary output of at least 30 ml/hr is a sensitive measure of adequacy of circulating volume to other vital areas of the body.)
11. Place a continuous FHR monitor, and observe for signs of fetal compromise.
12. Weigh daily, and assess for edema.
13. Administer cardiac glycosides, diuretics, vasodilators, anticoagulants, and antibiotics as ordered.
14. Administer oxygen as ordered.
15. Administer salt-poor intravenous fluids as ordered for maternal hydration to run only at a specifically ordered rate via infusion pump.
16. Inspect the site of arterial catheter insertion at least once each shift for signs of infection such as redness or drainage.
17. Prepare for delivery. If vaginal birth is to be attempted, prepare for epidural anesthesia and shortened second-stage labor with forceps. If cesarean birth is planned, prepare for epidural anesthesia.
18. Notice the level III nursery.
19. Continue postpartum hemodynamic monitoring for a minimum of 24 to 72 hours.
20. Provide photographs of delivered infant for mother, and encourage early family contact.
21. Refer to nursing specialists for critical care assistance.
22. Refer to social service representative or chaplain for psychosocial or spiritual assistance.

- **RISK FOR FEAR** related to potential intensive care, neonatal intensive care, or general threats to well-being of mother or baby.
  DESIRED OUTCOME: The mother and her family will verbalize fears and anxieties related to critical events and begin to identify strategies for dealing with them.
  INTERVENTIONS
  1. Take family and mother, if able, for a tour of the level III nursery.
  2. Encourage family participation in newborn visits and care.
  3. Facilitate and encourage exploration of feelings regarding maternal and newborn outcomes.
  4. Refer to intensive care nursery parent support group.
  5. Refer to social services for assistance with home care.
  6. Refer for and assist with follow-up with physician specialists.
  7. Provide education for medication and medical follow-up.

- ■ **RISK FOR ANTICIPATORY GRIEVING** related to potential loss or actual loss of the pregnancy or death of the fetus or newborn.
  DESIRED OUTCOMES: The family members will identify and discuss fears for maternal and fetal well-being. If loss occurs, they will work through the normal grief stages within a normal period.
  INTERVENTIONS
    1. Discuss loss- and grief-related issues in the antepartum period as appropriate.
    2. Include family members in the decisions made for medical management.
    3. Provide support and follow-up as indicated in Chapter 6.

CONCLUSION

The primary goal of nursing care for the pregnant woman and her family when cardiac disease complicates the pregnancy is to reduce potential risks of complications. This is accomplished by education of the woman and her partner; routine assessment of all systems involved; referral to appropriate nursing, nutritional, social, and medical experts; and facilitation of patient participation in decisions. Identification of fears and solutions helps the family to maintain desired control of care. Anticipatory guidance assists in preliminary planning for potential problems and their solutions. The nurse is often in the best position to advocate for the family and coordinate the multidisciplinary team.

BIBLIOGRAPHY

Brar H and others: Umbilical cord acid base changes associated with perinatal cardiac failure, *Am J Obstet Gynecol* 158(3):511-516, 1988.

Burlew B: Managing the pregnant patient with heart disease, *Clin Cardiol* 13(11):757-762, 1990.

Capeless E, Clapp J: Cardiovascular changes in early phase of pregnancy, *Am J Obstet Gynecol* 161(6):1449-1452, 1989.

Clark S: Cardiac disease in pregnancy, *Obstet Gynecol Clin North Am* 18(2):237-256, 1991.

Creasy R, Resnik R, editors: *Maternal-fetal medicine: principles and practice,* ed 3, Philadelphia, 1994, Saunders.

Dennison R: Understanding the four determinants of cardiac output, *Nurs 90,* pp 35-41, July 1990.

Few B: Dioxin immune fab, *MCN Am J Matern Child Nurs* 12:431-432, Nov/Dec 1987.

Fleschler R, Sala D: Pregnancy after organ transplantation, *J Obstet Gynecol Neonatal Nurs* 24(5):413-422, 1995.

Forster R, Joyce T: Spinal opioids and the treatment of the obstetric patient with cardiac disease, *Clin Perinatol* 16(4):955-974, 1989.

Garite T: Sinusoidal pattern from anemia, *Contemp OB/GYN,* pp 42-46, May, 1988.

Gonik B: Intensive care monitoring of the critically ill pregnant woman. In Creasy R, Resnik R, editors: *Maternal-fetal medicine: principles and practice,* ed 3, Philadelphia, 1994, Saunders.

Hatcher R and others: *Contraceptive technology,* ed 15, New York, 1990, Irvington.

Jordan E, Pugh L: Pregnancy after cardiac transplantation: principles of nursing care, *Obstet Gynecol Neonatal Nurs* 25(2):131-135, 1996.

Kendrick J: Open mitral commisurotomy during pregnancy: a case study, *J Obstet Gynecol Neonatal Nurs* 20(3):243-252, 1991.

Kennedy B: Mitral stenosis: implications for critical care obstetric nursing, *Obstet Gynecol Neonatal Nurs* 24(5):406-412, 1995.

Lawrence R: *Breast feeding: a guide for the medical profession,* ed 3, St Louis, 1989, Mosby.

Mashini I and others: Serial noninvasive evaluation of cardiovascular hemodynamics during pregnancy, *Am J Obstet Gynecol* 156(5):1208-1213, 1987.

Metcalf J and others: *Heart disease and pregnancy: physiology and management,* Boston, 1986, Little, Brown.

Rokey R and others: Inaccurate noninvasive mitral valve area calculation during pregnancy, *Obstet Gynecol* 84(6):950-955, 1994.

Schmidt J and others: Peripartum cardiomyopathy, *J Obstet Gynecol Neonatal Nurs* 18(6):465-472, 1989.

Shime J and others: Congenital heart disease in pregnancy: short and long term implications, *Am J Obstet Gynecol* 156(2):313-332, 1987.

Simpson W and others: Acute pericarditis complicated by cardiac tamponade during pregnancy, *Am J Obstet Gynecol* 160(2):415-416, 1989.

Sullivan J, Ramanathan K: Management of medical problems in pregnancy: severe cardiac disease, *N Engl J Med* 313:304, 1985.

Ueland K: Cardiac diseases. In Creasy R, Resnik R, editors: *Maternal-fetal medicine: principles and practice,* ed 3, Philadelphia, 1994, Saunders.

Wooldridge J, Jackson J: Injection techniques affect incidence and extent of bruising and induration following subcutaneous heparin injection, *Heart Lung* 17:476-482, 1988.

CHAPTER

11

Renal Disease

Of the various physiologic alterations in pregnancy, those affecting the urinary tract are the most striking. Improvements in our knowledge related to pregnancy care have meant better care for pregnant women with renal disease. This chapter focuses on urinary tract infection (UTI), chronic renal disease, pregnancy in the dialysis patient, and acute renal failure in pregnancy.

INCIDENCE

Infection

Asymptomatic Bacteriuria

Asymptomatic bacteriuria occurs in 2% to 10% of the pregnant population (Creasy, Resnik, 1994). During pregnancy, if the bacteriuria is left untreated, 40% of women will develop symptoms of UTI. Approximately 30% of women with untreated asymptomatic bacteriuria will develop pyelonephritis during pregnancy.

Symptomatic Bacteriuria

Symptomatic bacteriuria occurs in another 1% to 1.5%. Women with a history of previous UTI and current bacteriuria are 10 times more likely to develop symptoms during pregnancy than women without either feature (Creasy, Resnik, 1994).

Acute Renal Failure

Acute renal failure rarely occurs during pregnancy, but it can be triggered by various complications of pregnancy.

Renal Disease

The incidence of renal disease in pregnancy varies with the form it takes.

Renal Calculi

Renal calculi rarely occur in pregnancy. Less than 1 in 1000 pregnancies will require surgery to correct this problem.

Lupus

Lupus is exacerbated during pregnancy in 40% of women who are affected by the disease. If, before the pregnancy, renal involvement was present, the renal status may deteriorate during or immediately after the pregnancy.

Acute Glomerulonephritis

Acute glomerulonephritis during pregnancy is extremely rare, occurring in 1 of 40,000 pregnancies. This is attributed to the usual failure to ovulate in women with the disease.

Diabetic Renal Disease

Diabetic renal disease is seen more frequently now that better control can be established and it is known that pregnancy does not adversely affect diabetes. Kimmelstiel-Wilson disease is, however, rarely seen in pregnancy, probably because of the failure of ovulation associated with the disease.

Polycystic Kidney Disease

Because polycystic kidney disease does not generally become evident until after the age of 40 years, it is also rarely seen in pregnancy. It is associated with autosomal dominant genetic transmission. Therefore there is a 50% chance of its transmission to each child born to a parent before the disease becomes evident in that parent.

Following Renal Transplant

In the past, pregnancy following kidney transplant was extremely rare, probably not only because of the renal status, but also secondary to advanced maternal age by the time of transplant. Recent reports of women successfully completing pregnancy on continuous ambulatory peritoneal dialysis (Hou, 1987) have given a more optimistic outlook for transplantation potential and pregnancy prognosis (Davison, Lindheimer, 1994). Immunosuppressive drug therapy must be considered antenatally and postpartum (Fleschler, Sala, 1995).

ETIOLOGY
Infection

The cause of UTI is often bacteria from the gastrointestinal tract contaminating the perineal area. Often the organism implicated is *Escherichia coli.* It is more common when contaminants from the rectal area are brought forward across the urethral meatus during perineal hygiene. It can also occur from trauma to the meatus during sexual intercourse forcing perineal contaminants into the urethra. Bacteria may migrate from the urethra into the bladder and proliferate before the next urination. Bacteria may also pass into the dilated ureters during pregnancy and migrate into the kidney itself, causing inflammation of the tubules. Occasionally other perineal organisms, such as yeast, are introduced into the bladder and cause infection.

Staphylococcal or streptococcal bacteria can enter the blood in the kidney and result in renal tissue reaction to the organism or to its toxins. However, these organisms rarely cause infection during pregnancy.

Acute Renal Failure

Acute renal failure can be precipitated by hemorrhagic shock caused by placenta previa, abruptio placentae, uterine rupture, operative trauma, or postpartum uterine atony. Endotoxic shock in the cases of chorioamnionitis, pyelonephritis, or puerperal sepsis can also precipitate acute renal failure. Urinary tract obstruction is a third cause. A urinary obstruction can be caused by polyhydramnios, ureter calculi, pelvic or broad ligament hematoma, or damage to the ureters during a cesarean delivery.

Renal Disease

Renal disease can be caused by a UTI before or during pregnancy, can be the result of other diseases such as diabetes, or can occur in pregnancy from complications such as hypertensive disorders of pregnancy.

NORMAL PHYSIOLOGY

The kidneys fulfill several functions essential for the body. They excrete water, electrolytes, and nitrogenous waste products. They perform a major function in acid-base balance and are active in the renin-angiotensin-aldosterone system. The kidney also produces erythropoietin, which aids in stimulating red blood cell production.

The kidneys have the largest blood supply of any organ in the body. Renal blood flow accounts for 20% to 25% of the cardiac output. The blood supply to each kidney is supplied by a renal artery, which branches finally into the afferent arteriole, leading into the glomerulus. From the glomerulus the efferent arteriole leads out via branches into the renal vein.

The filtration of the blood through the glomerulus is the result of four forces acting on the capillaries: the permeability of the capillary walls, the hydrostatic pressure in the glomerular capillaries, the hydrostatic pressure in the glomerular capsule, and the osmotic pressure of the circulating plasma proteins. It is the pressure within the glomerular capillaries that determines the filtration rate. Glomerular filtration produces a protein-free filtrate of plasma. The glomeruli act as ultrafilters with microscopic pores. The microscopic pores do not normally allow the larger protein or glucose molecules through but rather send them along the circulatory route to the tubules. The major excretory product into urine is sodium.

The tubules act on the glomerular filtrate to produce urine. Substances are reabsorbed from the glomerular filtrate either actively or passively. Substances such as water passively follow sodium that is actively reabsorbed into the urine. Urea, a nitrogenous waste product, diffuses passively. Glucose is actively reabsorbed against the concentration gradient after being freely filtered in the glomerulus.

The tubule cells also secrete a number of substances, such as potassium, hydrogen, ammonium (NH_4), and organic anions and cations. As the glomerular filtrate flows through the proximal tubule, sodium is actively reabsorbed and chloride follows passively. Water follows with the change in osmotic pressure. As it reaches the loop of Henle in the tubule, the fluid volume is reduced by 80%. As the fluid flows through the thin, descending loop of Henle, water is removed passively because of the hypertonicity of the interstitial tissues. As the fluid enters the distal convoluted tubules, it becomes hypotonic.

If circulating antidiuretic hormone is elevated, the distal tubule is permeable to water and the urinary fluid then becomes isotonic to the interstitial fluid. Chloride, sodium, and passive osmotic diffusion of water further reduce the urinary fluid volume as it enters the collecting duct, where it changes from an isotonic to a hypertonic fluid. The urinary fluid and sodium removed in the loop of Henle return to the general circulation.

If the antidiuretic hormone level is low, the distal tubule is not permeable to water and the urinary fluid remains hypotonic. It loses its solutes and increases its hypotonicity. The ultimate outcome is that the urine is both dilute and increased in volume.

The kidney regulates acid-base balance by maintaining plasma bicarbonate between 26 and 28 mEq/L in response to the respiratory system's maintenance of carbonic acid at 1.3 to 1.4 mEq/L. Organic anions in the urine accept hydrogen ions, producing carbonic acid, which is in turn broken down into water and carbon dioxide. Ammonia (a combination of nitrogen and three hydrogen ions) takes on another hydrogen ion and becomes NH_4 and then is excreted in the urine. In this way the kidney serves as an efficient buffering mechanism.

During pregnancy a number of alterations occur in renal function. Secondary to prostaglandin E_2, renal blood flow increases, vascular resistance decreases, and glomerular filtration rate increases 30% to 50% over that in the nonpregnant state. Because of this increased filtration rate, nitrogenous waste products such as creatinine, urea, and uric acid are cleared in greater quantities. Therefore urine clearance levels are higher and serum levels are lower than in nonpregnant women.

As the filtrate enters the tubules, considerable changes in the mechanisms controlling salt and water excretion occur. Progesterone normally causes increased salt loss. In pregnancy this is countered by a rise in aldosterone to two to three times nonpregnant levels. As a result, sodium is actually retained in the tissues in larger amounts, thus aiding in the necessary volume expansion of pregnancy.

The healthy pregnant woman also excretes larger amounts of sugar in her urine. This is not related to the blood glucose levels but rather to an intermittent tubular failure to reabsorb glucose.

Amino acid excretion is known to be increased in pregnancy. This is thought to be caused by a partial failure of the normal reabsorptive mechanisms. The increased excretion of amino acids is related to high levels of cortisol in pregnancy.

Water-soluble vitamins, such as ascorbic acid, nicotinic acid, and folates, are also excreted at higher levels in the urine. This increased excretion is caused by failure of the tubules to reabsorb and can be serious when folate and protein intake is marginal.

Another important consideration of the high nutrient content of the urine is acknowledging its value as a culture medium for bacteria. Progesterone enhances the potential for UTI by relaxing the musculature of the bladder and the ureters. The dilation of the ureters, especially on the right side, is further compromised by the obstruction of the gravid uterus. All these factors contribute to the likelihood of urinary stasis of a fluid rich in nutrients, which substantially increases the potential for ascending UTI.

The activity of the renin-angiotensin system is greatly increased in pregnancy. Progesterone stimulates the increased plasma level of the enzyme renin. It is generally assumed that the maternal kidney is primarily responsible for this increase, although it is believed that the uterus is also a source of renin (Creasy, Resnik, 1994).

Renin then acts to form angiotensin, which in turn increases the production of aldosterone. The aldosterone increase preserves sodium and facilitates blood volume expansion. The sensitivity to the presser effects of renin-angiotensin is low during pregnancy, and normally the blood pressure does not rise.

PATHOPHYSIOLOGY

When infection from urinary bacteria ascends the urinary tract, the renal tubules can become inflamed. The inflammatory process leads to a decrease in tubular function. Reabsorption of sodium into the urinary fluid and secretion of buffering substances are affected adversely if large localized areas become inflamed. Sodium will then be retained in body tissues, and water will remain compartmentalized in tissues or in the intravascular space, which can cause edema or increased cardiac afterload.

Secretion of buffering substances may also be reduced. When buffering substances, such as potassium, ammonia, and organic ions, are deficient in quantity, free hydrogen ions cannot be absorbed. The blood pH will reflect the increased carbonic acid with a tendency toward acidemia. Concurrent conditions such as diabetes can complicate potential acidemia because of nephropathy or metabolic failures inherent in the disease.

Hypertensive renal disease, diabetic nephropathy, pregnancy-induced hypertension, and glomerulonephritis can be differentiated by the specific histology of the lesion in the kidneys. Lesions can be either in the glomeruli or in the tubules. Some affect the vasculature surrounding or comprising the glomeruli and tubules; others affect the cells within the glomeruli or tubules. When the vasculature of the renal tissues is damaged and blood supply to the kidneys is compromised, renin activity increases and blood pressure rises. Pregnancy sometimes initially improves the blood pressure because of the vasodilating effect of progesterone. However, this may be counteracted by a continuation of sensitivity to the presser effect, and preeclampsia may become superimposed.

If the glomeruli are damaged, filtration rate cannot increase to meet the demands of pregnancy. Nitrogenous waste cannot be removed from the bloodstream in sufficient quantities and builds up in abnormal amounts in the bloodstream. Creatinine, uric acid, and urea levels rise in the serum and fall in the urine.

Increased excretion of nitrogenous waste into the sweat and saliva can produce a characteristic ammonia odor. This can also cause itching and irritation of the skin.

If tubular cells or the surrounding vasculature is damaged, the primary tubular functions are affected. Because the tubules serve as the major sodium pump, it is this function that is dramatically decreased. Sodium cannot be pulled into the urine fluid in the proximal tubule, and therefore water cannot follow. Urine output will then reflect this in a reduced volume, with sodium remaining elevated in the blood and water increasing in the intravascular space. Sodium and water will therefore be increased in the tissues and result in edema.

If proteins are lost into the glomerular filtrate because of damage to the micropores, osmotic pressure changes and fluid is lost from the intravascular space into the tissue more readily. Because pregnancy favors increased spillage of protein, a marginal kidney function can cause greater likelihood of spillage of large quantities of protein into the urine.

SIGNS AND SYMPTOMS

Infection

Bladder Infection

Bladder infection may be heralded by frequency, dysuria, and urgency of urination or suprapubic or low back pain.

Kidney Infection

Pyelonephritis is usually present when fever, chills, nausea, vomiting, malaise, and flank pain occur.

Renal Disease

Chronic renal disease from other origins can be associated with generalized edema and proteinuria, increased blood pressure, and decreased urinary volume. These symptoms rarely worsen during pregnancy unless hypertensive disorders of pregnancy are superimposed on an impaired renal function.

Nitrogenous Waste

Symptoms of increased nitrogenous waste products in the bloodstream include mental confusion, apathy, and itching of the skin. Urinary output may be diminished, and the specific gravity will be low.

Electrolyte Imbalance

Symptoms of electrolyte imbalance, especially potassium, sodium, and calcium excesses or deficits, can appear.

Potassium excess. Potassium excess occurs when the plasma potassium is above 5.6 mEq/L. Signs include tachycardia and later bradycardia, electrocardiogram (ECG) changes with a high T wave and depressed ST segment, and oliguria, abdominal distention, or diarrhea.

Potassium deficit. Potassium deficit occurs when the plasma potassium is below 4 mEq/L. Signs include anorexia, abdominal distention, muscle weakness, hypotension, and dysrhythmias. Severe hypokalemia can cause heart block.

Sodium excess. Sodium excess occurs when the plasma sodium is greater than 147 mEq/L. Signs include a specific gravity of urine above 1.030; restlessness; dry, sticky mucous membranes; oliguria; hypertension; tachycardia; and edema. Severe hypernatremia can cause convulsions.

Sodium deficit. Sodium deficit does not occur.

Calcium excess. Calcium excess occurs when plasma calcium levels are above 5.5 mEq/L. Signs include drowsiness, headaches, irritability, muscle weakness, hypertension, anorexia, and flank pain. Severe hypercalcemia may cause heart block.

Calcium deficit. Calcium deficit occurs when plasma calcium levels are less than 4.5 mEq/L. Signs include irritability, twitching around the mouth, feeling of numbness, muscle spasms, hypotension, dysrhythmias, and diarrhea. Severe hypocalcemia may cause convulsions.

Base bicarbonate deficit. Primary base bicarbonate deficit can occur because of the inability of the tubules to secrete buffers. Metabolic acidosis may develop. Signs include urine pH below 6.0, plasma pH below 7.35, disorientation, and shortness of breath or deep, rapid breathing.

Fluid Imbalance

If renal tissues are severely damaged from hypertensive lesions, diabetic nephropathic lesions, or infectious processes, the loss of intravascular osmotic pressure can produce systemic and pulmonary edema. Signs and symptoms of pulmonary edema are sudden in onset and include shortness of breath, rales, frothy sputum, and decreased pO_2.

Other Signs of Severe Renal Damage

Other signs of severe renal damage include serum potassium excess, which can lead to cardiac dysrhythmias, dilation of the myocardium, and cardiac arrest. Serum calcium levels may also be low, with similar cardiac effects. Loss of buffering can lead to signs of metabolic acidosis, including a compensatory increase in respiratory rate.

MATERNAL EFFECTS

Infection in the urinary tract may predispose the woman to preterm labor. The exact mechanism is not clear, and the cause-and-effect relationship is controversial (Creasy, Resnik, 1994). Certainly, repeated UTIs increase the likelihood of the same organisms infecting the fetal membranes.

Severe, chronic renal impairment usually causes infertility, so it is rarely seen in pregnant women. Chronic renal impairment does not usually deteriorate during pregnancy unless severe preeclampsia or eclampsia is superimposed on the disease. If that occurs, lesions in the kidneys caused by preeclampsia or eclampsia can compromise what function is left and precipitate total renal failure (Creasy, Resnik, 1994).

FETAL AND NEONATAL EFFECTS

Because of the loss of water from the plasma volume, circulation to the uterus can be diminished. The fetus can suffer nutritionally from the resultant deficiency. Intrauterine growth retardation is common in the fetus of a woman with renal disease. If hypertension is also present, arterial resistance to blood flow into the intervillous space can cause chronic hypoxemia of the fetus. Depending on the severity and chronicity of hypoxia, the fetus can suffer central nervous system damage and face potential demise.

DIAGNOSTIC TESTING
Infection

The diagnosis of asymptomatic or symptomatic bacteriuria is made by obtaining a clean-catch urine specimen and doing a quantitative urine culture. A bacteria count of the same species greater than 10^5/ml of urine is significant. A presumptive diagnosis can be made on urinalysis with bacteria greater than 20 in centrifuged urine or white blood cells greater than 5 to 10 on high-power field (hpf) when symptoms are present. All pregnant women should be screened for asymptomatic bacteriuria with a quantitative urine culture early in their prenatal care.

Significant bacteriuria may represent either bladder or kidney infection. The differentiation is made by the symptoms presented. However, asymptomatic pyelonephritis can occur, just as bladder infection can be asymptomatic. Asymptomatic pyelonephritis should be suspected when urine cultures detect recurrent or persistent infection despite antibiotic therapy. It is for this reason that urine cultures should be repeated after a course of antibiotic therapy.

Renal Disease

When disease or complications of pregnancy exist and there is renal impairment, renal function studies are usually done to ascertain the degree of impairment. It is therefore common to do renal function studies for baseline data in pregnant women who have class D or greater diabetes, have systemic lupus, have a history of chronic renal disease or chronic hypertension, or develop pregnancy-induced hypertension. Such laboratory studies include 24-hour urine collection for creatinine clearance, serum creatinine, serum uric acid, blood urea nitrogen (BUN), and total urinary protein. Laboratory values differ in pregnancy beginning as early as 8 to 10 weeks of gestation. This should be considered when interpreting the results. Table 11-1 describes differences between nonpregnant and pregnant normal values.

Renal biopsy for diagnosis of a specific renal lesion is

TABLE 11-1 Renal function studies

Study	Nonpregnant normal value	Pregnant normal value
Blood urea nitrogen (BUN)	10-16 mg/dl	8.7 ± 1.5 mg/dl
Serum creatinine	0.67-1.2 mg/dl	0.6-1.28 mg/dl
Uric acid	4.2 ± 1.2 mg/dl	3 ± 0.17 mg/dl
Urinary creatinine clearance	100 mg/dl	140 mg/dl
24-hr urinary protein	Not different	Not greater than 300 mg/24 hr

Modified from Good Samaritan Regional Medical Center Laboratory Manual, Phoenix, 1989.

contraindicated during pregnancy because of the increased blood flow to the kidney. Increases in capillary pressures predispose the kidney to greater potential for hemorrhage, which can lead to further kidney damage.

The differentiation of chronic hypertension versus pregnancy-induced hypertension is made on the basis of persistent hypertension before 20 weeks of gestation. If preeclampsia does not develop, the differentiation can be made based on the existence or absence of generalized edema and proteinuria. Concurrent hypertension is not manifested by generalized edema nor often by proteinuria.

Other diagnostic studies, such as renal ultrasound, can aid in the diagnosis of obstruction of the ureters or pyelonephritis. Radiographic studies, such as the intravenous pyelogram, have rarely been used in pregnancy since the advent of sophisticated ultrasonic examinations.

USUAL MEDICAL MANAGEMENT AND PROTOCOLS FOR NURSE PRACTITIONERS
General Management

Treatment of renal disease in pregnancy depends on the nature of the disease.

Infection

UTI is treated with antibiotics. Asymptomatic bacteriuria and symptomatic bacteriuria are treated primarily with ampicillin because *Escherichia coli* is usually the causative organism. Antibiotic therapy must be continued in maximum doses for 10 to 14 days. High doses are required during pregnancy because of increased excretion caused by greater renal blood flow. If reculture demonstrates continued bacterial growth, the course of antibiotics must be reinstituted for 6 weeks. Reculture is again done, and if it is positive, an antimicrobial such as nitrofurantoin can be continued for the duration of the pregnancy (Creasy, Resnik, 1994). If infection has been recurrent during the pregnancy or if acute pyelonephritis occurs, a postpartum intravenous pyelogram is often done to rule out an obstruction in the urinary tract (see Chapter 24).

Acute Renal Failure

Treatment of sudden, acute renal failure in the pregnant woman resembles that of the nonpregnant population. The aim of treatment is to retard the development of uremic symptoms and restore acid-base balance, electrolyte balance, and volume homeostasis. The choice of hemodialysis or peritoneal dialysis depends on the experience of staff and the availability of staff consultation. If acute renal failure occurs during pregnancy, termination of the pregnancy is usually necessary for the mother's safety.

Chronic Renal Disease

The treatment for chronic renal disease is more complicated. The hypertension that is frequently associated with the disease requires control with an antihypertensive drug. The urinary output and fluid intake must be closely monitored to prevent fluid overload. Salt solutions must be administered with great caution because of the inability to excrete large quantities of salt and the potential for overwhelming edema, especially in the lungs. Diuretics can be used to aid in excretion of retained fluid, and electrolyte balance must then be closely monitored. If acidosis occurs, lack of an adequate buffering system in the kidneys can create further problems when salt solutions must be administered for their alkalinizing effects. Because the production of erythropoietin is suppressed in chronic renal failure, it is not uncommon to find an associated anemia in pregnancy. Coupled with the tendency for hemodilution on hemoglobin measurement, the anemia can be quite severe, causing shortness of breath, easy fatigue, and failure of fetal growth. These signs may be initially overlooked and attributed to other causes. Increased folic acid and iron supplementation will assist normal physiology and counteract some pathologic findings.

The effects of hypertension, loss of protein, and retention of sodium and water can create a life-threatening situation for the mother. If the fetus has little chance of surviving, the choice for termination of the pregnancy should be offered to the mother. If the maternal condition is likely to deteriorate, the risks and benefits of continuing the pregnancy should be discussed with the woman and her family. For the pregnancy that continues, fetal evaluation will be ordered. Ultrasound examinations may be done every 2 weeks from 24 weeks on. Nonstress tests (NSTs) and contraction stress tests (CSTs) are usually done weekly after 26 weeks. Daily fetal activity charts should also be kept.

End-Stage Renal Disease

Recent attempts at managing pregnancy complicated by end-stage renal disease with continuous ambulatory peritoneal dialysis (CAPD) have provided improved success in pregnancy outcome (Elliott and others, 1991). The advantages of CAPD are that there are not wide swings in blood chemistries proving to be fatal to most pregnancies and, during dialysis, there are not vast differences in blood pressure and circulating volume to the uterus and placenta as are seen with hemodialysis. Most patients who become pregnant with end-stage renal disease do so accidentally and without the advantage of preconceptual management considerations. Therefore both surgical termination of pregnancy and spontaneous fetal loss probably cause fetal loss rates to be artificially high.

When CAPD is used to manage a high risk pregnancy complicated by end-stage renal disease, the route of delivery requires special consideration. An emergency abdominal incision will in all likelihood permanently scar the peritoneum such that the peritoneal membrane is not able to be used for dialysis. Therefore a cesarean birth is best preplanned. An extraperitoneal incision, low in the abdominal wall, will cause the least amount of peritoneal scarring and disruption of the integrity of the peritoneal membrane. With CAPD, fetal surveillance and testing also become more complicated. It is easiest to conduct NSTs during the brief 10 to 15 minutes that the abdominal cavity is most empty of dialysate. This occurs at the end of draining and the beginning of the immediate refilling phase during the next new exchange.

Abdominal size and growth will restrict the amount of dialysate used in each exchange. Hence the frequency and the concentration of dialysate solution will be adjusted to accommodate pregnancy growth. Dialysate is a ready route to deliver $MgSO_4$ and insulin. Because diabetes can be the precipitating cause of renal disease, the addition of insulin to the dialysate may make euglycemia easier to maintain. Likewise, preterm labor is a common complication with CAPD, and the addition of $MgSO_4$ to the dialysate makes preterm labor easier to control and manage than intravenous administration of $MgSO_4$ (Elliott and others, 1991).

Drug Therapy

Antihypertensive Agents

The hypertensive pregnant woman with renal disease is treated with antihypertensives and diuretics. The antihypertensive of choice is usually methyldopa (Aldomet) or hydralazine. Home instruction should include information about possible side effects such as light-headedness or extreme lethargy. Both drugs should be taken at the same times each day.

Diuretics

Diuretics are often used if fluid retention is contributing to hypertension. They also help to prevent pulmonary edema. Any diuretic can cause electrolyte imbalance. The pregnant woman should be instructed especially to report signs of potassium deficit and to help prevent this condition with an increased dietary intake of potassium. Bananas and citrus fruits are high in potassium.

Antimicrobials

Antimicrobials will be prescribed for UTIs. It is important, for maintenance of blood levels, to administer them at evenly spaced intervals. The woman should be instructed to drink more fluids and to take the entire prescription. In the hospital setting, when antimicrobials are given intravenously, the site should be inspected for an inflammatory reaction. The site should also be changed every 48 hours to prevent phlebitis.

Tetracyclines are contraindicated for use in pregnancy because of rare maternal acute fatty liver necrosis. In addition, they bind with calcium orthophosphates and cause a permanent yellow staining of the fetal dentition. Chloramphenicol is not used in pregnancy because of the fatal gray syndrome that occurs in infants born of mothers receiving the drug. Sulfonamides and nitrofurantoin are contraindicated somewhat in the last trimester; this is because of their potential for increasing levels of fetal bilirubin.

NURSING PROCESS

PREVENTION

Prevention of symptomatic UTIs is greatly aided by nursing interventions. Pregnant women should be educated to practice correct perineal hygiene and to report any indication of vaginitis or a UTI. Routine evaluation of the urine should be carried out at each office visit. The voided specimen should be fresh, not saved from home, and should be evaluated for protein, nitrites, or leukocyte esterase, which are produced in increased amounts when bacterial growth is significant. If protein is 1+ or more in the absence of pregnancy-induced hypertension or nitrites are evident, a clean-catch or sterile catheterized specimen should be obtained for urinalysis, culture, and sensitivity studies. The pregnant woman should be encouraged to drink at least 3000 ml of fluid every 24 hours.

Prevention of complications from existing renal disease is also important. A careful history should include questions regarding repeated UTIs, hypertension when not pregnant, and renal function studies if hypertension, diabetes, or collagen vascular diseases have been previously diagnosed. This information will help in screening those women at risk for complications such as preeclampsia, pulmonary edema, uteroplacental insufficiency, and progression of existing renal disease.

NURSING DIAGNOSES/COLLABORATIVE PROBLEMS AND INTERVENTIONS

GENERAL CARE: INFECTION

■ **RISK FOR URINARY TRACT INFECTION** related to changes in vaginal pH, dilation of the ureters, stasis of urine, improper perineal hygiene, insufficient oral intake of fluids, or increased susceptibility secondary to history of UTI or pyelonephritis.

DESIRED OUTCOMES: The patient will be free of infection as evidenced by absence of dysuria, urgency, frequency, and flank pain. The urine will be free of nitrites, be clear, have a normal odor, and have a protein level less than 2+.

INTERVENTIONS
1. Do dipstick urine test for protein, nitrites, and/or leukocyte esterase each antepartum office visit and at least weekly for hospitalized patients.
2. Assess for symptoms of burning, frequency, and flank pain at each visit and if patient presents with signs of preterm labor.
3. Educate as to the importance of drinking a variety of fluids other than high acid and carbonated beverages in amounts of at least 8 to 10 ounces every waking hour.
4. Teach to empty bladder at least every 2 hours while awake and to void after intercourse.
5. Instruct to perform perineal hygiene front to back.
6. Educate about the importance of reporting signs of UTI immediately.
7. Collect all urine specimens for urinalysis by clean catch or catheter.
8. Educate regarding prophylactic antibiotic therapy if previous history of pyelonephritis.

GENERAL CARE: RENAL DISEASE

■ **ALTERED HEALTH MAINTENANCE** related to lack of knowledge of signs and symptoms of fluid and electrolyte imbalance caused by decreased renal function or diuretic therapy and lack of understanding of needed drug therapy.

DESIRED OUTCOMES: Patient will verbalize understanding of the signs and symptoms of fluid and electrolyte imbalance and the importance of reporting their development promptly. She will also verbalize understanding of prescribed medications as to purpose, dosage, schedule, and potential side effects.

INTERVENTIONS

1. Alert patient and family of the signs and symptoms of fluid and electrolyte imbalance.
2. If drug therapy is prescribed, teach patient and family about the purpose, dosage, schedule, and potential side effects.
3. Discuss the importance of increased nutritional needs of pregnancy considering needed dietary restrictions such as decreased sodium, increased potassium, and increased or decreased protein.
4. Teach patient to monitor own blood pressure.
5. Instruct as to the importance of reporting any signs of fluid or electrolyte imbalance or medicine-induced side effects.
6. Refer for appropriate nutritional counseling.

■ **RISK FOR INFECTION** related to increased susceptibility secondary to disease process and drug therapy.

DESIRED OUTCOME: Patient will be free of infection as evidenced by normothermia, clear breath sounds, and dysuria.

INTERVENTIONS

1. Assess breath sounds. (The respiratory system is a common site for an infection.)
2. Do dipstick urine test for protein, nitrites, and/or leukocyte esterase at each office visit or at least weekly for hospitalized patients.
3. Assess for symptoms of burning, frequency, and flank pain.
4. Stress the importance of adjusting activities to avoid fatigue.
5. Educate as to the importance of avoiding infections.
6. Teach signs of preterm labor and how to recognize it.
7. If the patient has a renal disorder, avoid the use of a urinary catheter if at all possible because of the increased risk of a UTI. If indwelling catheter is necessary, a triple-lumen catheter may be used so that an antibacterial irrigating solution can constantly be infused.
8. If patient develops an infection, be prepared to administer antibiotics.

■ **RISK FOR FLUID VOLUME EXCESS** related to pyelonephritis, superimposed preeclampsia, or renal failure.

DESIRED OUTCOME: The patient will remain normovolemic as evidenced by urine output greater than 30 ml/hr or 120 ml/4 hr, gradual weight gain of ¾ to 1 pound per week during the second and third trimesters, and no edema of face, hands, or abdomen.

INTERVENTIONS
1. Weigh at each antepartum visit or daily if hospitalized.
2. Evaluate level of edema.
3. Report abnormal weight gain and evidence of pathologic edema.
4. In the presence of renal failure, fluid intake should equal output unless the patient is febrile. (Then 100 ml of additional fluid is needed for every degree (C) of elevation.)

- **RISK FOR IMPAIRED FETAL GAS EXCHANGE** related to maternal UTI, renal failure, superimposed maternal hypertension, or pre-term labor.
  DESIRED OUTCOMES: The fetus will remain active and grow normally for gestational age. The fetal heart rate (FHR) will remain between 110 and 160 bpm. The biophysical profile will continue to be over 6 with a negative CST and a reactive NST.
  INTERVENTIONS
  1. Teach fetal movement counts after 24 weeks of gestation.
  2. Carry out ordered fetal surveillance studies.
  3. Report nonreassuring FHRs and fetal heart patterns.

- **RISK FOR INEFFECTIVE COPING (INDIVIDUAL OR FAMILY)** related to life-threatening diagnosis for mother or unborn infant (see Chapters 5 and 6).

- **RISK FOR ALTERED PARENTING** related to life-threatening diagnosis or illness of the mother or neonate (see Chapters 5 and 6).

- **RISK FOR FEAR** related to life-threatening illness in the mother and the potential effects on the baby (see Chapter 5).

CRITICAL CARE: ACUTE RENAL FAILURE

- **POSSIBLE COMPLICATION OF A PREGNANCY OR DELIVERY: ACUTE RENAL FAILURE** precipitated by hemorrhagic shock, endotoxic shock, or a urinary obstruction.
  DESIRED OUTCOME: Acute renal failure will be prevented or managed appropriately as evidenced by urine output greater than 30 ml/hr, a BUN level between 7.2 and 10.2 mg/dl, and a serum creatinine level between 0.6 and 0.8 mg/dl.
  INTERVENTIONS
  1. Prevent acute renal failure by assisting in replacement of blood and fluids in the event of massive hemorrhage.
  2. Report early signs of an infection.

3. Carefully evaluate intake and output of any high risk patient.
4. Refer to such diagnostic data as BUN and serum creatinine levels. (They are frequently the earliest signs of acute kidney failure.)
5. If acute renal failure develops, be prepared to use invasive hemodynamic monitoring and kidney dialysis.

CRITICAL CARE: RENAL DISEASE

■ **POTENTIAL COMPLICATIONS OF RENAL DISEASE: RENAL COMPROMISE, HYPERTENSIVE DISORDERS OF PREGNANCY, OR DISSEMINATED INTRAVASCULAR COAGULATION (DIC)**
DESIRED OUTCOME: Complications of renal disease will be prevented or managed appropriately as evidenced by urine output greater than 30 ml/hr, normotension, regular pulse rate and less than 100 bpm, serum creatinine between 0.6 and 1.2 mg/dl, normal platelets, and proteinuria less than 2+.
INTERVENTIONS
1. Assess for signs of superimposed preeclampsia by evaluating blood pressure at each antepartum visit or daily if hospitalized.
2. Assess for signs of hemorrhage and coagulopathy.
3. Assess respirations and breath sounds if possibility of renal compromise.
4. Assess for signs of fluid/electrolyte and acid-base imbalances.
5. Report any signs of preeclampsia or fluid/electrolyte or acid-base imbalances to the attending physician.
6. Report abnormal blood chemistries to the attending physician.
7. Perform dialysis as ordered.
8. Weigh with each dialysis exchange.
9. Report any signs of abnormal fluid retention if patient is on dialysis.
10. Administer appropriate salt-poor intravenous fluids if pyelonephritis or signs of renal failure are present.
11. Teach patient CAPD if ordered.
12. Refer patient to nurse clinician/specialist for education regarding dialysis.

CONCLUSION

The primary aim for care of the pregnant woman with bacteriuria is prevention of symptomatic UTI and preterm labor. Prophylactic administration of antibiotics with instructions for increased oral fluids and proper perineal hygiene is most effective.

Prompt treatment of renal tract infection and medical response to maternal renal failure can prevent life-threatening events for the mother and intrauterine growth restriction or intrauterine fetal death. Although there are few reports of successful pregnancy when end-stage maternal renal disease is present, some promise in recent years has been reported with medical management, which includes maternal CAPD and vigilant fetal surveillance. Pregnancy after renal transplant has been quite successful if the original medical condition is stabilized and carefully monitored.

BIBLIOGRAPHY

Barcelo P and others: Successful pregnancy in primary glomerular disease, *Kidney Int* 30:194, 1986.

Becker G and others: Effect of pregnancy on moderate renal failure in reflux nephropathy, *Br Med J* 294:796, 1986.

Campbell-Brown M and others: Is screening for bacteriuria in pregnancy worthwhile? *Br Med J* 294:579, 1987.

Challah S and others: Successful pregnancy in women on regular dialysis treatment and women with a functional transplant. In Andreucci V, editor: *The kidney in pregnancy,* Boston, 1986, Martinus Nijhoff.

Cousins L: Pregnancy complications among women with diabetic complications, *Obstet Gynecol Surv* 42:140, 1987.

Creasy R, Resnik R, editors: *Maternal-fetal medicine: principles and practice,* ed 3, Philadelphia, 1994, Saunders.

Cunningham F: Urinary tract infections complicating pregnancy, *Clin Obstet Gynecol* 1:891, 1987.

Davison J: Can normal pregnancy damage your health? *Br J Obstet Gynecol* 94:385, 1987.

Davison J, Lindheimer M: Renal disorders. In Creasy R, Resnik R, editors: *Maternal-fetal medicine: principles and practice,* ed 3, Philadelphia, 1994, Saunders.

Elliott J and others: Dialysis in pregnancy: a critical review, *Obstet Gynecol Surv* 46(6):319-324, 1991.

Fleschler R, Sala D: Pregnancy after organ transplantation, *Obstet Gynecol Neonatal Nurs* 24(5):413-422, 1995.

Hou S: Peritoneal and hemodialysis in pregnancy, *Clin Obstet Gynecol* 1:1009, 1987.

Jungers P and others: Chronic kidney disease and pregnancy, *Adv Nephrol* 15:103, 1986.

Lindheimer M, Katz A, Ganeval D: Acute renal failure in pregnancy. In Brenner B, Lazarus J, editors: *Acute renal failure,* New York, 1988, Churchill Livingstone.

Maikranz P, Katz A: Acute renal failure in pregnancy, *Obstet Gynecol Clin North Am* 18(2):333-343, 1991.

Parving H and others: Effect of antihypertensive treatment on kidney function in diabetic nephropathy, *Br Med J* 294:1443, 1987.

CHAPTER

12

Connective Tissue Disease

U ntil the past 15 years, connective tissue disease was so difficult to diagnose and categorize that it was rare to see a pregnant woman with such a diagnosis. Connective tissue disorders, or collagen vascular disorders, are a group of diseases characterized by a connective tissue abnormality that is autoimmune mediated. The following are some of these diseases:

- Rheumatoid arthritis (RA)
- Multiple sclerosis (MS)
- Scleroderma
- Periarteritis nodosa (PAN)
- Polymyositis
- Myasthenia gravis
- Disseminated or systemic lupus erythematosus (SLE)

Box 12-1 gives a brief description of each of the autoimmune disorders just listed. Of these, SLE has some of the most serious consequences for pregnancy. It is multisystem in its effects; is most commonly manifested in the childbearing years; and can affect mother, fetus, and newborn. This chapter focuses on SLE.

INCIDENCE

According to some sources (Buyon, 1989; Friedman and others, 1991; Hollingsworth, Resnik, 1994; Lockshin, 1990) the incidence of SLE in women from their late 20s to early 40s may be as high as 1:1000 with more than 500,000 cases diagnosed each year. The

Box 12-1
Definitions and Descriptions of Connective Tissue Diseases

Rheumatoid arthritis (RA)

RA manifests itself clinically as selective inflammation of synovial joints associated with a tissue antigen. Pathologic findings consist of antigenic infiltration of the hinged synovial joints and a high titer of a rheumatoid factor antiglobulin antibody. Still disease is a juvenile form of this disorder, but RA otherwise manifests itself most often in the 35- to 40-year age bracket. It occurs more often in women than in men. With childbearing being postponed in some groups of women, it may be seen in a pregnant woman. It is known to have a variable deleterious effect on the pregnancy and the fetus (Dudley, Branch, 1990; Hollingsworth, Resnik, 1994).

Although RA is primarily a synovial inflammatory process, systemic, inflammatory nodules or granulomas may be seen on the cardiac valves, myocardium, pericardium, and pleura. It may also be manifested by rheumatoid arteritis with cerebral and cardiac thromboses. Such systemic effects may prove life threatening to both the pregnant woman and her unborn baby. Pregnancy does not, however, appear to contribute to the progression of the disease. Systemic manifestations are probably incidental to the pregnancy.

Multiple sclerosis (MS)

MS is a disorder in which multiple plaques of demyelination develop at various times and sites throughout the nervous system. Pathologic findings appear to be secondary to an autoimmune response. Pregnancy does not seem to affect the course of the disease, nor does MS affect the pregnancy outcome (Hollingsworth, Resnik, 1994). Provided that disability is not so severe as to limit ability to perform parenting tasks, there is no real reason to limit number of pregnancies nor a single pregnancy.

Scleroderma

Scleroderma is a rarely occurring connective tissue disorder that evokes a vasospastic, inflammatory reaction in small arterioles, especially the dermis. Clinical features include calcinosis, Raynaud phenomenon, esophageal hypermotility, sclerodactyly (scarring and stiffening of the digits), and generalized skin lesions. During pregnancy, symptoms are likely to worsen. Pregnant women are at high risk for obstetric complications from hypertension and fetal stress. A terminal stage of scleroderma may mimic the severe manifestations of preeclampsia and the HELLP (hemolysis, elevated liver enzymes, and low platelet count in association with preeclampsia) syndrome (Black, 1990; Hollingsworth, Resnik, 1994).

Box 12-1
Definitions and Descriptions of Connective Tissue Diseases—cont'd

Periarteritis nodosa (PAN)

PAN is usually a fatal immunoinflammatory process involving medium-size arteries. The disease, although extremely rare, is reported to result in maternal death (Hollingsworth, Resnik, 1994).

Polymyositis

Polymyositis is a diffuse autoimmune disorder of the muscles. It is so rare that there are few reports of the disease during pregnancy. Anecdotal reports state that, although a pregnancy complicated by polymyositis is difficult to manage, such pregnancies have resulted in normal, healthy newborns (Friedman and others, 1991; Hollingsworth, Resnik, 1994).

Myasthenia gravis

The clinical manifestations of myasthenia gravis include variable weakness and fatigue of skeletal muscles caused by defective neuromuscular transmission. The disorder is probably explained by the autoimmune basis and is characterized by a reduced number of acetylcholine receptors at the neuromuscular junction. It is more common in women than in men. It may appear for the first time during a pregnancy or shortly after. The effect of the disease on pregnancy varies and is unpredictable individually. The effects in the neonate may mimic the disease in the mother, but these effects are generally transient and do not predict disease in the adult. Pregnancy termination does not lead to benefit in those with worsening disease during pregnancy. In fact, the postpartum period may be the most dangerous time regardless of the length of the pregnancy. If preterm labor occurs, the use of magnesium sulfate is absolutely contraindicated. Magnesium sulfate interferes with the already defective neuromuscular transmission by altering the exchange of ions across the junction.

Systemic lupus erythematosus (SLE)

SLE is a multisystem inflammatory disorder characterized by autoimmune antibody production. This results in inflammation of connective tissue in various organs and systems in the body (Buyon, 1989; Friedman and others, 1991; Hollingsworth, Resnik, 1994; Lockshin, 1990) and hematologic disorders related to the antigen/antibody reactions in vessel walls (Carp and others, 1989; Gordon, Isenberg, 1990; McCormack and others, 1991; Petri and others, 1989).

prediction in the 1970s and early 1980s of 6:100,000 has been changed dramatically because of the improved ability to diagnose SLE by radioimmune assays. Women are affected 10 times more often than men. Because childbearing is frequently postponed in professional educated women, their incidence is higher. Whether a woman is pregnant or not, the disease is characterized by exacerbations and remissions. Survival after exacerbation is 90% in the first 5 years and 80% after 10 years. Survival generally depends on the degree of cardiac and renal involvement and insult.

ETIOLOGY

The exact cause of SLE is unknown. Evidence indicates it may be interrelated with immunologic, environmental, hormonal, and genetic factors (Springhouse Corporation, 1989). Predisposing factors include viral infections, physical or psychologic stress, exposure to sunlight, immunization, or pregnancy.

NORMAL PHYSIOLOGY

See discussion of normal physiologic adaptations in pregnancy described by systems and functions in Chapter 1.

PATHOPHYSIOLOGY

In SLE the body is unable to distinguish "self" from "nonself." An immunologic deficit allows antibodies to be formed that attack the body's own cells and proteins. More than 50 autoantibodies and antigen/antibody complexes collectively have been identified in the serum of affected individuals. This autoimmune response causes suppression of the body's normal immunity and damages body tissue. The autoimmune response may initially involve one organ system or every organ system. In pregnancy, inflammation of the connective tissue of the decidua can result in placental implantation and functioning problems.

SIGNS AND SYMPTOMS

Clinical manifestations depend on which system or systems are being attacked by the autoantibodies. The most common symptoms are fever, malaise, fatigue, weight loss, skin rashes, and polyarthralgia. Table 12-1 gives clinical manifestations specific to various systems.

MATERNAL EFFECTS

If the disease has been in remission for at least 6 months before conception and renal function is normal, optimal pregnancy

TABLE 12-1   Clinical manifestations of SLE

System	Clinical manifestations
General	Malaise
	Fatigue
	Fever
	Weight loss
Integumentary	Skin rashes, butterfly rash
	Skin ulcers
Musculoskeletal	Arthralgia
Cardiovascular	Pericarditis
	Myocarditis
	Endocarditis
	Tachycardia
Respiratory	Pleuritis
	Dyspnea
	Pneumonitis
Renal	Urinary tract infection
	Nephrotic syndrome characterized by:
	Hematuria
	Proteinuria
	Urine sediment and cellular casts
	Glomerular nephritis
	May progress to total kidney failure
Central nervous system	Emotional instability
	Seizure disorders
	Psychosis
	Headaches
	Irritability
	Depression
Gastrointestinal	Mucosal ulcers of mouth
	Anorexia
	Nausea/vomiting
	Diarrhea
	Constipation
Hematologic	Chronic anemia
	Thrombocytopenia
	Leukocytopenia
	Lupus anticoagulant
Ocular	Conjunctivitis
	Photosensitivity

SLE, Systemic lupus erythematosus.

outcome is as high as 88% (Hollingsworth, Resnik, 1994). If the disease is active at the time of conception, exacerbation of the disease is common (60%), especially involving the renal, cardiac, and central nervous systems (Cunningham and others, 1989). Such complications as spontaneous abortion, preeclampsia, HELLP (hemolysis, elevated liver enzymes, and low platelet count in association with preeclampsia) syndrome (see Chapter 20), and preterm labor are the most common. If the patient before conception had severe cardiac or renal damage, the pregnancy can be life threatening. The postpartum period is a potentially dangerous time for the mother, since the physical and emotional stress of labor and delivery may trigger an exacerbation of the disease (Hollingsworth, Resnik, 1994). Pneumonitis, unresponsive to treatment, may develop.

FETAL AND NEONATAL EFFECTS

SLE affects pregnancy by increasing the risk of spontaneous abortion by 40% to 80% (Friedman and others, 1991), depending on the severity of exacerbations and the length of remission before conception. The risk of an abortion is directly related to maternal cardiac and renal involvement.

After spontaneous abortion risk, premature birth remains the next major risk to the fetus/newborn. The risk is primarily the result of the malformation of the placenta and placental insufficiency in nutritional and respiratory functions for the fetus. The placenta has connective tissue as part of its makeup. Microangiopathic changes take place in the placenta, resulting in disruption of normal functioning. Intrauterine fetal death is also a significant risk if the pregnancy continues to an otherwise favorable gestation (Freidman and others, 1991).

In addition, the connective tissue inflammation and the anti–deoxyribonucleic acid (anti-DNA) in the mother can affect the fetus and the newborn. The manifestations of connective tissue degradation can cause fetal heart block through disruption or destruction of the connective tissue in the fetal heart. Further, it can cause fetal developmental abnormalities. The neonate may exhibit a transient lupus complex with problems requiring up to 10 to 12 months of treatment before disappearing.

MEDICAL DIAGNOSIS

Before radioimmune assays, SLE was difficult to impossible to definitively diagnose. Now, two tests are standard for the diagnosis

TABLE 12-2 Antibody tests used to assess SLE exacerbations

Antibody tests	Results and significance
Anti-DNA	Positive: indicates disease activity Negative: indicates remission
Anti-LA (anti-SSB)	Positive: associated with nephritis; high correlation with neonatal lupus and congenital heart block
Anticentromere	Positive: associated with scleroderma
Anticardiolipin, lupus anticoagulant, prolonged partial thromboplastin time and prothrombin time	Positive: associated with vascular thrombosis
Antiribonucleoprotein (n-RNP)	Positive: associated with mixed connective tissue disease

of SLE. They are fluorescent antinuclear antibody test (ANA) and total serum complement (C_3, C_4).

During pregnancy antibody tests are helpful when assessing for exacerbations and in determining degree of multisystem involvement. Table 12-2 gives the various antibody tests used.

During pregnancy if the fetus is diagnosed with congenital heart block and the mother has not previously been diagnosed with lupus, she should have a complete SLE workup. In addition, certain clinical manifestations indicate a need to investigate a pregnant woman's predisposition for SLE and the lupus anticoagulant:

1. Recurrent fetal losses
2. Connective tissue disorder
3. Thrombotic events
4. Prolonged coagulation studies
5. Positive autoantibody tests
6. Thrombocytopenia

USUAL MEDICAL MANAGEMENT

Medical management is complicated by the various, sometimes vague, clinical manifestations of connective tissue disorders. Combined with this is the fact that both maternal and fetal well-being may be seriously threatened by pregnancy with renal or cardiac complications (Hollingsworth, Resnik, 1994).

Women with connective tissue disorders should be counseled about planning pregnancy and the importance of being at least 6 months in remission before conception. After conception a pregnancy complicated with SLE or other connective tissue disease requires very close supervision of both the pregnant woman and the fetus.

Medical Assessment

Maternal

Maternal assessment includes the following aspects:

1. Blood pressure and pulse
2. Complete blood count (CBC), platelet count
3. Blood urea nitrogen (BUN), creatinine
4. Glucose
5. Partial thromboplastin time (PTT) and, if prolonged, specific tests for lupus anticoagulant
6. ANA, anti-DNA, anti-Rho, C_3, C_4

Fetal

Fetal assessment includes the following aspects:

1. Serial ultrasounds to evaluate growth
2. Fetal surveillance studies using nonstress tests (NSTs), contraction stress tests (CSTs), or biophysical profiles

Drug Therapy

During pregnancy the goal is to keep drug therapy to a minimum. Patients who have a mild form of the disease or are experiencing a remission require minimal to no medication. The usual drug therapy when indicated includes an antiinflammatory drug, especially prednisone and aspirin.

Prednisone

The most common antiinflammatory drug used in the treatment of SLE is prednisone. Usual dose is 10 to 80 mg daily administered every 12 hours. High doses of prednisone for long periods may inhibit neonatal steroid production. Short-term therapy for SLE flare in pregnancy is less likely to do this.

Aspirin

Aspirin is a nonsteroidal antiinflammatory drug. Usual dose is 80 mg daily. Low-dose salicylate theoretically selectively inhibits the synthesis of thromboxane while allowing for the continued production of the vasodilator prostacyclin. It is also reported to help in preventing the more severe forms of pregnancy-induced hypertension (PIH) (see Chapter 20).

Ibuprofens

Ibuprofens may be used to control some of the inflammatory processes, as well as relieve arthritic pain. Ibuprofens include prostacyclin inhibitors as well. Premature closure of the patent ductus leading to intrauterine fetal death and interference with the production of amniotic fluid have been reported fetal side effects. These problems seem to be associated with gestation beyond 33 weeks or drug-related gestation.

Antimalarial Drugs

Antimalarial drugs are used to suppress mild SLE, especially when associated with skin lesions or rashes. The usual dose of chloroquine is 250 mg one or two times daily.

Azathioprine or Cyclophosphamide

Azathioprine and cyclophosphamide (Cytoxan) are immunosuppressant drugs that may be used in conjunction with corticosteroids (prednisone).

Other Treatments

Other treatment and management depend on clinical manifestations. For example, if the major threat to maternal well-being stems from cardiac problems related to valvular problems, a cardiology consultation may be sought. Medical management is directed at treatment and stabilization. If the primary clinical characteristics are arthritic in nature, a rheumatologist may be consulted. If pulmonary problems, hypertension, coagulation defects, or renal problems are the presenting complications, internists with specialty practice in those fields of medicine may be consulted (see Chapters 9 to 11, 18, and 20).

Lupus nephritis has recently been successfully managed in a number of cases in a large southwestern tertiary facility by a rarely attempted modality. Continuous ambulatory peritoneal dialysis has shown promise in facilitating a better pregnancy outcome and safeguards the maternal condition as well for a limited time (Elliott and others, 1991). Although the total number of between 12 and 20 successes is still only anecdotal, there are no reports worldwide of more than four previous attempts using this treatment in pregnancy complicated by end-stage renal disease. Even those reports do not include lupus nephritis among their anecdotes (see Chapters 11 and 20).

NURSING PROCESS

PREVENTION

Preventive nursing care focuses on early recognition and reporting of signs of SLE flare and common pregnancy complications precipitated by SLE. In an effort to do that, the family members and the woman need adequate information for her self-care. Collaboration with the medical management plan includes reinforcing preconceptual counseling, interpreting clinical information in lay terms, and vigilance in physical and psychosocial assessments for the family and the pregnant woman.

NURSING DIAGNOSES/COLLABORATIVE PROBLEMS AND INTERVENTIONS

■ **RISK FOR ALTERED HEALTH MAINTENANCE** related to exacerbation of the disease because of pregnancy.

DESIRED OUTCOMES: The patient will have been in remission for at least 6 months before conception and will stay in remission during the pregnancy. To optimize health, the patient will implement health-promoting practices. She will deliver a healthy newborn.

INTERVENTIONS

Antepartum

1. Discuss with the patient and her family the possible effects of SLE on pregnancy and the possible effects of pregnancy on SLE.
2. Emphasize to the patient the importance of a balance between activity and adequate rest.
3. Assess nutritional status, normal food intake, and understanding regarding nutritional needs.
4. Teach or reinforce information regarding special dietary needs as indicated by her disease and emphasize a nutritious diet to decrease risks.
5. Discuss implications of drug therapy if indicated. Teach the patient and family about the self-administration of all prescribed medications.
6. Instruct regarding skin care such as washing with a mild soap, avoiding sun exposure, using sunscreens, and avoiding products that cause side effects.

7. Discuss health-promoting practices to prevent infections and the importance of notifying physician on the first signs of an infection.
8. Educate patient and family about the early signs of an SLE flare and the importance of reporting them immediately.
9. Refer to the Lupus Foundation of America and to a high risk pregnancy support group.

Postpartum

1. Discuss the importance of birth control and the effects of various birth control methods on the disease. (Oral contraceptives may stimulate drug-induced SLE, and an intrauterine device may increase the risk of an infection. Therefore the barrier methods carry the least risk to the patient.)
2. Support breast-feeding or bottle-feeding decisions.

- **POTENTIAL COMPLICATION OF SLE: SUPPRESSED IMMUNITY AND MULTISYSTEM FAILURE, ESPECIALLY RENAL, CARDIAC, AND CENTRAL NERVOUS SYSTEM FAILURE** related to the autoimmune response of SLE.

DESIRED OUTCOMES: The complications of SLE will be minimized and managed as measured by a normal blood pressure, pulse, platelet count, and serum creatinine. No protein, blood, or white blood cells will be found in the urine, and its specific gravity will remain between 1.010 and 1.030. Chest sounds will remain clear. The biophysical profile will be greater than 6, the NST will be reactive, and there will be no decelerations on a CST.

INTERVENTIONS

Antepartum screening each visit

1. Measure the blood pressure in the same arm and in the same position each visit, and determine the mean arterial pressure.
2. Assess pulse for regularity and rhythm.
3. Assess respiratory rate, and auscultate lung fields.
4. Assess weight gain.
5. Screen for dyspnea, edema, and chest pain.
6. Discuss with the patient how she feels and whether she has experienced any headaches or mood change differences other than expected mood changes of pregnancy.
7. Assess for signs of renal involvement by checking urine for protein and specific gravity. (Specific gravity measures retention of urea solutes.)
8. Assess for signs of a urinary tract infection.
9. Be prepared to obtain serum creatinine levels and hematologic studies as indicated and ordered.

Intrapartum

1. Evaluate cardiac function by assessing for signs of congestive heart failure, blood pressure, and pulse rate for dysrhythmias.
2. Evaluate renal function by assessing urinary output, specific gravity, and proteinuria every 4 hours in the presence of hypertension.
3. Evaluate pulmonary function by assessing breath sounds every 4 hours and determining if chest pain develops. If tocolytics are used or if the patient has a positive history of pulmonary, cardiac, or renal involvement, the pulmonary assessment should be done more often.
4. Be prepared to institute prompt treatment of early pulmonary problems with antibiotics, bronchodilators, intravenous heparin, or diuretics as appropriate.
5. Evaluate the hematologic function by assessing for signs of disseminated intravascular coagulation (DIC).
6. Closely observe for late-onset preeclampsia.
7. If there is a positive history of central nervous system (CNS) involvement, evaluate the CNS function by assessing for seizure activity, unexpected mood swings, or transient changes in level of consciousness.
8. If either cardiac or renal complications are severe or if preeclampsia is superimposed, prepare for invasive hemodynamic monitoring. If noninvasive monitoring is ordered instead, use electrocardiogram (ECG) and conventional blood pressure monitoring to assess the hemodynamic status (see Chapters 10 and 20).

Postpartum

1. Continue the same assessment as was carried out during intrapartum period.
2. Assess for early signs of maternal infection by checking temperature every 4 hours.
3. Assess breath sounds for early evidence of pneumonia.
4. Assess for hematoma formation and lack of wound healing (episiotomy or cesarean incision).

■ **RISK FOR NONCOMPLIANCE** related to alterations in CNS function or to inability to cope with the effects of a chronic, life-threatening illness.

   DESIRED OUTCOMES: The patient and at least one family member will actively participate in decisions for care. The patient will seek information aimed at self-monitoring and self-care.

INTERVENTIONS
1. Assess patient's ability and willingness to follow directions and to perform appropriate activities of daily living.
2. Provide information for informed decisions.
3. Interpret information to the patient and her support person in terms they are most likely to understand.

■ **RISK FOR INFECTION** related to the use of immunosuppressant and antiinflammatory drugs and the effects of the disease when active.
   DESIRED OUTCOMES: The patient will optimize health by practicing health-promoting activities. If an infection develops, she will report it immediately. Signs of infection will respond to early treatment.
   INTERVENTIONS
   1. Teach or reinforce health-promoting practices.
   2. Educate patient and family members about the early signs of infection and the importance of reporting early signs of an infection.

■ **RISK FOR PAIN AND SELF-CARE DEFICIT** related to onset of exacerbation of arthritic symptoms.
   DESIRED OUTCOME: Patient will verbalize relief from pain or tolerance of the pain.
   INTERVENTIONS
   1. Administer antiinflammatory medications or teach patient about self-administration of antiinflammatory medications.
   2. Teach patient alternative methods of pain management such as relaxation techniques, biofeedback, and self-medication or hypnosis. Encourage use of heat packs to relieve joint pain and stiffness.
   3. Encourage receptivity to alternate methods to supplement medical methods of pain relief.
   4. Communicate belief in patient's ability to cope with pain. Use praise and honest appraisal of successes.

■ **RISK FOR POWERLESSNESS** related to perceived lack of control over chronicity of disease and potential effects on the pregnancy outcome.
   DESIRED OUTCOMES: The patient will verbalize a renewed interest in and belief in her ability to manage her disease and participate in her care. The family will demonstrate effective coping styles.

INTERVENTIONS

1. Encourage active participation in decisions for care.
2. Provide information that encourages selection of available options.
3. Express confidence in family members' ability to cope with the need for stringent adherence to the medical management of the pregnancy and complications.
4. Enhance the patient's self-image, if needed, by encouraging her to take an interest in her appearance, by providing helpful cosmetic tips, such as the use of hypoallergenic makeup, and by referring her to a hairdresser who specializes in scalp disorders.
5. Recognize life-style of helplessness if presented with family with a learned helplessness.

■ **RISK FOR INEFFECTIVE COPING** related to chronicity of the maternal disorder, fear for well-being, and previously developed ineffective coping skills.

DESIRED OUTCOME: The family will develop an appropriate, effective coping style and will be able to continue to provide for basic needs of all members of the family even if mother is hospitalized for an extended time.

INTERVENTIONS

1. Assess specific fears and anxieties.
2. Assess family coping styles and ability to cope with the effects of chronic illness.
3. Refer for psychosocial evaluation and support as needed.
4. Provide information and encourage its use to develop new coping skills.
5. Encourage the mother and her partner to remain close to each other even during extended hospitalization.

■ **RISK FOR ALTERED FETAL TISSUE PERFUSION AND IMPAIRED FETAL GAS EXCHANGE** related to maternal connective tissue disorder and the effects on the placental perfusion and function.

DESIRED OUTCOMES: The fetus will remain active, and its heart rate will be maintained at a baseline between 110 and 160 beats/min with normal variability and reactivity and no decelerations. Growth will not fall below the tenth percentile for gestational age as evidenced on ultrasound. The biophysical profile will continue to be greater than 6, NSTs reactive, and CSTs negative.

INTERVENTIONS
1. Instruct patient in the importance of procedure of fetal movement counts beginning at 24 weeks of gestation.
2. Perform some combination of NSTs, CSTs, biophysical profiles, or placental Doppler flow study as ordered.
3. Be prepared to schedule for ultrasound evaluation of fetal growth every 2 to 3 weeks after 24 weeks of gestation. Measure fundal height between ultrasound evaluations.
4. Teach patient prevention and recognition of preterm labor.
5. Refer to a perinatal home care program that offers comprehensive services (i.e., antenatal testing, prenatal evaluation, patient education).

■ **RISK FOR DYSFUNCTIONAL GRIEVING** related to anticipatory grieving for potential loss of the pregnancy and known threats to the maternal well-being.
DESIRED OUTCOMES: The family will seek and accept offered support. In the face of pregnancy or fetal loss, the family will progress through the four phases of bereavement in 1 to 2 years and by that time will be ready for reinvestment in the family and their future together.
INTERVENTIONS
1. Refer to support group.
2. Provide adequate information about true chances for survival of fetus or newborn.
3. Keep mother and her partner together when hospitalized.
4. Use Worden's counseling principles (see Chapter 6).
5. Recognize complicated grief, and make appropriate referrals (see Chapter 6).

Because connective tissue disorders and specifically SLE are multisystem disorders, for specific nursing care related to effects on each system see related chapters.

CONCLUSION

Connective tissue disease greatly complicates management of both the disease and the pregnancy. The complications, although not insurmountable, require close supervision. The keys to a successful outcome for mother and baby are as follows:
1. Accurate diagnosis of the specific disease and the systems involved
2. Preconceptual counseling to attempt pregnancy only after at least 6 months of remission

3. Vigilance during the pregnancy for progression of the disease, effects on the fetus, and the development of pregnancy-related maternal complications

With better, more accurate diagnostic laboratory evaluations available through radioimmune assays, closer and more adequate follow-up can now be provided. Nursing care must be directed at early detection of signs and symptoms, education of the mother and involved family members, and careful evaluation of the fetal status. If the pregnancy fails despite good care, grief support and referrals can aid the childbearing family affected by maternal connective tissue disorders.

BIBLIOGRAPHY

Black C: Systemic sclerosis and pregnancy, *Baillieres Clin Rheumatol* 4(1):105-124, 1990.

Buyon J: Neonatal lupus and congenital complete heart block: manifestations of passively acquired autoimmunity, *Clin Exp Rheumatol* 7(suppl 3):199-203, 1989.

Buyon J: Systemic lupus erythematosus and the maternal fetal dyad, *Baillieres Clin Rheumatol* 4(1):85-103, 1990.

Buyon J and others: Serum complement values to differentiate between lupus activity and preeclampsia, *Am J Med* 81:194, 1986.

Cameron J: Pathogenesis and treatment of lupus nephritis, Renal Unit, Guy's Campus UMDS, London, *Nippon Jinzo Gakkai Shi* 33(5):443-446, 1991.

Carp H and others: Fetal demise associated with lupus coagulant: clinical features and results of treatment, *Gynecol Obstet Invest* 28(4):178-184, 1989.

Cunningham F, MacDonald P, Gant N: *Williams' obstetrics,* ed 8, Norwalk, Conn, 1989, Appleton & Lange.

Derue G and others: Fetal loss in systemic lupus: association with anticardiolipin antibodies, *J Obstet Gynecol* 5:207, 1985.

Dudley D, Branch D: Pregnancy in the patient with rheumatic disease: the obstetrician's perspective, *Baillieres Clin Rheumatol* 4(1):141-156, 1990.

Elder M, Myatt L: First use of nafazatrom, a new antithrombic drug, in pregnancy, *Lancet* 1:1350, 1984.

Elliot J and others: Dialysis in pregnancy: a critical review, *Obstet Gynecol Surv* 46(6):319-324, 1991.

Feinstein D: Lupus anticoagulant, thrombosis, and fetal loss, *N Engl J Med* 313:1348, 1985.

Friedman S and others: Pregnancy complicated by collagen vascular disease, *Obstet Gynecol Clin North Am* 18(2):213-234, 1991.

Gordon T, Isenberg D: Organ specific and multisystemic autoimmune disease: part of the spectrum which may coexist in the same patient, *Clin Rheumatol* 9(3):401-403, 1990.

Hollingsworth J, Resnik R: Rheumatologic and connective tissue disorders. In Creasy R, Resnik R, editors: *Maternal-fetal medicine: principles and practice,* ed 3, Philadelphia, 1994, Saunders.

Hughes G and others: The anticardiolipin syndrome, *J Rheumatol* 13:486, 1986.

Lewis J and others: Immunologic mechanisms in the maternal fetal relationship, *Mayo Clin Proc* 61:655-665, 1986.

Lockshin M: Pregnancy associated with SLE, *Semin Perinatol* 14(2):130-138, 1990.

McCormack M and others: Anti-platelet antibodies: a prognostic marker in pregnancies associated with lupus nephritis, *Br J Obstet Gynaecol* 98(3):324-325, 1991.

Mintz G and others: Prospective study of pregnancy in systemic lupus erythematosus: results of a multidisciplinary approach, *J Rheumatol* 13:4, 1986.

Petri M, Watson R, Hochberg M: Anti-Ro antibodies and neonatal lupus, *Rheum Dis Clin North Am* 15(2):335-360, 1989.

Rapaport S: *Introduction to hematology,* Philadelphia, 1987, Lippincott.

Springhouse Corporation: *Professional guide to diseases,* ed 3, Springhouse, Pa, 1989, The Author.

Wallenberg H and others: Low dose aspirin prevents pregnancy induced hypertension and preeclampsia in angiotensin sensitive primigravidae, *Lancet* 1:1, 1986.

Watson R and others: Fetal wastage in women with anti-Ro (SSA) antibody, *J Rheumatol* 13:90, 1986.

CHAPTER

13

Pulmonary Disease and Respiratory Distress

Pregnancy complicated with pulmonary disease can be dangerous to both maternal well-being and fetal outcome. Understanding alterations in pulmonary physiology during pregnancy and the additional changes in immune responses can assist in anticipation of problems and prevention of complications in chronic and acute pulmonary disease. This chapter reviews the management of cystic fibrosis, asthma, infections, and respiratory emergencies, such as adult respiratory distress syndrome (ARDS), pulmonary embolism, and amniotic fluid embolism.

INCIDENCE

Pulmonary diseases have become more prevalent in the general population and in pregnancy.

CYSTIC FIBROSIS

As women with cystic fibrosis live longer and with improved quality of life, they face the new complication of pregnancy. The median age of survival of women with cystic fibrosis is about 29 years, and the disease occurs in 1 of 2000 births. Because of abnormally dense cervical mucus, women with cystic fibrosis are thought to have lower fertility (ACOG, 1996).

ASTHMA

The incidence of asthma is 4% in the general population and may complicate 0.4% to 1.3% of all pregnancies (Mabie, 1996; Niswander, Evans, 1995). The severity of the disease is unchanged in 50% of pregnant women with asthma, is improved in 29%, and is worse in 22%. This effect varies between pregnancies of an individual woman. Most recent studies have shown that with good control of the disease and its complications, perinatal morbidity and mortality are approximately the same as for the general pregnant population (ACOG, 1996; Niswander, Evans, 1995).

INFECTIONS

Respiratory infections that may have a significant effect on pregnancy outcome include bronchitis, pneumonia, and tuberculosis. Bronchitis progressing to pneumonia complicates 0.1% to 1% of all pregnancies. Co-infection with human immunodeficiency virus (HIV) will further worsen the prognosis (ACOG, 1996). The importance of bronchitis is in distinguishing it from pneumonia (Niswander, Evans, 1995). Tuberculosis, once considered rare in the United States, is now increasing in women of childbearing years. In endemic areas it may occur in 0.1% of pregnancies. Endemic areas include birth in a country with high tuberculosis prevalence or residence in a long-term facility, such as a prison or mental health facility.

RESPIRATORY EMERGENCIES

Respiratory emergencies are rare in pregnancy and include pulmonary embolism, amniotic fluid embolism, and ARDS. All are generally secondary to other physiologic complications. Pulmonary embolism may occur in as many as 24% of untreated or inadequately treated deep vein thromboses (DVTs), or it may occur as a complication of septic pelvic thrombophlebitis, or, even more rare, ovarian vein thrombosis (Creasy, Resnik, 1994).

Amniotic fluid embolism is an obstetric catastrophe and occurs rarely. However, when it occurs, there is a reported 80% to 85% maternal mortality (Niswander, Evans, 1995).

ARDS in pregnancy is also very rare. The outcome for mother and fetus is variable and depends on underlying cause and the extent of other organ or system involvement.

RESPIRATORY INFECTIONS

Etiology

Infections

Infections are frequently identified as caused by viruses, influenza, *Haemophilus, Streptococcus, Mycoplasma, Chlamydia,* or tuberculosis. These infections may also cause respiratory complications in women already compromised by asthma or cystic fibrosis. The etiology of pulmonary emboli is usually DVT, whereas the etiology of amniotic fluid emboli is unknown. ARDS is often preceded by respiratory sepsis.

Normal Physiology

In pregnancy the following alterations in respiratory anatomy and physiology occur:

1. The lower ribs flare out, and the subcostal angle, as well as the transverse diameter of the chest, increases.
2. The diaphragm rises by about 4 cm.
3. Progesterone stimulates the respiratory centers to produce hyperventilation and a sensation of dyspnea.
4. Because of hyperventilation, there is a decrease in alveolar CO_2 tension and the pCO_2 relative to respiratory alkalosis.

Pathophysiology

Infections of the respiratory system, asthma, and cystic fibrosis can all lead to obstruction of the airway and alveoli. The obstruction causes inability to clear CO_2 and results in hypercarbia. Patients with obstructive pulmonary disease may also be unable to breathe in sufficient amounts of oxygen. Hypoxia is the major threat to the fetus because the maternal-fetal placental unit depends on a passive system of oxygen uptake and the fetus grows in a lower pO_2 than its host, the mother. Therefore the fetus becomes more readily hypoxic with a lower percent of decrease in maternal pO_2.

Infectious agents invade and inflame the respiratory structures and mucous membranes. Inflammation of these structures causes an increase in mucus production in an effort to repair itself. The mucus contains protein and other substrates as cells shed and provides a good medium for bacterial or viral growth. As respiratory effort increases, there is a concomitant loss of moisture through increased breathing. The loss of moisture in turn causes the mucus to become drier and more viscous and thus obstructs the airways (ACOG, 1996; Creasy, Resnik, 1994).

Signs and Symptoms

Dyspnea

Dyspnea is experienced by most women at some time during a normal pregnancy. It may be a normal response to the anatomic pressure of the gravid uterus against the diaphragm and the conscious awareness of an increase in respiratory rate. Dyspnea is also a classic symptom of respiratory disease and distress, especially when coupled with prolonged expiratory phase hypoxemia.

Because respiratory physiology in a normal pregnancy tends toward respiratory alkalosis, hypoxemia is initially not accompanied by a corresponding increase in CO_2 (hypercarbia). Hypercarbia generally occurs in severe hypoxemia.

Leukocytosis

The complete blood count (CBC) may show an increase in leukocytes, with a left shift on differential if there is a bacterial infection. If mycoplasmal pneumonia is present, an increase in the sedimentation rate is common also. Hemoconcentration may also be seen.

Cough

A productive cough may be seen in cystic fibrosis as a normal part of the disease. If it produces thick, dark, bloody or rusty sputum, infection is probably superimposed. Productive cough in an asthmatic pregnant woman should be treated as an infection in the respiratory tract. Any thick or colored mucus that is produced with coughing is presumed to be a sign of infection.

Other signs and symptoms of infection include the following:
1. Fever
2. Sudden onset of chills
3. Chest pain, pleuritic pain

Assessment

Assessment may reveal the following:
1. Bronchial breath sounds
2. Chest dullness
3. Decreased breath sounds
4. Rales, crackles
5. Egophony, whispered pectoriloquy

A chest x-ray film may show infiltration and either segmental or lobar consolidation.

MATERNAL EFFECTS
Cystic Fibrosis

Maternal mortality from cystic fibrosis is the same as for the nonpregnant population at the same age. It therefore appears that cystic fibrosis has no unusually beneficial or detrimental effect on the pregnant woman.

Asthma

Asthma in pregnancy seems to have no consistent effect on the pregnancy. One review of more than 1000 pregnant women with asthma revealed that 48% experienced no effect, 29% showed improvement, and 23% showed deterioration of asthma during pregnancy.

Infections

Bronchitis poses little threat to pregnant women except that it may more readily progress to pneumonia and must be differentiated from pneumonia (ACOG, 1996). Pneumonia frequently is accompanied by a productive cough. Because of the anatomic accommodations to the respiratory system in pregnancy, forceful coughing to raise sputum may be more difficult. It is also more likely to cause painful separation of the cartilage between ribs and occasionally a spontaneous pneumothorax (Creasy, Resnik, 1994).

Adult Respiratory Distress Syndrome

ARDS can be the final result of several different obstetric complications, including inhalation of gastric contents during anesthesia and disseminated intravascular coagulation (DIC), as seen in preeclampsia, eclampsia, abruptio placentae, dead fetus syndrome, and amniotic fluid embolism. All these can be fatal to the mother.

FETAL EFFECTS

The greatest fetal threat is hypoxemia secondary to any condition that leads to acute respiratory emergencies. Chronic respiratory disease, such as asthma, can result in growth retardation. A true respiratory emergency, such as pulmonary embolism or amniotic fluid embolism, may necessitate emergency cesarean delivery at the same time that maternal resuscitation is being attempted. If maternal hypoxia and respiratory acidosis occur, the fetal brain is vulnerable to the resultant fetal hypoxia. Depending on the degree of hypoxia and the timing of the event in fetal gestational

TABLE 13-1   Arterial blood gas values in pregnant and nonpregnant women

	pH	pO_2 (mm Hg)	pCO_2 (mm Hg)
Pregnant	7.4	100-105	30
Nonpregnant	7.4	93	35-40

age, the fetus may suffer some degree of irreversible brain damage or death.

DIAGNOSTIC TESTING

Diagnostic testing is the same for pregnant women as for non-pregnant women. The following tests are routine when respiratory compromise is evident:

1. CBC
2. Sputum culture
3. Chest x-ray film, with abdominal shield
4. Arterial blood gases (Table 13-1)
5. Pulmonary function tests (Table 13-2)

In addition, if DVT is suspected, a Doppler flow study or a contrast dye venogram may be done. If an amniotic fluid embolism is suspected, coagulation blood studies are ordered during the critical care recovery, after initial resuscitation.

USUAL MEDICAL MANAGEMENT AND PROTOCOLS FOR NURSE PRACTITIONERS
Cystic Fibrosis

1. Preconceptual counseling to be in optimal physical condition
2. Genetic counseling and carrier testing of the father
3. Consultation with a pulmonary specialist or, ideally, a specialist in cystic fibrosis
4. Dietary consultation
5. Close monitoring of the pregnant woman for pulmonary infection
6. Prompt and vigorous treatment of pulmonary infections with antibiotics, fluids, and respiratory therapy
7. Closely monitored nutrition and weight gain
8. Early screening for diabetes because of its more frequent occurrence

TABLE 13-2 Comparison of pulmonary values in pregnant and nonpregnant women

Definition of terms	Nonpregnant	Pregnant	Clinical significance
Tidal volume (VT) = amount of air moved in one normal respiratory cycle	450 ml	600 ml	
Respiratory rate (RR) = number of respirations per min	16/min	Slight increase	
Minute ventilation = volume of air moved per min; $VT \times RR$	7.2 L	9.6 L	Increased O_2 available to fetus
Forced expiratory volume in 1 sec (FEV_1)	80%-85% of vital capacity	Unchanged	Valuable to measure because there is no change
Peak expiratory flow rate (PEFR)		Unchanged	Valuable to measure because there is no change
Forced vital capacity (FVC) = maximum amount of air that can be moved from maximum inspiration to maximum expiration	3.5 L	Unchanged	If over 1 L, pregnancy usually tolerated well
Residual volume (RV) = amount of air that remains in lung at end of a maximal expiration	1000 ml	Decreases to approx. 800 ml	Improves gas transfer from alveoli to blood

Asthma

Persons with asthma have hyperesponsive airways to such stimuli as allergens, viruses, air pollutants, exercise, and cold air. The hyperactivity is manifested by bronchospasm, mucosal edema, and mucus plugging in the airways, with hyperinflation of the lungs. Because of the inflammation in airway mucosa, measurement of forced expiratory volume (FEV) or peak expiratory flow rate (PEFR) (see Table 13-2) can help to quantify objectively the degree of obstruction. Measurement of these two values is also useful in monitoring the effectiveness of treatment (ACOG, 1996). Change in the treatment plan is based on the three zones in Table 13-3. Refer to Table 13-3 for the treatment plan, according to the three zones.

Usually, a pregnant woman with asthma has had previous episodes and knows when she is experiencing an acute attack. Therefore with an exacerbation, a good history of similar attacks and effective therapy should be obtained. Medications that may be used are summarized in Table 13-4. A good objective physical examination should include the following:

1. Answers to the following questions:
   a. General appearance: is the patient cyanotic?
   b. Can the patient speak in complete sentences without shortness of breath?
   c. Can she walk across a room?
   d. Is she using accessory muscles?
2. The following additional data:
   a. Temperature and respiratory rate
   b. Laboratory values for forced expiratory volume (FEV) or peak expiratory flow rate (PEFR) (these should be repeated after bronchial dilation treatment)
   c. Arterial blood gas determination

When bursts of corticosteroids are given either intravenously or orally, antibiotics should be given concurrently (see Table 13-4). Because of the increased circulating blood volume in pregnancy, by 26 weeks of gestation, dosing of medications should be adjusted upward to get therapeutic levels of corticosteroids and antibiotics.

If the weeks of gestation are equal to or greater than 24 weeks, the fetus should be monitored during the acute phases initially by 12 to 24 hours of electronic fetal monitoring (EFM) and then by nonstress tests (NSTs) twice weekly when stable. The fetus should also be evaluated by ultrasound for growth rate every 2 to 4 weeks. If the woman is hypoxemic, she should be monitored for contractions twice daily during the acute phase and should be

TABLE 13-3 Treatment plans by zone

	Green zone	Yellow zone	Red zone
Peak expiratory flow	80%-100% of personal best	70%-80% of personal best (upper yellow zone) = trouble 50%-60% of personal best (lower yellow zone) = danger	<50% of personal best
Exacerbation	<2/wk; uses albuterol (Proventil) rarely	>1-2/wk; albuterol (Proventil) MDI is refilled every 2 wk	Daily; uses albuterol (Proventil) frequently
Signs and symptoms	Few	Cough and wheeze	Constant
Exercise tolerance	Good	Diminished	Poor
Nocturnal waking	<2/wk	2-3/wk	Nightly
Work attendance	Good	Diminished	Poor

Treatment	Beta-agonist (2 puffs) before trigger such as exercise or bid prn for symptom exacerbation	Bronchodilators as often as necessary for comfort	Antiinflammatory medication at maximum
	If need beta-agonist >1-2 times/day, then add regular use of inhaled steroid	Boost antiinflammatory medications to maximum	Start oral prednisone
	Be alert to environmental triggers	May try cromolyn	Albuterol (Proventil) SVN treatment $\times 3$ or MDI $\times 4$-6 puffs
		Oral prednisone burst for nonresponders	Provider evaluation in office or emergency room; ambulance for cyanosis or persistent respiratory distress
		Check peak expiratory flow bid; if <70% after 2 days, notify primary care physician	Use IV steroids if necessary
			SVN's maximum frequency
			Once crisis is over, reevaluate:
			Management program regarding triggers
			Compliance
			Antiinflammatory drug
			Coverage

MDI, Metered dose inhaler; *SVN*, small-volume nebulizer.

TABLE 13-4 Medications and dosages for asthma during pregnancy

Drug class	Medication	Dose
Inhaled beta-agonists	Albuterol (Proventil) inhaler (metered dose)	2.5 mg/2.5 ml normal saline
Subcutaneous beta-agonists	Terbutaline	2 puffs (0.25 mg each) every 4 hr
Intravenous cortico-steroids	Methylprednisolone	60-80 mg IV every 6-8 hr
	Hydrocortisone	2.0 mg/kg IV bolus, then 0.5 mg/kg every hr
Oral corticosteroids	Prednisone	60-120 mg per day in divided doses, then tapered over several days to 5 mg qd × 2-4 days
Antiinflammatory inhalation	Cromolyn	2 puffs qid
	Beclomethasone	2-5 puffs bid to qid

Data from American College of Obstetricians and Gynecologists (ACOG): *ACOG Techn Bull,* no. 224, June 1996.

taught self-palpation and home monitoring for preterm labor during ambulatory care and home care.

Pneumonia

Pneumonia is an inflammation of the lower respiratory tract, including the alveoli and bronchioles. It may be caused by bacterial or viral invasion or chemical contact with the respiratory tract. Co-infection with HIV or tuberculosis may worsen the prognosis for mother and fetus.

A chest x-ray film and both blood and sputum cultures are usually obtained to diagnose the extent of infection and the organism or organisms responsible. If atypical bacterial infection is suspected, cold agglutinins are used to test for mycoplasma pneumonia (ACOG, 1996).

Usually therapy is started with a broad-spectrum antibiotic, and then, once the specific causative organism or organisms are detected and reported with sensitivity, more specifically directed antibiotic therapy is used. For gram-negative and *Staphylococcus aureus* infection, usually a third-generation cephalosporin and an aminoglycoside are used in combination. For mycoplasmal pneumonia, the erythromycins are used. Antibiotic therapy in pregnancy usually requires high doses because of increased blood volume and dilution.

For viral pneumonias the course may be complicated by a secondary bacterial infection. Although broad-spectrum antibiotics, such as cephalosporins, may work for the secondary infection, antivirals, such as amantadine, are not used in pregnancy except in fulminant respiratory failure. Amantadine is both embryotoxic and teratogenic in animal studies and is therefore reserved for life-threatening disease in the pregnant woman. Acyclovir is currently recommended for varicella pneumonia in pregnant women.

Tuberculosis

Treatment regimens for tuberculosis include the following:

1. Absence of active disease with less than 2 years converted PPD (purified protein derivative [tuberculin]) status is treated with 300 mg/day of isoniazid, starting after the first trimester and for 6 to 9 months.

2. Women younger than 35 years with an unknown duration of PPD positivity should receive 300 mg/day of isoniazid for 6 to 9 months postpartum.

3. For women older than 35 years, no isoniazid is used in the absence of active disease.

4. Active disease in pregnancy is treated immediately with dual-agent therapy for a full 9 months. The standard regimen is isoniazid, 300 mg/day, combined with rifampin, 600 mg/day. If resistance to isoniazid is identified, ethambutol, 2.5 g/day, is substituted.

5. Pyridoxine (vitamin B_6) is supplementary at 50 mg/day and is essential for all patients.

Although isoniazid, ethambutol, and rifampin have been used in pregnancy with no adverse fetal effects, antituberculosis agents that may *not* be used include streptomycin, kanamycin, ethionamide, capreomycin, cycloserine, and pyrazinamide (ACOG, 1996).

Antituberculosis agents should not be used concurrently in the newborn if the postpartum mother is being treated and is breast-feeding. Antituberculosis agents cross over in breast milk and will reach sufficient levels in the newborn and infant for the duration of breast-feeding (ACOG, 1996).

NURSING PROCESS

PREVENTION

Pregnant women with chronic diseases, such as cystic fibrosis and asthma, should be counseled preconceptually to have their disease under good control and continue good management and avoidance of exposure to environmental agents that may exacerbate or trigger disease response.

Pregnant women should be counseled during early pregnancy to avoid exposure to crowds of people during influenza season and other acute respiratory disease outbreaks and to avoid exposure to people infected with HIV and tuberculosis. Because of the depressed immune response in normal, healthy pregnancy, pregnant women are more susceptible to contracting infections than their nonpregnant counterparts.

NURSING DIAGNOSES/COLLABORATIVE PROBLEMS AND INTERVENTIONS

- **POTENTIAL COMPLICATION: RESPIRATORY INFECTIONS** related to altered immune response pregnancy

  DESIRED OUTCOMES: The patient with chronic disease will be in remission for 3 to 6 months before conception. The pregnant woman will exhibit health-promoting behaviors and avoid exposure to acute respiratory infections. The pregnant woman will seek early and prompt treatment if signs and symptoms of upper respiratory infection are present.

  INTERVENTIONS
  1. Discuss the risks of exposure with the woman and her family.
  2. Encourage early treatment of upper respiratory signs and symptoms.
  3. Encourage health-promoting behaviors such as the following:
     a. Avoid crowds during high infection incidence.
     b. Use a cool mist humidifier at night to help respiratory tract stay healthy.
     c. Drink at least 8 oz of nutritious liquid or water each hour of the day while awake.

- **RISK FOR ACTUAL RESPIRATORY INFECTION** related to presence of concurrent chronic disease such as asthma, cystic fibrosis, active tuberculosis, and positive HIV status

DESIRED OUTCOME: The patient will seek and receive early and prompt treatment and will therefore recover without long-term sequelae or fetal distress.

INTERVENTIONS

1. Respond to detected or reported signs and symptoms that warrant with chest x-ray film and sputum and blood cultures.
2. Treat with appropriate oral or intravenous antibiotics, when necessary.
3. Have baseline function studies in early pregnancy available for comparison in disease states. Seek and keep referrals/collaboration with pulmonary specialists.
4. Use SVNs with beta-agonists and antiinflammatories and corticosteroids as needed.
5. Monitor for contractions and fetal heart rate response in the acute phases after 24 weeks of gestation.
6. Teach women with chronic respiratory tract disease how to self-detect and prevent preterm labor.
7. Monitor fetal growth with ultrasound evaluation every 2 to 3 weeks.

■ **POTENTIAL COMPLICATION: FETAL HYPOXIA** related to degree and duration of maternal hypoxemia

DESIRED OUTCOMES: The fetus will have a baseline heart rate in the normal range for gestation, between 110 and 160 beats/min. The fetus will have the presence of gestationally appropriate short-term and long-term variability. The fetus will be delivered after 32 weeks of gestation, ideally after 37 weeks, and before 41 weeks.

INTERVENTIONS

1. Obtain nonstress tests (NSTs) every 3 or 4 days at onset of symptoms or by 32 weeks if chronic disease is present.
2. Perform ultrasound evaluation 2 to 3 weeks after onset of acute symptoms and until full recovery or delivery, for growth rate and amniotic fluid index.
3. Teach mother to do fetal movement counts once or twice daily after 24 weeks and for duration of pregnancy.
4. Teach the pregnant woman to self-detect signs of preterm contractions.
5. Teach the pregnant woman the importance of adequate calories and nutrients. Make appropriate referrals to a dietitian, the WIC (women, infants, and children) program, and specialists in high risk pregnancy.

CONCLUSION

Respiratory disease in pregnancy can complicate the pregnancy, as pregnancy can complicate the management of acute or chronic respiratory disease. These complications require early health-promoting activities, prompt response and supervision, and close collaboration with pulmonary specialists.

BIBLIOGRAPHY

American College of Obstetricians and Gynecologists (ACOG): Pulmonary disease in pregnancy, *ACOG Techn Bull,* no. 224, June 1996.

Corbett J, Yares P: Beta$_2$ agonists and maintenance drugs in the treatment of asthma, *MCN Am J Matern Child Nurs,* 19, Nov/Dec 1994.

Creasy R, Resnik R: *Maternal fetal medicine: principles and practice,* ed 3, Philadelphia, 1994, Saunders.

Kokenour N, Queenan J, Hobbins J: *Protocols for high risk pregnancies,* ed 3, Boston, 1996, Blackwell Science.

Mabie W: Asthma in pregnancy, *Clin Obstet Gynecol* 39(1):56-69, 1996.

Mays M, Leiner S: Asthma: a comprehensive review, *J Nurse Midwifery* 40(3):256-268, 1995.

Niswander K, Evans A: *Manual of obstetrics,* Boston, 1995, Little, Brown.

Surratt N, Troiana N: Adult respiratory distress in pregnancy: critical care issues, *J Obstet Gynecol Neonatal Nurs* 33(9):773-780, 1994.

V

Complications in Pregnancy

Various complications can develop during the course of a pregnancy and can affect the health and well-being of the mother and fetus as well as the outcome of the pregnancy. With early recognition and the advanced technology of today, the incidence of maternal and perinatal mortality and morbidity resulting from complications is declining. To continue to reduce maternal mortality and further decrease maternal morbidity related to complications, the perinatal nurse needs an in-depth understanding of complications of pregnancy.

The next 10 chapters present a physiologic and pathologic basis for the most common complications of pregnancy. Nursing care, which provides a basis for early recognition and effective management, is discussed.

CHAPTER

14

Spontaneous Abortion

Spontaneous abortion is a natural termination of pregnancy before the fetus has reached viability. A fetus of less than 20 weeks of gestation and weighing less than 350 to 500 g, depending on the state of residence (ACOG, 1993), is not considered viable. Spontaneous abortion is further divided into "early" and "late." An early abortion occurs before 12 weeks of gestation, and a late abortion occurs between 12 and 20 weeks of gestation. Seventy-five percent of early abortions occur before 8 weeks of gestation during the embryonic phase of development, with minimal losses occurring between 8 and 14 weeks (Goldstein, 1994). A spontaneous abortion is commonly referred to as a *miscarriage*. This term is preferred in talking with patients because the word *abortion* is frequently associated with induced abortions.

INCIDENCE

Spontaneous abortion occurs in approximately 15% to 20% of all clinically apparent pregnancies, with a recurrence loss of 25% to 47% (ACOG, 1995). Unrecognized early pregnancy losses occur more frequently. Therefore approximately 50% to 75% of all human conceptions are aborted (Boklage, 1990; Simpson, 1990).

ETIOLOGY
Sporadic Abortions

Nonrecurring Genetic Abnormality

Early abortions are likely to be caused by a nonrecurring genetic abnormality of the embryo (Cunningham and others, 1997). Several studies substantiate the fact that 50% to 60% of most early abortions, before 12 weeks of gestation, have a chromosomal abnormality (Simpson, 1990). The majority of these chromosomal abnormalities are related to numeric error occurring during meiotic cell division of the ovum or sperm or early mitotic cell division of the zygote or blastocyst. If two sperm penetrate one ovum, this can also lead to a chromosomal abnormality. The chromosomal makeup of both parents is usually normal.

Teratogenic Agents

Exposure to various teratogenic agents, such as high-dose radiation (Cunningham and others, 1997), chemicals, cytotoxic drugs (Heppard, Garite, 1996), cocaine (Brent, Beckman, 1994), alcohol (Pietrantoni, Knuppel, 1991), smoking (Brent, Beckman, 1994), moderate to heavy caffeine consumption (Armstrong and others, 1992), and extreme hyperthermia (Rogers, Davis, 1995), can cause placental vascular compromise and embryonic damage leading to a spontaneous abortion.

Systemic Infections

Viruses that are known to cause congenital malformations and stimulate abortions are rubella, cytomegalovirus (CMV), coxsackievirus, active genital herpes, and toxoplasmosis if contracted during pregnancy. It is not known whether the organism itself or the toxins liberated by the organism cause the fetal death (Summers, 1994).

Aging Gamete After Ovulation

Research has indicated that the more time the gamete (sperm or ovum) spends in the fallopian tube before fertilization, the greater the risk of an abortion (Cunningham and others, 1997).

Recurrent Abortions

Genetic Abnormalities

Parental structural chromosome abnormalities account for approximately 2% to 3% of recurrent abortions.

Incompetent Cervix

An incompetent cervix is a weak, structurally defective cervix that spontaneously dilates around 16 weeks of gestation.

Endometrial Infections

The T mycoplasma organisms such as *Ureaplasma urealyticum* and *Mycoplasma hominis,* commonly found in the vagina, may cause a spontaneous abortion if the organism moves into the endometrium (Cunningham and others, 1997). A causal relationship has also been demonstrated between the presence of organisms such as *Treponema pallidum, Chlamydia trachomatis, Neisseria gonorrhoeae,* and *Streptococcus agalactiae* and increased risk of a spontaneous abortion (ACOG, 1995).

Uncontrolled Systemic Diseases

Systemic diseases that are not well controlled, such as diabetes, systemic lupus, sickle cell anemia, hypertensive cardiovascular disease, phenylketonuria, and thyroid imbalance, can cause an abortion.

Uterine Abnormalities

Uterine disorders that may elicit an abortion are structural uterine defects that interfere with the growth and development of the embryo or fetus. The uterine defect may be the result of a congenital defect or an acquired defect secondary to diethylstilbestrol (DES) exposure.

Maternal Age

There appears to be a significantly increased risk of a spontaneous abortion in women older than 36 years (Dickey and others, 1992).

Failed Immunologic Protection

A form of immune rejection has been considered for a long time as a possible cause of spontaneous abortion. This could be caused by a maternal immune response that attacks the foreign paternal antigens on the trophoblast or fetal tissue or by failure of the immunoprotective mechanisms to be stimulated (Scott, 1994). One example of this occurs when the mother and father are genetically similar and share a significant number of human leukocyte antigens (HLAs) but are different enough to arouse the mother's immune system defenses. The mother's immune system then fails to produce the immunoglobulin G (IgG)–blocking antibody that protects the embryo and fetus against maternal lymphocytes

(Peterson, Scott, 1990). If the mother's immune system fails to produce suppressor cells, the embryonic or fetal tissue will be reabsorbed. This is another example of failed immunologic protection and causes a *blighted ovum.*

Autoimmune Factor

In various connective tissue diseases, such as systemic lupus erythematosus (SLE), spontaneous abortions occur more frequently. Many of these patients have an antiphospholipid syndrome characterized by significant levels of antiphospholipid antibodies. Two most common such antibodies are lupus anticoagulant and anticardiolipin antibodies that cause vascular endothelium damage and block the release of prostacyclin. Placental thrombosis and vascular insufficiency occur, causing subsequent fetal death (ACOG, 1995).

Luteal Phase Defects

Some spontaneous abortions are related to a luteal phase defect (LPD). This occurs when the corpus luteum fails to secrete significant amounts of progesterone to maintain the endometrial lining of the uterus and the pregnancy (Carp and others, 1990). It is the cause of approximately 35% of recurrent pregnancy losses (Heppard, Garite, 1996).

NORMAL PHYSIOLOGY
Embryo/Placenta Development

The gametes (sperm and ovum) undergo developmental changes before fertilization. During the maturation process, the number of chromosomes is reduced to 23, which is half the original number. This process is called *meiosis.* When fertilization takes place and a mature sperm enters the mature ovum, the 23 chromosomes from each gamete pair up to form a new cell with 46 chromosomes called the *zygote.* This new cell begins mitotic cell division. When the zygote has developed into a solid ball of cells, it is called a *morula.* As maturation continues, the morula develops into a *blastocyst.* At this stage an outer layer of cells called the *trophoblast,* which will form the placenta and fetal membranes, and an inner cluster of cells called the *embryoblast,* which will form the embryo, are present. On approximately the sixth day after fertilization, the blastocyst is ready to implant into the endometrium of the uterus. This is accomplished as the trophoblast cells begin to secrete a proteolytic enzyme that digests an opening a few cells wide and burrows its way into the uterine lining. A small amount of blood may be lost at this time, which can cause mild vaginal spotting. The opening is closed by a blood clot at first and then regenerated epithelium.

After the blastocyst is implanted into the endometrium of the uterus, the endometrium is called the *decidua*. The decidua is usually divided into three parts. The part of the decidua lying directly beneath the implanted blastocyst is called *decidua basalis*. This is where the placenta will primarily grow. The part of the decidua that covers the buried blastocyst is called *decidua capsularis,* and the remainder of the decidua that is not in direct contact with the blastocyst is called *decidua vera.*

After ovulation, when the mature ovum is released from the ovary, the ovary enters its luteal phase. During this time it excretes high levels of progesterone and some estrogen to prepare and maintain the endometrium for the fertilized ovum. Both hormones stimulate the glandular cells of the endometrium to secrete mucus and glycogen and increase the blood supply to the endometrium to facilitate an adequate nutritional environment for the implanted blastocyst/embryo/fetus. These hormones also facilitate the maintenance of pregnancy by keeping the myometrium quiet so that implantation can take place. For the corpus luteum to continue its production of progesterone and estrogen, the trophoblastic tissue must secrete human chorionic gonadotropin (HCG) until the placenta is mature enough to take over the production of hormones. This hormone maintains the corpus luteum for about the first 8 weeks of gestation.

Placental Immunology

Why the mother's body does not reject the blastocyst remains a mystery. On the surface of all body cells are structural antigens. The lymphocyte white blood cells are able to identify these antigens as either familiar or unfamiliar (foreign) and manufacture antibodies to destroy them if they are identified as foreign. Because the antigens are determined genetically, half the antigens on fetal cells come from each parent. Therefore half the antigens should be foreign to the mother's body.

Currently it is unknown what mechanism or mechanisms prevent the rejection of the fetus. Some of the latest research is beginning to indicate that first the mother's body must be able to recognize foreign paternal antigens on the products of conception. Second, appropriate immunoprotective mechanisms must be initiated.

Immunoabsorbence

The placental tissue that comes in contact with maternal decidua should contain human leukocyte antigen (HLA) class I antigens that can stimulate the T cell–killing mechanism (Scott and others, 1987). Therefore the normal placenta can destroy potentially harmful antipaternal HLA antibodies (Peterson, Scott, 1990) that are normally produced by the mother (Carp and others, 1990).

Immunosuppression

When foreign paternal antigens are recognized by the mother, a cell-mediated immune response is stimulated and suppressor cells develop that promote trophoblast growth and protect the embryo/fetus by rendering maternal antibodies harmless against paternal-originated antigens (Peterson, Scott, 1990).

Immunoregulation

When foreign paternal antigens are recognized by the mother, a humoral immune response is stimulated as well as a cellular response. Various blocking or enhancing antibodies are produced that destroy paternal lymphocytes that enter the maternal blood-stream. This decreases the immune response of the mother toward the embryo or fetus (Peterson, Scott, 1990).

Cervical Changes

An important structure that facilitates pregnancy maintenance is the cervix. The cervix must resist the forces of gravity and intrauterine pressure for 9 months of pregnancy and then become soft and distensible, allowing the fetus to pass through to the vagina. The pregnancy is maintained primarily because of the formation of a sphincterlike structure that forms at the internal cervical os (Parisi, 1994). This develops because of the distending muscular isthmus above and the cervix below, which is composed primarily of connective tissue (ground substance) plus collagen with scattered smooth muscle fibers (Huszar, Walsh, 1991). During pregnancy, collagen fibers are laid down in an orderly fashion among the connective tissue, which gives the cervix strength to remain firm and closed. At the end of pregnancy, rearrangement of the collagen fibers takes place so the fibers become more separable, promoting softening of the cervix (Cabrol, 1991). Numerous cervical glands line the cervical canal. During pregnancy, hyper-trophy and hyperplasia of the cervical glands occur as well, forming the mucous plug.

PATHOPHYSIOLOGY
Embryo/Fetal/Placental Effect

Death of the embryo or failure of the embryo or placenta to develop normally is usually the first step in the sequence of events that leads to a spontaneous abortion. Hemorrhage into the decidua basalis results, which causes necrotic changes at the site of implantation. Infiltration of leukocytes follows. Because of the absence of a functioning fetal circulation, the chorionic villi often become edematous and resemble a hydatidiform mole. At the same time, hormonal levels of progesterone and estrogen drop, causing decidual sloughing, which results in vaginal bleeding. The uterus becomes irritable, and uterine contractions result.

Cervical Incompetence

An incompetent cervix contains more smooth muscle than a normal cervix (Rechberger and others, 1988), and collagen concentration is less than normal. Cervical resistance is lowered. This is usually caused by one of two factors: a congenital defect or past cervical trauma.

Congenital Defect

With a congenital defect the lower genital tract is structurally abnormal. A common cause is exposure to DES.

Cervical Trauma

Cervical trauma is usually the result of mechanical trauma such as excessive dilation for curettage, cervical biopsy, or cervical lacerations acquired during a previous delivery.

SIGNS AND SYMPTOMS
Vaginal Bleeding

The classic sign of a spontaneous abortion is vaginal bleeding. At first it is usually dark spotting related to the decreased hormonal levels of progesterone and estrogen that cause the decidua (endometrium) to begin to slough. It may progress to frank, bright red bleeding as the products of conception begin to separate, opening up uterine blood vessels.

Abdominal Pain

Pain may be manifested in different ways. It may be rhythmic or persistent, and it may present as a low backache or as pelvic pressure or tenderness over the uterus.

CLASSIFICATION

Spontaneous abortions are classified into seven clinical types: threatened, inevitable, complete, incomplete, missed, septic, and recurrent (Fig. 14-1). Table 14-1 gives signs and symptoms manifested by each type.

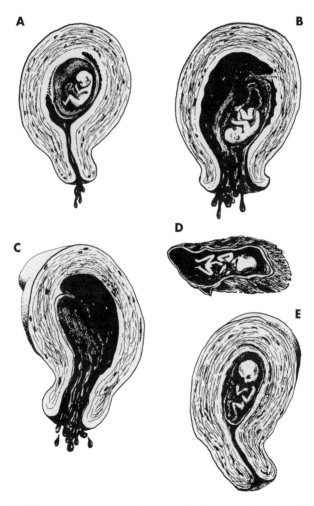

FIG. 14-1 Types of spontaneous abortions. **A,** Threatened abortion. **B,** Inevitable abortion. **C,** Complete abortion. **D,** Incomplete abortion. **E,** Missed abortion.

From Lowdermilk D, Perry S, Bobak I: *Maternity and women's health care,* ed 6, St Louis, 1997, Mosby.

TABLE 14-1 Clinical classification of spontaneous abortions

Classification	Definition	Manifestations
Threatened	Condition in which continuation of pregnancy is in doubt	Vaginal bleeding or spotting, which may be associated with mild cramps of back and lower abdomen Closed cervix Uterus that is soft, nontender, and enlarged appropriate to gestational age
Inevitable	Condition in which termination of pregnancy is in progress	Cervical dilation Membranes may be ruptured Vaginal bleeding Mild to painful uterine contractions
Complete	Condition in which products of conception are totally expelled from uterus	
Incomplete	Condition in which fragments of products of conception are expelled and part is retained in uterus	Profuse bleeding because retained tissue parts interfere with myometrial contractions
Missed	Condition in which embryo or fetus dies during first 20 wk of gestation but is retained in uterus for 4 wk or more afterward	Amenorrhea or intermittent vaginal bleeding, spotting, or brownish discharge No uterine growth No fetal movement felt Regression of breast changes
Septic	Condition in which products of conception become infected during abortion process	Elevated temperature of 100.4° F (38° C) or greater Foul-smelling vaginal discharge
Recurrent	Condition in which two or more successive pregnancies have ended in spontaneous abortion	

MATERNAL EFFECTS

The major contributions to maternal death surrounding a spontaneous abortion are related to two potential complications that rarely occur today: hemorrhage and infection. *Hemorrhage* may be related to a delay in seeking medical treatment or to perforation of the uterus during surgical treatment. *Infection* may be related to a delay in diagnosing a septic abortion or to inappropriate use of antibiotics.

FETAL EFFECT

Death of the fetus always occurs as the result of a spontaneous abortion. It may be the actual cause of the abortion.

DIAGNOSTIC TESTING

When vaginal bleeding occurs during the first 20 weeks of pregnancy, careful evaluation must be made to determine whether it is a threatened abortion or the bleeding is related to another cause. About 20% of all patients experience some vaginal bleeding during the first trimester, and only about half of these actually abort (Cunningham and others, 1997). Therefore consideration must be given to other possible causes of vaginal bleeding, which can be related to one of the following:

- Lesions of the cervix or vagina or cervical polyps that bleed because of increased vascularity of the vagina and cervix during pregnancy
- A hydatidiform mole
- An ectopic pregnancy
- Carcinoma of the cervix
- Normal implantation of the blastocyst into the endometrium

The evaluation to differentiate among the various possible causes of vaginal bleeding usually includes inspecting the vagina and cervix by a speculum examination to rule out vaginal or cervical lesions or cervical polyps and a Pap smear to rule out carcinoma. Pelvic ultrasound examination is usually done to determine if there is an intrauterine gestational sac. This rules out an ectopic pregnancy. A gestational sac, if present, should be identifiable with ultrasound by 6 weeks from the last menstrual period. Real-time ultrasounds can be used to document lack of heart movement, which indicates fetal death. Quantitative beta-HCG assays are helpful in determining the state of the fetus. Serial doubling of quantitative beta-HCG assays strongly indicates a healthy pregnancy.

If the patient presents with signs of an inevitable abortion, tests are not usually necessary to make the diagnosis. Any patient with a history of cervical trauma or painless second-trimester abortion should be examined weekly during the second trimester for an incompetent cervix.

Refer to Box 14-1 for a nurse practitioner workup summary.

USUAL MEDICAL MANAGEMENT AND PROTOCOLS FOR NURSE PRACTITIONERS

Most often, when vaginal bleeding is definitely related to a spontaneous abortion, treatment centers around determining the cause, if possible, keeping the couple informed, and providing emotional support instead of attempting to sustain the pregnancy. This protocol is based on the following factors:

- In an early threatened abortion, the embryo or fetus is usually dead before the bleeding begins.
- Approximately 60% of all early abortions are associated with chromosomal anomalies and are nature's way of preventing the birth of a genetically defective child.
- In late abortions, after 12 weeks of gestation, maternal factors are usually the cause and death does not usually precede the vaginal bleeding. However, if the pregnancy is maintained, the bleeding itself can increase perinatal mortality or the risk of developing congenital abnormalities.
- Controlled studies have also failed to prove that bed rest, hormones such as progesterone, or sedatives have any effect on the outcome of a threatened abortion.
- Administration of medications during organogenesis (weeks 3 to 8) exposes the embryo to possible teratogenic effects.

Threatened Abortion

When a threatened abortion is diagnosed, an assessment is done to determine the probable outcome. Prompt evacuation of the uterus must be carried out if any of the following findings are present:

- Bleeding has become excessive.
- Any part of the products of conception has been lost.
- The cervix shows signs of dilation.
- Signs and symptoms of an intrauterine infection are present.
- There is a definite diagnosis of a dead fetus with ultrasound.

To assess for the presence of one of these negative findings, a medical workup is done that usually includes the following:

- A pelvic examination to determine signs of dilation
- A blood count for red blood cells, hemoglobin, and hematocrit

Box 14-1

Nurse Practitioner Workup Summary

Evaluation of amount of blood loss
  Subjective report
  Vital signs
  Orthostatic blood pressure changes
      Check orthostatic blood pressure if condition permits. To do this, take the patient's blood pressure and pulse while she is supine. Retake these vital signs after the patient has been in a standing position for 5 minutes. A decrease in systolic blood pressure of 10 mm Hg or an increase in the pulse rate of 10 beats/min or more is interpreted as an indication of significant blood loss.
  Pulse pressure
      The diastolic blood pressure reflects the amount of systemic vasoconstriction present; the pulse pressure (difference between systolic and diastolic pressure) indicates stroke volume; the systolic pressure denotes the interrelationship between the level of vasoconstriction and the stroke volume. A narrowing of the pulse pressure (normal 30 to 40 mm Hg) is an early sign of hypovolemia.
  Hypothenar refilling
      Squeeze the hypothenar area of the hand (the fleshy elevation of the ulnar side of the palm) for 1 to 2 seconds. Normal blood volume is indicated by initial blanching with return to the normal pink coloration within 1 to 2 seconds. A blood volume deficit of 15% to 25% will be indicated by delayed refilling.
Menstrual history
  Last normal menstrual period (LNMP), frequency, duration, and flow
Gynecologic history
  Contraceptive history
  Sexually transmitted disease
Obstetric history
Checking for history of a coagulation disorder
Physical examination
  Abdominal examination
      Auscultation
      Percussion
      Palpation (tender area last)
      Rebound tenderness
      McBurney point
      Iliopsoas
      Obturator test
      Murphy sign

Continued

Box 14-1
Nurse Practitioner Workup Summary—cont'd

Vaginal speculum examination to determine the following:
  Source of the bleeding: rule out cervical or vaginal causes such as polyps, cervical or vaginal lesions, vaginal infection, vaginal trauma, cervical pregnancy, cervical cancer, or pelvic inflammatory disease
  Amount of vaginal bleeding
  Cervical status: opened or closed
  Presence of tissue at the cervix
Bimanual vaginal examination
  Assess the uterine size and determine the presence of an adnexal mass or tenderness
Diagnostic data
  Quantitative serum human chorionic gonadotropin (HCG)
  Complete blood cell count and serology
  Blood type and platelet count
  Vaginal ultrasound
  Urine for culture and sensitivity

---

to aid in the determination of the amount of blood lost and the presence or absence of anemia

- A blood count for white blood cells to determine whether an infection is present
- Vaginal ultrasound, serial serum quantitative beta-HCG assays, and serum progesterone values to determine if the fetus is alive; indicators of fetal well-being: a well-formed gestational ring with central echoes from the embryo, serum progesterone greater than 10 ng/ml, and serial doubling of quantitative beta-HCG assays

If the assessment does not reveal a negative finding, the patient is usually managed as an outpatient with frequent physician's visits and instructions to limit her activity and abstain from intercourse. If an intrauterine device (IUD) is in place and the string is visible, it is usually removed. Further treatment depends on the signs and symptoms that develop.

Inevitable, Complete, or Incomplete Abortion

Once the cervix begins to dilate, there is no hope for the pregnancy and an abortion becomes inevitable. If part of the products of conception is lost, the abortion becomes incomplete, and if all the products of conception are lost, the abortion is complete.

From the time an abortion becomes inevitable until it becomes complete, naturally or with surgical intervention, there is a high risk for complications such as hemorrhage or an infection. The risk of hemorrhage usually correlates with the gestational age of the pregnancy. For the first 6 weeks the placenta is very tentatively attached to the decidua of the uterus. Therefore if a spontaneous abortion occurs before 6 weeks of gestation, the bleeding usually takes the form of a heavy menstrual period. Between 6 and 12 weeks of gestation, the chorionic villi of the placenta begin to grow into the decidua of the uterus, and by week 12 or shortly after, the chorionic villi have deeply penetrated into the decidua. If a spontaneous abortion occurs after the placenta has completed its penetration process (week 12), the fetus is usually expelled before placental separation. Bleeding is usually held in check by the placenta until it is separated and then by uterine contractions if the separation is complete. Therefore the most severe bleeding is seen between 6 and 12 weeks of gestation because the placenta can detach before expulsion of the fetus, or severe bleeding can result after 12 weeks of gestation if the placenta does not separate completely and parts are retained. Thus if the gestational age is known, the risk of bleeding can be more easily estimated.

The risk of infection usually depends on many factors, such as the nutritional state of the patient, perineal hygiene, and whether anything, except a sterile speculum, entered the vagina after dilation began.

According to Nielsen and Hahlin (1995), expectant management to allow spontaneous resolution was found to be just as safe a treatment plan for first-trimester spontaneous abortion as was a dilation and curettage (D & C). Complications were similar between the two treatment groups with less incidence of pelvic inflammatory disease (PID) in the expectant management group. However, prompt evacuation of the uterus may be indicated in the presence of excessive cramping, heavy bleeding, or emotional instability. This is usually carried out by curettage, vacuum aspiration, or injection of oxytocin intravenously followed by curettage. If vacuum aspiration is used to remove the products of conception, a vacuum aspirator suction curet is inserted through the dilated cervix after the patient is anesthetized. The vacuum aspirator is moved gently over the surface of the uterine wall in a systematic pattern so as to cover all the uterine cavity, and the products of conception are collected in a vacuum container. When curettage is done, a sharp curet, a spoon-shaped instrument, is gently moved in downward strokes over the uterine wall to remove the products of conception and the necrotic decidua.

These procedures can be done in an outpatient setting or in the hospital. The woman is usually hospitalized if gestational age is 12 weeks or greater or if severe bleeding or signs of infection are present. If time permits, a history and physical examination are usually performed and a complete blood count is done. A tube of blood is usually held for typing and cross matching in case a transfusion becomes necessary. A dilute solution of intravenous (IV) oxytocin is often started before the surgery to reduce blood loss and decrease the risk of uterine perforation by causing the uterus to contract and thicken. A preoperative medication of 5 to 10 mg of diazepam (Valium) may be ordered. The procedure can be done with a paracervical block, especially if an outpatient setting is used, or with the patient under a light general anesthesia. If the procedure is done with the patient under local anesthesia, the patient may experience some cramping sensations during the procedure.

If the bleeding is severe, the patient's vital signs must be stabilized before surgery. This is usually accomplished by infusing 1 to 2 L of a crystalloid solution such as lactated Ringer's solution intravenously with 30 U of oxytocin per 1000 ml. If lactated Ringer's solution with oxytocin is used, the IV infusion is usually set to infuse at 200 ml/hr or more. This large dose of oxytocin is needed during the first half of pregnancy because the uterus is less sensitive to oxytocin at this time because of the low levels of estrogen present to potentiate its effect. If this is not effective, an erythrocyte infusion or another appropriate blood component may be used. If signs of infection are present or develop, antibiotic therapy is usually initiated.

If the cervix is not partially dilated, dilation is usually accomplished slowly by placing *Laminaria* dilators or a prostaglandin suppository or gel in the cervix before the evacuation procedure. *Laminaria* tents, such as *Laminaria digitata* or *Laminaria japonica,* are natural cervical dilators made from seaweed, the stems of which have been peeled, dried, and sterilized. Synthetic alternatives are being used more frequently. Dilapan, a hygroscopic cervical dilator, and Lamicel, an alcohol polymer sponge impregnated with 450 mg of magnesium sulfate and compressed into a tent, are two commonly used synthetic dilators. Inserted into the full length of the cervical canal, the dilators absorb cervical fluids and swell, dilating the cervix slowly (Fig. 14-2). The patient may experience cramping, which is easily

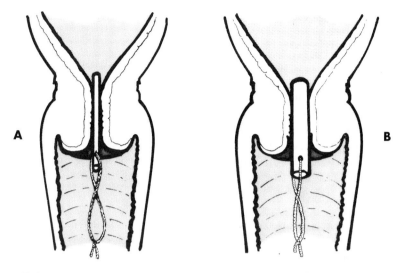

FIG. 14-2 A, Properly inserted laminaria. **B,** Laminaria after 8 hours of absorbing cervical fluid, causing it to swell and dilate cervix gradually.
Illustration by Vincenza Genovese, Phoenix.

controlled with a mild analgesic. Then at the time of surgery or before the evacuation procedure the *Laminaria* dilators are removed. Serial applications of prostaglandin gel or vaginal suppositories placed in the cervix can accomplish the same result. Because both methods dilate the cervix slowly, they decrease the risk of cervical trauma, which can occur with mechanical dilators.

If all the embryonic or fetal and placental tissue can be identified and there are no signs of bleeding or an infection, the abortion is complete and no surgical intervention is necessary. However, some physicians believe that all abortions should be considered incomplete until curettage is performed to remove the necrotic decidual tissue. Therefore some physicians routinely do curettage after all abortions.

Missed Abortion

Most missed abortions will terminate spontaneously. However, if there are no signs of a spontaneous abortion at the time a missed abortion is diagnosed, the physician usually evacuates the uterus as soon as possible because of the following potential problems:

1. Psychologic stress related to carrying a dead fetus
2. Sepsis
3. Disseminated intravascular coagulopathy (DIC), a coagulation defect with hypofibrinogenemia, increased fibrin, and

decreased platelets; this occurs because the dead products of conception release thromboplastin into the maternal circulation, stimulating this process (see Chapter 18)

The techniques used for the evacuation usually depend on the length of pregnancy. Pregnancies up to 16 weeks of gestation are usually terminated by prostaglandin E_1 vaginal suppositories or dilation and evacuation by curettage or vacuum aspiration. Vacuum aspiration is preferable to curettage during the first 10 weeks of gestation; there is less chance of perforation, bleeding, or infection. After 16 weeks the likelihood of uterine perforation, cervical lacerations, hemorrhage, incomplete removal of the products of conception, and infection is the usual reason given for not using curettage or vacuum aspiration. Various prostaglandin preparations are used from 16 to 20 weeks of gestation.

Prostaglandins can be administered orally, parenterally, into the amniotic sac, or as a vaginal suppository. The oral method is not used because of the extremely uncomfortable side effects, such as severe gastrointestinal distress. All other routes are used to induce contractions and cause the uterus to expel the products of conception. Side effects that the patient may experience are nausea, vomiting, diarrhea, fever, dizziness, headache, and hypertension. Rare side effects are bronchospasm, cardiac dysrhythmias, chest pain, and hyperventilation.

Intraamniotic injection of hypotonic saline is rarely used because of the reduced volume of amniotic fluid, which makes the procedure too difficult. The hypertonic saline solution can also further increase the risk of developing a coagulation defect.

Dilation of the cervix should take place before any of these methods of evacuation. A *Laminaria* tent or intravaginal prostaglandins are usually the treatment of choice to dilate the cervix without risk of its injury.

Recurrent Spontaneous Abortion

Some recurrent abortions occur by chance; others are related to a maternal or paternal cause. Treatment should focus on identifying the cause and treating accordingly.

Chromosomal Disorder

When a couple repeatedly loses an embryo or fetus early in gestation, a chromosomal disorder of the father or mother may be the cause. A genetic history should be taken, karyotyping is recommended, and genetic counseling should follow as indicated.

Uterine Defect

Uterine defects are occasionally the cause of late recurrent spontaneous abortions. During curettage for a spontaneous abortion, the uterine cavity should be closely examined for any abnormalities.

Incompetent Cervix

Treatment for recurrent abortions caused by an incompetent cervix is usually cerclage, a surgical procedure in which a purse-string suture is placed around the cervix to reinforce it. This procedure is usually performed around 14 to 16 weeks of gestation before cervical dilation or effacement takes place and any bleeding or cramping is present.

Luteal Phase Defect

If no structural defects of the cervix or uterus or chromosomal abnormality can be found, the woman should be tested for a luteal defect or an immunologic cause. When an endometrial biopsy, done late in the menstrual cycle, indicates inadequate production of progesterone by the corpus luteum, a luteal defect may be the cause. Supplemental natural progesterone suppositories can be beneficial. The usual dose is 25 mg twice per day. To be most effective, the progesterone should be started at the time of ovulation and continued until week 12 of gestation (ACOG, 1995). It has been effective when started as soon as the pregnancy is suspected in some cases.

Immunologic Factors

After two or three spontaneous abortions for which no cause can be determined, the couple should be tissue typed to identify the antigens on the white blood cells (called *human leukocyte antigen [HLA] typing*). If the couple is found to share a significant number of antigens, it is currently thought that the mother's body might not be stimulated into making a blocking antibody and is rejecting the products of conception. Women found to have this problem have been treated by immunization with paternal or third-party leukocytes (Coulam and others, 1994). It is thought that immunization tricks the mother's body into producing the blocking antibodies (Branch, 1992).

Endometrial Infections

After a recurrent spontaneous abortion, endometrial cultures for *U. urealyticum* should be obtained. If the cultures are positive, the couple should be treated with doxycycline, 250 mg twice daily for 10 days.

Autoimmune Factor

A patient who has a lupus anticoagulant or an anticardiolipin antibody may be given prednisone, 40 to 60 mg/day, and aspirin, 75 to 80 mg/day, as soon as the pregnancy is determined. Prednisone is given to inhibit platelet aggregation and aspirin to restore the normal thromboxane/prostacyclin ratio (Branch and others, 1992). Refer to Chapter 12.

NURSING PROCESS

PREVENTION

Because teratogenic agents increase the risk of a spontaneous abortion, preventive measures should be taken to avoid this risk. These measures should be instituted before pregnancy by maintaining a healthful life-style, including a nutritious diet, no smoking, no drinking alcoholic beverages, and receiving available immunizations against infectious diseases. When pregnancy is diagnosed, instructions given to expectant mothers should include ways they can decrease their chance of contacting an infection, such as eating nutritiously, avoiding fatigue, and avoiding people with infections. They should also be instructed, if they eat meat, to cook it well; if they have a pet cat or bird, to leave the cleaning of the litter area to someone else; and if they work in the yard, to use gloves to avoid contact with the toxoplasmosis virus. Instructions should be provided regarding the avoidance of x-rays and medications, especially nonprescription ones, unless ordered by their obstetrician.

NURSING DIAGNOSES/COLLABORATIVE PROBLEMS AND INTERVENTIONS

- **POTENTIAL COMPLICATION: HEMORRHAGE** related to partially detached placenta or surgical intervention.
  DESIRED OUTCOME: The signs and symptoms of hemorrhage will be minimized or managed as measured by stable vital signs, a blood loss less than 250 ml, urine output greater than 30 ml/hr or 120 ml/4 hr, and a hematocrit maintained between 30% and 45%.
  INTERVENTIONS
    1. Obtain a history of onset, duration, amount, color, and consistency of bleeding.
    2. Obtain a history regarding associated symptoms, prior bleeding episodes, and activity at onset of bleeding.

3. Record visual blood loss in cubic centimeters of blood stained on pad in a certain period of time, or weigh saturated pads, linen protectors, or linen (1 g = 1 ml).

4. Record blood pressure, pulse, and respirations as indicated (depends on severity).

5. Observe for passage of tissue or clots.

6. Observe for signs of shock.

7. Keep an accurate record of intake and output.

8. Refer to such laboratory data as hemoglobin, hematocrit, and red blood cell count.

9. Determine gestational age by estimated date of delivery (EDD).

10. Save all tissue and clots expelled for examination.

11. If bleeding is severe or the hemoglobin or hematocrit is low, start an IV line with an 18-gauge intracatheter and normal saline to be prepared for blood component therapy or blood administration as ordered. Start another IV line to administer a crystalloid solution such as lactated Ringer's solution as ordered. Most patients can be stabilized with a crystalloid solution (Naef, Morrison, 1995). Prepare for type and cross match, and have oxytocin available. Usual dose is 10 units in 500 ml of 0.9% (normal) saline or D5W solution to infuse at 20 to 40 gtt/min (Zatuchni, Slupik, 1996).

12. Notify physician if the blood pressure drops, pulse or respirations increase, more than one pad is saturated with blood in 1 hour, urinary output drops below 30 ml/hr or 120 ml/4 hr, or the hematocrit is less than 30% or hemoglobin less than 11 g. Be prepared to intervene based on percentage of blood loss. Refer to Table 17-3 for guidelines for blood component replacement.

13. Assist with medical management based on diagnosis.

If no signs of an inevitable, incomplete, or missed abortion are found, the following interventions apply:

1. Provide discharge instructions that include the importance of limiting activity, abstaining from intercourse, and returning for a reevaluation appointment.

2. Instruct as to the importance of notifying physician immediately if bleeding becomes more than a period or persists, if cramps develop, or if a fever develops.

3. Encourage patient to continue to take her prenatal vitamins and eat foods high in protein, iron, and fiber.

4. If the patient asks, discuss the prognosis (50% chance) of the threatened abortion resulting in a spontaneous abortion (Cunningham and others, 1997).

If signs of an inevitable, incomplete, or missed abortion are present, the following interventions apply:

1. Prepare for surgical or medical intervention as applicable.
2. Explain procedure to patient.
3. Surgically prepare patient.

If curettage or vacuum aspiration is to be used, the following interventions apply:

1. Have patient empty bladder before procedure.
2. Be prepared to start an IV line so that oxytocin can be administered to facilitate uterine contractions during or after the procedure.
3. If cervix is not dilated, be prepared to assist with some form of cervical dilation.
4. Administer an antiemetic or analgesic as ordered.
5. Explain sensations that may be experienced during the procedure.

If prostaglandins are used, the following interventions apply:

1. Observe for side effects such as nausea/vomiting, diarrhea, drug-related fever, or a blood pressure change.
2. If intraamniotic prostaglandins are used, be prepared for and assist with amniocentesis.
3. If prostaglandin vaginal suppositories or gel is used, be prepared to assist with insertion.
4. Assess for uterine contractions.
5. Provide comfort measures.

After evacuation be prepared to give ergonovine maleate (Methergine), 200 µg orally every 6 hours for 6 doses if bleeding is heavy.

- **RISK FOR INFECTION**   related to open uterine blood vessels, dilated cervix, or surgical intervention.

  DESIRED OUTCOME: The signs and symptoms of an infection will be minimized or managed as measured by normothermia, absence of foul-smelling vaginal discharge, and the white blood cell count between 4500 and 10,000/mm^3.

  INTERVENTIONS

  1. Check the temperature every 4 hours for 48 hours.
  2. Check vaginal discharge for an odor every shift.
  3. Refer to laboratory data such as white cell count.
  4. Teach the patient the importance of perineal care after each voiding, and encourage patient to change perineal pads often.
  5. Keep bed linen clean and dry.

6. If signs of an infection develop, be prepared to administer antibiotics as ordered.
7. Discharge instructions include appropriate perineal care: shower only for first 2 weeks; no use of tampons, douching, or sexual intercourse for 2 weeks; and notification of physician if an elevated temperature or a foul-smelling vaginal discharge develops.

■ **ANTICIPATORY GRIEVING** related to loss of an anticipated infant and possible threat to fertility (see Chapter 6).
DESIRED OUTCOME: The patient and the family members will verbalize their feelings of grief appropriately and identify any problems as they work through the grief process.
INTERVENTIONS

1. Assess significance of the loss to all family members and level of guilt or blame. Guilt is commonly experienced after a spontaneous abortion (Frost, Condon, 1996). Counsel the patient and her family as to frequency of a spontaneous abortion and its possible etiologies.
2. Encourage the patient and her family to express their feelings and concerns openly.
3. Assess the family's communication pattern and support systems.
4. Acknowledge, permit, and assist individual family members to identify feelings of relief, sadness, distress, or neutrality toward the loss.
5. Provide physical care such as a back rub or nourishment as needed.
6. Consider any significant cultural beliefs or values. Refer to a pastor, priest, or chaplain per family's request for spiritual assistance to work through their grief.
7. Refer to a support group such as Resolve Through Sharing or Compassionate Friends if available.
8. Refer to psychologic support or counseling if indicated.
9. Provide family with a list of helpful publications such as a 1997 pamphlet, *Understanding Miscarriage: Coping With the Loss* by Krames Communications (800-333-3032); *When Pregnancy Fails* by Susan Borg and Judith Lasker; *Death of a Dream* by Donna and Rodger Ewy; *After a Loss in Pregnancy* by Nancy Barezin; *Ended Beginnings* by C. Panuthos and C. Romeo; and *Empty Arms: Coping After Miscarriage, Stillbirth and Infant Death* by I. Sherokee. (Refer to Chapter 6.)

10. Discuss with the family the importance of grieving the loss before getting pregnant again. Many parents try to lessen their grief by planning and getting pregnant. According to Frost and Condon (1996), another pregnancy inhibits mourning and delays resolution.

- **RISK FOR ALTERED HEALTH MAINTENANCE** related to lack of knowledge regarding risk factors and preventive measures.
  DESIRED OUTCOME: The patient and her family will be able to identify health promotion measures that decrease one's risk of a spontaneous abortion and state reasons for a diagnostic and genetic workup to determine possible cause, if needed.
  INTERVENTIONS
  1. Discuss with the couple the cause, if known, or otherwise explain possible reasons for a spontaneous abortion.
  2. If this is their second or third spontaneous abortion, they should be encouraged to have a diagnostic and genetic workup to attempt to determine the cause. This might include the following:
     a. Karyotyping of abortus
     b. Karyotyping of parents
     c. Late luteal phase biopsy
     d. Thyroid panel
     e. Fasting blood sugar
     f. Endometrium cultures for *U. urealyticum*
     g. A hysterosalpingogram or hysteroscopy to rule out uterine anomaly
     h. Ruling out autoimmune disease with tests for lupus anticoagulant or anticardiolipin antibodies
  3. If the couple asks, discuss the prognosis of a subsequent abortion (35% risk after the initial abortion with a 50% risk with consecutive abortions [Portnoi and others, 1988]).
  4. Teach the couple the importance of using contraception of choice through two normal menstrual periods, at least, to allow time for the woman's body to recover. (After an abortion, the woman usually ovulates during the next cycle [Donnet and others, 1990], but there is a significantly increased risk of endometrial abnormalities for the next two cycles [Nakajima and others, 1991].)
  5. Develop and consistently use a self-administered, matter-of-fact, nonjudgmental questionnaire to obtain life-style behaviors such as patterns of smoking, alcohol consumption, caffeine intake, recreational drug use, nonprescription medication use, and occupation.

6. Analyze the responses for potential risk.
7. Motivate family to want to make life-style changes to improve health-related behaviors by providing them with information about health risks and possible effects on pregnancy outcome.
8. Provide supportive counseling to aid the family in making changes and help them to build self-esteem and overcome feelings of guilt. Avoid using threatening statements that make them feel guilty.
9. Assess patient's immunization record and encourage immunization for rubella if rubella titer is less than 1:10.
10. Provide instructions regarding ways to decrease the chance of contracting an infection, such as eating nutritiously, preventing fatigue, avoiding people with infections, cooking meat well, and leaving the cleaning of the pet cat or bird area to someone else to avoid contact with the toxoplasmosis virus.
11. Provide instructions regarding the pregnant woman avoiding x-rays and medications, especially nonprescription drugs, unless ordered by her obstetrician.
12. Make appropriate community referrals to resources that enable implementation of the family's goals.

- **RISK FOR ACUTE PAIN** related to uterine cramping or surgical intervention.
  DESIRED OUTCOME: The patient will verbalize relief from discomfort with ordered analgesia.
  INTERVENTIONS
  1. Observe for restlessness and discomfort at least two times per shift.
  2. Use natural pain-relieving techniques, such as relaxation and positioning in the most comfortable position.
  3. Administer a narcotic or nonsteroidal antiinflammatory analgesic as needed for pain relief.
  4. Instruct patient to report to nurse when uncomfortable.
  5. Notify physician if ordered analgesic is ineffective.

- **POTENTIAL COMPLICATION: ANEMIA** related to blood loss.
  DESIRED OUTCOME: The signs and symptoms of anemia will be minimized or managed as measured by maintaining a hemoglobin between 11 and 14 g/dl.
  INTERVENTIONS
  1. Assess for fatigue level.
  2. Refer to laboratory data such as hemoglobin.

3. Provide discharge instructions as to the importance of eating food high in iron and protein to promote tissue repair and red blood cell replacement. Foods high in iron include meat and plant foods such as legumes, dried fruits, whole grains, and green, leafy vegetables. Iron from plant foods is less well absorbed by the body, but absorption can be improved by eating these foods along with a food high in vitamin C.

4. Instruct the patient also to notify physician if feelings of fatigue persist beyond 2 weeks.

- **POTENTIAL COMPLICATION: DIC** related to retention of a dead fetus.

  DESIRED OUTCOME: The signs and symptoms of DIC will be minimized or managed as measured by normal clotting factors.

  INTERVENTIONS
  1. Observe for nose or gum bleeding, oozing from IV sites, or petechiae.
  2. Refer to such laboratory data as fibrinogen, platelets, partial thromboplastin time, and clotting time.
  3. If DIC develops, see DIC nursing diagnoses and collaborative problems in Chapter 18.

- **POTENTIAL COMPLICATION: D SENSITIZATION** in a D-negative mother carrying a D-positive fetus.

  DESIRED OUTCOME: The mother's body will not develop antibodies against the D-negative factor.

  INTERVENTIONS
  1. Determine mother's blood type and Rh factor.
  2. If mother is Rh negative, be prepared to administer Rho (D) immune globulin (RhoGAM) (HypRho-D). (The usual dose is 50 µg for a gestation of 12 weeks or less and 300 µg if the gestational age is greater than 12 weeks.)

CONCLUSION

Many times a spontaneous abortion is nature's way of eliminating a chromosomally defective fetus. These defects can be caused by an unpreventable, nonrecurring genetic abnormality or by a preventable teratogenic agent. The nurse can have an impact on lowering the incidence of spontaneous abortion by implementing an education program. This program should include the effects of alcohol, smoking, infections, x-rays, cocaine, and other teratogenic agents on the developing fetus. In these and other cases in which the cause is unpreventable, the nurse should provide adequate emotional support so the parents will not be left with emotional scars because of anxiety or guilt over their failure to maintain the pregnancy to term.

In some cases the cause is related to a maternal defect. The nurse should work with the health care team in recognizing these cases and then make appropriate referrals to facilitate treatment so that a recurrent abortion will not occur.

BIBLIOGRAPHY

American College of Obstetricians and Gynecologists (ACOG): Diagnosis and management of fetal death, *ACOG Techn Bull,* no. 176, 1993.

American College of Obstetricians and Gynecologists (ACOG): Early pregnancy loss, *ACOG Techn Bull,* no. 212, 1995.

Armstrong B, McDonald A, Sloan M: Cigarette, alcohol, and coffee consumption and spontaneous abortion, *Am J Public Health* 82:85, 1992.

Boklage E: Survival probability of human conceptions from fertilization to term, *Int J Fertil* 35:189-194, 1990.

Branch D: Immunologic aspects of pregnancy loss: alloimmune and autoimmune considerations. In Reece E and others, editors: *Medicine of the fetus and mother,* Philadelphia, 1992, Lippincott.

Branch D and others: Outcome of treated pregnancies in women with antiphospholipid syndrome: an update of the Utah experience, *Obstet Gynecol* 80:614-620, 1992.

Brent R, Beckman D: The contribution of environmental teratogens to embryonic and fetal loss, *Clin Obstet Gynecol* 37(3):646-670, 1994.

Cabrol D: Cervical distensibility changes in pregnancy, term, and preterm labor, *Semin Perinatol* 15(2):133-139, 1991.

Carp H and others: Recurrent miscarriage: a review of current concepts, immune mechanisms, and results of treatment, *Obstet Gynecol Surv* 45(10):657-669, 1990.

Coulam C, Stern J: Endocrine factors associated with recurrent spontaneous abortion, *Clin Obstet Gynecol* 37(3):730-744, 1994.

Coulam C and others: A worldwide collaborative observational study and meta-analysis on allogenic leukocyte immunotherapy for recurrent spontaneous abortion, *Am J Reprod Immunol* 23:55-72, 1994.

Cunningham F and others: *Williams' obstetrics,* ed 20, Stamford, Conn, 1997, Appleton & Lange.

Dickey R and others: Relationship of small gestational sac-crown-rump length differences to abortion and abortus karyotypes, *Obstet Gynecol* 79:554, 1992.

Donnet M and others: Return of ovarian function following spontaneous abortion, *Clin Endocrinol* 33:13-20, 1990.

Egarter C and others: Gemeprost for first trimester missed abortion, *Arch Gynecol Obstet* 256:29, 1995.

Frost M, Condon J: The psychological sequelae of miscarriage: a critical review of the literature, *Aust NZ J Psychiatry* 30:54-62, 1996.

Goldstein S: Embryonic death in early pregnancy: a new look at the first trimester, *Obstet Gynecol* 84:294-297, 1994.

Heppard M, Garite T: *Acute obstetrics: a practical guide,* ed 2, St Louis, 1996, Mosby.

Huszar G, Walsh M: Relationship between myometrial and cervical functions in pregnancy and labor, *Semin Perinatol* 15(2):97-117, 1991.

Lowdermilk D, Perry S, Bobak I: *Maternity and women's health care,* ed 6, St Louis, 1997, Mosby.

Lyon D: Critical pathways in the management of first-trimester bleeding and pain, *The Female Patient* 20(2):19-27, 1995.

Naef R, Morrison J: Transfusion therapy in pregnancy, *Clin Obstet Gynecol* 38(3):547-557, 1995.

Nakajima S and others: Endometrial histology after first trimester spontaneous abortion, *Fertil Steril* 55(1):32-35, 1991.

Neilsen S, Hahlin M: Expectant management vs. D&C for first-trimester spontaneous abortion, *Lancet* 345:84-86, 1995.

Parisi V: Cervical incompetence. In Creasy R, Resnik R, editors: *Maternal-fetal medicine: principles and practice,* ed 3, Philadelphia, 1994, Saunders.

Patton P: Anatomic uterine defects, *Clin Obstet Gynecol* 37(3):705-721, 1994.

Peterson C, Scott J: Immunologic factors in reproductive failure, *Obstet Gynecol Rep* 2:234-254, 1990.

Pietrantoni M, Knuppel R: Alcohol use in pregnancy, *Clin Perinatol* 18(1):93-111, 1991.

Portnoi M and others: Karyotypes of 1,142 couples with recurrent abortion, *Obstet Gynecol* 72:31-34, 1988.

Rechberger T, Uldbjerg N, Oxlund H: Connective tissue changes in the cervix during normal pregnancy and pregnancy complicated by cervical incompetence, *Obstet Gynecol* 71:563-567, 1988.

Rogers J, Davis B: How risky are hot tubs and saunas for pregnant women? *MCN Am J Matern Child Nurs* 20(3):137-140, 1995.

Scott J: Recurrent miscarriage: overview and recommendations, *Clin Obstet Gynecol* 37(3):768-773, 1994.

Scott J, Rote N, Branch D: Immunologic aspects of recurrent abortion and fetal death, *Obstet Gynecol* 70:645-656, 1987.

Silver R, Branch D: Recurrent miscarriage: autoimmune considerations, *Clin Obstet Gynecol* 37(3):745-760, 1994.

Simpson J: Genetic causes of spontaneous abortion, *Contemp Obstet Gynecol* 35(9):25-40, 1990.

Summers P: Microbiology relevant to recurrent miscarriage, *Clin Obstet Gynecol* 37(3):722-729, 1994.

Zatuchni G, Slupik R: *Obstetrics and gynecology drug handbook,* ed 2, St Louis, 1996, Mosby.

CHAPTER

15

Ectopic Pregnancy

An ectopic pregnancy develops as the result of the blastocyst implanting somewhere other than in the endometrium of the uterus. Sites of an ectopic pregnancy (Fig. 15-1) are the fallopian tube, ovary, cervix, or abdominal cavity. The majority of ectopic pregnancies (95%) are located in the fallopian tube, with 1% located on an ovary, less than 1% on the cervix, and 3% to 4% in the abdominal cavity (Minnick-Smith, Cook, 1997).

Of all tubal ectopic pregnancies, 90% are located in the ampulla, or largest portion of the tube. The next most common site is the isthmus, or the narrow part of the tube that connects the interstitium to the ampullar portion. Three percent are located in the interstitium or muscular portion of the tube adjacent to the uterine cavity. Rarely does the ectopic pregnancy locate in the fimbria or terminal end of the tube (Cunningham and others, 1997). The outcome and gestational length of the ectopic pregnancy will be influenced by its location in the fallopian tube.

INCIDENCE

The incidence of ectopic pregnancy in the United States is approximately 1 of every 50 to 60 pregnancies (Cowan, 1993), with the number increasing each year worldwide (Centers for Disease Control and Prevention, 1995). Women older than 35 years, teenagers, nonwhites, and women who have a history of infertility are at a greater risk of experiencing an ectopic pregnancy (Bernstein, 1995).

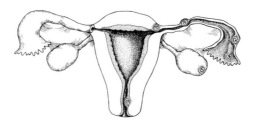

FIG. 15-1 Common sites for an ectopic pregnancy.

ETIOLOGY
Previous Tubal Infections

Previous pelvic infections caused by certain sexually transmitted diseases, such as *Chlamydia* and gonorrhea, postpartum endometritis, and postabortal uterine infections can predispose to a tubal infection (Cunningham and others, 1997; Phillips and others, 1992). A tubal infection can damage the mucosal surface of the fallopian tube, causing intraluminal adhesions that interfere with the transportation of the fertilized ovum to the uterine cavity (Brunham and others, 1992).

Previous Tubal or Pelvic Surgery

During surgery, if blood is allowed to enter the fallopian tubes, tubal adhesions can result from the irritation of the mucosal surface. Salpingectomy, for previous ectopic pregnancy or for treatment of an inflammatory process, and salpingoplasty, for infertility or for previous ectopic pregnancy, are the surgeries that most frequently cause tubal adhesions. Occasionally irritation results from an appendectomy. A previous cesarean delivery slightly increases the risk of a future ectopic pregnancy (Hemminki, Merilainen, 1996).

Hormonal Factors

Altered estrogen/progesterone levels or inappropriate levels of prostaglandins or catecholamines can interfere with normal tubal motility of the fertilized ovum. For example, a luteal phase defect leading to a low progesterone level can cause weak propulsive force in the tube (Guillaume and others, 1995).

Contraceptive Failure

Ectopic pregnancies occur with the use of an intrauterine device (IUD) in approximately 5 per 1000 users each year (Hatcher,

1994.) This appears to occur more often with the use of the Progestasert IUD as compared with the copper IUD (Hatcher and others, 1994). The cause is unknown but may be related to altered tubal motility or a tubal infection. There is a 5% increased risk for an ectopic pregnancy with the progestin-only pill but no increase with Norplant or Depo-Provera contraceptives (Hatcher and others, 1994). When the morning-after pill has been used and fails, there is a 10 times increased risk of an ectopic pregnancy because of its high estrogen level, which interferes with tubal motility (Cunningham and others, 1997).

Stimulation of Ovulation

There is an increased incidence of an ectopic pregnancy associated with ovulation-stimulating drugs, such as human menopausal gonadotropin and clomiphene citrate. These drugs alter the estrogen/progesterone level, which can affect tubal motility.

Infertility Treatment

There is an increased risk of an ectopic pregnancy with in vitro fertilization (IVF) or gamete intrafallopian transfer (GIFT), since underlying tubal damage is frequently one of the causative factors predisposing a woman to this type of infertility treatment.

Environmental Effect

Maternal cigarette smoking at the time of conception was found by both Coste and others (1991) and Phillips and others (1992) to be associated with an increased risk of an ectopic pregnancy. Secondhand smoking was not associated with an increased risk.

Transmigration of Ovum

Migration of the ovum from one ovary to the opposite fallopian tube can occur by an extrauterine or intrauterine route. This can delay transportation of the fertilized ovum to the uterus. Then trophoblastic tissue is present on the blastocyst before it reaches the uterine cavity, and therefore the trophoblastic tissue implants itself on the wall of the fallopian tube.

NORMAL PHYSIOLOGY

The fallopian tube wall is very muscular and narrow and contains very few ciliated cells at the interstitial area. In the ampullar area the fallopian tube becomes less muscular, the luminal size increases, and the ciliated cells are more abundant.

The fimbriated end of the fallopian tube serves to pick up the ovum when it is released from the ovary. Then the fallopian tube has the unique function of moving the ovum and sperm in opposite directions almost simultaneously, by peristaltic (muscular contractions) and ciliated activity. This tubal activity is initiated by two or more adjacent pacemakers in the ampullar and isthmic areas of the fallopian tube by sending out myoelectrical activity in either direction. The net directional movement in the fallopian tubes will vary during the menstrual cycle. During menstruation the net directional force is toward the uterus starting from the ampullar area to prevent menstrual blood reflux into the tubes (Pulkkinen, Talo, 1987). This is stimulated primarily by estrogen-induced prostaglandins. Just before ovulation, the directional force from the ampullar area is inward, to pick up the released ovum from the ovary and move it into the ampullar area of the fallopian tube. At the same time the directional force from the uterine area is the opposite, to facilitate sperm mobility toward the ovum (Pulkkinen, Talo, 1987). This is influenced by estrogen primarily. After fertilization the directional force varies in the ampullar area, which delays ovum transport. Approximately 5 days after ovulation, the net directional force from the middle of the ampullar area is inward through the isthmus, to transport the ovum to the uterus. This is influenced by increasing progesterone and prostaglandin E_2. Appoximately 7 days after ovulation, the myoelectrical activity becomes variable again, moving in both directions from each of the pacemakers (Pulkkinen, Talo, 1987).

The fertilized ovum should reach the uterine cavity in 6 to 7 days—just about the time the trophoblast cells begin to secrete the proteolytic enzyme and start to develop the threadlike projections called *chorionic villi* that initiate the implantation process.

The uterus is normally prepared by estrogen and progesterone to accept the fertilized ovum, now called a *blastocyst.* As the chorionic villa invade the endometrium, the villi are held in check by a fibrinoid zone. The uterus is also supplied with an increased blood supply capable of nourishing the products of conception.

PATHOPHYSIOLOGY
Tubal Ectopic Pregnancy

Because most ectopic pregnancies initially implant in a fallopian tube, the pathophysiology will focus on tubal ectopic pregnancies. The blastocyst burrows into the epithelium of the tubal wall, tapping blood vessels, by the same process as normal implantation into the uterine endometrium. However, the environment of the tube is quite different because of the following factors:

1. Resistance to the invading trophoblastic tissue by the fallopian tube is decreased.
2. Muscle mass lining the fallopian tubes is decreased; therefore their distensibility is greatly limited.
3. The blood pressure is much higher in the tubal arteries than in the uterine arteries.
4. Decidual reaction is limited; therefore human chorionic gonadotropin (HCG) is decreased and the signs and symptoms of pregnancy are limited.

It is because of these characteristic factors that termination of a tubal pregnancy occurs gestationally early by an abortion, spontaneous regression, or rupture, depending on the gestational age and the location of the implantation (Table 15-1). If the embryo dies early in gestation, spontaneous regression often occurs. If spontaneous regression fails to occur, usually an ampullar or fimbriated tubal pregnancy ends in an abortion and an isthmic or interstitial pregnancy ends in a rupture (Caspi, Sherman, 1987).

A tubal abortion (Fig. 15-2) occurs primarily because of separation of all or part of the placenta. This separation is caused by the pressure exerted by the tapped blood vessels or tubal contractions. With complete separation, the products of conception are expelled into the abdominal cavity by way of the fimbriated end of the fallopian tube, and unless there is an injured blood vessel, the bleeding stops. With an incomplete separation, bleeding continues until complete separation takes place, and the blood flows into the abdominal cavity, collecting in the rectouterine cul-de-sac of Douglas.

Tubal rupture (Fig. 15-3) results from the uninterrupted invasion of the trophoblastic tissue or tearing of the extremely

TABLE 15-1 Tubular pregnancy

Type	Duration (weeks)	Usual method of termination
Ampullar	6-12	Tubal abortion
Fimbriated	6-12	Tubal abortion
Isthmic	6-8	Tubal rupture
Interstitial	12-14	Tubal rupture

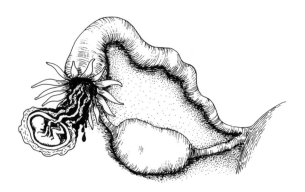

FIG. 15-2 Tubal abortion.

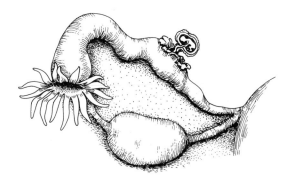

FIG. 15-3 Tubal rupture.

stretched tissue. In either case the products of conception are completely or incompletely expelled into the abdominal cavity or between the folds of the broad ligaments by way of the torn tube.

The duration of the tubal pregnancy depends on the location of the implanted embryo or fetus and the distensibility of that part of the fallopian tube. For instance, if the implantation is located in the narrow isthmic portion of the tube, it will rupture very early, within 6 to 8 weeks; the distensible interstitial portion may be able to retain the pregnancy up to 14 weeks. An ampullar or fimbriated tubal pregnancy is usually lost between 6 and 12 weeks of gestation.

The outcome of the pregnancy at the time of the interruption depends on the age of the embryo or fetus and whether the rupture is complete or incomplete. In rare cases, when the abortion occurs very early in the pregnancy and the placenta is initially separated completely from the tubal wall, the trophoblastic tissue will reimplant in the abdominal cavity and the placenta and embryo or fetus will continue to grow. This leads to the development of a secondary abdominal pregnancy. Usually only a small amount of blood is lost at this time.

If the rupture is incomplete, in rare cases, the ruptured part of the placenta will reattach to some surrounding abdominal tissue. This leads to the development of a tuboabdominal, tuboovarian, or a broad ligament pregnancy. In most instances, however, the embryo or fetus dies at the time of the abortion or rupture. If not surgically removed, it can be absorbed if small or, if too large to be absorbed, it can mummify or calcify. When the bleeding is slight, no problems result. However, in most cases blood vessels are torn open and bleeding is profuse. This blood and the lost products of conception collect in the cul-de-sac of Douglas, causing severe pain and hypovolemia. A real emergency is present, which can end in maternal death if the bleeding is not quickly stopped.

Abdominal Ectopic Pregnancy

An abdominal pregnancy almost always results from an implantation secondary to a tubal rupture or abortion through the fimbriated end of the fallopian tube. In these cases the placenta continues to grow following attachment to some abdominal structure, usually the surface of the uterus, broad ligaments, or ovaries. However, it can be any abdominal structure, including the liver, spleen, or intestines. Because the invading trophoblastic tissue is not held in check, it can erode major blood vessels at any time and cause severe bleeding. Fetal movements are also very painful because they are not cushioned by the myometrium.

Cervical Ectopic Pregnancy

In very rare cases the fertilized ovum bypasses the uterine endometrium and implants itself in the cervical mucus. Painless bleeding begins shortly after implantation, and surgical termination is usually required before the fourteenth week of gestation.

SIGNS AND SYMPTOMS

Before Rupture

Abdominal Pain

Abdominal pain occurs close to 100% of the time. It is usually first manifested by a dull, lower quadrant, unilateral pain caused by tubal stretching; this is followed by a sharp, colicky tubal pain caused by further tubal stretching and stimulated contractions. It progresses to a diffuse, constant, severe pain generalized throughout the lower abdomen (McIntyre-Seltman, Andrews-Detrich, 1995).

Delayed Menses

A history of a late period for approximately 2 weeks or a lighter than usual or irregular period is reported by 75% to 90% of the patients (Stabile, Grudzinskas, 1990).

Abnormal Vaginal Bleeding

Mild to intermittent dark red or brown vaginal discharge occurs in 50% to 80% of the cases related to uterine decidual shedding secondary to decreased hormones (Stabile, Grudzinskas, 1990; Weckstein, 1987).

Absence of Common Signs of Pregnancy

Absence of common signs of pregnancy is secondary to decreased pregnancy hormones and occurs 75% of the time (Weckstein, 1987).

Abdominal Tenderness

Abdominal tenderness occurs in more than 75% of the cases (Cunningham and others, 1997).

Palpable Pelvic Mass

A pelvic mass is palpable in approximately 50% of the cases (McIntyre-Seltman, Andrews-Detrich, 1995). It may be in the opposite abdominal quadrant from the ectopic growth related to a corpus luteum cyst (Cunningham and others, 1997).

Rupture

Exacerbation of the pain occurs during rupture in an ectopic pregnancy.

After Rupture

Faintness/Dizziness

Faintness and dizziness occur in the presence of significant bleeding.

Generalized, Unilateral, or Deep Lower Quadrant Acute Abdominal Pain

Abdominal pain is caused by blood irritating the peritoneum.

Referred Shoulder Pain

Referred shoulder pain is related to diaphragmatic irritation from blood in the peritoneal cavity (McIntyre-Seltman, Andrews-Detrich, 1995).

Signs of Shock

Shock is related to the severity of the bleeding into the abdomen.

Afebrile State

In the beginning usually no signs of an infection are present.

MATERNAL EFFECTS

Ectopic pregnancies account for approximately 10% of all maternal deaths (Berg and others, 1996). They are the second leading cause of maternal mortality, but they are the number one cause of maternal mortality in the first trimester of pregnancy (Centers for Disease Control and Prevention, 1995). Hemorrhage is the cause of death in 85% to 89% of the cases (Atrash and others, 1990; Stock, 1990) and occurs more frequently with an interstitial or abdominal ectopic pregnancy. Infection is the cause of 5% of the deaths, and anesthesia complications cause 2% of the deaths (Cunningham and others, 1997).

FETAL AND NEONATAL EFFECTS

Death is almost certain for the fetus in an ectopic pregnancy. From 5% to 25% of abdominal ectopic pregnancies will reach viability (Martin, McCaul, 1990). However, it is not recommended to continue an abdominal pregnancy if diagnosed early because of the extreme risk of hemorrhage at any time during the pregnancy. The risk of fetal deformity is also high; 20% to 40% of the fetuses that live beyond 20 weeks of gestation will have such deformities as facial asymmetry, severe neck webbing, joint deformities, and hypoplastic limbs (Ombelet and others, 1988). These are pressure deformities caused by oligohydramnios.

DIAGNOSTIC TESTING

Early diagnosis before extrauterine rupture or abortion can decrease maternal mortality from hemorrhage and simplify the management of an ectopic pregnancy. However, because this condition mimics other diseases (Table 15-2) and no one diagnostic tool is specific for detecting an early ectopic gestation, early diagnosis is difficult. However, by using HCG levels, progesterone levels, and transvaginal ultrasound, laparoscopy and

Text continued on p. 388

TABLE 15-2 Pelvic pain: differential diagnosis

	Ectopic (unruptured/ ruptured*)	Spontaneous abortion	Ovarian cyst
Chief complaint workup	Abdominal pain	Slight to severe vaginal bleeding	Abdominal pain
Associated symptoms			
P: provocative What causes the symptoms? What makes symptoms better or worse?	Sex and activity increase symptoms		Dyspareunia
Q: quality or quantity How does the pain feel?	Dull pain/*deep acute abdominal pain*	Crampy	Dull
R: region or radiation Where are the symptoms? Do symptoms spread?	Unilateral or bilateral lower quadrant/ *generalized deep/ referred shoulder pain related to diaphragmatic irritation*	Pressure pain, generalized or localized	Unilateral
S: severity scale How severe are the symptoms?	Vague, crampy/*severe*	Mild to severe	Crampy pain
T: timing When did the symptom begin? Association with menses?	Continuous		
Review of systems (ROS) General	Absence of common signs of pregnancy No GI symptoms *Vertigo/fainting*		Flatulence, bloating/ indigestion
History of recent surgery/pregnancy Sexual history STD exposure/diagnosis Contraceptive use	IUD, mini pill		
Complete menstrual history	Delayed menses/ amenorrhea		Menstrual irregularities
Vital signs	Increased temperature initially *After rupture: decreased BP and increased pulse if bleeding continuous and rapid*	Signs of shock equal to obvious bleeding	

PID, Pelvic inflammatory disease; *STD*, sexually transmitted disease; *CVA*, cerebrovascular accident; *CMT*, cervical motion tenderness; *ESR*, erythrocyte sedimentation rate; *CBC*, complete blood count; *GI*, gastrointestinal; *IUD*, intrauterine device; *BP*, blood pressure; *WBC*, white blood cell; *LH*, luteinizing hormone; *OC*, oral contraceptive; *BUS*, Bartholin, urethral, and Skene glands; *RLQ*, right lower quadrant; *RUQ*, right upper quadrant; *N/V*, nausea and vomiting.
*Signs and symptoms of ruptured ectopic pregnancy are in *italics*.

Salpingitis/PID	Appendicitis	Urinary tract infection	Pyelonephritis	Cholelithiasis during pregnancy
Lower abdominal and pelvic pain	Abdominal pain Coughing increases pain	Pain on urination; pelvic heaviness May have had recent intercourse	Pain on urination; general malaise	Abdominal pain
Pelvic pressure, back pain radiating down one or both legs		Burning pain at end of urination Urinary frequency	Burning pain at end of urination Urinary frequency	Lancinating, cramping, colicky or steady up to 1 hr
Bilateral or unilateral	Usually generalized or unilateral RLQ pain	Lower pelvic area	Lower back pain	Originating in mid portion of epigastrium, radiating to RUQ of abdomen and back
Mild to severe	Severe		Dysuria	
Usually following onset or cessation of menses	Sudden onset	Hesitancy in urination		Pain of abrupt onset
Generally no GI upset or appetite loss	History of anorexia; N/V		Chills, N/V, uterine contractions	Anorexia; N/V
+ + IUD; OC		Possible use of diaphragm		
May have a high fever	Low grade fever (100.2°-100.6° F)		Fever	

Continued

TABLE 15-2 Pelvic pain: differential diagnosis—cont'd

	Ectopic (unruptured/ ruptured)*	Spontaneous abortion	Ovarian cyst
Complete physical examination			
CVA tenderness			
Abdomen			
Auscultation			
Percussion			
Palpation (tender area last)	Lower abdominal tenderness/*after rupture severe generalized tenderness*	No abdominal tenderness	
Rebound tenderness			
McBurney point			
Iliopsoas			
Obturator test			
Murphy sign			
Pelvic			
Speculum examination	*After rupture may be a bulging cul-de-sac*		
Cervix	Slightly softened	Cervix closed or dilated	
Discharge	Dark red or brown	Vaginal bleeding mild to severe	
Obtain endocervical cultures			
Palpate uterus	Slightly softened		Enlarged ovaries palpated 50% of the time
Check CMT	+	−	
Palpate adnexal area	+	−	Unilateral adnexal tenderness
Rectovaginal palpation			
Diagnostic data			
ESR			
CBC with differential	Increased WBC count (15,000/mm^3)		
Other			LH elevated
Ultrasound	Rule out intrauterine pregnancy after 6 wk		+/− for ovarian cyst
Pregnancy test	+	+	− unless pregnant also
Urine culture and sensitivity			

Salpingitis/PID	Appendicitis	Urinary tract infection	Pyelonephritis	Cholelithiasis during pregnancy
		−	+	
Bilateral tenderness with deep/light	Abdominal guarding/muscular rigidity		Question if contractions present if pregnant	Localized tenderness
+	Rebound tenderness + +			+ suggests perforation
+BUS				
Purulent discharge May be + gonorrhea/*Chlamydia*	No vaginal discharge			
+ + if abscess is present		− −		
↑ ↑ WBC with left shift	Elevated shift to left			↑ WBC; ↑ amylase; ↑ alkaline phosphates 96% accurate in diagnosis of stone (Heppard, Garite, 1996)
	↑ WBC might be present if pregnant; − bacteria	+ nitrites; cloudy; hematuria; + WBC; + bacteriuria	+ nitrites; cloudy; hematuria; + WBC; + bacteriuria	

other surgical interventions are less likely. For a summary of the diagnostic tests results and interpretation, refer to Table 15-3.

Serum Progesterone Levels

Serum progesterone levels are being used to determine who needs further testing. In a normal pregnancy, the corpus luteum produces an increased amount of progesterone for the first 8 to 10 weeks. Then the placenta takes over the production of progesterone. In an ectopic pregnancy, progesterone levels are usually decreased to less than 10 to 15 ng/ml (Catlin, Wetzel, 1991). Serum progesterone levels above 25 ng/ml most often indicate a normal intrauterine pregnancy. Levels below 5 ng/ml indicate nonviability related to a spontaneous abortion or an ectopic pregnancy. Values between 5 and 25 ng/ml are not conclusive and indicate the need for further testing (Carson, Buster, 1993; Stovall, 1996; Stovall, Ling, 1993).

Serial Serum Beta–Human Chorionic Gonadotropin Levels

The fertilized ovum and the chorionic villi produce HCG, which maintains the corpus luteum to produce progesterone and estrogen. This maintains the pregnancy until the placenta is mature enough to assume that role at around 10 weeks of gestation. In a normal pregnancy, HCG is present in detectable levels (50 mIU/ml) in the maternal serum 8 to 10 days after fertilization. Early in pregnancy, levels double every 1.2 to 1.5 days. Levels normally double every 48 hours from 3 to 6 weeks following conception, rising well above 6000 mIU/ml and then gradually decreasing after 10 weeks. In an ectopic or spontaneous abortion, beta-HCG levels rise slower than normal (Carson, Buster, 1993). In an ectopic pregnancy they usually plateau at about 6 weeks and then gradually diminish (Lyon, 1995). In a spontaneous abortion or tubal abruption HCG levels fall rapidly (Lyon, 1995). Thus serial beta-HCG levels 48 hours apart aid in the differentiation between a normal and an abnormal pregnancy.

Vaginal Ultrasound

The usefulness of ultrasound in the diagnosis of an ectopic pregnancy is improving continuously. In the past it was useful only in diagnosing an intrauterine pregnancy, which would rule out an ectopic pregnancy. One exception was in the case of an advanced abdominal pregnancy. In these cases it would show a fetal head outside the uterus. With the more sophisticated real-time equipment and an expert technician, characteristic changes of an ectopic pregnancy can be picked up with pelvic ultrasound. With

TABLE 15-3 Diagnostic tests

Test	Results	Interpretation
Serum progesterone	>25 ng/ml	Normal intrauterine pregnancy
	>5 ng/ml but <25 ng/ml	Undetermined viability
	<5 ng/ml	Nonviable
Beta-HCG	Detected in the serum 8-10 days after fertilization	Normal intrauterine pregnancy
	First 2-3-wk after conception, beta-HCG levels double every 1.2-1.5 days	
	3 wk after conception, beta-HCG doubles every 48 hr until week 10	
	Beta-HCG levels after 10 wk start decreasing sharply	
	Prolonged doubling time or beta-HCG levels plateau at around 6 wk and then diminish	May indicate an ectopic pregnancy or a spontaneous abortion
Transvaginal ultrasound	Visible intrauterine pregnancy after beta-HCG levels are >2000 mIU/ml	Normal intrauterine pregnancy, 5-6 wk of gestation
	Pulsating fetal heart within the sac	Normal intrauterine pregnancy, 7-8 wk of gestation
	Pseudogestational sac without fetus found in uterus and/or cystic mass found in tubes	Ectopic pregnancy

HCG, Human chorionic gonadotropin.

transvaginal ultrasound, the location of the gestational sac of an early ectopic pregnancy can be visualized with 82% to 84% accuracy (Kivikoski and others, 1990; Stiller and others, 1989). Therefore transvaginal ultrasound is becoming an important diagnostic tool in an ectopic pregnancy before rupture because the probe can be placed closer to the pelvic structures. When HCG levels are 2000 mIU/ml or greater, a normal intrauterine pregnancy should be visible with transvaginal ultrasound (Lyon, 1995; Nyberg, Hill, 1992). Therefore when HCG levels are greater than 2000 mIU/ml with no visible intrauterine pregnancy, ectopic pregnancy is very likely. Many times, a cystic mass may be visualized in the tubes or outside the uterine cavity and an ectopic pregnancy can be confirmed before rupture (Cunningham and others, 1997). If an ectopic sac is identified, it is measured for size and attempts are made to determine any fetal cardiac activity. This will ascertain the selection of therapy. However, there is a 20-day window between the initial presence of HCG when a pregnancy is diagnosed and when the gestational sac can be visualized with vaginal ultrasound. During this 20-day window it is very hard to diagnose an ectopic pregnancy before signs of rupture.

Abdominal Ultrasound

Abdominal ultrasound will be used if vaginal ultrasound is unavailable. When HCG levels are 6000 mIU/ml or greater, a normal intrauterine pregnancy should be visible with abdominal ultrasound (Cunningham and others, 1997).

Culdocentesis

Culdocentesis can be used to diagnose intraperitoneal bleeding if a ruptured ectopic pregnancy is suspected. The procedure involves passing a needle through the cul-de-sac of Douglas to aspirate fluid from the peritoneal cavity (Fig. 15-4). Nonclotted blood will be withdrawn in the presence of a ruptured ectopic pregnancy since blood in the abdomen first undergoes clotting and subsequent fibrinolysis, after which it fails to clot. However, with the availability of sensitive HCG tests and transvaginal ultrasound, the value of culdocentesis is limited and it is seldom used.

Laparoscopy

If no intrauterine pregnancy is found on ultrasound and the patient is experiencing escalating pain, signs of pelvic irritation related to blood, or any signs of hemodynamic instability, a laparoscopy should be done. An endoscope is inserted through a small

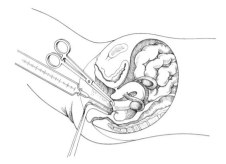

FIG. 15-4 Culdocentesis.

abdominal incision to visualize the peritoneal cavity for an ectopic implanted pregnancy.

Curettage

Curettage may be used in differentiating a spontaneous abortion from an ectopic pregnancy before 6 weeks of gestation when an intrauterine pregnancy is not yet visible. In the presence of rapidly falling beta-HCG levels and progesterone less than 5 ng/ml, a curettage can be done. Ectopic pregnancy can be ruled out if chorionic villi are noted histologically or HCG levels fall significantly 24 hours after the procedure (Brumsted, 1996). Otherwise, the pregnancy is assumed to be extrauterine.

MEDICAL TREATMENT

Tubal Ectopic Pregnancy Before Rupture

Surgical Treatment

The type of surgical management depends on the location and cause of the ectopic pregnancy, the extent of tissue involvement, and the patient's wishes for future fertility. The choice of treatment for an unruptured ampullar or fimbriated tubal pregnancy is a salpingostomy, in which a longitudinal incision is made over the pregnancy site and the products of conception are gently and very carefully removed to prevent or control the bleeding (Leach, Ory, 1989; Paulson, Sauer, 1990). The fallopian tube incision is allowed to close by secondary intention. If the fallopian tube incision is closed with sutures, the procedure is called a *salpingotomy.* Segmental resection and subsequent end-to-end anastomosis are recommended if the ectopic pregnancy is located in the proximal isthmus portion of the tube (Cunningham and others, 1997). If residual trophoblastic tissue remains after conservative surgical treatment, methotrexate, 5 mg orally three times per day for 5 days (Minnick-Smith, Cook 1997), or methotrexate, 50 mg/m^2 intramuscularly for one dose (Bengtsson and others, 1992; Hoppe and others, 1994), is being used successfully.

Nonsurgical Treatment

Methotrexate, a type of chemotherapy, has been successfully used as an alternative to surgery in some cases. It is a folic acid antagonist that interferes with deoxyribonucleic acid (DNA) synthesis and cell multiplication (Carson, Buster, 1993) causing dissolution of the ectopic mass (Leach, Ory, 1989). Criteria for its use follow (Maiolatesi, Peddicord, 1996; Minnick-Smith, Cook, 1997; Stovall, 1995):

- Hemodynamically stable with no signs of severe abdominal pain, weakness, dizziness, syncope, orthostatic hypotension, tachycardia, or falling hematocrit
- Ectopic sac less than 3.5 cm in diameter
- Fetus not alive as indicated by no cardiac activity
- Liver function studies within normal limits
- Normal kidney function as indicated by normal serum creatinine and blood urea nitrogen (BUN)
- No evidence of peptic ulcer disease
- No evidence of leukopenia (blood leukocytes above 3500/mm^3)
- No evidence of thrombocytopenia (platelet count above 100,000/mm^3)

Methotrexate dosing takes several forms:

- Single-dose method: methotrexate, 50 mg/m^2 intramuscularly, with follow-up on days 4 and 7 and then weekly until HCG titers drop to less than 15 mIU/ml. If beta-HCG fails to drop 15% by day 7, methotrexate dose may be repeated (Alexander and others, 1996; Maiolatesi, Peddicord, 1996).
- Multiple-dose method: methotrexate, 1 mg/kg intramuscularly every other day (even days), and leucovorin, 0.1 mg/kg intramuscularly every other day (odd days), until beta-HCG levels drop at least 15% in a 48-hour period; or maximum of four doses each (Minnick-Smith, Cook, 1997).

Tubal Ectopic Pregnancy After Rupture

Following a ruptured tubal pregnancy, a salpingectomy (removal of the affected fallopian tube) is the most common surgical treatment. Occasionally a salpingo-oophorectomy (removal of the affected fallopian tube and adjacent ovary) is performed if the blood supply to the ovary is affected or the ectopic pregnancy involved the ovary. Otherwise, preservation of the ovary is recommended. If the couple does not wish to have more children, a hysterectomy may be done if the woman's condition is stable.

Abdominal Ectopic Pregnancy

For an abdominal pregnancy, hemorrhage is a serious possibility because the placenta can separate from its attachment site at any time. Abdominal surgery to remove the embryo or fetus is usually done as soon as an abdominal pregnancy is diagnosed. Unless the placenta is attached to abdominal structures that can be removed, such as the ovary or exterior of the uterus, or the blood vessels that supply blood to the placenta can be ligated, the placenta is left without being disturbed (Martin, McCaul, 1990). If the placenta is removed, large blood vessels would be opened and there would not be a constricting muscle such as the uterus to apply a sealing pressure. If left intact, the placenta is usually absorbed by the body, but unfortunately it may cause such complications as infection, abscesses, adhesions, intestinal obstruction, paralytic ileus, post-partum preeclampsia, and wound dehiscence. These complications are less life threatening than the hemorrhage that could result if the placenta is removed.

Cervical Ectopic Pregnancy

Because of the risks of uncontrollable hemorrhage and urinary tract injury, surgical management is the last alternative treatment for a cervical ectopic pregnancy. Methotrexate is being success-fully used. The agent is injected directly into the gestational sac or given systematically as outlined earlier (Dotters and others, 1995). If methotrexate is contraindicated and surgical management is necessary, several methods are used to diminish the risk of hemorrhage. Such treatments include a cerclage and local injection of vasopressin before evacuation (Bachus and others, 1990), inflation of a 30-ml Foley catheter bulb in the cervix and vaginal packing following curettage (Thomas and others, 1991), or uterine artery embolization (Saliken and others, 1994).

NURSING PROCESS

PREVENTION

An ectopic pregnancy is closely associated with tubal scarring. Preventing tubal scarring is the key to prevention of an ectopic pregnancy. Safe sex to prevent a sexually transmitted disease

(STD) should be a routine part of well-woman care. Screening for *Chlamydia* and gonorrhea should be included in the yearly gynecologic examination for at-risk women. An STD should be treated effectively to prevent pelvic inflammatory disease (PID). However, if PID develops, rapid treatment can decrease the chance of tubal scarring. When a woman chooses an IUD or progesterone-only oral contraceptive, signs of PID should be included in the teaching. Because a correlation exists between cigarette smoking and an increased risk of an ectopic pregnancy, women during their childbearing years should be encouraged to avoid smoking. If an elective abortion is desired, it should always be carried out only by medically prepared professionals. These measures can decrease the chance of tubal defects and thereby decrease the incidence of an ectopic pregnancy. Because of the increasing incidence of ectopic pregnancy, health professionals should consider the possibility in any woman who presents with any type of abdominal discomfort during her childbearing years.

ASSESSMENT

Because of the high maternal mortality associated with an undiagnosed ectopic pregnancy until after rupture or tubal abortion, it is very important for nurses to be alert to signs and symptoms of this complication of pregnancy. Therefore any woman during her childbearing years who experiences irregular vaginal spotting associated with a dull, aching pelvic pain, with or without signs of pregnancy, should be evaluated for a possible ectopic pregnancy. The following areas should be explored:

- **Risk Factors:** A history of any PID, previous ectopic pregnancies, elective abortions, or prior infertility disorders should be determined; they can increase the patient's risk for a tubal defect.
- **Pain:** If an ectopic pregnancy is suspected, a detailed history should include questions regarding the type of abdominal pain. The pain caused by an unruptured ectopic pregnancy can be a unilateral, cramplike pain related to tubal distention by the enlarging embryo or fetus. At the time of tubal rupture many patients experience a sudden, sharp, stabbing pain in the lower abdomen. Blood in the peritoneum can cause a dull aching or severe, generalized pain. If the blood touches the diaphragm, it usually causes referred shoulder pain. Many times, movement of the body will aggravate the pain.
- **Vaginal Bleeding:** Assess for the presence of vaginal bleeding, and obtain a menstrual history. Vaginal bleeding is

usually related to the sloughing of the endometrial lining related to decreasing progesterone and estrogen levels and can present as continuous or intermittent vaginal bleeding in small or large quantities. It usually differs from the patient's normal period. Pad counts should be kept to determine the amount and type of vaginal bleeding.

- **Syncope:** Assess for the presence of any signs of syncope. When an ectopic pregnancy ruptures or aborts, blood is lost into the peritoneal cavity. At this time the patient can experience a feeling of faintness or weakness related to hypovolemia. If the bleeding is not continuous, the depleted blood volume is restored to near normal in 1 or 2 days by hemodilution and the faint or weak feeling subsides. If the bleeding is profuse, the patient can go into shock quickly.
- **Vital Signs:** To assess the amount of intraperitoneal blood loss, the patient's vital signs should be checked as frequently as the situation indicates.

NURSING DIAGNOSES/COLLABORATIVE PROBLEMS AND INTERVENTIONS

- **FEAR** related to risk of mortality and possible treatment alternatives.
  DESIRED OUTCOME: The patient and her family will be able to communicate their fears and concerns openly.
  INTERVENTIONS
    1. Assess family's anxiety over maternal well-being because 10% of pregnancy-related deaths are caused by ectopic pregnancy (Berg and others, 1996).
    2. Assess family's level of guilt such as their feeling as to what they did to cause this to happen.
    3. Assess family's coping strategies and resources.
    4. Explain all diagnostic and treatment modalities and reasons for each in understandable terms.
    5. Prepare patient for serial beta-HCG levels, progesterone levels, or transvaginal ultrasound. If transvaginal ultrasound diagnostic procedure is ordered, have patient empty her bladder before the procedure.
    6. Prepare patient for a culdocentesis, if this diagnostic procedure is ordered, by explaining the procedure. (A sterile speculum is inserted into the vagina, the cervix is steadied with a tenaculum, and a 16- to 18-gauge needle is inserted into the cul-de-sac so any fluid that is present can be aspirated for evaluation.) Position patient in a semi-Fowler's position to allow any intraperitoneal blood, if present, to

pool in the cul-de-sac. Just before the procedure, prepare the external genitalia with povidone-iodine (Betadine).

7. Prepare the patient for the medical or surgical procedure.

- **ACUTE PAIN** related to stretching of the tube, severe abdominal bleeding secondary to tubal rupture, or surgical treatment.

  DESIRED OUTCOME: The patient will verbally and nonverbally express reasonable comfort.

  INTERVENTIONS
  1. Assess the type and location of pain.
  2. Maintain position of comfort.
  3. Limit movement, and support patient.
  4. Provide reassurance.
  5. Instruct regarding use of relaxation and breathing techniques to reduce pain if pain medication cannot be administered.
  6. Administer pain medication as ordered if needed.
  7. Notify physician regarding any change in the amount or type of pain the patient experiences.

- **POTENTIAL COMPLICATION: HEMORRHAGE** caused by ectopic rupture/abortion or surgical treatment.

  DESIRED OUTCOME: The signs and symptoms of hemorrhage will be minimized or managed as measured by stable vital signs, urinary output of 30 ml/hr or greater, absence of signs of shock, and hematocrit maintained between 30% and 45%.

  INTERVENTIONS
  Preoperative
  1. Check vital signs as indicated (depending on severity).
  2. Check orthostatic blood pressure if condition permits. To do this, take the patient's blood pressure and pulse while she is supine. Retake these vital signs after the patient has been in a standing position for 5 minutes. A decrease in diastolic blood pressure of 10 to 20 mm Hg or an increase in the pulse rate of 10 to 20 beats/min or more is interpreted as a positive indication of significant blood loss.
  3. Check amount of vaginal bleeding.
  4. Check for signs of shock, such as tachycardia, drop in blood pressure, and cool, clammy skin. (During pregnancy, signs of shock are not manifested until there has been at least a 30% blood volume loss [Heppard, Garite, 1996].)
  5. Check state of mental acuity/level of consciousness.
  6. Keep an accurate record of intake and output. Urinary output during pregnancy is the best noninvasive indicator

of circulatory volume. Diminished cardiac output causes a shunting of blood away from the skin, kidneys, and skeletal muscles to ensure blood delivery to the heart and brain.

7. Start an IV infusion with an 18-gauge intracatheter, and maintain as ordered. Fluid replacement may reverse impending, shock by increasing capillary blood flow, and thereby cardiac output increases. (Lactated Ringer's solution is one of the best volume expanders [ACOG, 1994].)

8. Obtain blood as ordered for a complete blood count, prothrombin time, partial thromboplastin time, platelet count, Rh antibody screen, and type and cross match for 2 to 4 units of packed red blood cells.

9. Administer oxygen at 8 to 10 L/min by mask as needed.

10. Carry out such preoperative protocol as giving the patient nothing by mouth, giving no enemas or cathartics since they could stimulate a tubal ectopic pregnancy to rupture, being prepared to insert a Foley catheter as ordered, and getting the permit signed for surgery.

11. Notify the attending physician of any changes in vital signs, decreasing urinary output, an orthostatic blood pressure that falls 10 to 20 mm Hg or more, or a change in mental acuity.

12. If the patient presents in shock, be prepared to assist with central line placement. The internal jugular and subclavian veins are less likely to be collapsed.

13. Be prepared to administer blood component therapy if the hemoglobin level is below 8 g/dl or the patient is manifesting signs of shock. Refer to Table 17-3 for guidelines for blood component replacement.

Postoperative

1. Check blood pressure, pulse, and respirations every 15 minutes for eight times; every 30 minutes for two times; every hour for two times; every 4 hours for two times; and then routinely.

2. Assess vaginal bleeding by pad count.

3. Check dressing every hour for four times and then every shift for bleeding.

4. Refer to laboratory work, such as hemoglobin and hematocrit.

5. Keep an accurate intake and output record.

6. Assess for cyanosis.

7. Reinforce or change dressing as needed.

8. Carefully administer IV fluids as ordered.

9. Once the gastrointestinal tract resumes normal function, instruct regarding the importance of a high-protein, high-iron diet for body repair and replacement of blood loss.

10. Notify physician if blood pressure drops to less than 90 mm Hg systolic, pulse rises to greater than 120 beats/min, or anemia develops.

Medical management

1. Review how the medication or medications work. Be prepared to discuss the advantages of this type of management, such as an 85% to 94% successs rate (Carson, Buster, 1993; Henry, Gentry, 1994; Stovall, Ling, 1993), cost effectiveness, patient's ability to return to normal activities quicker than when surgery is done, and possible preservation of tubal patency.

2. Explain adverse side effects such as nausea, vomiting, transient stomatitis, oral ulcers, gastritis, and gastrointestinal bleeding.

3. Provide emotional support for the patient and her family.

4. Be prepared to obtain baseline levels such as a complete blood count, BUN, creatinine, platelet count, liver function studies, blood type, and Rh.

5. Prepare patient for possible increase in abdominal pain related to tubal absorption, which usually lasts 4 to 12 hours, sometime between 5 and 10 days after initial dose of medication.

6. Prepare patient as to the importance of follow-up that includes beta-HCG titers until zero because of continued inflammation of the ectopic site until spontaneous absorption is complete.

7. Teach patient the importance of refraining from consuming alcohol, taking a vitamin supplement with folic acid, or having sexual intercourse until the ectopic pregnancy is resolved to decrease the risk of medication side effects or exacerbating the rupture of the ectopic pregnancy.

8. Teach patient to report signs of ectopic rupture immediately, such as severe, sharp, stabbing, unilateral abdominal pain.

9. Encourage patient to avoid sun exposure related to the photosensitivity of the drug during treatment and avoid the use of aspirin and all nonsteroidal antiinflammatory drugs because they worsen the gastrointestinal effects.

10. Validate with the couple that this is a loss of a pregnancy and it is acceptable to grieve over the loss.

- **RISK FOR INFECTION** related to blood being an ideal medium for bacterial growth.

  DESIRED OUTCOME: The patient's temperature will remain normal, incision will approximate without redness or drainage, vaginal discharge will be without odor, and the white blood cell count will remain less than $16,000/mm^3$.

  INTERVENTIONS
  1. Check temperature every 4 hours.
  2. Refer to laboratory work, such as white blood cell count.
  3. Check incision for redness, swelling, and drainage every shift.
  4. Administer prophylactic antibiotics as ordered.
  5. Notify the physician if the temperature increases or any signs of infection develop.

- **ANTICIPATORY GRIEVING** related to loss of an anticipated infant and possible threat to fertility.

  DESIRED OUTCOME: The patient and family members will verbalize their feelings of grief appropriately and identify any problems as they work through the grief process.

  INTERVENTIONS
  1. Assess level of loss and desire for future childbearing.
  2. Encourage the patient and her family to express their feelings and concerns openly.
  3. Discuss with the patient and family the chances of recurrence (12% to 18% risk, according to Stabile and Grudzinskas [1990]) and infertility problems (50% risk according to Leach and Ory [1989]).
  4. Teach the couple the importance of using a contraceptive of choice for at least three menstrual cycles to allow time for the woman's body to recover.
  5. Refer to a support group, such as Resolve Through Sharing, if available.
  6. Refer to a pastor, priest, or chaplain per family's request.
  7. Refer to Chapter 6.

- **OTHER POTENTIAL POSTOPERATIVE COMPLICATIONS:** paralytic ileus, urinary tract infection, pneumonia, anemia, pulmonary edema, D sensitization, persistent ectopic pregnancy, or adhesions.

  DESIRED OUTCOME: Postoperative complications will be minimized or managed as measured by no burning on urination, hematocrit maintained between 30% and 45%, breath sounds clear, bowel sounds active, abdomen soft, and beta-HCG levels at zero in 2 weeks postoperatively.

INTERVENTIONS

1. Assess for burning on urination.
2. Auscultate lung fields every shift for rales, and observe for coughing or dyspnea.
3. Auscultate bowel sounds every shift.
4. Assess for passage of flatus.
5. Palpate abdomen for hardness and rigidity.
6. Have patient turn, cough, and deep breathe every 2 hours.
7. Have patient use an inspiratory incentive spirometer every hour while awake.
8. Give patient nothing by mouth until bowel sounds are present. Then introduce clear liquids until patient passes flatus. Then advance to soft or regular diet.
9. Have patient do leg exercises every hour while awake until ambulating well.
10. Have patient do abdominal tightening every hour while awake until normal gastrointestinal activity returns.
11. Encourage and assist with ambulation as soon as ordered.
12. If patient is D negative, be prepared to administer Rho (D) immune globulin (RhoGAM) (HypRho-D).
13. Administer steroids as ordered to decrease inflammation that would increase the risk of adhesions.
14. Once the gastrointestinal tract resumes normal function, instruct regarding the importance of six to eight glasses of fluid per day to decrease the risk of a urinary tract infection.
15. Notify physician if abdominal distention develops, signs of infection manifest, or anemia develops.

CONCLUSION

The ultimate goal for nursing intervention is prevention of complications that can cause tubal or uterine defects. These set the stage for an ectopic pregnancy. If an ectopic pregnancy develops, the goal is to prevent complications during the treatment. Therefore efforts are best directed at prevention of future impairment of fertility through patient education. Education should include information for self-detection of signs of infections contributing to ectopic pregnancy. Efforts should also be directed at detecting and reporting early signs of an ectopic pregnancy so that diagnosis before a rupture or abortion can be made. Thus the complication of hemorrhage, which is the major cause of maternal death, can be prevented.

BIBLIOGRAPHY

Alexander J and others: Treatment of the small unruptured ectopic pregnancy: a cost analysis of methotrexate versus laparoscopy, *Obstet Gynecol* 88(1):123-127, 1996.

American College of Obstetricians and Gynecologists (ACOG): *Blood component therapy,* ACOG Tech Bull, no. 199, 1994.

Atrash H and others: Maternal mortality in the United States, 1979-1986, *Obstet Gynecol* 76:1055-1060, 1990.

Bachus K and others: Conservative management of cervical pregnancy with subsequent fertility, *Am J Obstet Gynecol* 162:450, 1990.

Bengtsson G and others: Low-dose oral methotrexate as second-line therapy for persistent trophoblast after conservative treatment of ectopic pregnancy, *Obstet Gynecol* 79:589-591, 1992.

Berg C and others: Pregnancy-related morality in the United States, 1987-1990, *Obstet Gynecol* 88:161, 1996.

Bernstein J: Ectopic pregnancy: a nursing approach to excess risk among minority women, *J Obstet Gynecol Neonatal Nurs* 24(9):803-810, 1995.

Brumsted J: Managing ectopic pregnancy nonsurgically, *Contemp OB/GYN* 40(3):43-56, 1996.

Brunham R and others: *Chlamydia trachomatis* associated ectopic pregnancy: serologic and histologic correlates, *J Infect Dis* 165:1075, 1992.

Carson B, Buster J: Ectopic pregnancy, *N Engl J Med* 329(16):1174-1181, 1993.

Caspi E, Sherman D: Tubal abortion and infundibular ectopic pregnancy, *Clin Obstet Gynecol* 30(1):155-163, 1987.

Catlin A, Wetzel W: Ectopic pregnancy: clinical evaluation, diagnostic measures, and prevention, *Nurse Pract* 16(1):38-46, 1991.

Centers for Disease Control and Prevention: Ectopic pregnancy—United States, 1990-1992, *MMWR Morb Mortal Wkly Rep* 44(3):46-48, 1995.

Coste J, Job-Spira N, Fernandez H: Increased risk of ectopic pregnancy with maternal cigarette smoking, *Am J Public Health* 81(2):199-201, 1991.

Coste J and others: Risk factors for ectopic pregnancy: a case-control study in France, with special focus on infectious factors, *Am J Epidemiol* 133:839, 1993.

Cowan B: Ectopic pregnancy, *Curr Opin Obstet Gynecol* 5(6):328-332, 1993.

Cunningham G and others: *Williams' obstetrics,* ed 20, Norwalk, Conn, 1997, Appleton & Lange.

Dotters D and others: Successful treatment of a cervical pregnancy with a single low dose methotrexate regimen, *Eur J Obstet Gynecol Reprod Biol* 60:187, 1995.

Grosskindky C and others: hCG, progesterone, alpha-fetoprotein, and estradiol in the identification of ectopic pregnancy, *Obstet Gynecol* 81:705-709, 1993.

Guillaume A and others: Luteal phase defects and ectopic pregnancy, *Fertil Steril* 3:30, 1995.

Hatcher R and others: *Contraceptive technology 1994-1996,* ed 16, New York, 1994, Irvington Publishers.

Hemminki E, Merilainen J: Long-term effects of cesarean sections: ectopic pregnancies and placental problems, *Am J Obstet Gynecol* 174:1569-1574, 1996.

Henry M, Gentry W: Single injection of methotrexate for treatment of ectopic pregnancies, *Am J Obstet Gynecol* 171:1584-1587, 1994.

Heppard MCS, Garite TJ: *Acute obstetrics: a practical guide,* ed 2, St Louis, 1996, Mosby.

Hoppe D, Bekkar B, Nager C: Single-dose systemic methotrexate for the treatment of persistent ectopic pregnancy after conservative surgery, *Obstet Gynecol* 83:51-54, 1994.

Kivikoski A, Martin C, Smeltzer J: Transabdominal and transvaginal ultrasonography in the diagnosis of ectopic pregnancy: a comparative study, *Am J Obstet Gynecol* 163:123-128, 1990.

Leach R, Ory S: Modern management of ectopic pregnancy, *J Reprod Med* 34(15):324-338, 1989.

Lyon D: Critical pathways in the management of first-trimester bleeding and pain, *Female Patient* 20(2):19-27, 1995.

Maiolatesi C, Peddicord K: Methotrexate for nonsurgical treatment of ectopic pregnancy: nursing implications, *J Obstet Gynecol Neonatal Nurs* 25(2):205-208, 1996.

Martin J, McCaul J: Emergent management of abdominal pregnancy, *Clin Obstet Gynecol* 33(3):438-447, 1990.

McIntyre-Seltman K, Andrews-Detrich L: Ectopic pregnancy. In Niswander K, Evans A, editors: *Manual of obstetrics,* ed 5, Boston, 1995, Little, Brown.

Minnick-Smith K, Cook F: Current treatment options for ectopic pregnancy, *MCN Am J Matern Child Nurs* 22(1):21-25, 1997.

Naef R, Morrison J: Transfusion therapy in pregnancy, *Clin Obstet Gynecol* 38(3):547-557, 1995.

Nolan T, Gallup D: Shock in ectopic pregnancy, *Female Patient* 14(10):66-74, 1989.

Nyberg D, Hill L: Normal intrauterine pregnancy: sonographic development and hCG correlation. In Nyberg D and others, editors: *Transvaginal ultrasound,* St Louis, 1992, Mosby.

Ombelet W, Vandermerwe J, Van Assche F: Advanced extrauterine pregnancy: description of 38 cases with literature survey, *Obstet Gynecol Surv* 43:386, 1988.

Paulson R, Sauer M: Conservative surgical treatment of ectopic pregnancy, *J Reprod Med* 35(1):22-24, 1990.

Phillips R and others: The effect of cigarette smoking, *Chlamydia trachomatis* infection, and vaginal douching on ectopic pregnancy, *Obstet Gynecol* 79:85, 1992.

Pulkkinen M, Talo A: Tubal physiologic consideration in ectopic pregnancy, *Clin Obstet Gynecol* 30(1):164-172, 1987.

Reinhardt M: Emergency! ectopic pregnancy rupture, *Am J Nurs* 94(7):41, 1994.

Saliken J and others: Embolization of the uterine arteries before termination of a 15-week cervical pregnancy, *Can Assoc Radiol J* 45:399, 1994.

Stabile I, Grudzinskas J: Ectopic pregnancy: a review of incidence, etiology and diagnostic aspects, *Obstet Gynecol Surv* 45(6):335-347, 1990.

Stiller R, Haynes de Regt R, Blair E: Transvaginal ultrasonography in patients at risk for ectopic pregnancy, *Am J Obstet Gynecol* 161:930-933, 1989.

Stock R: Ectopic pregnancy: a look at changing concepts and problems, *Clin Obstet Gynecol* 33(3):448-453, 1990.

Stovall T: Medical management should be routinely used as primary therapy for ectopic pregnancy, *Clin Obstet Gynecol* 38:34-36, 1995.

Stovall T, Ling F: Ectopic pregnancy: diagnostic and therapeutic algorithms minimizing surgical intervention, *J Reprod Med* 38(10): 807-811, 1993.

Stovall T: Imaging—conservative treatment of ectopic gestation. In Jaffe R and others, editors: *Imaging in infertility and reproductive endocrinology,* Philadelphia, 1996, Lippincott-Raven.

Thomas R, Gingold B, Gallagher M: Cervical pregnancy: a report of two cases, *J Reprod Med* 36:459, 1991.

Weckstein L: Clinical diagnosis of ectopic pregnancy, *Clin Obstet Gynecol* 30(1):236-244, 1987.

CHAPTER

16

Gestational Trophoblastic Disease

G estational trophoblastic disease is a spectrum of pregnancy-related trophoblastic proliferative disorders. The benign hydatidiform mole represents the beginning of the disease continuum, and metastatic gestational trophoblastic tumor, also referred to as *choriocarcinoma,* is at the end of the continuum. Malignant nonmetastatic gestational trophoblastic tumor is somewhere in the middle.

HYDATIDIFORM MOLE

A hydatidiform mole is a benign proliferative growth of the trophoblast in which the chorionic villi develop into edematous, cystic, avascular, transparent vesicles that hang in a grapelike cluster (Fig. 16-1). There are two categories of hydatidiform moles: complete and partial.

The *complete moles* are characterized as follows:
- Generalized areas of the chorionic villi become hyperplastic, edematous, and avascular.
- There is no embryo or fetus and amniotic sac.
- A diploid karyotype is present that is most often a 46,XX chromosomal pattern of paternal origin; a sperm with 23,X chromosomes duplicates itself because it fertilizes an ovum

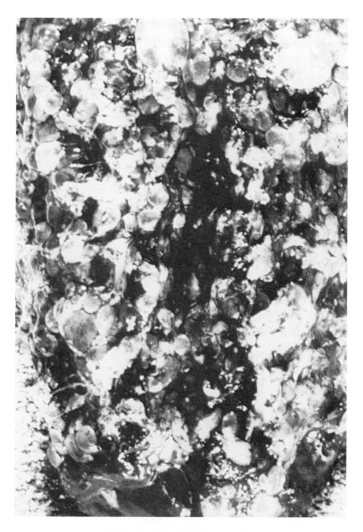

FIG. 16-1 Hydatidiform mole.

that contains no genetic material or the genetic material is inactive (Berkowitz and others, 1996; Ko and others, 1991). Occasionally (6% to 10% of the time) the karyotype is 46,XY. In these cases, two sperm have fertilized an ovum without genetic material (Berkowitz and others, l996).

The *partial moles* are characterized as follows:

• Localized areas of chorionic villi become hyperplastic, edematous, and avascular.

- There is an embryo or fetus and an amniotic sac, usually with multiple congenital anomalies.
- A triploid karyotype of 69,XXY, 69,XXX, or 69,XYY chromosomes is present in most of the cases: one set of chromosomes of maternal origin and two sets of paternal origin. In these cases, two sperm have fertilized an apparently normal ovum (Berkowitz and others, 1996; Wolf, Lage, 1995).
- A diploid karyotype is present in a few of the cases (Berkowitz and others, 1996).

Incidence

The incidence of a hydatidiform mole in the United States is 0.6 to 1.1 per 1000 pregnancies (Palmer, 1994). In many other countries, especially in some southeast Asian countries and in the Far East, the incidence is much higher (Cunningham and others, 1997). There is a 1% to 2% increased risk of a repeat occurrence of hydatidiform mole (Berkowitz and others, 1994; Loret de Mola, Goldfarb, 1995) and a 75 times greater risk associated with a maternal age more than 40 years (Berkowitz and others, 1996; Semer, Macfee, 1995).

Etiology

The cause of a hydatidiform mole is unknown, but it is theorized that an ovular defect, stress, or a nutritional deficiency (especially in carotene) may contribute to its development (Berkowitz and others, 1996).

Normal Physiology

Normally one sperm fertilizes one ovum and each contributes 23 chromosomes to form a new cell called a *zygote.* The zygote begins to grow immediately by undergoing a series of rapid mitotic cell divisions to form a solid mass of cells called a *morula.* As cellular activity continues, fluid begins to form in the center of the morula and causes the cells to rearrange until there is one single layer of cells lining the periphery and an inner cluster of cells. The single layer of cells, called the *trophoblast,* will grow and develop into the placenta, and the inner cluster of cells, called the *embryoblast,* will develop into a fetus. The umbilical cord will eventually connect the two structures.

The placenta is formed by the trophoblast cells sending out threadlike projections termed *chorionic villi* into the endometrium of the uterus. As the chorionic villi grow, they erode areas of the endometrium, forming intervillous spaces that fill with maternal blood. Invasion is normally held in check by the endometrium.

Inside the chorionic villi, blood vessels and connective tissue begin to form. These blood vessels will connect with the blood vessels inside the umbilical cord.

Pathophysiology

What actually causes the proliferation of the placenta to occur is unknown. In any case the trophoblastic tissue absorbs fluid from the maternal blood. Fluid then begins to accumulate in the chorionic villi because of inadequate or absent fetal circulation. As the pooling of fluid continues, vesicles are formed out of the chorionic villi.

Signs and Symptoms: Complete Mole

Characteristic symptoms of a complete hydatidiform mole are given below.

Abnormal Uterine Bleeding

Abnormal uterine bleeding, which is intermittent or continuous, usually not profuse, and often brownish in color, occurs in approximately 95% of cases. This is usually related to the lack of circulatory integrity of molar tissue (Rose, 1995). When the molar tissue starts separating from the uterus, bright red bleeding may result.

Variable Uterine Size

A uterus larger than expected for the estimated gestational age occurs in approximately 50% of the cases (Berkowitz and others, 1991; Cunningham and others, 1997).

Ovarian Enlargement

Bilateral ovarian enlargement caused by theca lutein cysts occurs in 50% of cases and may cause abdominal pain. This is usually related to the elevated levels of human chorionic gonadotropin (HCG) (Osathanond and others, 1986).

Hyperemesis Gravidarum

Hyperemesis gravidarum occurs in approximately 25% of cases (Berkowitz, Goldstein, 1988).

Preeclampsia

Signs and symptoms of preeclampsia, such as proteinuria, hypertension, and edema developing before week 24 of gestation, occur in approximately 30% of cases (Berkowitz, Goldstein, 1988; Cunningham and others, 1997).

Passage of Vesicles

Passage of grapelike vesicles occurs in approximately 50% of cases.

Absence of Fetus

Inability to detect a fetal heart rate (FHR) after 10 to 12 weeks of gestation, inability to palpate fetal parts even though the uterus is at or above the umbilicus, and lack of fetal movement after 16 to 20 weeks of gestation are common findings.

Respiratory Distress

Respiratory distress, a condition that may be caused by a trophoblastic pulmonary embolus, occurs in 2% of cases (Berkowitz and others, 1991).

Signs and Symptoms: Partial Mole

A partial mole does not exhibit as often the preceding clinical symptoms. It may present with signs of an incomplete or missed abortion, which include irregular vaginal bleeding, no FHR, or a uterus that is small for dates (Berkowitz and others, 1996).

Maternal Effects

Maternal effects of hydatidiform mole include the following:

1. Preeclampsia (approximately a 30% risk of developing a gestational hypertensive disorder before 24 weeks of gestation [Cunningham and others, 1997])
2. Bleeding
3. Anemia
4. Hyperemesis gravidarum
5. Intrauterine infection or sepsis
6. Uterine rupture
7. Rupture of ovarian cysts
8. Trophoblastic embolism
9. Emotional trauma
10. Gestational trophoblastic tumor

Following surgical evacuation of a complete mole, there is a 20% risk of developing a persistent gestational trophoblastic tumor (Berkowitz, Goldstein, 1995; Wolf, Lage, 1995). This risk increases 40% to 50% if there was marked trophoblastic proliferation before evacuation as evidenced by a high serum HCG level, excessively enlarged uterus, or theca-lutein cysts (Berkowitz, Goldstein, 1995). Women older than 40 years have a 37% to 56% risk, with the risk increasing with age. Following a partial mole there is only a 2% to 4% risk of developing a nonmetastatic gestational trophoblastic tumor (Berkowitz, Goldstein, 1995; Berkowitz and others, 1996).

Fetal Effects

The embryoblastic tissue of the complete hydatidiform mole never develops into a fetus. The embryoblastic tissue of the partial hydatidiform mole is always abnormal and never matures. A living child can be delivered from a hydatidiform molar pregnancy. These are twin gestations, and only one of the gestational sacs is affected by the molar changes. According to Vejerslev (1991), 60% of the fetuses progress to approximately 28 weeks of gestation with a 70% survival rate.

Diagnostic Testing

Diagnostic tests used to validate a hydatidiform mole include ultrasound and serial beta-HCG immunoassay. *Ultrasound* is the most accurate tool for diagnosing the presence of a mole. A characteristic pattern of multiple diffuse echoes is shown in place of, or along with, an embryo or a fetus.

HCG hormone is secreted by the trophoblast tissue starting at about the time of implantation. In a normal pregnancy, HCG levels gradually increase until around 8 to 10 weeks of pregnancy and then the levels plateau at around 6.6 mIU/ml. Between 10 and 12 weeks the levels begin to decline sharply. In a molar pregnancy the beta-HCG titers are persistently high or rising beyond the normal peak (Ozturk, 1991).

Usual Medical Treatment

Immediate Evacuation

The uterus is usually emptied by suction curettage followed by sharp curettage of the molar implantation site (Bloss and Miller, 1995) unless the patient is no longer interested in childbearing; then an abdominal hysterectomy might be performed. Even if the ovaries are enlarged or cystic, they do not have to be removed; they usually regress spontaneously with the reduction of HCG.

Hemorrhage, perforation of the uterus, infection, and respiratory insufficiency are the four primary complications of surgery. Oxytocin infusion is begun at the beginning of surgery to promote myometrial contractions, which will decrease bleeding and thicken the uterine wall to reduce the risk of perforation of the uterus. Dilation of the cervix is usually accomplished with the patient under general anesthesia unless the cervix is long and closed; then one of the cervical ripening methods may be used to dilate the cervix.

D-negative women may become sensitized following the evacuation of a hydatidiform mole. Therefore they should receive D immune globulin within 72 hours following the surgery to prevent D isoimmunization.

Follow-up Assessment

Because of the existing risk of a gestational trophoblastic tumor developing, these patients should be instructed regarding the importance of a follow-up assessment. When the patient obtains this assessment, early detection of a tumor is possible and treatment is most effective. The follow-up assessment may include the following:

- A baseline beta-HCG determination level, chest x-ray film, and ultrasound scan of the abdomen
- Biweekly serum HCG values are drawn until the beta-HCG level drops to normal and remains normal for 3 consecutive weeks, then monthly for 6 months, and then every 2 months for a total of 1 year
- Regular pelvic examinations to assess uterine and ovarian regression and to observe changes in the vagina that would indicate gestational trophoblastic tumor
- Regular chest x-ray films to detect pulmonary metastasis
- Assessments for such symptoms as dyspnea, cough, and pleuritic pain (these symptoms may indicate pulmonary metastasis); a dull headache, behavioral change, or dizzy spells (may indicate cerebral metastasis); right upper quadrant pain or jaundice (may indicate liver metastasis); and vaginal bleeding (may indicate vaginal metastasis)
- Advice to the patient to avoid becoming pregnant during the follow-up assessment, which usually lasts for about 1 year, since the HCG of the gestational trophoblastic tumor cannot be distinguished from the HCG of pregnancy

Prophylactic Chemotherapy

Some obstetricians recommend prophylactic chemotherapy, but its use is controversial. There is no evidence that such therapy improves long-term prognosis, and it may cause toxicity that occasionally leads to death (Bloss, Miller, 1995). Chemoprophylaxis should be considered only if the patient is at high risk for developing a gestational trophoblastic tumor and the probability of the patient adhering to the follow-up program is poor. Indications of high risk are excessive uterine enlargement, high preevacuation HCG levels, prominent theca-lutein ovarian cysts, maternal age older than 40 years, or repeated molar gestations (Berkowitz and others, 1996; Goldstein, Berkowitz, 1995).

Coexisting Hydatidiform Mole With a Normal Fetus

An amniocentesis is usually performed to determine the fetal karyotype. If the karyotype is normal and the woman's condition is stable, continuation of the pregnancy may be attempted. If the karyotype of the fetus is abnormal, uterine evacuation is recommended (Cunningham and others, 1997; Urbanski and others, 1996). If continuation of the pregnancy is the plan, the patient is usually placed on limited activity to minimize vaginal bleeding and monitored closely for pregnancy-induced hypertension, the HELLP (hemolysis, elevated liver enzymes, and low platelet count in association with preeclampsia) syndrome, preterm labor, anemia, and pulmonary edema (Urbanski and others, 1996).

GESTATIONAL TROPHOBLASTIC TUMOR

Gestational trophoblastic tumor is persistent trophoblastic proliferation. It may develop following a hydatidiform mole, an abortion, or an ectopic or normal pregnancy. Gestational trophoblastic tumor is divided into nonmetastatic, metastatic low risk, and metastatic high risk disorders (Soper, 1997).

Etiology

Approximately 50% of these tumors follow a hydatidiform mole. The risk of occurrence following an ectopic pregnancy or a spontaneous abortion is approximately 25%, with 25% following an apparently normal term pregnancy (Cunningham and others, 1997; Soper, 1997). It has been reported to occur after attempts at in-vitro fertilization (Tanos and others, 1994).

Signs and Symptoms

After any type of delivery, the following signs may indicate a gestational trophoblastic tumor:

- Irregular bleeding: continuous or intermittent irregular bleeding related to uterine subinvolution caused by the presence of trophoblastic tissue
- Metastatic vaginal or vulvar tumors
- Bloody sputum related to pulmonary metastasis
- Intraperitoneal hemorrhage caused by perforation of the uterus as the result of continuous trophoblastic growth through the uterus

Maternal Effects

There is virtually a 100% cure rate following nonmetastatic and low risk metastatic gestational trophoblastic tumor if treated early and appropriately. The risk of maternal mortality is 10% following high risk metastatic gestational trophoblastic tumor (ACOG, 1993), usually the result of hemorrhage or pulmonary insufficiency.

Diagnostic Testing

Follow-up Program

After a hydatidiform mole or anytime abnormal postdelivery bleeding occurs, an intense follow-up program will be implemented to facilitate early detection of a gestational trophoblastic tumor (see usual medical management below). Once a diagnosis is made, the stage of the tumor must be determined (Soper, 1997; Soper and others, 1994). Refer to Table 16-1.

Serial Human Chorionic Gonadotropin Levels

Serial HCG levels should be measured to rule out gestational trophoblastic tumor, and rarely is curettage done to assess for malignant tissue. Persistent or rising HCG levels in the absence of a pregnancy indicate a gestational trophoblastic tumor.

Computed Tomography

Computed tomography (CT scan) is used to check for brain, lung, liver, and pelvic metastases.

Usual Medical Management

Treatment for gestational trophoblastic tumor with chemotherapy is instituted whenever the serum level of HCG rises or plateaus for more than 2 consecutive weeks or if signs of metastasis are detected during examinations.

Nonmetastatic Gestational Trophoblastic Tumor

Single-agent chemotherapy such as methotrexate or actinomycin D is usually effective (Berkowitz and others, 1996; Lurain, Sciarra, 1991).

Low Risk Metastatic Gestational Trophoblastic Tumor

Treatment usually starts with methotrexate, single-agent chemotherapy that is 80% to 90% effective (Berkowitz, Goldstein, 1995). Combination chemotherapy, such as methotrexate, actinomycin D, and cyclophosphamide, is required in 14% of cases. Resec-

TABLE 16-1 Classification of gestational trophoblastic neoplasia

Type	Description
Nonmetastatic	Neoplasm confined to uterus Cure rate virtually 100%
Metastatic	Neoplasm has spread outside uterus
Low risk/good prognosis	Neoplasm present less than 4 mo Serum HCG level less than 40,000 mIU/ml No liver, brain, or peritoneal metastases Metastases limited to lungs or vagina No prior chemotherapy Cure rate virtually 100%
High risk/poor prognosis	Neoplasm present more than 4 mo Serum HCG level more than 40,000 mIU/ml Liver, brain, or peritoneal metastases Failed prior chemotherapy Neoplasm following term pregnancy Cure rate 65%-90% depending on type of chemotherapy used

Modified from Soper J: *Contemp OB/GYN* 42(3):36-54, 1997.

tion of resistant tumors may be necessary in 12% of cases (DuBeshter, 1991).

High Risk Gestational Trophoblastic Tumor

Multiagent chemotherapy, which includes a combination of etoposide, methotrexate, actinomycin D, cyclophosphamide, and Oncovin (vincristine sulfate) (EMA-CO regimen), has been found to be the most effective in cases of high risk gestational trophoblastic tumor (Laurain, 1994; Newlands and others, 1991; Surwit, Childers, 1991).

Follow-up

After the initial treatment, serum beta-HCG levels are evaluated every 1 to 2 weeks. As long as the HCG level is regressing, further chemotherapy is withheld. A plateau or rise in the level indicates a need for additional chemotherapy. When beta-HCG is undetectable for 3 consecutive weeks, remission has occurred. Serial beta-HCG levels will be checked monthly for 6 months and then bimonthly for 6 months or a variation of this. To check the serial beta-HCG levels, the patient should avoid getting pregnant during the follow-up program.

NURSING PROCESS

PREVENTION

Because the cause of a hydatidiform mole is unknown, there is no known prevention. However, malnutrition or stress might play a part in influencing its development; therefore instructions should be given to all patients planning a pregnancy regarding the importance of stress management and a balanced diet high in protein and vitamin A.

ASSESSMENT

- **Hydatidiform Mole:** To detect a hydatidiform mole early, the nurse should observe for signs of a mole at each prenatal visit during the first 20 weeks of gestation. Signs such as uterine bleeding, uterine size small or large for dates, hyperemesis gravidarum, signs of preeclampsia before 24 weeks of gestation, passage of grapelike vesicles, or inability to detect FHR with a Doppler FHR device after 10 to 12 weeks of gestation should be brought to the attention of the obstetrician or health care provider immediately.
- **Gestational Trophoblastic Tumor:** Because a gestational trophoblastic tumor may develop following a normal delivery or an abortion, all patients should be taught the importance of reporting any unusual bleeding following any reproductive event. In these cases, HCG levels should be determined to detect early a gestational trophoblastic tumor.

NURSING DIAGNOSES/COLLABORATIVE PROBLEMS AND INTERVENTIONS

- **POTENTIAL COMPLICATION: HEMORRHAGE** related to trophoblastic invasion or uterine rupture.
  DESIRED OUTCOMES: The signs and symptoms of hemorrhage will be minimized or managed as measured by distal pulses; stable vital signs; orientation to person, place, and time; urinary output greater than 30 ml/hr; and no signs of bleeding.

INTERVENTIONS (ACOG, 1990)

1. Monitor for evidence of hemorrhage such as vital signs, abdominal pain, uterine status, and vaginal bleeding.
2. Start intravenous (IV) infusion with an 18-gauge intracatheter.
3. Prepare for surgery according to preoperative protocol, and type and cross match 2 to 4 units of packed red blood cells as ordered.
4. Postoperative IV infusions with oxytocin added are usually continued initially to facilitate uterine contractions and decrease uterine bleeding.
5. Do not massage a boggy uterus if ovaries are enlarged since it can cause ovarian rupture.
6. Notify physician of first signs of bleeding.
7. Postoperatively, methylergonovine maleate (Methergine) should not be used because it can precipitate a hypertensive crisis.

■ **RISK FOR INFECTION** related to invasive qualities of a hydatidiform mole or surgical intervention.
DESIRED OUTCOME: The patient will remain infection free postoperatively as indicated by her temperature remaining below 38° C (100° F), absence of foul-smelling vaginal discharge, and a white blood cell count between 4500 and 10,000/mm^3.
INTERVENTIONS

1. Assess for indicators of infection by checking temperature every 4 hours and assessing vaginal discharge for a foul odor.
2. Monitor laboratory data, especially white blood cell count.
3. Teach the importance of perineal care.
4. Administer antibiotics at the first sign of an infection as ordered.
5. Notify physician if temperature is greater than 38° C or if foul-smelling vaginal discharge develops.

■ **POTENTIAL COMPLICATION: RESPIRATORY COMPROMISE** related to trophoblastic emboli, fluid overload, cardiac failure caused by gestational hypertension, or a thromboembolism.
DESIRED OUTCOME: Signs and symptoms of respiratory compromise will be minimized or managed as measured by normal breath sounds (absence of adventitious breath sounds), pH 7.35 to 7.45, PaO$_2$ equal to or greater than 80 mm Hg, and PaCO$_2$ less than 45

mm Hg (or arterial blood gas results consistent with patient's baseline parameters).

INTERVENTIONS

1. Auscultate breath sounds postoperatively.
2. Monitor patient for signs and symptoms of hypoxia: restlessness, agitation, and changes in level of consciousness.
3. Monitor serial arterial blood gas values if ordered.
4. Administer oxygen as prescribed.
5. Notify physician of first signs of respiratory compromise, such as decreased breath sounds or an increase in adventitious breath sounds, changes in level of consciousness, decreasing PaO_2, or increasing $PaCO_2$.

- **RISK FOR ALTERED URINARY ELIMINATION** (oliguria) related to the antidiuretic effect of oxytocin.

  DESIRED OUTCOME: The patient will maintain a urinary output greater than 120 ml/4 hr.

  INTERVENTIONS

  1. Monitor intake and output.
  2. Administer oxytocin intravenously as ordered, and monitor flow rate closely.
  3. Notify attending physician if urine output drops below 120 ml/4 hr.

- **FEAR** related to the possible development of a gestational trophoblastic tumor, future threat to family planning, and financial concern regarding long-term medical care.

  DESIRED OUTCOME: The patient and family members will be able to communicate their fears and concerns openly.

  INTERVENTIONS

  1. Provide time for the patient and her family to express their concerns regarding the possible outcome and inconvenience to the mother and family during the treatment and long-term follow-up assessment. Encourage them to vent any feelings, fears, and anger they may be experiencing.
  2. Assess family's support system and coping mechanisms.
  3. Provide information to the family regarding the disease process, plan of treatment, and risk for the patient.
  4. Explain all treatment modalities and reasons.
  5. Keep patient informed of health status and results of tests.
  6. Discuss risk of a gestational trophoblastic tumor based on whether the patient had a partial or complete mole.

7. Refer to social services for financial concerns if the family is without health benefits.

- **ANTICIPATORY GRIEVING** related to loss of an anticipated infant, state of wellness, and possible threat to fertility.
  DESIRED OUTCOME: The patient and her family will verbalize their feelings of grief appropriately and identify any problems as they work through the grief process.
  INTERVENTIONS
  1. Assess significance of the loss to all family members and level of guilt or blame.
  2. Assess family's communication pattern and support systems.
  3. Reaffirm with the family their losses, and let them know you are aware that these are real.
  4. Provide physical care such as a back rub or nourishment as needed.
  5. Consider any significant cultural beliefs or values.
  6. Spiritual assistance might help the family to work through their grief. Refer to the chaplain or family's own clergy.
  7. Refer to psychiatric services when deemed necessary.

- **RISK FOR ALTERED HEALTH MANAGEMENT** related to follow-up assessment and chemotherapy regimen if metastasis occurs.
  DESIRED OUTCOME: The patient and her family will verbalize compliance, outline the proposed follow-up assessment, and use a contraceptive method during the follow-up care.
  INTERVENTIONS
  1. Assess the patient's and family's understanding of the disease and risks of an ongoing gestational trophoblastic tumor.
  2. Explain the disease and plan of treatment.
  3. Educate about the importance of the follow-up assessment to detect early a gestational trophoblastic tumor when it is almost 100% curable.
  4. Educate about the importance of avoiding pregnancy during the follow-up assessment to prevent masking the HCG rise of a gestational trophoblastic tumor.
  5. Teach that any effective contraceptive method may be used except an intrauterine device (IUD) because of bleeding irregularities associated with the IUD. Oral contraceptives are the preferred method since they are highly effective (Deicas and others, 1991).

6. Explain the treatment program if a gestational trophoblastic tumor develops.

7. Future family planning can be facilitated when the couple is reassured that even following chemotherapy, they can anticipate a normal reproductive outcome in the future with no increased risk of congenital fetal malformations (Ayhan and others, 1990; Berkowitz and others, 1994). The risk of a repeat molar pregnancy is 1% (Berkowitz and others, 1994). After two molar pregnancies, the risk is about 20% (Berkowitz and others, 1996).

■ **POTENTIAL COMPLICATION: D SENSITIZATION** in a D-negative mother carrying a D-positive fetus.

DESIRED OUTCOME: The mother's body will not develop antibodies against the D-negative factor.

INTERVENTION

1. Determine mother's blood type and Rh factor.

2. If mother is Rh negative, be prepared to administer Rho (D) immune globulin (RhoGAM) (HypRho-D). (The usual dose is 1 vial, which equals approximately 300 µg.)

CONCLUSION

The goals of the nurse in treating patients who have had a hydatidiform mole are twofold. First, the nurse must impress them with the importance of the follow-up assessment. To determine if a gestational trophoblastic tumor is going to occur, serum beta-HCG levels should be checked closely. The beta-HCG levels should progressively decline and by 10 to 12 weeks be nondetectable. Second, the nurse must help the patient work through the loss of an expected baby, a defective pregnancy, the fear of the development of proliferative trophoblastic disease, and the fear of recurrence in subsequent pregnancies.

The goal of management of a gestational trophoblastic tumor is early detection when there is an almost 100% cure rate with appropriate treatment. To detect early all gestational trophoblastic tumors, it must be kept in mind that they may occur after any reproductive event, and therefore any abnormal bleeding should be evaluated as a possible indication of this disorder.

BIBLIOGRAPHY

American College of Obstetricians and Gynecologists (ACOG): Diagnosis and management of postpartum hemorrhage, *ACOG Techn Bull,* no. 143, 1990.

American College of Obstetricians and Gynecologists (ACOG): Management of gestational trophoblastic disease, *ACOG Techn Bull,* no. 178, 1993.

Ayhan A and others: Pregnancy after chemotherapy for gestational trophoblastic disease, *J Reprod Med* 35(5):522-524, 1990.

Berkowitz R and others: Subsequent pregnancy experience in patients with gestational trophoblastic disease—New England Trophoblastic Disease Center, 1965-1992, *J Reprod Med* 39:228, 1994.

Berkowitz R, Goldstein D: Diagnosis and management of the primary hydatidiform mole, *Obstet Gynecol Clin North Am* 15(3):491-501, 1988.

Berkowitz R, Goldstein D: Gestational trophoblastic disease. In Ryan K, Berkowitz R, Barbieri R: *Kistner's gynecology—principles and practice,* St Louis, 1995, Mosby.

Berkowitz R, Goldstein D, Bernstein M: Evolving concepts of molar pregnancy, *J Reprod Med* 36(1):40-44, 1991.

Berkowitz R, Goldstein D, Bernstein M: Update on gestational trophoblastic disease, *Contemp OB/GYN* 40(4):21-29, 1996.

Bloss J, Miller D: Gestational trophoblastic disease. In Hankins G and others: *Operative obstetrics,* Norwalk, Conn, 1995, Appleton & Lange.

Cunningham G, MacDonald P, Gant N: *Williams' obstetrics,* ed 20, Norwalk, Conn, 1997, Appleton & Lange.

Deicas R and others: The role of contraception in the development of postmolar gestational trophoblastic tumor, *Obstet Gynecol* 78:221, 1991.

DuBeshter B: High risk factors in metastatic gestational trophoblastic tumor, *J Reprod Med* 36(1):9-13, 1991.

Goldstein D, Berkowitz R: Prophylactic chemotherapy of complete molar pregnancy, *Semin Oncol* 22:157, 1995.

Ko T and others: Restriction fragment length polymorphism analysis to study the genetic origin of complete hydatidiform mole, *Am J Obstet Gynecol* 64:901-906, 1991.

Laurain J: High-risk metastatic gestational trophoblastic tumors: current management, *J Reprod Med* 39:217, 1994.

Loret de Mola J, Goldfarb J: Reproductive performance of patients after gestational trophoblastic disease, *Semin Oncol* 22:193, 1995.

Lurain J, Sciarra J: Study and treatment of gestational trophoblastic diseases at the John I. Brewer Trophoblastic Disease Center, 1962-1990, *Eur J Gynaecol Oncol* 12:425, 1991.

Newlands E and others: Results with the EMA/CO etoposide, methotrexate, actinomycin D, cyclophosphamide, vincristine regimen in high risk gestational trophoblastic tumors, 1979-1989, *Br J Obstet Gynaecol* 98:550, 1991.

Osathanond R and others: Hormonal measurements in patients with theca lutein cysts and gestational trophoblastic disease, *J Reprod Med* 31:179, 1986.

Ozturk M: Human chorionic gonadotropin, its free subunits and gestational trophoblastic disease, *J Reprod Med* 36(1):21-26, 1991.

Palmer J: Advances in the epidemiology of gestational trophoblastic disease, *J Reprod Med* 39:155, 1994.

Rose P: Hydatidiform mole: diagnosis and management, *Semin Oncol* 22:149, 1995.

Semer D, Macfee M: Gestational trophoblastic disease: epidemiology, *Semin Oncol* 22:109, 1995.

Soper J: Staging and prognostic factors in gestational trophoblastic disease, *Contemp OB/GYN* 42(3):36-54, 1997.

Soper J and others: Evaluation of prognostic factors and staging in gestational trophoblastic tumor, *Obstet Gynceol* 84:969, 1994.

Surwit E, Childers J: High risk metastatic gestational trophoblastic disease, *J Reprod Med* 36(1):45-48, 1991.

Tanos V and others: Recurrent gestational trophoblastic disease following in vitro fertilization, *Hum Reprod* 9:2010, 1994.

Urbanski T and others: Caring for a woman with a hydatidiform mole and coexisting pregnancy, *MCN Am J Matern Child Nurs* 21(2):85-89, 1996.

Vejerslev L: Clinical management and diagnostic possibilities in hydatidiform mole with coexistent fetus, *Obstet Gynecol Surv* 46:577, 1991.

Wolf N, Lage J: Genetic analysis of gestational trophoblastic disease: a review, *Semin Oncol* 22:113, 1995.

CHAPTER

17

Placental Abnormalities

About 4% of all pregnant women experience some type of vaginal bleeding during the third trimester of pregnancy (Lockwood, 1996). The major causes of this bleeding are abruptio placentae and placenta previa. This chapter focuses on these two main causes and contrasts the treatments of both. Other causes of third-trimester bleeding are heavy bloody show, cervical carcinoma, polyps, infection of the cervix or vagina, placenta accreta, and vasa previa. Placenta accreta and vasa previa will be briefly covered in this chapter as well.

ABRUPTIO PLACENTAE

An abruptio placentae is the premature separation, either partial or total, of a normally implanted placenta from the decidual lining of the uterus after 20 weeks of gestation. It is normally classified into one of three categories: mild, moderate, or severe (Table 17-1). Some medical personnel refer to a grade of 1, 2, or 3 instead. Mild abruptio placentae is a grade 1, moderate a grade 2, and severe a grade 3. There is also a grade 0 given when no antepartum symptoms were manifested but on examination of the placenta after delivery a small area of adherent clot at the periphery of the placenta is noted (Green, 1994). Maternal bleeding in any class can be marginal, concealed, or both (Fig. 17-1) depending on whether

T A B L E 17-1 Comparison of three classifications of abruptio placentae

	Mild: grade 1	Moderate: grade 2	Severe: grade 3
Definition	Less than one sixth of placenta separates prematurely	From one sixth to one half of placenta separates prematurely	More than one half of placenta separates prematurely
Incidence	48%	27%	24%
Signs and symptoms	Total blood loss less than 500 ml	Total blood loss 1000-1500 ml	Total blood loss more than 1500 ml
	15% of total blood volume	15%-30% of total blood volume	Greater than 30% total blood volume
	Dark vaginal bleeding (mild to moderate)	Dark vaginal bleeding (mild to severe)	Dark vaginal bleeding moderate to excessive
	Vague lower abdominal or back discomfort	Gradual or abrupt onset of abdominal pain	Usually abrupt onset of uterine pain described as tearing, knifelike, and continuous
	No uterine tenderness	Uterine tenderness present	Uterus boardlike and highly reactive to stimuli
	No uterine irritability	Uterine tone increased	
Hypovolemia	Vital signs normal	Mild shock	Moderate to profound shock common
		Normal maternal blood pressure	Decreased maternal blood pressure
		Maternal tachycardia	Maternal tachycardia significant
		Narrowed pulse pressure	Narrowed pulse pressure
		Orthostatic hypotension	Orthostatic hypotension severe
		Tachypnea	Significant tachypnea
Disseminated intravascular coagulopathy (DIC)	Normal fibrinogen of 450 mg/dl	Early signs of DIC common	DIC develops usually unless condition is treated immediately
		Fibrinogen 150-300 mg/dl	Fibrinogen less than 150 mg/dl
Fetal effects	Normal fetal heart rate pattern	Fetal heart rate shows nonreassuring signs of possible fetal distress	Fetal heart rate shows signs of fetal distress and death can occur

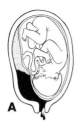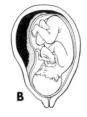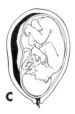

FIG. 17-1 Classification of abruptio placentae. **A,** Marginal or apparent. **B,** Central or concealed. **C,** Missed or combined.

it is trapped in the uterus. Maternal bleeding is classified as one of the following:

- Marginal or apparent: the separation is near the edge of the placenta, and the blood is able to escape.
- Central or concealed: the separation is somewhere in the center of the placenta, and the blood is trapped.
- Mixed or combined: part of the separation is near the edge, and part is concealed in the center area.

Incidence

The incidence of abruptio placentae is 1 in 200 pregnancies (Cunningham and others, 1997).

Etiology

The actual cause of an abruptio placentae is unknown. Conditions frequently associated with abruptio placentae are as follows:

1. Pregnancy-induced or chronic hypertension: this is the most common cause of an abruption and is more likely to result in a more severe abruption (Morgan and others, 1994).
2. Previous abruption: there is a 10% increased risk after one abruption and a 25% risk of recurrence after two abruptions (Cunningham and others, 1997).
3. Trauma: a placental abruption may result from a direct blow to the abdomen, most commonly as the result of a motor vehicle collision or maternal battering.
4. Cigarette smoking: smoking causes approximately 40% of abruptions by vasoconstriction of the spiral arteriole, which can lead to decidual necrosis (Voigt and others, 1990). However, there is a significant dose-dependent relationship between cigarette smoking and abruptio placentae (Floyd and others, 1991).

5. Cocaine: cocaine causes vasoconstriction and hypertension, which can interfere with placental adherence to the uterine wall (Janke, 1990; Peters, Theorell, 1991).
6. Premature rupture of membranes: a 5% risk of developing an abruptio placentae following premature rupture of membranes exists (Major and others, 1995), and a greater risk exists if sudden uterine decompression results from the rupture of membranes in multiple gestations or polyhydramnios (Ananth and others, 1996).

Normal Physiology

The blastocyst normally implants into the endometrium, now called the *decidua,* by sending out threadlike projections called *chorionic villi* from the trophoblast cells. These villi open up intervillous spaces, which fill with maternal blood. These spaces are supplied by the spiral arteries. At the same time the trophoblast cells send out anchoring cords to attach themselves to the uterus.

Pathophysiology

An abruptio placentae is theoretically thought to be caused by degeneration of the spiral arterioles that nourish the decidua (endometrium) and supply blood to the placenta, causing decidua basalis necrosis. When this process takes place, rupture of that blood vessel occurs and bleeding quickly results because the uterus is still distended and cannot contract sufficiently to close off the opened blood vessels. Separation of the placenta takes place in the area of the hemorrhage. If the tear is at the margin of the placenta or if it separates the membranes from the decidua, vaginal bleeding is evident. Otherwise, the blood is concealed between the placenta and the decidua. If it is concealed, pressure can build up enough for blood to be forced through the fetal membranes into the amniotic sac or into the myometrial muscle fibers, which is called *Couvelaire uterus.* This increases uterine tone and irritability. Clotting occurs simultaneously with the hemorrhage because the decidual tissue is rich in thromboplastin. This leads to the formation of a retroplacental or a subchorionic hematoma, causing the release of large quantities of thromboplastin into the maternal circulation. This can lead to disseminated intravascular coagulopathy (DIC).

Signs and Symptoms

Classic Manifestations

The classic manifestations of an abruptio placentae are as follows:
- Dark vaginal bleeding (80%)
- Uterine hypertonus (17%)

- Uterine contractions (17%)
- Abdominal or low back pain
- Uterine tenderness
- Fetal distress signs or fetal death
- Signs of hypovolemia beyond those expected on the basis of observed external blood loss

The presence and degree of each sign are related to the amount of concealed blood trapped behind the placenta and the degree of separation. If the separation occurs at the margin of the placenta, the blood usually tears the membranes away from the decidua and escapes externally. The blood appears dark because it has had some time to begin clotting. If the separation is in the center of the placenta, blood is trapped behind the placenta. Concealed blood causes pressure and myometrial contractions, and this results in abdominal pain and uterine tenderness. With no way to escape, pressure builds up and can force blood into the myometrial tissue of the uterus, causing increased uterine irritability. Increasing uterine size and decreasing serial hematocrits are other signs of concealed bleeding. If some of this trapped blood is forced through the fetal membranes into the amniotic cavity, the amniotic fluid will be bloody.

Mild Abruptio Placentae: Grade 1

Mild forms of abruptio placentae usually develop gradually and produce mild to moderate dark vaginal bleeding without uterine tenderness. Signs of fetal distress are absent, and the mother's vital signs remain stable. There are no signs of DIC. This type of abruption can be self-limiting or can progress into a more advanced form.

Moderate Abruptio Placentae: Grade 2

A moderate abruptio placentae can develop gradually or abruptly and produce persistent abdominal pain accompanied by visible dark vaginal bleeding. The uterus may be very tender on palpation and may remain firm between contractions if the mother is in labor. This can make auditory appraisal of the fetal heart rate (FHR) difficult. Fetal distress may be present depending on the extent of placental separation and the amount of maternal blood loss. Signs of shock may be present.

Severe Abruptio Placentae: Grade 3

A severe abruptio placentae usually develops suddenly, causing excruciating, unremitting abdominal pain often referred to as *knifelike* or *tearing*. The uterus is often boardlike and tender and fails to relax. Profuse bleeding results, although it may not be evident vaginally if the blood is trapped behind the placenta. In this case the uterus will show signs of enlarging. Shock can ensue, although the signs of shock may not be in proportion to the amount of visible blood loss. Signs of fetal distress are usually evident, and fetal death may result.

Posteriorly Implanted Abruptio Placentae

In a few instances, when an abruptio placentae occurs in a posteriorly implanted placenta, no signs of uterine tenderness and pain are manifested. In these cases the classic signs are only vaginal bleeding and backache.

Complications

Shock

Shock results as the body attempts to protect the vital organs, especially the brain and heart, from a reduction of effective circulating blood volume. When blood is lost from the vascular system, venous return is diminished and consequently cardiac output is reduced. Physiologic compensatory mechanisms are then activated. The decrease in arterial pressure initiates powerful sympathetic reflexes that stimulate vasoconstriction of the arterioles and venules in the kidneys, liver, lungs, gastrointestinal tract, muscles, skin, and uterus. Blood is then redistributed to the heart and brain from these areas.

The heart and respiratory rates increase in an attempt to compensate by delivering increased volume and better oxygenated blood to the vital organs. A slower compensatory mechanism is activated that stimulates the absorption of fluid from the intestinal tract and stimulates the kidneys to increase reabsorption of sodium and water. Therefore the results are classic signs of hypovolemic shock, which include hypotension; oliguria; rapid, thready pulse; shallow, irregular respirations; cold and clammy skin; pallor; syncope; and thirst. Should severe bleeding continue, the compensatory mechanisms cannot keep up with tissue needs, and cardiac deterioration, loss of vasomotor tone, and release of toxins by ischemic tissue result; cellular death ensues.

Because of the normally increased maternal blood volume during pregnancy, the classic signs of shock are not always present until after the fetal circulation is affected. During pregnancy, signs of shock usually do not present until after 30% of maternal blood volume is lost. Shunting of blood away from the placenta occurs before this 30% blood loss. Refer to Table 17-2 for manifested symptoms of blood loss.

TABLE 17-2 Manifested symptoms of blood loss

Percent of blood loss	Manifested symptoms	Treatment
15% = 1 unit	Minimal tachycardia Normal blood pressure Normal pulse pressure Normal respiratory rate Normal capillary refill	Stabilize with crystalloid
15%-30% = 2-3 units	Tachycardia Increased blood pressure, especially diastolic Decreased pulse pressure Delayed hypothenar refilling Orthostatic blood pressure changes Tachypnea	Usually successful stabilizing with crystalloid
30%-40% = 3-4 units	Significant tachycardia Decreased blood pressure, especially systolic Decreased pulse pressure Significant tachypnea Oliguria Syncope, shortness of breath, headaches, chest pain	Infuse 1-2 L of a crystalloid solution Then infuse blood component therpay such as erythrocytes
40% or greater = >4 units	Marked tachycardia Significant depression of blood pressure Narrow pulse pressure Significant tachypnea Oliguria Syncope, shortness of breath, headaches, chest pain Skin cold and pale	Infuse 1-2 L of crystalloid solution Then infuse blood component therapy such as erythrocytes Whole blood Infuse platelets and fresh frozen plasma after several units of whole blood

Modified from data in Naef R, Morrison J: *Clin Obstet Gynecol* 38(3):547-557, 1995.

Disseminated Intravascular Coagulopathy

Abruptio placentae is the most common cause of DIC. Clinically significant DIC occurs in 10% of all cases of abruptio placentae (Green, 1994). Of the total number of cases, 30% will develop severe maternal and fetal complications related to DIC while the fetus remains alive (Cunningham and others, 1997). In these cases the clotting will become intravascular as well as retroplacental. This coagulation defect usually occurs in patients with a severe, concealed abruptio placentae related to one or more of the following:

- Depletion of the clotting factors, especially platelets, fibrinogen, and prothrombin
- Thromboplastin from the decidua and placenta entering the maternal circulation and activating the clotting mechanism throughout the body
- Activation of the anticoagulant effect stimulated by the presence of increased fibrin degradation products; when a coagulation defect occurs, hypofibrinogenemia results and massive bleeding occurs (see Chapter 18)

Other Complications

Renal failure can develop if shock, vascular spasms, or DIC has occurred. Pituitary necrosis (Sheehan syndrome) occasionally results from the same conditions that cause renal failure. To assess for pituitary necrosis, lactation should not be suppressed with medication in patients who experienced hypovolemic shock, vascular spasms, or DIC until after the onset of lactation. In the presence of pituitary necrosis, lactation will not occur since pituitary hormones regulate lactation.

Maternal Effects

In fewer than 1% of cases, maternal death occurs from hemorrhagic shock. This low maternal mortality is mainly because of the availability of blood replacement therapy. However, maternal morbidity is significant. Because of the potential for massive bleeding, the patient is at high risk for developing shock and DIC at any time before delivery. In rare cases a fetal-to-maternal hemorrhage may occur, which can cause the Rh-negative mother to become sensitized.

During the postpartum period, mothers who had experienced an abruptio placentae are at an increased risk of anemia, development of an infection related to prolonged separation of the placenta, a postpartum hemorrhage related to a poorly contracted uterus caused by blood infiltrating the uterus, and DIC. Other complications that can develop as a result of ischemia are renal failure and pituitary necrosis (Sheehan syndrome).

Fetal and Neonatal Effects

Perinatal mortality ranges from 15% to 30% (Fretts and others, 1992; Queenan, 1995). The most common effects are fetal hypoxia, neonatal prematurity, and small for gestational age.

Fetal Hypoxia

Fetal hypoxia is caused by uteroplacental insufficiency resulting from placental separation or decreased uterine perfusion resulting from maternal hypovolemia, uterine hypertonus, or, less often, fetal hemorrhage. Total anoxia may develop.

Neonatal Prematurity

The neonate is frequently premature since the fetus must be delivered early because of fetal distress or preterm labor.

Small for Gestational Age

Even if the bleeding and separation stop, the decreased placental surface area that remains intact may not be adequate to meet the increased needs of the growing fetus (Voigt and others, 1990).

Neurologic Defects

The infant who survives is at increased risk of a neurologic defect such as cerebral palsy (Spinillo and others, 1993).

Diagnostic Testing

Diagnosis usually is made on the basis of presenting symptoms and a physical assessment. Severe abruptio placentae and moderate abruptio placentae are easier to diagnose; a patient presents with one or more of the classic symptoms. Mild abruptio placentae is more difficult to diagnose; it is easily confused with a placenta previa, because vaginal bleeding may be the only presenting symptom. Therefore ultrasound is usually used to rule out a placenta previa and is accompanied by a clinical examination to rule out other less common causes of third-trimester bleeding. Recently a thrombomodulin, an endothelial cell marker, has been found to be elevated in the serum of women experiencing a placental abruption (Magriples and others, 1996). However, at present, no diagnostic method is available to determine the degree of placental separation.

Usual Medical Management and Protocols for Nurse Practitioners

Treatment of an abruptio placentae depends on the severity of blood loss, fetal maturity, and fetal well-being.

Expectant Management

If the abruptio placentae is mild with no signs of hypovolemia or anemia, gestational age of the fetus is determined first. With an immature fetus of less than 36 weeks of gestation without signs of fetal distress, expectant management is usually the treatment. The components of expectant management (ACOG, 1994) are as follows:

1. Closely observe for signs of concealed or external bleeding.
2. Do continuous FHR monitoring until 72 hours without bleeding, hypertension, or an abnormal FHR pattern.
3. Monitor for preterm uterine contractions, which can be stimulated by prostaglandin release from placental separation. If preterm uterine contractions occur, in select cases a tocolytic agent, preferably magnesium sulfate, may be used (Cunningham and others, 1997). Beta-sympathomimetics can cause maternal tachycardia and thereby falsely indicate hemorrhage. Calcium channel blockers can cause hypotension and thereby adversely affect maternal perfusion of the uterus.
4. Hospitalize, in a facility that can immediately intervene by cesarean delivery, since the placenta may further separate at any time and, very quickly, seriously compromise the fetus unless delivery can be performed immediately. Corticosteroids to accelerate fetal lung maturity may be part of the plan

Emergency Management

If the abruptio placentae is moderate to severe, the following are the objectives of treatment:

1. Restore blood loss quickly.
2. Continuously monitor the fetus.
3. Correct coagulation defect if present.
4. Expedite delivery.

Maternal volume status must be monitored continually with (1) an indwelling Foley catheter to determine urine output and (2) serial hematocrits every 2 to 3 hours. If urine output drops below 30 ml/hr despite vigorous volume replacement, a central venous pressure (CVP) catheter is needed to determine intravascular volume status.

Fluid replacement is usually accomplished with a crystalloid solution, such as lactated Ringer's, and blood component therapy as soon as it is available. IV lactated Ringer's solution and blood are usually administered at a rate adequate to maintain the hematocrit at 30% or greater and urinary output at 30 ml/hr or greater. In rare instances the patient's blood loss is rapid and massive, leading to severe shock. In such cases, volume expanders or immediate transfusions with type O, Rh-negative blood may be given until properly matched blood is available. Oxygen should be administered with face mask because it will increase oxygen tension and increase oxygen delivery to end-organs.

The fetus must be monitored continuously until delivery takes place. It should be kept in mind that a maternal heart beat may be picked up through the fetal scalp electrode in the event of fetal death. Therefore the FHR should be compared with the maternal pulse. If a coagulation defect develops (fibrinogen level less than 150 mg/dl), replacement of the clotting factors is the usual treatment. This can be accomplished by the administration of cryoprecipitate or fresh frozen plasma to replace fibrinogen and a platelet transfusion if the platelet count is below 50,000/mm^3. Heparin was once used to treat DIC in the presence of an abruptio placentae, but it is no longer an acceptable treatment. Within 24 hours following delivery, the coagulation defect normally corrects itself. The platelet count may not return to return to a normal level for 2 to 4 days. Refer to Table 17-3 for guidelines for blood component replacement.

Delivery

Delivery should be effected if the abruption is moderate to severe, if the fetus is older than 36 weeks, or at any time fetal distress is noted. If the fetus is mature and in a cephalic presentation, a vaginal delivery may be attempted with continuous fetal monitoring in an environment where a cesarean delivery can be performed immediately. If the woman is not in labor and nonreassuring signs of fetal stress are absent, vaginal delivery can be initiated by an amniotomy or a labor stimulant such as oxytocin, provided that the patient is in a tertiary care center where rapid emergency measures can be initiated if further abruption occurs with contractions. If the fetus in not in a cephalic presentation or if, during the induction of labor, bleeding increases, the uterus fails to relax between contractions, fetal distress occurs, or labor fails to progress actively, a cesarean birth will be performed.

In the presence of a severe abruptio placentae, if the fetus is

Text continued on p. 436

TABLE 17-3 Guidelines for blood component replacement

Conditions	Blood component	Volume per unit	Dose	Effect	Administration
Acute blood loss	Volume expansion with crystalloid solutions (lactated Ringer's and NS) Other volume expanders Albumin Hydroxyethyl starch Dextran Purified protein fractions	1000 ml	Depends on amount of blood lost		If bleeding stops and blood pressure rises after 1-2 L, blood components may not be necessary
Acute blood loss Hgb 7 g/dl or less Hct 21% or less Symptomatic Syncope Shortness of breath Chest pain Oliguria Tachycardia	Volume expansion with crystalloid solutions Packed RBCs to restore oxygen-carrying capacity	250 ml	Depends on Hgb/Hct levels and amount of continued bleeding	1 unit will increase Hgb 1 g/dl and Hct 3%	Packed RBCs have a Hct of 70% and therefore increased viscosity; if need to infuse rapidly, mix with 200 ml of NS per unit

Indication	Product	Volume	Dose	Effect	Comments
Deficiency in clotting factors (II, V, VII, IX, XI) indicated by PT or PTT 1.5 × normal or greater PT >18 sec PTT >55 sec	Fresh frozen plasma	250 ml	Normal dose: 2 bags	1 unit will increase each clotting factor by 2%-3%	
Platelet count <50,000/mm³ with active bleeding or surgery schedules Abnormal function as indicated by normal platelet count with bleeding time >9 min	Platelet transfusions	50 ml	1 unit × 10 kg of body weight Minimum of 6 units	1 unit will increase platelet count 5000-10,000/mm³	Do not use a platelet count RBC leukocyte-depleting filter because most of the platelets will also be removed Approximately 0.5 ml of RBCs are present in platelet transfusions; if ABO and CDE (Rh) type-specific

Continued

Data from American College of Obstetricians and Gynecologists (ACOG): *ACOG Techn Bull*, no. 199, 1994; Naef R, Morrison J: *Clin Obstet Gynecol* 38(3):547-557, 1995.

NS, Normal saline; *Hgb*, hemoglobin; *RBCs*, red blood cells; *Hct*, hematocrit; *PT*, prothrombin time; *PTT*, partial thromboplastin time.

TABLE 17-3 Guidelines for blood component replacement—cont'd

Conditions	Blood component	Volume per unit	Dose	Effect	Administration
					platelets are not available, a D-negative woman can be sensitized with D-positive platelets; administer RhoGAM (one dose needed for every 15 ml of RBCs)
Deficiency in one or more of the following clotting factors: Fibrinogen (<200 mg/dl)	Cypoprecipitate contains factors VIII and XIII, fibrinogen, fibronectin, von Willebrand factor	40 ml	For hypofibrinogenemia: 1 bag × 5 kg of body weight	1 unit will increase fibrinogen 10 mg/dl	

Factor VIII or XIII			
von Willebrand factor			
Fibronectin			
Total blood loss exceeds 25% of total blood volume	Packed RBCs and fresh frozen plasma or whole blood	500 ml	All blood products should be administered through a Y type blood administration set with a filter designed to remove debris; only normal saline should be infused through the same line

alive, a cesarean birth should be performed as soon as possible. If the fetus is dead, a vaginal delivery is preferred unless bleeding cannot be controlled.

PLACENTA PREVIA

Placenta previa occurs when the placenta attaches to the lower segment of the uterus, near or over the internal os, instead of in the body or fundal segment of the uterus. It is normally classified into one of three categories depending on the degree of coverage of the cervix (Fig.17-2):

1. Marginal: the placenta is near but does not cover any part of the internal os.
2. Partial: the placenta implants near and partially covers the internal os.
3. Total: the placenta completely covers the internal os.

Incidence

The incidence of placenta previa is approximately 1 in 200 pregnancies, or a 0.5% risk (Iyasu and others, 1993).

Etiology

The actual cause of placenta previa is unknown. However, it is frequently associated with endometrial scarring, impeded endometrial vascularization, and increased placental mass.

Endometrial Scarring

Endometrial scarring can result from a previous placenta previa, an abortion, cesarean delivery, increased parity, or closely spaced pregnancies (Green, 1994). Subsequent pregnancies, after a cesarean delivery, have a 50% greater likelihood of a placenta previa complication (Taylor and others, 1994).

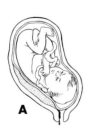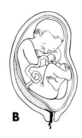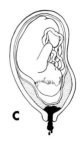

FIG. 17-2 Classifications of placenta previa. **A,** Marginal placenta previa. **B,** Partial placenta previa. **C,** Total placenta previa.

Impeded Endometrial Vascularization

Factors that interfere with adequate blood supply to the endometrium, such as a medical condition of hypertension or diabetes, a uterine tumor, drug addiction, smoking, or advancing maternal age, can cause placenta previa (Cunningham and others, 1997; Handler and others, 1994).

Increased Placental Mass

A multiple pregnancy leads to more than one placenta and therefore may increase the risk of placenta previa.

Normal Physiology

The blastocyst normally implants into the upper anterior portion of the uterus, where the vascular blood supply is rich. After implantation of the blastocyst, the trophoblastic tissue sends out threadlike projections, the chorionic villi, that grow into the decidua (endometrium). At first these chorionic villi surround the blastocyst, but soon after, the portion of the chorionic villi in contact with the decidua basalis proliferates to form the placenta, and the villi, in contact with the decidua capsularis, atrophy.

The chorionic villi are of two types. One type opens up intervillous spaces, which fill with maternal blood to form an area of exchange between the embryonic or fetal and maternal circulatory systems. Another type of villi forms anchoring cords to stabilize the placenta and embryo or fetus in the uterus. The chorionic villi growth is normally confined to the endometrium because of the fibrinoid layer of Nitabuch, which separates the decidua from the myometrium and stops chorionic villi growth.

Pathophysiology

With placenta previa the blastocyst implants itself in the lower uterine segment, over or very near the internal os. A large percentage of placentas that initially implant low migrate upward (Lavery, 1990; Lockwood, 1990). There are two current theories as to why placental migration takes place. According to the first theory, the growth of the lower uterine segment from 0.5 to 5 cm causes movement of the placenta away from the cervical os (Lavery, 1990). The second theory postulates that the chorionic villi have the ability to grow in one area and to remain dormant in another (Lockwood, 1990).

The decidua basalis is less developed in the lower segment of the uterus. The fibrinoid layer of Nitabuch, which stops chorionic villi growth, may be absent. Therefore placental tissue may come into direct contact with the myometrium and a placenta accreta, increta, or percreta may develop.

Signs and Symptoms

Bleeding

Normally, during the latter half of pregnancy, the lower uterine segment elongates as the fundal segment of the uterus hypertrophies. Toward the end of the pregnancy, the cervix begins to efface and dilate. When the placenta is implanted in the lower uterine segment over or around the internal cervical os, separation or tearing of portions of the placenta can occur with subsequent bleeding. Usually, the greater the percent of placenta covering the os, the earlier the first episode of bleeding occurs. Because the normal uterine changes occur very gradually until labor begins, the initial bleeding episode is usually slight and ceases spontaneously as clot formation occurs. This is not always the case, however. The bleeding is usually painless and bright red in color without associated uterine tenderness because the blood is not trapped behind the placenta. Recurrence is unpredictable and can take place at any time.

Vital Signs

Vital signs may be misleadingly normal even in the presence of severe blood loss. This is related to the normal increase of 40% to 50% in the circulatory blood volume during pregnancy. In fact, after week 32 of gestation, the pregnant patient can lose 30% of her blood volume without exhibiting signs of shock. The blood supply to the placenta is affected before a 30% decrease in the maternal blood volume. Refer to Table 17-2 for manifested symptoms of blood loss.

Fetal Distress

FHR is usually normal unless the placental exchange is compromised by excessive blood loss, maternal shock, or major placental detachment.

Fetal Malpresentation

The presenting part of the fetus usually remains high even in late pregnancy because the placenta occupies the lower uterine segment. For this same reason, the risk of malpresentations, such as transverse, oblique, or breech lie, increases.

Maternal Effects

Maternal mortality is less than 1% (Green, 1994).

Hemorrhage and Hypovolemic Shock

Placenta previa can cause maternal hemorrhage and hypovolemic shock.

Placenta Accreta/Increta/Percreta

The risk of placenta accreta, increta, or percreta is 5% to 10% with any placenta previa, and if the woman had a previous cesarean delivery, the risk is 10% to 35% (Chattophadhyay and others, 1993). It can be as high as 65% in a pregnancy following multiple cesarean deliveries and a history of placenta previa (Lavery, 1990; Zahn, Yeomans, 1990).

Preterm Delivery

The risk of preterm delivery is 40% with placenta previa (Lockwood, 1990).

Premature Rupture of Membranes

The risk of premature rupture of membranes is 11% with placenta previa (Lockwood, 1990).

D Sensitization

A D-negative woman can become sensitized during any antepartum bleeding episode (Green, 1994).

Puerperal Hemorrhage

Puerperal hemorrhage can occur even in the presence of a firmly contracted uterus. This is because the lower uterine segment does not have the contractility of the upper uterine segment, and, as a consequence, there is less compression of the open vessels, resulting from the removal of the placenta. This risk of hemorrhage is further increased by the larger than normal surface area denuded by the removal of the placenta.

Puerperal Anemia

Puerperal anemia is the result of increased blood loss.

Puerperal Infection

The opened blood vessels are near the cervical os and can become infected easily.

Fetal and Neonatal Effects

Perinatal mortality is less than 10% with a placenta previa (Queenan, 1995).

Prematurity

Prematurity is the greatest cause of mortality.

Malpresentation

The risk of malpresentation is 35% with placenta previa (Green, 1994).

Small for Gestational Age

Small size for gestational age occurs if the placental exchange is chronically compromised (Wolf and others, 1991).

Congenital Abnormalities

The risk of central nervous system, cardiovascular, respiratory, or gastrointestinal tract abnormalities increases with placenta previa (Green, 1994).

Neonatal Anemia

Anemia is in proportion to maternal blood loss.

Velamentous Inserted Umbilical Cord

Because the velamentous umbilical vessels are partially not covered with Wharton jelly as they course through the placenta, they are more vulnerable to compression that can lead to intrauterine hypoxia. Refer to the section in this chapter on vasa previa.

Vasa Previa

In the presence of a vasa previa, fetal mortality is 50% to 60% with intact membranes, but when membranes rupture, mortality may be as high as 75% to 100% with this condition (Carlan, Knuppel, 1990). Refer to the section in this chapter on vasa previa.

Diagnostic Testing

Determining Placental Location

When any pregnant woman complains of vaginal bleeding after 20 weeks of gestation, placenta previa should be considered. To diagnose a placenta previa, the location of the placenta must be determined. If the patient is not bleeding profusely, ultrasound is the preferred method, with a 95% accuracy rating. First, a transabdominal scan is done with a full bladder. Then it is repeated with an empty bladder to decrease false-positive results (Cunningham and others, 1997). When the transabdominal scan provides inconclusive data, a transvaginal ultrasonography facilitates diagnosis. Occasionally if the fetus is 36 or more weeks of gestation, a double-setup vaginal examination may be used. A double-setup vaginal examination is done by taking the patient to an operating room prepared for immediate cesarean birth and doing the vaginal examination with blood available for transfusion. However, double-setup vaginal examination is practiced less often because ultrasound is so highly accurate, safe, and easily done.

Ruling Out Other Causes of Bleeding

A speculum examination is usually done to rule out other causes of bright red vaginal bleeding such as cervicitis, cervical polyps, heavy show, or cervical carcinoma.

Determining Gestational Age

An amniocentesis may be included in the diagnostic workup to determine fetal lung maturity. If the lecithin/sphingomyelin (L/S) ratio is $2:1$ or phosphatidyl glycerol (PG) is present, indicating fetal pulmonary lung maturity, delivery is probably the treatment of choice.

Early Diagnosis of Placenta Previa

An asymptomatic placenta previa, which is identified before the latter half of the third trimester, has a 90% chance of changing to a normal placenta (Queenan, 1995). Therefore the patient should be observed with serial ultrasound every 6 to 8 weeks to determine if the placenta previa will persist.

Usual Medical Management and Protocols for Nurse Practitioners

Expectant Management

Treatment of placenta previa depends on the gestational age and the extent of bleeding. If the gestational age is less than 36 weeks, the bleeding is mild (less than 250 ml), and the patient is not in labor, the treatment of choice is expectant management. The sole purpose is to allow the fetus time to mature to improve perinatal mortality from prematurity. When expectant management is chosen, it usually includes the following:

- Hospitalization with complete bed rest for 72 hours in an attempt to use the fetus as a tamponade and then bed rest with limited activity, such as bathroom privileges.

- Pad check every hour to determine amount of vaginal bleeding.
- Continuous fetal monitoring to facilitate early detection of fetal distress during bleeding episodes; otherwise, assessment every 4 hours with a Doppler FHR device or fetoscope.
- Weekly nonstress tests (NSTs) and biophysical profiles are usually done to determine fetal well-being. These tests may be ordered more frequently as determined by the severity of the bleeding.
- IV infusions with a 16- to 18-gauge needle, unless bleeding is minimal; then a heparin lock may be left in place and changed as needed.
- Maternal blood sample available at all times in the blood bank for immediate type and cross match for blood component therapy. Periodic blood component therapy may be given to maintain hemoglobin at 10 g/dl or greater. Refer to Table 17-3 for guidelines for blood component replacement.
- Antepartum steroids such as betamethasone (Celestone) or dexamethasone to enhance fetal pulmonary maturity may be ordered between 25 and 33 weeks of gestation.
- Amniocentesis is usually performed between 34 and 36 weeks of gestation to determine fetal lung maturity.
- Monitor for signs of preterm uterine contractions stimulated by prostaglandin release from placental separation with tocolytic therapy, preferably magnesium sulfate.
- If patient is allowed to return home after stabilization, should be instructed to limit activity and avoid douching, enemas, or coitus. She must be within 15 minutes of the hospital, have a telephone, have ready access to transportation, and have close supervision by family in the home. Discharge is not the most desirable choice of care but may be necessary for social or financial reasons. Fetal activity charts should be kept daily, and an NST or biophysical profile should be done weekly or more often if intrauterine growth restriction (IUGR) is suspected or there is ongoing vaginal bleeding.

Delivery

Expectant management is terminated as soon as the fetus is mature, excessive bleeding occurs, active labor begins, or any other obstetric reason to terminate the pregnancy develops, such as an intraamniotic infection.

If the bleeding is profuse, the gestational age is 36 or more weeks, the L/S ratio is 2:1, or PG is present, immediate delivery is usually the treatment of choice. Cesarean delivery is the accepted method of delivery in almost all placenta previa cases. Only if the fetus is dead, the fetus has anomalies incompatible with life, or the delivery has already advanced with an engaged fetal head would vaginal delivery be attempted.

• • •

Table 17-4 compares placenta previa and abruptio placentae.

PLACENTA ACCRETA

Placenta accreta is an uncommon condition in which the chorionic villi adhere to the myometrium. Its more advanced forms are placenta increta and placenta percreta. Placenta increta is invasion of the chorionic villi into the myometrium, and placenta percreta is growth of the chorionic villi through the myometrium. This causes the placenta to adhere abnormally to the uterus. The abnormal placental adherence may involve a single cotyledon (focal), a few cotyledons (partial adherence), or all the cotyledons (total adherence).

Etiology

Placenta accreta can occur if there is an inadequate or absent decidua basalis and fibrinoid layer of Nitabuch. Predisposing factors are those that contribute to an abnormal decidua (endometrium). These factors include prior uterine surgery such as cesarean delivery and women who have a current placenta previa.

Diagnosis

Antepartum

Usually there is no clinical evidence until after delivery. However, in a placenta percreta, hemorrhage may present because of chorionic villi growth through the myometrium, opening up a major blood vessel. In 5% of cases the abnormal growth of the chorionic villi into the myometrium will cause the uterus to rupture. This occurs 60% of the time before labor (Zahn, Yeomans, 1990).

Postpartum

Placenta accreta is usually diagnosed soon after delivery when the placenta fails to normally separate from the uterine wall and spontaneously deliver. In a focal or partial adherence the placenta may separate only partially, opening blood vessels while leaving part of the placenta attached. Profuse hemorrhage results because the uterus cannot contract. In a totally adhering placenta, there is no bleeding until attempts are made to manually remove it.

Text continued on p. 448

TABLE 17-4 Comparison of placenta previa and abruptio placentae

Parameter	Placenta previa	Abruptio placentae
Description	Implantation of placenta in lower segment of uterus near or over internal os	Premature separation of normally implanted placenta after 20 wk of gestation
Classification	Marginal: placenta implanted near but does not cover any part of internal os	Mild: less than one sixth of placenta is separated, there is mild to moderate bleeding, and no uterine tenderness; maternal vital signs and FHR normal
	Partial: placenta implants near and partially covers internal os	Moderate: one sixth to one half of placenta is separated; abdominal pain; increased uterine tone; maternal vital signs may show mild hypovolemia, and FHR may indicate distress
	Total: placenta completely covers internal os	Severe: over one half of placenta is separated; profuse bleeding, persistent and severe abdominal pain, and increased uterine tenderness; signs of shock or coagulopathy frequently present with fetal distress or death resulting
Etiology	Unknown: theoretic considerations include a defective vascularization of decidua resulting from uterine scarring or interference with adequate blood supply to endometrium; increased placental mass; early or late ovulation	Unknown: theoretic considerations include degeneration of spiral arteriole, which causes rupture of involved blood vessels and bleeding; bleeding under placenta separates placenta from decidua

Associated conditions:	Multiparity more than five children	Gestational hypertensive disorder
	Previous placenta previa	Previous abruption
	Prior uterine scar related to previous abortion or cesarean birth	Trauma from motor vehicle collision or maternal battering
	Smoking or drug addiction	Cigarette smoking
	Uterine tumor	Cocaine use
	Multiple pregnancy	PROM
Signs and symptoms	Painless, bright red bleeding; onset of bleeding usually slight to moderate and ceases spontaneously	Painful, dark red bleeding unless only marginal; onset of bleeding is slight to profuse and usually continues
	Presenting part high or displaced	Presenting part engaged
	Uterus soft and nontender	Uterus tender or rigid (moderate to severe abruption)
	During labor, uterus relaxes between contractions	During labor, uterus usually has increased resting tone
	Blood usually clots normally	Clotting defects may be present
Diagnosis	Ultrasound	According to signs and symptoms
	No vaginal examination except under double setup	
Treatment	If initial bleeding episode is slight and gestational age less than 37 weeks, expectant management is usual choice of treatment:	In presence of mild abruptio placentae and gestational age less than 36 wk, expectant management is usual choice of treatment:
	Close observation of fetal well-being and amount of bleeding	Close observation of fetal well-being and amount of bleeding

FHR, Fetal heart rate; *PROM*, premature rupture of membranes.

Continued

TABLE 17-4 Comparison of placenta previa and abruptio placentae—cont'd

Parameter	Placenta previa	Abruptio placentae
	Limited physical activity	Limited physical activity
	No douches, enemas, or sexual intercourse	Serial hematocrits to assess concealed bleeding
	Delivery when fetus is mature or hemorrhage dictates	Delivery when fetus is mature or hemorrhage dictates; in presence of mild abruptio placentae, with gestational age of 36 wk or greater, delivery is usual choice of treatment
	When bleeding is profuse, gestational age greater than 36 wk, or L/S ratio 2:1 or greater, delivery is choice of treatment; if placenta previa is:	In presence of moderate to severe abruptio placentae:
	Marginal, a vaginal delivery may be attempted	Restore blood loss
	Partial or complete, a cesarean delivery is performed	Correct coagulation defect if present
		Facilitate delivery:
		Vaginal delivery is attempted if there is no evidence of fetal or maternal distress with fluid and blood replacement, fetus is in cephalic presentation, labor progresses actively, or fetus is dead
		Cesarean delivery is indicated for severe abruptio if fetus is alive, fetal or maternal distress develops with fluid and blood replacement, labor fails to progress actively, or fetal presentation is not cephalic

Maternal outcome	Less than 1% maternal mortality	Less than 1% maternal mortality
Maternal complications	Hemorrhage and hypovolemic shock Placenta accreta/increta/percreta Premature rupture of membranes D sensitization Puerperal infection Puerperal anemia Puerperal hemorrhage	Hemorrhage and hypovolemic shock DIC D sensitization Couvelaire uterus Puerperal infection Puerperal anemia Puerperal hemorrhage Puerperal DIC Renal failure Pituitary necrosis
Fetal outcome	Perinatal mortality 12%-24%	Perinatal mortality 25%-35%
Fetal/neonatal complications	Prematurity Intrauterine hypoxia Malpresentation Small for gestational age Congenital abnormalities Velamentous inserted umbilical cord Vasa previa Neonatal anemia	Prematurity Intrauterine hypoxia Small for gestational age Central nervous system malformations

L/S, Lecithin/sphingomyelin; *DIC*, disseminated intravascular coagulation.

Resulting tears in the placenta or partial removal then causes profuse hemorrhage.

Maternal and Fetal Effects

The fetus is rarely affected by this condition unless uterine rupture or extensive bleeding occurs during the pregnancy. The mother is at extreme risk of hemorrhage. Shock and even death can occur but are uncommon with aggressive treatment.

Usual Medical Management

Treatment depends on the number of cotyledons involved and the depth of penetration. In a focal accreta, the one cotyledon can usually be gently removed from the myometrium. The increased bleeding that results is treated with massage and oxytocin. With more extensive involvement, treatment begins with immediate blood replacement therapy and nearly always prompt hysterectomy. Conservative treatment may be attempted in some cases if preservation of fertility is desired. Conservative management may include leaving the placenta totally or partially in place followed possibly by antibiotic therapy and methotrexate; placental removal and oversewing the uterine defects; localized resection and uterine repair; or curettage of the uterine cavity (Benedetti, 1994).

VASA PREVIA

Vasa previa is a rare developmental disorder of the umbilical cord that may occur with a velamentous inserted umbilical cord. Velamentous inserted umbilical cord is a condition in which the umbilical blood vessels leave the placenta separated and are not protected with Wharton jelly as they course between the amnion and chorion before uniting to form the umbilical cord (Fig. 17-3). Vasa previa occurs when velamentous vessels cross the region of

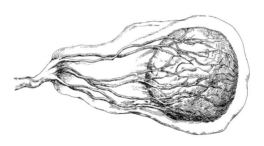

FIG. 17-3 Velamentous inserted umbilical cord.

the internal os and occupy a position ahead of the presenting part. These vessels are very easily compressed or ruptured, which causes immediate fetal distress or death.

Etiology

One presumable cause of vasa previa is postulated to be the result of the blastocyst failing to implant with the area of the embryonic disk first into the endometrium. This causes the umbilical cord and the placenta to lie opposite each other. Another possible cause may be the result of one side of the placenta growing toward the vascularized uterine fundus and the other side remaining dormant (Lockwood, 1990).

Maternal Effects

Vasa previa presents no danger to the mother since her circulatory system is not involved.

Fetal Effects

Death

If one of the umbilical vessels ruptures, death is virtually certain. When the fetal membranes rupture, 75% to 100% of the time velamentous umbilical vessels will rupture as well (Carlan, Knuppel, 1990).

Fetal Deformities

Umbilical vessels without Wharton jelly are very easily compressed. Compression would affect the blood flow to the fetus. Resultant chronic fetal hypoxia leads to fetal growth defects in 25% of the cases (Cunningham and others, 1997).

Signs and Symptoms

Occasionally the umbilical vessels may be felt during a vaginal examination in the membranes, and the vessels have been visualized directly with ultrasound. However, most often the first sign of vasa previa is vaginal bleeding at the time the membranes rupture.

Diagnosis

Vasa previa should be suspected if the FHR drops during a vaginal examination and then returns to baseline. In the presence of vaginal bleeding when vasa previa is suspected, a Kleihauer-Betke or APT (alum-precipitated toxoid) test should be run to determine if the blood is of fetal origin.

Treatment

Once a vasa previa is confirmed in the presence of a live fetus, emergency cesarean delivery should be carried out. If the fetus is dead, the mother should be delivered vaginally.

NURSING PROCESS

PREVENTION

Because inadequate blood supply to the decidua (endometrium) before implantation may be the underlying cause of a placenta previa and inadequate blood supply to the decidua during pregnancy may be the underlying cause of an abruptio placentae, any condition that would decrease the uterine blood supply should be avoided if possible. Because cigarette smoking decreases uterine blood supply, it should be avoided by the childbearing mother. Adequate contraceptive instructions should be given so that couples can plan the time and number of their children, preventing therapeutic abortions and closely spaced pregnancies. Hypertensive disorders of pregnancy should be monitored closely for an abruptio placentae since hypertensive disorders increase the risk of an abruptio placentae. Use of the street drug cocaine is known to cause transient acute hypertensive episodes, which can initiate abruption of the placenta, so cocaine should be avoided altogether during pregnancy (Peters, Theorell, 1991).

ASSESSMENT

INITIAL ASSESSMENT

When any patient experiences bleeding during the last half of pregnancy, the first nursing responsibility is to gather a data base to assess the cause of the bleeding and the severity of the condition. There is one exception to the rule. If the bleeding is life threatening, immediate care must be implemented without a complete data base. If possible, the following data should be obtained:

1. The patient's perception of what is happening
2. When the bleeding started and its frequency
3. The amount, color, and consistency of the blood present (The bleeding is usually bright red with placenta previa and dark with an abruption.)
4. The patient's activity just before and at the time the bleeding started
5. What self-treatment, if any, was used by the patient (If tampons are being used to collect the bleeding, there is concealed bleeding.)

6. Whether any pain or uterine contractions accompanied this bleeding and whether the uterus feels firm or tender to touch

7. Whether the uterus is contracting, to determine if the patient is in labor

8. Whether any previous bleeding episodes occurred during this pregnancy

9. The estimated delivery date (EDD), to determine appropriate management

10. Vital signs and FHR

11. Fundal height, to recognize continued concealed bleeding

12. A clot observation test for DIC if the bleeding is moderate to severe

13. Fetal presentation and state of engagement if near term by abdominal palpation (Transverse or oblique lie is common with a placenta previa because the placenta usually interferes with engagement.)

ONGOING ASSESSMENT

When the diagnosis of mild abruptio placentae or placenta previa is confirmed and expectant management is ordered, a continuous assessment plan for hemorrhage, fetal distress, level of maternal anxiety, and signs of labor must be implemented.

- **Hemorrhage:** Further bleeding can be assessed by visually inspecting the amount of external bleeding present on the pads, bed protectors, or linen. Measurable terms are used in describing the amount of blood lost such as how many cubic centimeters of the pad is stained with blood in a certain period of time. A standard of how many milliliters of blood makes a 1-cm^3 stain should be set by each health care facility. This is because all perineal pads do not have the same absorbency (Luegenbiehl and others, 1990). When the nurse changes the pad, it can be weighed to obtain a more accurate assessment by applying the conversion that 1 ml of blood weighs 1 g. Marking the fundal height on the abdomen and then observing for a change and observing serial hematocrits can facilitate early detection of concealed blood loss. Taking frequent vital signs, observing for other signs and symptoms of shock, and keeping an accurate intake and output record are also important monitors of bleeding.
- **Fetal distress:** Fetal well-being should be monitored closely by evaluating FHR with a fetal monitor or a Doppler FHR device, carrying out NSTs, and assisting with a biophysical profile as ordered.

- **Signs of labor:** The uterus should be palpated with each set of vital signs to assess for uterine contractions, tenderness, and rigidity. The patient should be instructed to notify the nurse if she experiences any uterine contraction, abdominal pain, tenderness, or hardness. Uterine irritability increases the likelihood of bleeding as well as indicates labor.
- **Level of maternal anxiety:** Parents are usually very concerned about the health and well-being of the baby and the mother's safety. They may also be experiencing some unusual fears or worries such as wondering what they might have done to cause this to happen. Therefore the expectant parents should be encouraged to express their feelings and concerns. In this way the nurse will know better how to individualize emotional support.

NURSING DIAGNOSES/COLLABORATIVE PROBLEMS AND INTERVENTIONS

- **POTENTIAL COMPLICATION: HEMORRHAGE** caused by premature separation of the placenta.

  DESIRED OUTCOMES: The signs and symptoms of hemorrhage will be minimized or managed as measured by stable vital signs, urinary output 30 ml/hr or greater, absence of signs of shock, hematocrit maintained between 30% and 45%, and a blood loss less than 250 ml.

  INTERVENTIONS

  Mild bleeding

  1. Assess blood loss by obtaining a history of onset, duration, amount, color, and consistency of bleeding; obtaining a history regarding associated symptoms, prior bleeding episodes, and activity at onset of bleeding; recording visual blood loss in cubic centimeters or weighing saturated pads, linen protectors, or linen (1 g = 1 ml); recording blood pressure, pulse, and respirations as indicated, depending on severity; determining pulse pressure, orthostatic blood pressure changes, and hypothenar refilling by blanching the fleshy elevation of the ulnar side of the palm of the hand (normal refill is 1 to 2 seconds); checking for abdominal pain, uterine tenderness, or rigidity; keeping an accurate intake and output record, and assessing urine specific gravity intermittently; monitoring such laboratory data as serial hematocrits; and observing fundal height changes.
  2. Do not perform vaginal or rectal examinations and do not give enemas or douches in the presence of vaginal bleeding.

In the presence of a placenta previa they can initiate further separation, and profuse bleeding would result. In the presence of an abruptio placentae, when delivery is not to be initiated immediately, no vaginal or rectal examinations should be carried out to avoid disturbing the injured placenta any further.

3. Implement bed rest with bathroom privileges.
4. Prevent constipation and excessive stool straining by educating as to the importance of a high-fiber diet. Administer a stool softener as ordered.
5. Decrease risk of anemia by educating as to the importance of foods high in iron. Administer ferrous gluconate as ordered between meals to facilitate the absorption of supplemental iron.
6. Establish an IV access with a 16- or 18-gauge IV catheter to allow for fluid and blood component therapy if necessary. Once bleeding has stopped and the hematocrit is within normal limits, a heparin lock may be placed.
7. Have a maternal blood sample in the blood bank at all times for immediate type and cross match for blood component therapy, and be prepared to transfuse to maintain hemodynamic stability. Be prepared to obtain such diagnostic data as a complete blood count, electrolytes, creatinine, and coagulation factors such as fibrinogen, platelet count, fibrin degradation products, prothrombin time (PT), and partial thromboplastin time (PTT).
8. Notify the physician of any change in the diagnostic data or patient's bleeding pattern.

Moderate to severe bleeding
1. Bed rest in a quiet environment will optimize the outcome. Activity and sensory stimulation can increase the bleeding and elevate the basal metabolic rate, which increases oxygen consumption. To facilitate tamponade with the fetal head, the head of the bed should be elevated 20 to 30 degrees. Encourage the mother to lie on either side to prevent pressure on the vena cava and further compromise of the fetal circulation.
2. If for any reason the patient must be positioned on her back, the uterus should be tilted to the left by placing a folded sheet under the patient's right hip to keep the gravid uterus off the vena cava.
3. Start an IV line immediately with a 16- or 18-gauge intracatheter to allow for blood administration, and blood

should be drawn for type and cross matching of 2 to 5 units of packed red blood cells. A lactated Ringer's solution can be administered until blood component therapy is available; it is a better volume expander than dextrose in water. Volume expanders can also be ordered while waiting for properly matched blood components. Prepare for blood component therapy as ordered by having 250 ml of normal saline available. Administer blood component therapy or volume expanders as ordered. Refer to Table 17-4 for guidelines for blood component replacement.

4. Fluid therapy is aimed at maintaining an adequate circulating blood volume and a hematocrit of 30% or greater.

5. If the patient is hemodynamically unstable despite apparently adequate fluid replacement or has an underlying renal, cardiac, or pulmonary disease, a triple-lumen Swan-Ganz catheter may be placed for a more accurate assessment of central venous pressure, pulmonary capillary wedge pressure, and cardiac output.

6. After stabilization of the patient with adequate blood component replacement, be prepared to facilitate delivery. Be prepared to assist with an amniotomy and administer a labor stimulant as ordered. Prepare patient for possible cesarean delivery.

7. Give patient nothing by mouth unless otherwise ordered.

8. Continue to assess for signs of bleeding as severity of condition indicates.

9. Report to the physician any change in the patient's bleeding pattern or failure to respond to treatment.

■ **POTENTIAL COMPLICATION: HYPOVOLEMIC SHOCK** causing inadequate organ blood flow and tissue oxygenation secondary to the hemorrhage.

DESIRED OUTCOMES: Hypovolemic shock will be minimized or managed as measured by stable vital signs, urinary output of 30 ml/hr or greater, normal peripheral pulses, normal motor function, and orientation to person, place, and time.

INTERVENTIONS

1. Monitor blood pressure, pulse, and respirations at frequent intervals.

2. Assess peripheral pulses.

3. Observe for indicators of decreased cerebral perfusion, such as restlessness or confusion.

4. Observe for signs of shock. During pregnancy, because of the increased blood volume, the classic early signs of shock, such as hypotension, tachycardia, and hyperpnea, are less pronounced. Therefore shock is more difficult to detect. In patients with an abruption, the signs of shock can ensue without notice, even more often than with a placenta previa. This is because the signs of bleeding may be masked if the bleeding is concealed behind the placenta.

5. Monitor urinary output hourly or as indicated by severity. Because of increased peripheral resistance, cerebral and cardiac perfusion may be preserved, but renal blood flow is often jeopardized since it is very sensitive to lack of perfusion. Therefore urinary output during pregnancy is the best noninvasive indicator of circulatory volume. Less than 30 ml/hr indicates decreased circulatory volume to the uterus.

6. If signs of shock develop, place patient in modified Trendelenburg position (only elevate legs) to increase blood return without contributing to respiratory impairment and administer oxygen at 8 to 10 L/min by mask.

7. Report first signs of shock or vital sign changes to physician.

Postpartum

1. If hypovolemic shock occurred, assess for the possible development of pituitary necrosis (Sheehan syndrome) by assessing for the onset of lactation.

2. Administer no lactation suppressant if patient experienced shock during pregnancy, labor, or delivery.

3. If patient is bottle feeding, explain the reason for the delay in initiating a lactation suppressant therapy.

4. Instruct patient to notify physician if onset of lactation does not occur by the fifth postpartum day.

- **POTENTIAL COMPLICATION: DISSEMINATED INTRAVASCULAR COAGULOPATHY (DIC)**
  DESIRED OUTCOMES: The signs and symptoms of DIC will be minimized or managed as measured by blood pressure and pulse within normal limits; presence of peripheral pulses; urinary output greater than 30 ml/hr or 120 ml/4 hr; normal motor function; orientation to time and place; and clotting factors within normal limits for pregnancy as manifested by clotting time between 8 and 12 minutes, fibrinogen levels of 450 mg/dl, platelets between 150,000 and 350,000/mm^3, and partial prothrombin time between 18 and 39 seconds.

INTERVENTIONS

1. Observe for signs of DIC such as oozing of blood from the IV site, easy bruising, or petechiae.
2. Monitor the patient's coagulation profile, which includes fibrinogen, platelet count, prothrombin time, partial thromboplastin time, and clotting time.
3. A simple clot observation test may be done every 30 to 60 minutes at the bedside by the nurse to assess for DIC. To carry this out, the nurse places 5 ml of venous blood in a test tube, hangs it in the room, and observes the time it takes to clot. If it does not form a clot within 8 to 12 minutes, a coagulation defect is usually present (see Chapter 18).
4. If DIC develops, refer to DIC nursing plan of care.
5. Report first signs of DIC to physician.

- **RISK FOR FLUID VOLUME EXCESS**   related to excessive replacement therapy.

  DESIRED OUTCOMES: The patient will maintain a urinary output greater than 30 ml/hr with clear breath sounds. If a Swan-Ganz catheter is in place, pulmonary capillary wedge pressure (PCWP) will be maintained between 10 and 15 mm Hg and central venous pressure (CVP) between 12 and 15 cm H_2O.

  INTERVENTIONS

  1. Assess for signs of pulmonary congestion, such as dyspnea, cough, or rales, by auscultating lung fields every shift.
  2. Keep an accurate input and output record.
  3. Monitor PCWP or CVP if a Swan-Ganz catheter or CVP line is in place. This is the most accurate way to determine the patient's fluid needs and prevent fluid overload.
  4. Notify the physician immediately of any signs of fluid overload or changes in the PCWP or CVP.

- **FEAR**   related to effect on health status and threat of fetal or neonatal death.

  DESIRED OUTCOME: The patient and her family will be able to communicate their fears and concerns openly.

  INTERVENTIONS

  1. Assess family's anxiety over maternal and fetal/neonatal well-being.
  2. Assess family members' level of guilt such as wondering what they might have done to cause this to happen.
  3. Assess the family's coping strategies and resources.

4. Encourage expectant parents to express their feelings, concerns, and labor experience.

5. Clarify any misconceptions. Explain that the cause of the condition is unknown but it is not related to patient's activity at time of occurrence.

6. Provide information to the patient and her family regarding the pregnancy complication, plan of treatment, and implications for mother and fetus in understandable terms. Discuss with the expectant parents the possibility of a cesarean delivery. The parents will then be more prepared if the event arises.

7. Explain all treatment modalities and reasons for each.

8. Keep parents informed of health status, results of tests, and fetal well-being. Focus the expectant parents on the positive signs of fetal well-being such as a normal FHR, fetal activity, and reactive NSTs.

9. Compliment the patient for her cooperation in adhering to medical therapy.

10. Refer to the social worker if inadequate coping is noted.

11. Refer to pastor, priest, or chaplain per parents' request.

- **RISK FOR ALTERED ROLE PERFORMANCE** related to prolonged hospitalization and treatment with bed rest.
  DESIRED OUTCOME: The patient will verbalize a plan that will take care of all her work- and family-related responsibilities during her absence.
  INTERVENTIONS
    1. Assess the patient's responsibilities to determine difficulties she will have in implementing prescribed bed rest.
    2. Teach the patient and her significant other about the importance of bed rest in the lateral position.
    3. Facilitate the family in problem solving if difficulties arise in implementing bed rest.
    4. Make needed referrals, such as to the social worker, if problems are identified.
    5. Encourage participation in her care and decision making as much as possible.

- **DIVERSIONAL ACTIVITY DEFICIT** related to the therapeutic treatment of bed rest.
  DESIRED OUTCOME: The patient will verbalize various appropriate activities she would like to do while maintaining bed rest.

INTERVENTIONS
1. Assess patient's interest in various diversional activities within the activity limit.
2. Provide crafts, reading, and puzzles that can be done in bed, or encourage patient to have these things brought in.
3. Provide classes in preparation for childbirth by way of video, the hospital television, or group classes that can be attended while reclining.
4. Refer to a diversional therapist or volunteer to provide reading materials, handicrafts, or other interesting things.

- **RISK FOR INFECTION** related to opened blood vessels near cervical os and premature separation of the placenta.
  DESIRED OUTCOME: The patient's temperature will remain normal, vaginal discharge will be without odor, and white blood cell count will remain less than 16,000/mm^3.
  INTERVENTIONS
  1. Check temperature four times daily until 48 hours after delivery; if greater than 39° C (100.4° F), check every 2 hours.
  2. Check vaginal discharge (lochia) for odor every shift.
  3. Use aseptic technique in care of patient.
  4. Explain perineal care and the importance of adequate hand washing.
  5. Notify the physician if the temperature is elevated over 39° C (100.4° F) or if any other signs of infection develop.

- **RISK FOR IMPAIRED FETAL GAS EXCHANGE** related to maternal bleeding or partially detached placenta, which cannot keep up with the growing needs as the fetus matures because of the decreased surface area available for perfusion.
  DESIRED OUTCOMES: The fetus will remain active, and its heart rate will be maintained at a baseline between 110 and 160 with normal variability, normal reactivity, and no decelerations. The biophysical profile will continue to be greater than 6.
  INTERVENTIONS
  1. Determine gestational age.
  2. Monitor FHR as indicated (depending on severity).
  3. Evaluate FHR for tachycardia, bradycardia, late or variable decelerations, and loss of long- or short-term variability.
  4. During labor, check uterine contractions for duration, frequency, and uterine resting tone. Observe amniotic fluid for meconium staining.

5. Keep patient positioned on left or right side; if must be on back, tilt uterus to the left by placing folded sheet under the right hip.

6. Administer oxygen as indicated with mask at 8 to 10 L/min.

7. Prepare the patient for fetal well-being and maturity studies as ordered. Biophysical profiles, ultrasound, NSTs, and amniocentesis are usually ordered on a frequent basis in an attempt to determine the optimal time for delivery.

8. Be prepared to intermittently assess blood to determine if it is of fetal origin by a Kleihauer-Betke analysis or APT (alum-precipitated toxoid) test because of the increased risk of a vasa previa associated with a placenta previa.

9. If vaginal bleeding occurs immediately following rupture of membranes, suspect vasa previa.

10. Notify physician if a baseline or periodic FHR change is noted or if there is a nonreactive NST or a biophysical profile of 6 or less.

11. During a trial of labor, notify the physician of a hypertonic uterus, increased signs of bleeding, a labor that progresses abnormally slowly, or any signs of fetal distress.

12. Once delivery is imminent, notify the intensive care nursery of a possible high risk infant.

■ **ALTERED NUTRITION: LESS THAN BODY REQUIREMENTS** related to decreased intake to overcome losses related to hemorrhage. *DESIRED OUTCOME:* The patient has adequate nutritional intake to replace hemorrhage loss as manifested by an adequate weight gain of ¾ to 1 pound per week during the last half of her pregnancy and hemoglobin maintained between 11 and 16 g/dl.
INTERVENTIONS

1. Obtain a nutritional assessment, and analyze for iron deficiency.

2. Monitor patient's hemoglobin levels.

3. Teach patient to eat foods high in iron (e.g., whole grains, green leafy vegetables, and legumes), vitamin C (e.g., citrus, strawberries, potatoes, and broccoli), and protein.

4. If an iron supplement is ordered, educate patient to take the iron tablets with meals to decrease adverse gastrointestinal symptoms and with vitamin C to enhance its absorption. Instruct patient that her stools may turn black and may be more formed.

5. Notify physician if hemoglobin drops below 11 g/dl.

- **POTENTIAL COMPLICATION: D SENSITIZATION** in a D-negative mother carrying an Rh-positive fetus.

  DESIRED OUTCOME: The mother's body will not develop antibodies against the D-negative factor.

  INTERVENTIONS
  1. Be prepared to monitor the D antibody titer with an indirect Coombs test at gestational weeks 24, 28, 32, 36, and 40 and after any bleeding episode if a fetal-maternal bleed is suspected.
  2. Be prepared to administer Rho (D) immune globulin (RhoGAM) (HypRho-D) intramuscularly in the deltoid as ordered at 28 weeks, following any suspected fetal-maternal bleed, and within 72 hours postpartum.
  3. If a transplacental bleed is suspected, be prepared to order a Kleihauer-Betke stain or APT test to assess the amount of fetal blood in the maternal circulation. A dose of Rho (D) immune globulin greater than the normal 300 μg is needed if the D-positive fetal bleed is greater than 15 ml.

CONCLUSION

The ultimate goal in the treatment of both an abruptio placentae and a placenta previa is early recognition and appropriate intervention to prevent hemorrhage and its resulting complications of shock, DIC, multisystem failure, and ultimately death to mother or fetus. At the same time, premature delivery should be avoided as long as intrauterine hypoxia is not present.

BIBLIOGRAPHY

American College of Obstetricians and Gynecologists (ACOG): *Antenatal corticosteroid therapy for fetal maturation,* Washington, DC, 1994, The Author.

Ananth C, Savitz D, Williams M: Placental abruption and its association with hypertension and prolonged rupture of membranes: a methodologic review and meta-analysis, *Obstet Gynecol* 88:309, 1996.

Benedetti T: Obstetric hemorrhage. In Gabbe S, Niebyl J, Simpson J: *Obstetrics: normal and problem pregnancies,* ed 3, New York, 1996, Churchill Livingstone.

Berg C and others: Pregnancy-related mortality in the United States, 1987-1990, *Obstet Gynecol* 88:161, 1996.

Carlan S, Knuppel R: Vasa praevia: approaches to detection, *Female Patient* 15(8):35-41, 1990.

Chattophadhyay S, Kharif H, Sherbeeni J: Placenta previa and accreta after previous cesarean section, *Eur J Obstet Gynecol Reprod Biol* 52:151, 1993.

Cunningham G, MacDonald P, Gant N: *Williams' obstetrics,* ed 20, Stamford, Conn, 1997, Appleton & Lange.

Droste S, Keil K: Expectant management of placenta previa: cost benefit analysis of outpatient treatment, *Am J Obstet Gynecol* 170:1252, 1994.

Floyd R and others: Smoking during pregnancy: prevalence, effects, and intervention strategies, *Birth* 18(1):48-53, 1991.

Fretts R and others: The changing pattern of fetal death, 1961-1988, *Obstet Gynecol* 79:25, 1992.

Green J: Placenta previa and abruptio placentae. In Creasy R, Resnik R, editors: *Maternal-fetal medicine: principles and practice,* ed 3, Philadelphia, 1994, Saunders.

Handler A and others: The relationship between exposure during pregnancy to cigarette smoking and cocaine use and placenta previa, *Am J Obstet Gynecol* 170:884, 1994.

Hurd W and others: Selective management of abruptio placentae: a prospective study, *Obstet Gynecol* 61:467-473, 1983.

Iyasu S and others: The epidemiology of placenta previa in the United States, 1979 through 1987, *Am J Obstet Gynecol* 168:1424, 1993.

Janke J: Prenatal cocaine use: effects on perinatal outcome, *J Nurse Midwifery* 35(2):74-77, 1990.

Lavery P: Placenta previa, *Clin Obstet Gynecol* 33(3):414-421, 1990.

Lockwood C: Placenta previa and related disorders, *Contemp OB/GYN* 35(1):47-68, 1990.

Lockwood C: Third-trimester bleeding. In Queenan J, Hobbins J, editors: *Protocols for high-risk pregnancies,* ed 3, Cambridge, England, 1996, Blackwell Science.

Luegenbiehl D and others: Standardized assessment of blood loss, *MCN Am J Matern Child Nurs* 15(4):241-244, 1990.

Magriples U and others: Thrombomodulin: a novel maker for abruptio placenta, *Am J Obstet Gynecol* 174:364, 1996.

Major C and others: Preterm premature rupture of membranes and abruptio placentae: is there an association between these pregnancy complications? *Am J Obstet Gynecol* 172:672, 1995.

Morgan M and others: Abruptio placentae: perinatal outcome in normotensive and hypertensive patients, *Am J Obstet Gynecol* 170:1595, 1994.

Mouer J: Placenta previa: antepartum conservative management inpatient vs. outpatient, *Am J Obstet Gynecol* 170:1685, 1994.

Nolan T, Gallup D: Shock in ectopic pregnancy, *Female Patient* 14(10):66-72, 1989.

Peters H, Theorell C: Fetal and neonatal effects of maternal cocaine use, *J Obstet Gynecol Neonatal Nurs* 20(2):121-126, 1991.

Queenan R: Third-trimester bleeding. In Niswander K, Evans A, editors: *Manual of obstetrics,* ed 5, Boston, 1995, Little, Brown.

Spinillo A and others: Severity of abruptio placenta and neurologic developmental outcome in low birth weight infants, *Early Hum Dev* 35:44, 1993.

Taylor V and others: Placenta previa and prior cesarean delivery: how strong is the association? *Obstet Gynecol* 84:55-57, 1994.

Voigt L and others: The relationship of abruptio placentae with maternal smoking and small for gestational age infants, *Obstet Gyencol* 75:771, 1990.

Wolf E and others: Placenta previa is not an independent risk factor for small-for-gestational-age infant, *Obstet Gynecol* 77:707, 1991.

Zahn C, Yeomans E: Postpartum hemorrhage: placenta accreta, uterine inversion and puerperal hematomas, *Clin Obstet Gynecol* 33(3):422-431, 1990.

CHAPTER

18

Disseminated Intravascular Coagulopathy

Disseminated intravascular coagulopathy (DIC) is not a primary disease but rather a secondary event activated by a number of severe illnesses. It is also called *consumptive coagulopathy* or *intravascular coagulation and fibrinolysis*. It occurs when a severe illness causes a generalized activation of the coagulation process. If coagulation factors are consumed faster than the liver can replace them, depletion occurs. At that point the process of fibrinolysis is activated in response to coagulation. The result is rampant coagulation and massive fibrinolysis at the same time.

INCIDENCE

The incidence of DIC is unknown.

ETIOLOGY

The following stimuli are known to activate the coagulation process (Anderson, 1994):
- Infusion of tissue extract from injured tissue
- Severe injury to endothelial cells
- Red cell or platelet injury seen in hemolytic processes

- Bacterial debris or endotoxins
- Immune reactions
- Thrombocytopenia
- Chemical and physical agents

NORMAL PHYSIOLOGY

The processes of clot formation and clot breakdown (fibrinolysis) must be understood to understand DIC. Clot formation and fibrinolysis are intertwined with the activation of factors maintaining a homeostasis under normal circumstances.

Whenever blood vessels or tissues become damaged and bleeding occurs, several factors attempt hemostasis. First, central nervous system (CNS) reflexes cause vascular spasms, reducing blood flow to the area. Second, platelets attempt to plug the break. Finally, clot formation occurs. Clot formation can be activated by intrinsic and extrinsic factors. The intrinsic factors exist within the vascular system and are activated with blood vessel damage. The extrinsic factors are within the tissue and are activated in response to tissue trauma. When either process is activated, prothrombin activator is formed. Prothrombin activator, along with calcium and phospholipids, acts as a catalyst to convert inactive plasma prothrombin into thrombin. The enzyme *thrombin* converts inactive plasma fibrinogen into fibrin. Fibrin, along with platelets, causes the red blood cells and plasma to mesh, and a clot is then formed (Fig. 18-1).

Fibrinolysis normally occurs simultaneously with clot formation as long as activators are present. Plasminogen, a plasma euglobulin, is activated into plasmin. Plasmin then breaks fibrin down into fibrin split products and fibrinogen into fibrinogen split products. This process consumes factors V, VIII, and XII (intrinsic factors) and prothrombin. Anticoagulants, antithrombin III, and heparin also facilitate fibrinolysis. Antithrombin III neutralizes thrombin, plasmin, and factors VII, IX, XI, and XII, which are intrinsic and extrinsic factors. Heparin greatly enhances the action of antithrombin III (Fig. 18-2) (Creasy, Resnik, 1994).

In pregnancy, fibrinogen, platelet adhesiveness, and factor VIII are increased. Antithrombin III and the activators for plasminogen are decreased. Plasminogen itself is increased. Therefore the equilibrium of coagulation and fibrinolysis is skewed toward procoagulation. Factors in pregnancy that can promote this include fetoplacental hormones, pregnancy-specific hormones, immunologic complexes, and entry of placental thrombin into maternal circulation through the vascular interfaces.

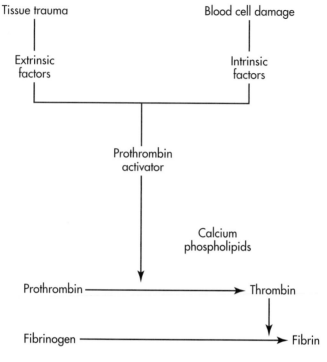

FIG. 18-1 Clot formation.

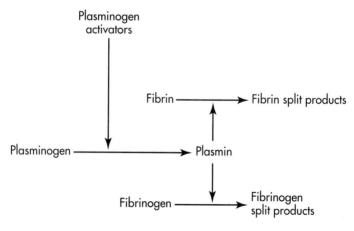

FIG. 18-2 Fibrinolysis.

PATHOPHYSIOLOGY

DIC occurs when factor consumption of the coagulation-fibrinolysis processes exceeds the liver's capacity to produce factors. When factors are depleted, equilibrium is disrupted and bleeding occurs because of deficient coagulation factors. The body continues to attempt clot formation in the presence of bleeding, which further depletes coagulation factors.

This disruption of the equilibrium of clot formation and breakdown can be triggered by severe illnesses, such as the following:

- Abruption of the placenta
- Intrauterine fetal death, especially if longer than 5 weeks in duration
- Preeclampsia/eclampsia
- Postpartum hemorrhagic sepsis
- Rapid, traumatic labor and delivery
- Amniotic fluid embolism

When the placenta separates from the wall of the uterus, a retroplacental clot forms. Part of the products of clot formation, and placental thrombin, can be pushed into the maternal circulation, and massive consumption of clotting factors results.

Amniotic fluid embolism causes an extravasation of amniotic fluid with vernix, squamous cells, and mucus into the maternal circulation. Maternal immunologic defenses attempt to wall off the huge quantities of these foreign substances. This attempt initiates a cascade of activation of both the coagulation and the fibrinolysis processes.

When the products of conception are retained after intrauterine fetal demise, thromboplastic material can seep into the maternal circulation. This infusion of tissue extract activates the overwhelming depletion of coagulation factors.

In preeclampsia and eclampsia, damage to vessel walls occurs secondary to vasospasm and hypoxia. The vessel wall damage causes products of cellular breakdown to come in contact with the surface of the platelets, and the coagulation-fibrinolysis process occurs simultaneously. Massive amounts of coagulation-fibrinolysis factors are then consumed by the process, and the liver is unable to replace factors as rapidly as is necessary (Leduc and others, 1992; Roberts, 1994).

Hemorrhage and shock can also precipitate disequilibrium of coagulation-fibrinolysis. Hypovolemia causes decreased cardiac output, decreased arterial pressure, and decreased systemic blood flow. This leads to decreased nutrition to the brain and vascular system. The hypoxic vascular endothelium triggers intravascular coagulation. Intravascular coagulation releases toxins that increase capillary permeability, further diminishing circulating volume. Brain anoxia results in cardiac depression and further compromises cardiac output (Young, 1990).

SIGNS AND SYMPTOMS

Early symptoms of DIC include ecchymoses and bleeding into the urine or at the site of an intravenous (IV) line. As DIC develops, these early signs may rapidly progress to the following severe signs of shock:

- Respirations progress from rapid and deep to rapid, shallow, and irregular and finally to barely perceptible.
- Pulse rate becomes rapid, weaker, irregular, and thready.
- Blood pressure may initially be normal but then begins falling until the systolic pressure is below 60 mm Hg or is not palpable.
- Skin color may then begin to pale and cool, progressing rapidly to being cold, clammy, and cyanotic.
- Urinary output initially remains stable and then quickly begins to decrease to less than 30 ml/hr.
- Level of consciousness changes from apprehension to increasing restlessness, lethargy, and finally coma.
- Central venous pressure and pulmonary artery wedge pressure drop.

Laboratory signs of DIC include hypofibrinogenemia, decreased platelet count, abnormal prothrombin and partial thromboplastin times, and an increase in fibrin and fibrinogen split products. Normal coagulation factor values are given below:

- Fibrinogen: 400 mg/dl
- Platelets: 150,000 to 400,000/mm^3
- Prothrombin time: 10 to 14 seconds
- Partial thromboplastin time: 18 to 38 seconds
- Fibrin split products: less than 10 mg/ml

MATERNAL EFFECTS

DIC can result in maternal death.

FETAL AND NEONATAL EFFECTS

DIC can result in fetal death or severe hypoxia. Possible neonatal sequelae to severe hypoxia are intracranial bleeding and brain death.

DIAGNOSTIC TESTING

The medical diagnosis is made from a history of predisposing conditions and the early signs of ecchymosis formation and bleeding from the IV site or urinary tract. Definitive diagnosis is made by the laboratory data previously listed.

USUAL MEDICAL MANAGEMENT AND PROTOCOLS FOR NURSE PRACTITIONERS

When DIC occurs in the antepartum period, the initial treatment is to empty the uterus by the most expeditious means. Blood replacement with packed cells, fresh frozen plasma, cryoprecipitate, and platelets is necessary to replace volume and depleted coagulation factors. Simultaneously, the primary disease must be stabilized and corrected.

Supportive measures for monitoring fluid replacement and cardiac output are necessary. These include cardiac monitoring, hemodynamic monitoring, and blood pressure recordings every 5 to 15 minutes. Because clinical signs of DIC may be rapid in onset, the emergency initially threatens the mother's life and fetal considerations are excluded. Once factor replacement is instituted for the mother, the fetus is often delivered before continuous monitoring of the fetal heart rate (FHR) can be initiated. Fetal delivery may be accomplished simultaneously with resuscitation of the pregnant woman. Two teams, one for trauma response and one for perinatal response, are usually required for this approach.

NURSING PROCESS

PREVENTION

When the mother has a condition that might predispose her to development of DIC, the nurse must be alert for early signs of ecchymosis and bleeding. A simple test to confirm possible early signs of DIC is the clot retraction test; 5 ml of blood is drawn into a test tube, capped, and taped to the bedside wall. If a clot has not formed and separated the serum from the cells within 8 to 10 minutes, DIC is possible and the physician should be notified.

ASSESSMENT

Early signs of disequilibrium of the coagulation-fibrinolysis process should be assessed in any diseases or conditions known to predispose the pregnant woman to DIC. Early signs include unusual ecchymosis formation; bleeding from the gums, IV insertion site, or other venous puncture sites; and blood in the urine.

If early signs are not recognized, late signs will be manifested, which include progressive changes in respiration, pulse, blood pressure, skin color, and urinary output; indications of mild to moderate shock; and acute renal failure (see Chapter 9).

In the recovery phase (2 to 7 days), the woman should also be observed for complications such as infection and transfusion hepatitis. These problems are usually readily remediable with medical management.

NURSING DIAGNOSES/COLLABORATIVE PROBLEMS AND INTERVENTIONS

- **POTENTIAL COMPLICATION: HYPOVOLEMIC SHOCK** related to rapid bleeding from abruptio placentae or placenta previa, accreta, increta, or percreta or related to a surgical procedure with DIC present.

  DESIRED OUTCOMES: Blood pressure will be within a normal range of 90/50 to 120/80; pulse rate will be 60 to 100 beats/min (bpm); respirations will be 12 to 24/min; urinary output will be greater than 30 ml/hr; and central venous pressure, pulmonary artery pressure, and pulmonary arterial wedge pressure will remain within normal limits.

  INTERVENTIONS *(Turner, 1991)*

    1. Observe patients who have complications precipitating DIC for early signs of shock.
    2. Perform bedside clot retraction test by placing 5 ml of blood in test tube and observing time for clot to form.
    3. Have IV line started with at least a 16-gauge angiocatheter and physiologic salt solution infusing.
    4. Prepare to transfuse rapidly with cryoprecipitate, packed cells, and fresh frozen plasma.
    5. Notify laboratory trauma support personnel for possible need for un-cross-matched blood and blood products.
    6. Notify intensive care or trauma team for assistance with fluid replacement and monitoring.
    7. Prepare to insert invasive hemodynamic lines.
    8. Report vital signs and hemodynamic monitoring data to the physician in charge of fluid replacement.

- **POTENTIAL COMPLICATION: DIC** related to a precipitating medical problem, such as third-trimester bleeding, placental implantation problems, pregnancy-induced hypertension (PIH), or HELLP (hemolysis, elevated liver enzymes, and low platelet count in association with preeclampsia) syndrome, and depletion of clotting factors.

DESIRED OUTCOMES: Normal clotting factors will be evidenced in laboratory data: there will be a normal clot formation time of 8 to 12 minutes; fibrinogen levels will be 400 mg/dl; platelet count will be 150,000 to 400,000/mm^3; and partial thromboplastin time will be 12 to 14 seconds.

INTERVENTIONS *(Roberts, 1994)*

1. Prepare to administer appropriate blood and blood products.
2. Start an IV line with at least a 16-gauge angiocatheter, and infuse physiologic salt solution.
3. Assist with insertion of invasive monitoring lines.
4. Notify trauma or intensive care team for assistance with fluid replacement.
5. Report vital signs, hemodynamic monitoring data, amount of continued bleeding, and laboratory data immediately to the physician in charge of fluid replacement therapy.
6. Administer oxygen, 8 to 10 L/min.

- **POTENTIAL COMPLICATION: ACUTE RENAL FAILURE** related to hypovolemic shock. See Chapter 11.

- **RISK FOR IMPAIRED FETAL GAS EXCHANGE** related to maternal hypovolemia and resultant diminished uteroplacental blood flow.
  DESIRED OUTCOMES: The newborn will have a 5-minute birth Apgar score of greater than 6; the newborn will have a birth cord pH greater than 7.19; and there will be an absence of persistent preterminal FHR patterns such as a sinusoidal pattern or persistent nonreassuring patterns of late decelerations or loss of short-term variability (STV).
  INTERVENTIONS
    1. Institute fetal monitoring as soon as maternal emergency is being managed by intensive care or trauma team. Labor nurse responsibility shifts to the fetus.
    2. Administer appropriate fluids to the mother.
    3. Position off back with a rolled towel under right hip.
    4. Administer oxygen at 8 to 10 L/min by face mask.
    5. Prepare for an emergent (agonal) cesarean birth if the mother is not immediately stabilized before delivery and the fetus is viable.
    6. Notify neonatal team.

- **RISK FOR INFECTION** related to depletion of normal immunologic factors with loss of blood and to increased risk of transfusion hepatitis.

  DESIRED OUTCOMES: No evidence of febrile condition or jaundice will be present during the first 2 to 7 days of recovery; prophylactic or therapeutic antibiotic administration will be begun at earliest sign of infection.

  INTERVENTIONS
  1. Report signs of infection to the physician.
  2. Administer antibiotics as ordered.
  3. Teach patient regarding self-administration of antibiotics and follow-up after discharge.

- **RISK FOR FAMILY GRIEF** related to poor neonatal outcome, death, or unexpected maternal long-term sequelae or death (see Chapter 6).

CONCLUSION

The primary goal of care of the pregnant woman with DIC is to prevent shock and its sequelae. Early recognition of conditions that predispose a woman to DIC can assist in prevention of maternal death or unexpected long-term sequelae, as well as promote a healthy newborn outcome. When a pregnant woman presents with a severe medical condition and has developed DIC, it is important to attempt rapid stabilization of the mother before attempting an emergency or agonal cesarean delivery.

BIBLIOGRAPHY

Anderson H: Maternal hematologic disorders. In Creasy R, Resnik R, editors: *Maternal-fetal medicine: principles and practice,* ed 3, Philadelphia, 1994, Saunders.

Creasy R, Resnik R, editors: *Maternal-fetal medicine: principles and practice,* ed 3, Philadelphia, 1994, Saunders.

Green J: Placental abnormalities. In Creasy R, Resnik R, editors: *Maternal-fetal medicine: principles and practice,* ed 3, Philadelphia, 1994, Saunders.

Leduc L and others: Coagulation profile in severe preeclampsia, *Obstet Gynecol* 79(1):14-18, 1992.

Roberts J: Pregnancy related hypertension. In Creasy R, Resnik R, editors: *Maternal-fetal medicine: principles and practice,* ed 3, Philadelphia, 1994, Saunders.

Turner G: Disseminating intravascular coagulation (DIC): nursing interventions, *Adv Clin Care (US)* 6(2):19-23, 1991.

Young L: DIC: the insidious killer, *Crit Care Nurse (US)* 10(10):23-26, 1990.

19

Hemolytic Incompatibility

Hemolytic incompatibility occurs when a pregnant woman is sensitized to produce immune globulin G (IgG) antibodies against fetal red blood cells usually from the CDE (Rh) or ABO blood system. The antibodies, returning to the fetal circulation, can cause erythrocyte destruction in the fetus and subsequent fetal anemia with liver failure and congestive heart failure (hydrops).

INCIDENCE

Despite routine use of postpartum D immune globulin, 1% to 2% of all D-negative women who are pregnant continue to become sensitized. Although D incompatibility is the most common and usually the most serious, other hemolytic incompatibilities do occur. Hemolytic disease is seen in 10% of the ABO blood group incompatibilities. ABO and D incompatibilities account for 98% of all hemolytic disease in the fetus. Of the remaining 2%, rare antibodies, such as C, c, E, e, Kell, or Duffy antibodies, are implicated. The pathophysiologic processes for all incompatibilities are similar.

ETIOLOGY

ABO incompatibility occurs when the mother's blood type is O and the fetal blood type is A, B, or AB. Compared with the CDE

(Rh) system, the ABO system is weakly antigenic to its own factors for two reasons. First, A and B antibodies do not cross the placenta. Second, fewer A and B antigenic sites exist on fetal red cells. Therefore there is only a 5% risk of an ABO incompatibility, and it seldom causes hydrops fetalis.

Rh incompatibility occurs primarily when the mother is D negative and the fetus is D positive. However, it can occur if the fetus has any antigen C, c, E, or e and the mother does not.

NORMAL PHYSIOLOGY
Blood Type Genetics

Each father and mother, having received their blood type half from each parent, can be said to be homozygous or heterozygous. Thus, in the ABO system, combinations occur. All persons with type O blood are homozygous. When the mother is type O, she is homozygous, having received an O from both parents. If the father is type O also, there are no antigenic possibilities for the fetal ABO system; the fetus must be type O. If the father is type A, he could be AO heterozygous or AA homozygous. If the father is type B, he could be BB homozygous or BO heterozygous. If the father is type AB, he is heterozygous. To understand the possible fetal blood types from heterozygous fathers with type A, B, or AB and homozygous O mothers or from homozygous type A or B fathers and homozygous O mothers, the following examples may be helpful:

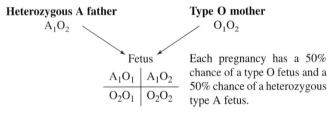

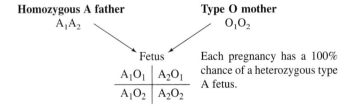

The heterozygous type A fetus carried by a type O mother has antigen A that can evoke antibody formation in the type O mother. Type B works the same way:

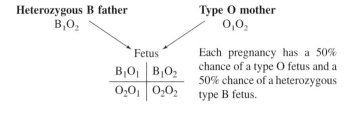

Each pregnancy has a 50% chance of a type O fetus and a 50% chance of a heterozygous type B fetus.

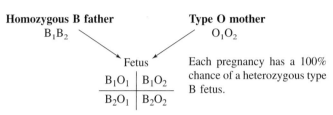

Each pregnancy has a 100% chance of a heterozygous type B fetus.

The heterozygous type B fetus has the B antigen, which can evoke antibody formation in the type O mother.

Type AB fathers are always heterozygous. Their children from a type O mother have the following chances:

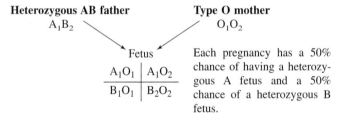

Each pregnancy has a 50% chance of having a heterozygous A fetus and a 50% chance of a heterozygous B fetus.

Because type AB fathers having children with type O mothers will always produce heterozygous A or heterozygous B children, each fetus has the potential of antigenic factors evoking antibody formation by the type O mother. All have antigenic factors that are relatively weak compared with the CDE blood system.

If a mother is D negative, she is always homozygous, having received the D-negative gene from both parents. The D-positive father may be D-positive heterozygous or D-positive homozygous. The following examples demonstrate this:

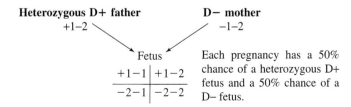

Each pregnancy has a 50% chance of a heterozygous D+ fetus and a 50% chance of a D− fetus.

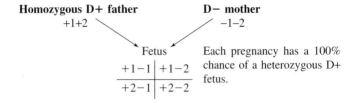

The D fetus has a strong D antigen on the surface of each red blood cell. These antigens will evoke antibody formation in the D mother. The degree of sensitivity to the fetal D antigen varies but is assumed to be related to the total number of D fetal red blood cells entering the maternal circulation.

ABO Blood Group System

The ABO blood group system has the following antigens:
1. A has antigen A.
2. B has antigen B.
3. AB has both antigens A and B.
4. O has none.

The person who does not have the AB antigen probably has the antibody against the respective antigen.

CDE (Rh) Blood Group System

More than 400 red cell antigens have been identified. The person who lacks a specific red cell antigen and is exposed to that antigen can potentially produce an antibody against that respective antigen. It is fortunate that many of these red cell antigens are rare and many have low immunogenicity capability. The greatest immunogenicity capability is seen with the D antigen. If the mother is Rh positive, she probably has the D antigen. If the mother is Rh negative, she does not have the antigen and is extremely vulnerable to the formation of anti-D antibodies if exposed to the D antigen. However, recognition of immunogenicity in the Rh system if factor E, c, C, or e (listed in order of frequency) is present is growing.

Placental Transport

The placenta provides a large area in which exchange of nutrients and waste can take place across the placental membrane. This membrane consists of fetal tissues that separate maternal and fetal blood. As the pregnancy advances, the placental membrane, which also serves as a barrier, becomes progressively thinner. Because of the thinning of this membrane, some fetal blood cells may pass into the maternal blood in the intervillous space. It has been established that small numbers of fetal erythrocytes pass into the maternal circulation normally throughout pregnancy. Typically a greater amount enters at the time of delivery when the separation of the placenta traumatically forces entry of cells through the ciliated, open maternal vessels. However, small separations of the placenta can occur during pregnancy or with any potentially traumatic procedure such as amniocentesis. In most instances the fetal-maternal transfusion is small enough to evoke no sensitivity or involves no incompatibilities from the CDE or ABO system.

PATHOPHYSIOLOGY

The pathophysiology for all the hemolytic incompatibilities is similar. D incompatibility, being the most common, will be used to describe the process of isoimmunization. Isoimmunization occurs when the mother is sensitive to the fetal cells; it is also called *sensitization* (Hecher and others, 1995).

Fetal erythrocytes, with the paternal D antigen, gain entry across the placental membrane into the intervillous blood, which is made up entirely of maternal blood. The fetal erythrocytes mix with the maternal blood and are then carried into the mother's circulation.

The breakthrough of fetal erythrocytes carrying the D antigen into the maternal circulation requires certain conditions favorable to sensitization of the mother and antibody formation. The widely dilated uteroplacental vessels facilitating blood flow also facilitate this process. Maximum maternal blood volume increasing between 28 and 32 weeks further facilitates dilation of these vessels. Changes in fetal blood pressure are responsive to changes in blood flow in the maternal circulation and presumably could increase the chance of a few fetal erythrocytes, under increased pressure, breaking into the intervillous space. For this reason, the second most likely time for D isoimmunization to occur in the mother is at approximately 28 weeks of gestation.

The most likely time for fetal erythrocytes to escape into maternal circulation is at the time of delivery. The wide open vessels at the site of placental separation allow rapid back pressure as the uterus relaxes, and large numbers of fetal erythrocytes can escape into the maternal circulation.

The formation of antibodies is gradual in the mother. Conditions favoring small areas of placental separation such as placenta previa, marginal abruption, or trauma to the placenta during amniocentesis can also favor the entry of increased numbers of fetal erythrocytes carrying the D antigen into the maternal circulation.

SIGNS AND SYMPTOMS

Evidence of antibody formation in the D-negative woman can be detected with an indirect Coombs test and positive identification of the specific antibody on a screen. A titer of 1:4 or greater is significant and indicates maternal sensitization.

In the fetus, signs of anemia and impending hydrops include the following:

- A baseline heart rate of 180 beats/min or greater
- Late decelerations, or loss of short-term variability with presence of regular sine-wave long-term variability (sinusoidal pattern) (Fig. 19-1)

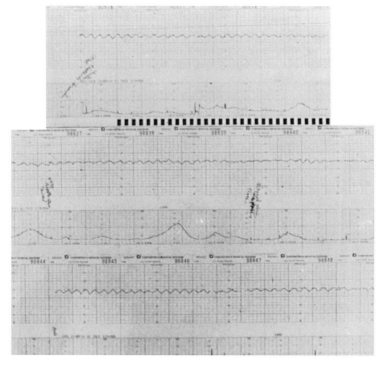

FIG. 19-1 *Top,* D-isoimmunized woman at 30 weeks of gestation. Nonstress test after fourth amniocentesis. *Middle and bottom,* The following day strip shows sinusoidal pattern.
Courtesy John Elliott, Good Samaritan Medical Center, Phoenix.

- Decreased fetal activity
- Ascites or congestive heart failure on ultrasound examination

MATERNAL EFFECTS

There are no physiologic negative effects on the well-being of the mother other than discomfort if polyhydramnios occurs with fetal hydrops. If the mother is sensitized and desires future pregnancies, she may experience significant psychologic difficulties. The various feelings evoked will depend on the circumstances leading to the isoimmunization.

FETAL AND NEONATAL EFFECTS

Harmful effects of D isoimmunization of the mother are seen as hemolysis of fetal erythrocytes. If the sensitization process begins in one pregnancy, the effects will be seen in future pregnancies.

The current pregnancy may be in jeopardy if the process of sensitization is undetected. This can occur if minute placental tissue fragments enter maternal circulation during an amniocentesis, at 28 weeks, or because of placenta previa or abruptio placentae. The current pregnancy may also be jeopardized because sensitization occurred inadvertently with a previous pregnancy.

Hemolysis of fetal erythrocytes can lead to various degrees of fetal anemia. When anemia becomes severe, large amounts of bilirubin, resulting from hemolysis of the erythrocytes, place an overwhelming burden on the fetal liver. As a result, swelling occurs in the liver and portal pressure increases, causing abdominal ascites and congestive heart failure. This phenomenon is called *hydrops fetalis* and can be fatal to the fetus if not corrected by intrauterine transfusion or by delivery so that exchange transfusion of the neonate can occur (Larrabee, Cowan, 1995).

Because of excessive bilirubin breakdown from rapid, increased hemolysis of fetal erythrocytes, the fetus attempts to excrete as much bilirubin as possible. It is excreted in abnormally large amounts into the amniotic fluid and gives it a characteristic yellow-brown appearance.

A fetal sign of hypoxia unique to hemolytic anemia or anemia from fetal-maternal hemorrhage is loss of short-term variability in the fetal heart rate (FHR). The pattern is that of regular smooth oscillations resembling a sine wave and is called a *sinusoidal pattern*. There are no accelerations or variation from the regular smooth oscillations around the baseline. A sinusoidal pattern (Fig. 19-1), if left untreated, will be terminal or may have serious consequences for neonatal outcome (Bowman, 1994).

DIAGNOSTIC TESTING
Antibody Screen

Diagnosis of a hemolytic incompatibility is made by routine pre-natal screening, which should be done in all patients, regardless of Rh factor, on the initial prenatal visit. The test that is used is an antibody screen or indirect Coombs test. The D-negative mother who is not sensitized at the beginning of the pregnancy is rescreened at 28 weeks. Transplacental transfusion at 28 weeks is the second most common time for sensitization to occur; the placental membrane becomes thin enough by this time for fetal red cells to cross.

Severity of Fetal Bleed

In the event a large fetal-maternal hemorrhage is suspected in the D-negative woman, a Kleihauer-Betke blood test on the mother is done. This test detects the amount of fetal cells that have entered the maternal circulation. If more than 15 ml of fetal cells have entered the maternal circulation, the usual D immune globulin dose of 300 mg is not sufficient to prevent sensitization.

Severity of Disease

If the mother has been D isoimmunized from a previous pregnancy, fetal erythroblastosis must be detected early to promote optimal fetal outcome by either early delivery or intrauterine transfusions. Unless previous obstetric history indicates earlier involvement, the fetal erythroblastosis is followed by serial maternal antibody titers beginning at 16 to 18 weeks. When the antibody titers are 1:16 or greater, serial amniocenteses or, in a level III perinatal center, percutaneous umbilical blood samplings are begun. (Refer to Chapter 4 for a description of the procedures.)

Amniocentesis

Bilirubin, a breakdown product of red blood cells, can be measured in the amniotic fluid. The breakdown product is identified as delta-OD 450. Liley, of Aukland, New Zealand, developed a graph for measuring the optical density of delta-OD in the amniotic fluid. He divided the levels of bilirubin optical density into "zones" of safety based on gestation. Levels of delta-OD should decrease with increasing gestation. If the level of bilirubin optical density for delta-OD is increased, it indicates abnormal erythrocyte destruc-tion (Creasy, Resnik, 1994).

Percutaneous Umbilical Blood Sampling

In percutaneous umbilical blood sampling (PUBS) a direct fetal blood sample is obtained from the umbilical cord vessels to evaluate the fetal hemoglobin and hematocrit. An anemic fetus is indicative of abnormal erthrocyte destruction (Sacher, Falchuk, 1990).

USUAL MEDICAL MANAGEMENT AND PROTOCOLS FOR NURSE PRACTITIONERS
Prevention

To prevent sensitization in unsensitized D-negative women, D immune globulin is used. D immune globulin is a specially prepared gamma-globulin that contains a specific concentration of D antibodies. These antibodies neutralize the D-positive fetal antigens that have entered the maternal circulation. For this reason D immune globulin cannot correct sensitization but can prevent it from occurring if given within 72 hours of the potential fetal-maternal red blood cell infusion.

Because the antibody formation in the mother is gradual, it is also apparently effective in preventing sensitization during pregnancy. When D immune globulin is given at 28 weeks of gestation to unsensitized women, the incidence of D isoimmunization has been further reduced. D immune globulin is also given any time a traumatic fetal-maternal bleed is likely to occur, such as after a genetic amniocentesis, a chorionic villi sampling, maternal abdominal trauma, termination of an ectopic pregnancy, or spontaneous or induced abortion (ACOG, 1990b).

The usual dose of D immune globulin is 300 mg at 28 weeks, at the time of any amniocentesis or PUBS, and within 72 hours after delivery. If a test such as the Kleihauer-Betke indicates that more than 30 ml of fetal blood or 15 ml of fetal red blood cells has entered the maternal circulation, a higher dose may be required to prevent sensitization. A first-trimester spontaneous or induced abortion, an ectopic pregnancy, or a chorionic villi sampling requires a minidose of 50 mg within 72 hours (ACOG, 1990b). There are no immune globulins for prevention of other blood group sensitization incompatibilities.

Treatment for Hemolytic Incompatibility

Follow-up

If a hemolytic incompatibility is present, the usual medical management depends on levels of bilirubin optical density in the amniotic fluid, which are obtained by serial amniocenteses or through direct evaluation of the fetal hemoglobin and hematocrit by way of PUBS. When the level of bilirubin is low for a particular gestational age or the hemoglobin and hematocrit are normal, the test is repeated in 3 weeks. If the bilirubin level rises or the hemoglobin and hematocrit levels decrease, evaluation may be repeated in 1 to 2 weeks. Extremely abnormal levels for a particular gestation indicate a need for intrauterine transfusion in the very immature fetus. Cesarean delivery may be necessary when this occurs after 34 weeks of gestation (ACOG, 1990a).

Fetal Surveillance

By 26 weeks of gestation, FHR monitoring should be started. A nonstress test may be done biweekly, a contraction stress test may be done weekly, or some combination of testing methods may be used. Between FHR monitorings, daily fetal activity charts should be kept by the mother. At the time of each evaluation, an ultrasound evaluation or biophysical profile may be done to further assess the fetus for presence of hydrops.

Intrauterine Transfusions

If the fetus becomes anemic anytime after 18 weeks of gestation, an intrauterine transfusion is indicated to allow more time in utero for the immature or nonviable fetus (ACOG, 1990a). The transfusion must be done by a specially skilled physician, usually a perinatologist, who has learned the procedure during postgraduate training in maternal-fetal medicine (see Chapter 4). The intrauterine transfusion can be performed intravascularly or intraperitoneally.

Intravascular transfusion. When an intravascular transfusion is performed, the percutaneous umbilical vein is used (PUBS). The mother is medicated with a uterine relaxant and an antianxiety or tranquilizer agent. The procedure is done under ultrasound direction. A 22-gauge spinal needle is guided through the mother's abdomen and the uterine wall into the umbilical vein in the umbilical cord. Either washed, packed O-negative blood or negative blood matched to the mother's blood type may be used (Doyle and others, 1993).

Intraperitoneal transfusion. The procedure for intraperitoneal transfusion is done under ultrasound direction. Approximately 50 to 150 ml of negative blood, cross matched to the mother, is used. It is spun down to increase the hematocrit to 70% to 80%. Rh-negative blood from a donor must be used because it contains no antibodies to the fetal Rh-positive blood.

The mother is given a narcotic or tranquilizer to quiet the baby for the procedure. After an abdominal scrub of the amniocentesis site and with the direction of ultrasound, a large-gauge intracatheter is inserted through the maternal abdomen, into the uterus, and into the fetal abdomen, just under the fetal diaphragm. The intracatheter tubing, the attached intravenous (IV) tubing, and the syringe for the blood are all preflushed with normal saline. A small amount of normal saline can be injected to view on ultrasound and confirm placement. The syringe with the specially prepared blood is connected to an infusion pump designed for constant speed infusion via syringe. Depending on fetal gestation, 50 to 150 ml of blood is infused over a 1- to 2-hour period. The fetus is monitored before and during the procedure if younger than 26 weeks of gestation. If the fetus is less than 26 weeks, frequent auscultation of the FHR is usually done. During the next 3 to 4 days, the fetal diaphragmatic lymph system absorbs the blood, and improvement in fetal anemia can be expected.

Outcome. Success of intrauterine transfusion generally depends on a number of factors. If the fetus is extremely immature or there is significant liver and congestive heart failure, the potential for improved fetal well-being is less likely and death in utero can ensue in a few days. The earlier the transfusions must be started, the greater the number required to gain maturity while maintaining fetal well-being. This puts the fetus at higher risk for intrauterine infection or premature rupture of membranes (Creasy, Resnik, 1994) and therefore interferes with the potentially successful outcome for the fetus.

NURSING PROCESS

PREVENTION

The nurse caring for the pregnant woman prenatally must recognize the importance of antibody screening in all pregnant patients not only for D incompatibility but also for any blood system incompatibility. Education of the patient regarding necessary prenatal laboratory work should include the need for antibody screening. Patients can be given this information in early prenatal classes as well as during early office visits.

In addition, the nurse should advocate screening of D (Rh)–negative women at 28 weeks of gestation for sensitization at that time. Regardless of the setting, the caregiver must be cognizant of the fetus of the D-negative woman. For instance, if a D-negative woman presents to a labor and delivery setting in premature labor at 28 weeks, the nurse should, in addition to caring for the woman's preterm labor, remember to care for her potentially D-positive fetus. D immune globulin should be given if the patient is D negative and unsensitized.

At the time of delivery, all D-negative women should be screened for sensitization if the baby is D positive. Unsensitized patients should receive D immune globulin within 72 hours after delivery. The nurse caring for the woman during this time is responsible for assuring that the workup for eligibility has been done and that the patient is educated regarding indications for the injection. Even when permanent sterilization is expected, the woman should be instructed regarding potential future problems should sterilization fail or should she ever choose to have a reversal of the sterilization after becoming sensitized with this pregnancy. If a D-negative woman becomes sensitized, she must know that emergency transfusions of D-positive blood when D-negative blood is not available will be impossible and would be dangerous to her well-being.

NURSING DIAGNOSES/COLLABORATIVE PROBLEMS AND INTERVENTIONS

- **RISK FOR ALTERED HEALTH MAINTENANCE** related to the D-negative mother's lack of knowledge regarding potential risk.

  DESIRED OUTCOME: The mother will verbalize understanding of the potential risk related to being D negative and of prevention protocol.

  INTERVENTIONS
  1. Increase the public's awareness of various potential times for sensitization to occur.
  2. Assess the D-negative woman's understanding of when sensitization can take place. Educate the patient in a reassuring manner regarding the use of D immune globulin at all recommended times.
  3. At the initial prenatal visit, determine the mother's blood type and screen for the presence of antibodies by an indirect Coombs test (antibody screen). The D-negative unsensitized pregnant woman should be screened around 28 weeks of gestation.
  4. Administer D immune globulin to D-negative unsensitized pregnant women intramuscularly following a miscarriage, amniocentesis, or chorionic villi sampling in the first trimester; at 26 to 28 weeks of gestation; in the event of a third-trimester bleed; and postpartum within 72 hours.

5. Prepare patient for such potential side effects as temporary soreness at the site of injection and a low-grade fever. In rare instances, an anaphylactic reaction occurs. It is for this reason that the patient should remain in the health care setting for 15 to 30 minutes following the injection.

6. Fill out an identification card confirming the injection, and give it to the patient to keep. Instruct her to keep it with her identification papers. Of women who receive D immune globulin antepartum prophylaxis, 15% to 20% will subsequently have passive acquired D antibodies at the time of delivery. This could lead to misinterpretation and withholding of eligible D immune globulin. In the event of confusion, the mother should be instructed to present her identification card (ACOG, 1990b).

7. Fill out appropriately the blood bank form. Return the form and empty ampule or syringe to the blood bank. In the event of an allergic reaction, the blood bank needs the information these provide.

8. Be prepared to discuss the issue of risk of transmission of human immunodeficiency virus (HIV) through D immune globulin. According to the American College of Obstetricians and Gynecologists (1990b), the risk is eliminated because the preparing process is effective in removing HIV particles.

■ **POTENTIAL FETAL COMPLICATION: ISOIMMUNIZATION** related to D-positive sensitization in a D-negative pregnant woman carrying a D-positive fetus and failure to receive D immune globulin to prevent isoimmunization.

DESIRED OUTCOMES: D incompatibility will be detected through routine antibody screening. Signs of fetal hydrops will be absent, or hydrops will be detected early so appropriate treatment will allow continuation of the pregnancy to more than 32 weeks of gestation.

INTERVENTIONS

Antepartum

1. Accurate information should be obtained regarding first day of last menstrual period, regularity of menstrual cycles, type of birth control used, date of a positive pregnancy test, and ultrasound to facilitate determining the estimated date of delivery. This will be invaluable in determining when necessary interventions should be instituted.

2. Prepare for ultrasound examinations at least every 3 weeks after 20 weeks of gestation when isoimmunization has already occurred.

3. Assess fetal growth with fundal height measurement. Concern for fetal growth should occur if fundal growth stops or decreases. If the fetus becomes anemic, the decreased oxygenation can lead to decreased growth rate. If the fetus becomes hydropic, fundal height can be abnormally large because of associated polyhydramnios.

4. Assess FHR for tachycardia at each prenatal visit after 10 weeks.

5. Teach mother to keep a daily fetal movement chart after 26 weeks of gestation. An active fetus can be assumed to be adequately oxygenated.

6. Instruct D-negative women regarding the timing of fetal evaluation and screening tests.

7. Explain special evaluation procedures and treatment.

8. Prepare and assist with monitoring FHR during evaluation of fetus by amniocentesis or PUBS. A baseline FHR should be determined before the procedure, and a 20- to 30-minute fetal monitoring strip should be run to assess FHR for signs of fetal compromise. Such signs include tachycardia, late decelerations, or absent long-term variability with the presence of short-term variability (sinusoidal pattern, Fig. 19-1).

9. Assist with intrauterine fetal transfusion.

10. Monitor FHR during and after treatment for isoimmunization, for evidence of sinusoidal FHR pattern, or for nonreassuring features such as persistent late decelerations or loss of long-term or short-term variability. Because of maternal sedation during intrauterine transfusion, baseline variability can be decreased and should be compared with the strip before premedication and with the strip 1 hour after.

11. Refer to a nurse specialist for patient education specific to tertiary-level care and referral.

Intrapartum

1. Monitor FHR continuously with an electronic fetal monitor during labor for nonreassuring or preterminal patterns or events. If fetal anemia has developed, labor can further stress the fetus.

2. Prepare the patient and her family for the possible necessity of a cesarean delivery if the fetus shows signs of hypoxia.

3. Refer signs of fetal stress to the physician immediately because these fetuses are very sensitive.

■ **FEAR** related to unpredictable outcome of the fetus.
DESIRED OUTCOME: The patient and family members will verbalize their fears and seek information to identify solutions for problems that develop.
INTERVENTIONS
1. Assess the mother and her family for level of anxiety related to fear for the fetus or infant and potential outcome.
2. Assess anxiety level for unrealistic fears regarding possible emergent surgery and infant status.
3. Determine the family's support system. Assess the couple's support of each other.
4. Keep the parents informed of the status of their fetus or neonate.

■ **RISK FOR INEFFECTIVE COPING** related to unresolved guilt, anger, or frustration if the D-negative woman has become sensitized.
DESIRED OUTCOME: The individuals of the family will demonstrate adequate coping skills and implement a plan to effectively work through their feelings.
INTERVENTIONS
1. Determine how the woman became sensitized. If the injection was overlooked or mistaken Rh results were reported with a previous pregnancy, anger may be unresolved. This can be true especially if the matter is under litigation. If the injection was omitted after a therapeutic abortion, guilt regarding the abortion may be overriding other feelings. When a previous pregnancy occurred before the routine use of D immune globulin, feelings of frustration with an event that could not be controlled and anxiety for the future or the present pregnancy will interact.
2. Evaluate how the woman and her family felt at the time sensitization took place, what means the family used to cope, and how they feel now.
3. Discuss the timing of fetal evaluation and screening tests and the possible treatment plan.
4. Discuss the patient's financial resources, such as insurance, to determine if the serial amniocenteses, ultrasounds, and possible intrauterine transfusions will place a financial burden on the family.

5. Make appropriate referrals based on expressed psychosocial and financial needs.

■ **RISK FOR ALTERED PARENTING** related to neonatal status and lack of early contact.
   DESIRED OUTCOME: The parents will demonstrate attachment behaviors such as calling the infant by name, making positive comments regarding the infant, seeking contact, wanting to touch, and showing interest in caretaking.
   INTERVENTIONS
   1. If the neonate is sick or premature, assess amount of parental attachment behaviors such as frequent visitation, early touching and stroking, calling the infant by name, and attempting to establish eye contact.
   2. Encourage and facilitate early and close contact with the nursery personnel.

■ **RISK FOR ANTICIPATORY OR ACTUAL GRIEF** related to unexpected neonatal outcome (see Chapter 6).

CONCLUSION

For the unsensitized D-negative woman, prevention is the primary goal. This can be accomplished (1) through antibody screening at the first prenatal visit; (2) at 26 to 28 weeks; and (3) by giving D immune globulin by 26 to 28 weeks of gestation, after delivery, with potential placental accidents, and after an abortion. Education regarding indications for D immune globulin and times of greatest risk can improve the future protection of D-negative women from unintentional isoimmunization. As yet there is no protective therapy for other hemolytic incompatibilities.

For the sensitized woman the primary goal is to promote an optimal neonatal outcome through close monitoring of fetal well-being and institution of therapy at the earliest safe time. High risk perinatal nurses should encourage the D-negative woman to seek information about new, proven methods of evaluation and treatment such as those described in Chapter 4.

BIBLIOGRAPHY

American College of Obstetricians and Gynecologists (ACOG): Management of isoimmunization in pregnancy, *ACOG Techn Bull,* no. 148, 1990a.

American College of Obstetricians and Gynecologists (ACOG): Prevention of D isoimmunization, *ACOG Techn Bull,* no. 147, 1990b.

Bowman J: Maternal blood group immunization. In Creasy R, Resnik R, editors: *Maternal-fetal medicine: principles and practice,* ed 3, Philadelphia, 1994, Saunders.

Bowman J, Pollack J, Penston L: Fetomaternal transplacental hemorrhage during pregnancy and after delivery, *Vox Sang* 51:117, 1986.

Caine M, Mueller-Huebach E: Kell sensitization in pregnancy, *Am J Obstet Gynecol* 154:85, 1986.

Creasy R, Resnik R, editors: *Maternal-fetal medicine: principles and practice,* ed 3, Philadelphia, 1994, Saunders.

Daffos F and others: Fetal blood sampling during pregnancy with use of a needle guided by ultrasound: a study of 606 consecutive cases, *Am J Obstet Gynecol* 153:655, 1985.

Doyle L and others: Sensorineural outcome at 2 years for survivors of erythroblastosis treated with fetal intravascular transfusions, *Obstet Gynecol* 81(6):931-934, 1993.

Grannum P, Capel J, Plaxe S: In-utero exchange transfusion by direct intravascular injection in severe erythroblastosis fetalis, *N Engl J Med* 314:1431, 1986.

Hecher K and others: Fetal venous, arterial, and intracardiac blood flows in red blood cell isoimmunization, *Obstet Gynecol* 85(1):122-128, 1995.

Larrabee K, Cowan M: Clinical nursing management of sickle cell disease and trait during pregnancy, *J Perinatal Neonatal Nurs* 9(2):29-41, 1995.

Lloyd T: Rh-factor incompatibility: a primer for prevention, *J Nurse Midwifery* 32(5):297-305, 1987.

Nickolades K and others: Have Liley charts outlived their usefulness? *Am J Obstet Gynecol* 155:90, 1986.

Sacher R, Falchuk S: Percutaneous umbilical blood sampling, *Crit Rev Clin Lab Sci* 28(1):19-35, 1990.

Seeds J, Bowes W: Ultrasound guided intravascular transfusion in severe rhesus immunization, *Am J Obstet Gynecol* 154:1105, 1986.

Steiner E and others: Percutaneous umbilical blood sampling and umbilical vein transfusions, *Transfusion* 30(2):104-108, 1990.

CHAPTER

20

Hypertensive Disorders

The specific terminology for hypertensive disorders of pregnancy is inconsistent. According to ACOG (1996) and the Working Group on High Blood Pressure in Pregnancy (1990), two etiologic disorders are involved. One disorder develops during pregnancy, labor, or the early postpartum period in a previously normotensive, nonproteinuric woman. The other disorder is related to a preexisting condition. Gestational hypertension includes hypertension or proteinuria that develops during pregnancy, generally after 20 weeks of gestation in the absence of a molar pregnancy or within 7 days postpartum and subsides after delivery. Chronic hypertensive disorders include chronic hypertension and chronic renal disease that preexisted before the pregnancy. Table 20-1 summarizes these classifications. This chapter focuses on gestational hypertensive disorders often referred to as *pregnancy-induced hypertension (PIH)* and particularly on preeclampsia and eclampsia. Of the gestational hypertensive disorders, preeclampsia and eclampsia pose the greatest threat to the fetus and cause the most complications to the mother. Transient gestational hypertension alone is usually benign (Working Group on High Blood Pressure in Pregnancy, 1990). Chronic hypertension is not as dangerous but does increase the risk for placental insufficiency, abruptio placentae, and superimposed preeclampsia/eclampsia.

TABLE 20-1   Classification of hypertensive states of pregnancy

Type	Description
Gestational hypertensive disorders: pregnancy-induced hypertension (PIH)	
Transient hypertension	Development of mild hypertension during pregnancy in previously normotensive patient without proteinuria or pathologic edema
Gestational proteinuria	Development of proteinuria after 20 wk of gestation in previously nonproteinuric patient without hypertension
Preeclampsia	Development of hypertension and proteinuria in previously normotensive patient after 20 wk of gestation or in early postpartum period; in presence of trophoblastic disease it can develop before 20 wk of gestation
Eclampsia	Development of convulsions or coma in preeclamptic patient
Chronic hypertensive disorders	
Chronic hypertension	Hypertension and/or proteinuria in pregnant patient with chronic hypertension
Superimposed preeclampsia/eclampsia	Development of preeclampsia or eclampsia in patient with chronic hypertension

INCIDENCE

Approximately 6% to 8% of all pregnant women will develop preeclampsia (ACOG, 1996). The strongest risk factors for preeclampsia are a primigravida younger than 19 years or older than 40 years (Roberts, 1994a) or a history of severe preeclampsia (Sibai and others, 1991). According to the American College of Obstetricians and Gynecologists (1996), other factors associated with a higher-than-normal incidence of preeclampsia follow:

- Familial history
- Preexisting vascular disease such as diabetes or chronic hypertension
- Exposure to a superabundance of chorionic villi such as in multiple gestation and hydatidiform mole
- Rh incompatibility
- Antiphospholipid syndrome

ETIOLOGY

The cause of preeclampsia remains unknown. However, there are many current theories as to its possible cause. A few of the more common theories are presented here.

Nutritional Deficiency

Protein not only promotes cellular growth but also is important in maintaining a normal serum osmotic pressure, in transporting lipids, and in converting fats to lipoproteins. Therefore protein could be significant in preventing edema and elevated blood pressure (Worthington-Roberts, Williams, 1997). A possible correlation between a low-protein diet and the development of preeclampsia is unknown. Because adequate calcium can decrease the vascular sensitivity to angiotensin by stimulating prostacyclin or nitric oxide synthesis, a calcium deficiency during pregnancy may trigger preeclampsia, according to several recent research studies (Belizan and others, 1991; Carroli and others, 1994; Sanchez-Ramos and others, 1994). A correlation may exist between adequate magnesium and a decreased risk of preeclampsia (Repke, 1991). Magnesium is known to cause vasodilation, but its ability to prevent preeclampsia is uncertain. In summary, no adequate data prove or disprove a strong association between nutritional deficiencies or supplementation and prevention of PIH.

Immunologic Deficiency

Another current theory being studied is immunologically based. According to Beer and Need (1985), preeclampsia might be the result of an overwhelming immune response, similar to organ rejection, activated by the woman's body against the placenta and fetus. This reaction is being proposed as the result of insufficient "blocking" or enhancing antibodies or insufficient B- and T-lymphocyte production to immunoprotect the expanding invasive trophoblast. These antibodies, if present, prevent the development of effector lymphocytes and humoral antibodies against the cytotrophoblast tissue. If effector lymphocytes and humoral antibodies are produced against the trophoblastic tissue, trophoblast invasion along the maternal spiral arteries does not occur and vasoconstriction of these arteries results. This may cause the disproportionate release of thromboxane, a vasoconstrictor prostaglandin, over prostacyclin, a vasodilator prostaglandin. This might partially explain why primigravidas, multigravidas who have changed partners, couples who used only barrier contraceptive methods (Robillard and others, 1994), and artificial donor-inseminated pregnancies (Need and others, 1983) are at greater risk for preeclampsia. All these variables limit the woman's exposure to the father's sperm, thereby preventing, blocking, or enhancing antibody formation.

Genetic Predisposition

Chesley and Cooper (1986) studied the possibility of preeclampsia being related to a single recessive gene, and they found that a high percentage of the daughters of mothers who had experienced preeclampsia also developed preeclampsia. Ward and associates (1993) found these women to carry the angiotensinogen gene variant T235, and Dizon-Townson and associates (1996) found a higher incidence of factor V in preeclamptic women. Other research has not reproduced these findings.

NORMAL PHYSIOLOGY

Even though the triggering factor of this disease remains unknown, much of the pathophysiology of the disease is understood. To understand the pathophysiology of preeclampsia, the nurse should be familiar with the normal physiologic changes of pregnancy. The normal physiologic changes of pregnancy that are affected by preeclampsia are summarized as follows.

Plasma Blood Volume

Plasma blood volume is increased 30% to 50%, and cardiac output is maximized.

Kidney Function

The normal glomerular filtration rate is increased by approximately 50%, and tubular reabsorption is enhanced.

Fluid Balance

Renin, angiotensin II, and aldosterone levels are increased. These substrates, along with increasing estrogen, facilitate the normal expansion of the blood volume by 40% to 50% above nonpregnant levels (Friedman, 1991).

Placentation

Between 10 and 16 weeks of gestation the muscular component of the uterine spiral arteries begins to be replaced by trophoblast. To further increase fetoplacental blood flow between 16 and 22 weeks of gestation, the trophoblast erodes the myometrial portions of the uterine spiral arteries so they widen and lose their vasoconstrictive properties.

Vasopressor and Vasodilator Balance

A delicate balance between vasodilator and vasopressor activity must be maintained during pregnancy to maintain a normotensive state. Prostacyclin is produced by the placenta and intact endothelium that line the blood vessel walls. It stimulates the renin-angiotensin-aldosterone cycle important for fluid balance. It is a potent vasodilator because of its resistance to the presser effects of angiotensin II. It prevents platelet clumping and promotes increased uteroplacental blood flow as well. Nitric oxide is another vasodilator substance very important in maintaining low basal blood vessel tone but at the same time weakening the action of vasoconstrictors (Ghabour and others, 1995) and inhibiting platelet aggregation (Lowenstein and others, 1994). Nitric oxide is derived from the endothelial blood vessel cells. A progressive increase in the ratio of antioxidant activity of vitamin E to lipid peroxides decreases the risk of endothelial damage and thereby aids in the production of prostacyclin and nitric oxide and lessens the production of vasopressors that are produced in greater amounts when the endothelial tissue is damaged (Wang and others, 1991a, 1991b).

Active vasopressors are thromboxane, endothelins (endothelin-1), and increased lipid peroxides. Thromboxane is a vasoconstrictor, a stimulant of platelet aggregation, and a uterine stimulating prostaglandin (Wang and others, 1991a, 1991b). Thromboxane is produced by the placenta and in less amount by the platelets. Endothelin-1 is increased normally during pregnancy (Branch and others, 1991; Clark and others, 1992; Nova and others, 1991). In the event of endothelial damage, endothelin-1 is produced in abnormally increasing amounts, which causes inactivation of nitric oxide (Zeeman, Dekker, 1992).

During pregnancy there is a progressive increase in the ratios of vasodilator to vasopressor substances, with the balance in favor of vasodilator substances. This is true for the prostacyclin/thromboxane ratio and the antioxidant activity of vitamin E/lipid peroxide ratio. Nitric oxide facilitates vasodilator substances by weakening the action of thromboxane and endothelin-1 (Ghabour and others, 1995). This balance is further facilitated by the progressive increase in the ratios of antioxidant activity of vitamin E and lipid peroxides, which enhances the endothelium of the placenta to produce greater amounts of prostacyclin relative to thromboxane (Wang and others, 1991a, 1991b).

Angiotensin Balance

Angiotensin II is a potent pressor substance that stimulates a rise in blood pressure. In normal pregnancy, even though the levels of angiotensin II are elevated, blood pressure does not rise. This is because healthy pregnant women have an increased resistance to the presser effects of angiotensin II (deJong and others, 1991; Gilstrap, Gant, 1990) related to increased levels of vasodilator prostacyclin (PGI_2) and nitric oxide, an endothelium-derived relaxing factor (Friedman, 1991). Angiotensin II in turn stimulates the synthesis of two vasodilators: prostacyclin and nitric oxide.

Vascular Response

To accommodate the increased blood volume, peripheral vascular resistance decreases during pregnancy related to two endothelium-derived substances: prostacyclin and nitric oxide (Zeeman, Dekker, 1992). The diastolic blood pressure normally drops 7 to 10 mm Hg during the first and second trimesters followed by a return to nonpregnant levels during the third trimester (Working Group on High Blood Pressure in Pregnancy, 1990).

Fluid Shifts

Fluid moves from the intravascular space to the extracellular space in the dependent limbs. The fluid shift is related to decreased plasma colloid osmotic pressure below 23 mm Hg secondary to the normal hemodilution of the blood. This is also related to the increased venous capillary hydrostatic pressure in the dependent limbs secondary to the gravid uterus pressing on the inferior vena cava, interfering with the blood returning to the heart. The net result is physiologic edema in the dependent limbs during the last trimester of pregnancy. Physiologic edema should disappear after 8 to 12 hours of bed rest.

PATHOPHYSIOLOGY

In preeclampsia it appears that the trophoblastic tissue of the placenta fails to migrate down the maternal spiral arteries and displace the musculoelastic structures of these arteries (Zuspan, 1991b). Therefore these arteries do not widen as they normally do to increase placental perfusion. The resulting placental ischemia stimulates the release of a factor or substance that is toxic to endothelial cells that line all blood vessels and provide blood vessel wall integrity (De Groot and others, 1995). With endothelial damage, there is less production of such vasodilators as prostacyclin and nitric oxide and an increased production of such vasopressors as thromboxane, endothelin-1, oxygen free radical, and lipid peroxides. As a result, there is a sevenfold increased production of thromboxane, a vasoconstrictor and stimulant of platelet aggregation, over prostacyclin, a vasodilator and inhibitor of platelet aggregation, causing a compensatory increased vascular sensitivity to angiotensin II (de Jong and others, 1991; Gilstrap, Gant, 1990; Wallenburg and others, 1991; Walsh, 1990). Decreased production of nitric oxide by terminal placental vessels, along with increased thromboxane, causes platelet adhesion to the surface of the trophoblast, resulting in intervillous thrombi (Ghabour and others, 1995), which further alters blood flow to the fetus. Damaged endothelial cells cause increased release of endothelin-1, which inactivates nitric oxide (Zeeman, Dekker, 1992). Increased production of oxygen free radicals and lipid peroxides results, which further inactivates the vasodilator effect of nitric oxide (Zeeman, Dekker, 1992) and further damages endothelium (Wang and others, 1991a, 1991b).

Multiple-organ endothelial cell injury ensues (Nova and others, 1991). Generalized vasospasm results, leading to poor tissue perfusion, increased total peripheral resistance with subsequent elevation of blood pressure, and increased endothelial cell permeability, which allows intravascular protein and fluid loss (Friedman, 1991). Vascular endothelial cell injury may initiate coagulation pathways as well (Roberts and others, 1991).

Resulting Pathophysiologic Changes

Other specific pathophysiologic changes result from preeclampsia; a discussion of these follows.

Uteroplacental Insufficiency

Uteroplacental perfusion is compromised 50%, even before preeclamptic symptoms, related to pathologic spiral arteriole lesions and a deficiency of prostacyclin (Usta, Sibai, 1996). The uteroplacental perfusion will be further reduced as the disease progresses. The fetal blood flow is further decreased related to constriction of umbilical vessels.

Renal Damage

In 70% of preeclamptic cases, glomerular endothelial damage, fibrin deposition, and resulting ischemia reduce renal plasma flow and glomerular filtration rate (Friedman, 1991). Protein, mainly in the form of albumin, is lost into the urine. Uric acid and creatinine clearance is decreased, and oliguria develops as the condition worsens. Therefore proteinuria and increased plasma uric acid levels are signs of preeclampsia, and oliguria is a sign of severe preeclampsia and kidney damage.

Fluid and Electrolyte Imbalance

Serum albumin is decreased as the result of serum protein lost into extracellular spaces by way of damaged capillary walls and in the urine. Decreased serum albumin causes a decrease in the plasma colloid osmotic pressure, an increase in intracellular edema, and failure of the normal expansion of the intravascular plasma volume (ACOG, 1996). Even though there is intravascular hemoconcentration, the production of renin, angiotensin, and aldosterone decreases, resulting in an increased hematocrit.

Worsening Pathophysiologic Changes

As preeclampsia progresses, the following systemic changes, which are signs that the condition is worsening, may occur.

Pulmonary Involvement

Pulmonary edema may develop and is related to one of three factors. The most common factor is volume overload as a result of left ventricular failure caused by extremely high vascular resistance, excessive fluid infusion during treatment of the disease, or postpartum diuresis. The other two factors are related to a further decreased colloid osmotic pressure or an endothelial injury that increases pulmonary capillary permeability, resulting in a fluid leak or a noncardiogenic pulmonary edema.

Central Nervous System Involvement

Endothelial damage to the cortical region of the brain, resulting in fibrin deposition, edema, and cerebral hemorrhage, may lead to hyperreflexia and severe headaches and can progress to seizure activity (eclampsia) (Gilstrap, Gant, 1990).

Ophthalmic Involvement

Visual changes, such as scotoma, photophobia, blurring, or double vision, can occur related to retinal arteriolar spasms caused by arteriolar narrowing (Wallenburg, 1989).

Hemodynamic Changes

The exact hemodynamic changes that may occur in the presence of preeclampsia remain unknown. Hemodynamic values ranging from normal to increased cardiac output, cardiac afterload, or systemic vascular resistance and decreased ventricular preload have been reported to occur (Sibai, Mabie, 1991; Working Group on High Blood Pressure in Pregnancy, 1990). However, in untreated preeclampsia, Wallenburg (1988) found a low wedge pressure, low cardiac output, and high systemic vascular resistance. Therefore it appears that the disparity in hemodynamic findings is related to various interventions before monitoring (Mabie, 1996).

Coagulation Involvement

Occasionally inappropriate activation of the coagulation system may result, and disseminated intravascular coagulopathy (DIC) develops.

Hepatic Involvement

Hepatic ischemia can lead to periportal hemorrhagic necrosis in the liver, which can cause a subcapsular hematoma. This occurs in approximately 10% of all preeclamptic patients (Sibai, 1996a). When hepatic ischemia does occur, it indicates a very severe form of the disease and the condition can advance to eclampsia very quickly. Warning signs of hepatic involvement such as right upper quadrant pain or epigastric pain can indicate impending eclampsia.

HELLP Syndrome Development

In 2% to 12% of preeclamptic cases, the HELLP syndrome, which is characterized by *h*emolysis of red blood cells, *e*levated *l*iver enzymes, and *l*ow *p*latelets, may develop (Martin and others, 1991; Sibai and others, 1993a; Weinstein, 1985). This cascade of events is the result of systemic capillary endothelial cell damage exposing the basement membrane, which activates platelet adherence and fibrin deposition. Platelets are then decreased, and red blood cells are torn trying to pass through the narrowed vessels and are deposited along with the fibrin. Activation of platelets results in release of more thromboxane, and endothelial damage leads to further reduction in prostacyclin production, thus setting up a vicious cycle (Barton, Sibai, 1991; Walsh, 1990). Hyperbilirubinemia (jaundice) may develop as a result of hemolysis of the red blood cells. At the same time, endothelial damage and fibrin deposition in the liver may lead to impaired liver function and can result in hemorrhagic necrosis, indicated by right upper quadrant tenderness or epigastric pain, nausea, and vomiting (Phelan,

Easter, 1990). Liver enzymes are elevated when liver tissue is necrotic. Normal blood pressure is found in approximately 10% to 20% of the patients with HELLP syndrome (Sibai and others, 1993a).

• • •

Fig. 20-1 summarizes the pathophysiologic changes of pre-eclampsia.

MATERNAL EFFECTS

Preeclampsia is a very serious disease and is the second leading cause of maternal mortality (ACOG, 1996). If preeclampsia is treated early and effectively, maternal mortality is very low. If the disease is allowed to progress to the HELLP syndrome or eclampsia, maternal mortality increases to as high as 15%. The most common causes of death are related to abruptio placentae; pulmonary edema; renal, hepatic, or respiratory failure; myocardial infarction; coagulopathy; and cerebral hemorrhage (ACOG, 1996; Heppard, Garite, 1996).

FETAL AND NEONATAL EFFECTS

Perinatal mortality related to mild preeclampsia ranges from 1% to 8%, increasing to an overall average of 15% in severe preeclampsia, with a higher incidence found with early onset and lower incidence if the onset develops after 37 weeks of gestation (Sibai and others, 1990). If the disease progresses into the HELLP syndrome or eclampsia or exists in the presence of preexisting chronic hypertension, perinatal mortality can be as high as 35% to 60% (Sibai, 1988). The majority of perinatal losses are related to placental insufficiency, which causes intrauterine growth restriction (IUGR), prematurity associated with preterm delivery, or abruptio placentae.

SIGNS AND SYMPTOMS
Cardinal Signs

The cardinal signs of preeclampsia are hypertension and proteinuria or overt generalized edema or both. Except in the presence of a hydatidiform mole, these signs develop after 20 weeks of gestation. An elevated blood pressure is usually the first sign to develop in the early stages of this disease; therefore the disease may be diagnosed without the presence of proteinuria.

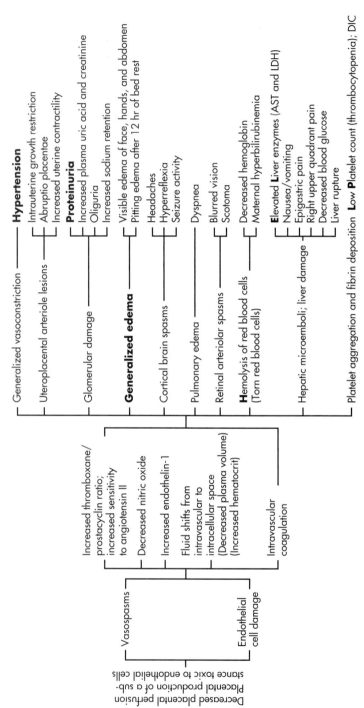

FIG. 20-1 Pathophysiologic changes of preeclampsia. *AST,* Aspartate transaminase; *LDH,* lactate dehydrogenase.

Hypertension

Hypertension is diagnosed if one of the following is present:
- The systolic blood pressure is 140 mm Hg or greater.
- The diastolic blood pressure is 90 mm Hg or greater.
- The mean arterial pressure (MAP) is 105 or greater, or an increase in MAP is 20 or more.

$$MAP = \frac{Systolic + (Diastolic \times 2)}{3}$$

Proteinuria

Proteinuria is diagnosed if one of the following is present:
- More than 0.3 g (300 mg) of protein per liter of urine is found in a 24-hour urine collection.
- More than 0.1 g (100 mg) of protein per liter is found in at least two random urine specimens collected on two or more occasions at least 6 hours apart when the specific gravity is 1.030 or less and the pH is less than 8. (This is indicated as +2 or greater on a dipstick.)

The following guidelines should be kept in mind when evaluating the urine for protein:
- Vaginal discharge, blood, amniotic fluid, and bacteria can contaminate the specimen and give a false-positive reading.
- The specimen should be obtained by either a voided midstream collection or catheterization to avoid contamination with vaginal discharge.
- Alkaline urine or very concentrated urine (specific gravity greater than 1.030) may give a false-positive reading (Davey, MacGillivray, 1988).
- Dilute urine (specific gravity less than 1.010) may give a false-negative reading.

Pathologic Edema

Pathologic edema must be differentiated from normal physiologic edema that occurs in approximately 80% of all pregnancies (McAnulty, and others, 1995). Pathologic edema is indicated by nondependent edema of the face, hands, or abdomen nonresponsive to 12 hours of bed rest or by a rapid weight gain of more than 2 pounds in 1 week.

Subjective Signs

Subjective signs of preeclampsia suggesting end-organ involvement are listed below:

- Headaches
- Visual changes, such as blurred vision
- Rapid-onset edema of the face or abdomen or pitting edema in the feet or legs after 12 hours of bed rest
- Oliguria
- Hyperreflexia
- Nausea or vomiting
- Epigastric pain

HELLP Syndrome Signs

Signs of the HELLP syndrome are as follows:

- Epigastric pain or right upper quadrant tenderness
- Nausea or vomiting
- Headache
- Malaise
- Jaundice
- Hematuria

Comparison of Mild and Severe Preeclamptic Signs

Preeclampsia is usually categorized in grades of either mild or severe for the purpose of treatment (Table 20-2).

TABLE 20-2 Comparison of mild and severe preeclampsia

	Mild	Severe
Blood pressure		
Systolic	140-160 mm Hg	>160 mm Hg
Diastolic	90-110 mm Hg	≥110 mm Hg
Proteinuria (24 hr)	0.3-4 g	≥5 g
Dipstick	+2/+3	+4
Urinary output	>30 ml/hr	<20 ml/hr
	>650 ml/24 hr	<500 ml/24 hr
Pulmonary edema	Not present	Can be present
Subjective signs	Not present	Can be present
HELLP syndrome signs	Not present	Can be present

HELLP, Hemolysis, elevated liver enzymes, and low platelet count in association with preeclampsia.

Eclampsia

If coma or convulsions occur, preeclampsia is then classified as eclampsia. Epigastric pain, hyperreflexia, and clonus are usually signs of an approaching convulsion. However, in the presence of only edema, some normal women have hyperreflexia.

DIAGNOSTIC TESTING
Diagnostic Signs

No diagnostic tests are available to detect preeclampsia. One must recognize signs and symptoms to detect its development. The most diagnostic symptom is a rise in blood pressure. To detect blood pressure diagnostic of early preeclampsia, one must consider two things. First, the blood pressure, mostly the diastolic pressure, normally drops slightly during the second trimester of pregnancy and then gradually returns to its original baseline level during the third trimester. Second, the systolic blood pressure is more affected by cardiac output changes. In contrast, the diastolic blood pressure is more affected by peripheral vascular resistance changes (Guyton, Hall, 1996). Therefore the diastolic blood pressure is the most diagnostic.

Screening for the presence of the antibody *antiphospholipid* has been found to aid in determining the risk of severity of the disease. Its presence indicates a higher diverse risk (Branch and others, 1992).

Obtaining Accurate Blood Pressure Readings

To obtain an accurate blood pressure reading, the blood pressure cuff must cover approximately 80% of the upper arm. Because position can lead to variability in the blood pressure reading, blood pressure should be measured in the same arm and with the patient in the same position each time. If the patient is sitting, her arm should rest on a table at heart level. If the patient is lying down, she should be at a 30-degree tilt on her left side and the blood pressure cuff should be on her right arm so the cuff is at the same level as the heart (Working Group on High Blood Pressure in Pregnancy, 1990). Controversy exists among health care providers as to which diastolic sound should be recorded: phase IV (the muffled sound) or phase V (the disappearance of sound). Several factors are to be considered. During pregnancy, Korotkoff phase V most accurately reflects intraarterial pressure (Brown and others, 1994). Therefore the National Heart, Lung and Blood Institute and others currently recommend that the Korotkoff phase V sound be used (Shennan and others, 1996; Wenger and others, 1993).

However, because of the high cardiac output state of pregnancy, the diastolic pressure falls to zero before the Korotkoff phase V is heard in 15% of pregnant women (WHO Study Group, 1987). Therefore, according to the Working Group on High Blood Pressure in Pregnancy (1990), the systolic and diastolic phase IV and V blood pressure readings should be recorded during pregnancy.

A second controversy exists as to the device used to take blood pressure. The question is whether blood pressure readings obtained by either the standard mercury sphygmomanometer (manual) or the automated blood pressure device (electronic) can be used interchangeably. Brown and others (1994) found the auscultatory (manual) systolic pressures were 7 to 10 mm Hg lower than the oscillatory (electronic) values. Auscultatory diastolic pressures were 5 to 7 mm Hg higher than oscillatory values. Therefore caution should be use when interpreting blood pressure values taken with different devices (Green, Froman, 1996).

Predictive Tests

Because the hypertensive disease process begins long before signs and symptoms appear, various researchers have attempted to develop a predictive test. More than 100 clinical biophysical and biochemical tests have been evaluated for predicting patients at risk for preeclampsia. Inconsistent and contradictory predictive abilities have limited their usefulness. After an extensive review of the literature, Dekker and Sibai (1991) concluded that there is currently no ideal predictive test.

USUAL MEDICAL MANAGEMENT AND PROTOCOLS FOR NURSE PRACTITIONERS

The only cure for preeclampsia is termination of the pregnancy. The goal of management is to prevent eclampsia and other severe complications while allowing the fetus to mature. Because fetuses are usually immature when the disease develops, the severity of the disease and the maturity of the fetus must be considered in determining when delivery should take place. If the pregnancy has progressed 36 weeks or more or fetal maturity is confirmed by a lecithin/sphingomyelin (L/S) ratio of 2 : 1, delivery is the treatment of choice after the condition is stabilized. If the pregnancy is less than 36 weeks of gestation or the fetus is immature, interventions will be instituted to attempt to arrest or improve preeclampsia and allow time for the fetus to mature. However, if the HELLP (hemolysis, elevated liver enzymes, and low platelet count in association with preeclampsia) syndrome develops, signs of impending eclampsia are present, or symptoms manifest indicating the condition is worsening, immediate delivery is necessary at any gestational age.

Expectant Management

The medical interventions depend on the severity of the disease and gestational age. In mild preeclampsia when the gestational age is 36 weeks or greater, the patient is usually treated with intravenous (IV) magnesium sulfate and oxytocin to induce labor. In mild preeclampsia when the fetus is immature, the patient is usually hospitalized with decreased activity to attempt to arrest the disease or at least stabilize the disease to allow the fetus time to mature without jeopardizing the mother's health. If the patient becomes normotensive with no significant proteinuria (less than 500 mg/24 hr), research has indicated similar outcomes with home management (either in a day care unit or with home health care) as with in-patient hospital care (Barton and others, 1994; Crawther and others, 1992; Tuffnell and others, 1992; Twaddle, Harper, 1992). Refer to Box 20-1 for home care guidelines for treatment of mild preeclampsia.

If the disease is severe, as indicated by worsening maternal symptoms, diagnostic tests showing evidence of end-organ dysfunction, or deterioration of the fetus, or if HELLP syndrome develops, the current treatment is to prevent convulsions with an anticonvulsant, control the blood pressure within a safe range with an antihypertensive agent, and frequently evaluate maternal and fetal well-being. Then expeditious delivery is initiated as the woman's condition indicates (Sibai, 1991). If the patient manifests a bleeding tendency, fresh frozen plasma and packed red blood cells are usually transfused.

Activity Restriction

Resting in bed in the lateral recumbent position takes the pressure of the gravid uterus off the inferior vena cava. This facilitates venous return, thereby increasing the circulatory volume, which increases renal blood flow and promotes diuresis. The release of angiotensin II is also decreased (Sibai, 1988). Blood pressure normally drops as a result, enhancing blood flow to the placenta and fetus. How much of the day should be spend in bed is currently controversial. According to Maloni (1996), there is lack of scientific support for the effectiveness of continuous bed rest when compared with maternal risks of bed rest. Refer to Chapter 1.

Box 20-1

Home Health Care for Mild Preeclampsia

Criteria selection

Blood pressure less than 150/100 mm Hg sitting and less than 140/90 mm Hg in the left lateral position

Proteinuria less than 500 mg/day

Platelet count more than 125,000/µl

Normal liver enzymes: AST less than 50 U/L; ALT less than 50 U/L; LDH less than 200 U/L

Serum creatinine less than 1.32 mg/dl

Reassuring fetal status with no intrauterine fetal growth restriction

No worsening signs present

A compliant patient

A reliable patient

Home care protocols

Limited home activity with 12 hours of sleep each night and rest periods during the day to facilitate renal and placental perfusion by mobilizing the movement of extracellular fluid back into the intravascular space

Balanced diet containing at least 60-70 g of protein; 1200 mg of calcium; adequate zinc and sodium (2-6 g); and 6 to 8 glasses of water per day

Blood pressure checked every 4-6 hours daily while awake

Daily weight at the same time each day

Urine for protein using first-voided specimen of the day

Instructed as to worsening signs and symptoms that should be reported immediately

    Headaches

    Changes in vision

    Epigastric pain or RUQ pain

    Increased edema

    Vaginal bleeding or changes in vaginal discharge

    Severe abdominal pain

    Sudden gush of fluid

Home health nurse visits two times per week with daily telephone contact

Weekly prenatal visits

Initial and frequent diagnostic laboratory assessments

    Creatinine clearance

    Serum creatinine

    Serum uric acid levels

    Platelet count

    Hematocrit

    Serum albumin

    Liver enzymes

Box 20-1
Home Health Care for Mild Preeclampsia—cont'd

Home care protocols—cont'd
Fetal surveillance
    Daily fetal movement charts
    Frequent evaluations with BPP, CST, NST, and/or AFI
    Fetal growth by ultrasound every 3 weeks
Hospital admission for worsening status

Developed from information in Grohar J: *J Obstet Gynecol Neonatal Nurs* 23(8):687-694, 1994.
AST, Aspartate transaminase; *ALT,* alanine transaminase; *LDH,* lactate dehydrogenase; *RUQ,* right upper quadrant; *BPP,* biophysical profile; *CST,* contraction stress test; *NST,* nonstress test; *AFI,* amniotic fluid index.

Diet

A high-protein diet of at least 60 g (NRC, 1989) and preferably 70 g (Zuspan, 1991a) is therapeutic in replacing the protein lost in the urine. Protein also increases the plasma colloid osmotic pressure. As the plasma colloid osmotic pressure increases, it pulls fluid from the intracellular spaces back into the circulatory system. Adequate calcium, magnesium, and vitamins are important also. Sodium intake should not exceed 6 g daily. In general, instruct the patient to salt foods to taste. An excessive salt intake can increase angiotensin II sensitivity and cause increased vasoconstriction. On the other hand, an inappropriate dietary sodium restriction below 2 g can further reduce the blood volume and decrease placental perfusion (Newman, Fullerton, 1990). However, if the patient has salt-sensitive chronic hypertension or renal disease and was on a sodium-restricted diet before pregnancy, she should continue on this diet during her pregnancy.

Pharmacologic Therapy

The following medications are commonly used in the treatment of preeclampsia.

Anticonvulsive Therapy

Magnesium sulfate is still the anticonvulsant drug of choice to prevent seizure activity (Eclampsia Trial Collaborative Group, 1995; Lucas, 1995; Sibai, 1996). Phenytoin may be used as an alternative therapy. For anticonvulsant therapy refer to the section on collaborative intervention later in this chapter.

Antihypertensive Therapy

Hydralazine (Apresoline) is the usual antihypertensive drug of choice if the diastolic blood pressure is more than 110 mm Hg. Labetalol hydrochloride (Normodyne) may be used when hydralazine is ineffective. Other antihypertensive agents being tried are nifedipine and verapamil. Nitroglycerin is not recommended because of potential fetal cyanide toxicity (Working Group on High Blood Pressure in Pregnancy, 1990). For antihypertensive therapy refer to the section on collaborative intervention later in this chapter.

Stimulant for Fetal Surfactant

The use of corticosteroids and thyrotropin-releasing hormone (TRH) to facilitate fetal lung maturity is recommended if delivery is imminent before 34 weeks of gestation (Cunningham and others, 1997; Heppard, Garite, 1996).

Sedatives

Sedatives are not recommended in the treatment of preeclampsia since they may mask maternal subjective symptoms and lead to fetal central nervous system (CNS) depression.

Diuretics

Diuretics, except in the presence of heart failure, are not used today. It has been shown that diuretics further decrease blood flow to the placenta by decreasing blood volume, disrupt the normal electrolyte balance, which can impair certain aspects of placental function (such as estrogen production), and create further stress on already compromised kidneys (Brown and others, 1988).

Blood Component Replacement

In the presence of severe persistent thrombocytopenia, fresh frozen plasma or packed red blood cells are usually infused. Platelet transfusions are ineffective because platelet consumption occurs soon after administration (Martin and others, 1990).

Diagnostic Tests

Diagnostic tests that can be helpful in evaluating the severity and rate of progression of PIH or HELLP syndrome and the mother's response to treatment are summarized in Tables 20-3 and 20-4.

TABLE 20-3 Summary of diagnostic tests affected by pregnancy-induced hypertension

Condition evaluated	Diagnostic test	Significant finding
Kidney involvement	BUN (blood urea nitrogen)	>10 mg/dl
	Creatinine	>2 mg/dl
Reduced blood volume	Hematocrit	>40%
Disseminated intravascular coagulopathy (DIC)	Fibrin split products (FSP)	>40 µg/ml
	Platelet count	<100,000/mm^3
	Bleeding time	Prolonged
	Fibrinogen	<300 mg/dl
Uteroplacental involvement	Biophysical profile (BPP)	<8
	Amniotic fluid index	<8 cm
Fetal lung immaturity	Lecithin/sphingomyelin (L/S) ratio	<2
	Phosphatidyl glycerol (PG)	Not present
Hepatic involvement	Albumin	<2.5

TABLE 20-4 Summary of diagnostic tests affected by HELLP

Condition evaluated	Diagnostic test	Significant finding
Hemolysis	Peripheral smear	Abnormal Schistocytes or burr cells present
	Bilirubin	>1.2 mg/dl
Hepatic involvement	Liver enzymes	
	AST (SGOT)	>72 U/L
	ALT (SGPT)	>50 U/L
	LDH (lactate dehydrogenase)	>600 IU/L
Thrombocytopenia	Platelet count	<100,000/mm^3
Red blood cell volume involvement	Hematocrit	<32%
	Hemoglobin	<10 g/dl
Renal involvement	Uric acid	>10 mg/dl
	Creatinine clearance	<130 ml/min

HELLP, Hemolysis, elevated liver enzymes, and low platelet count in association with preeclampsia; *AST,* aspartate transaminase; *SGOT,* serum glutamic oxaloacetic transaminase; *ALT,* alanine transaminase; *SGPT,* serum glutamic pyruvate transaminase.

Intensive Hemodynamic Monitoring

Intensive hemodynamic monitoring is not considered a standard of practice for severe preeclampsia or eclampsia according to the American College of Obstetricians and Gynecologists (1996). However, many clinicians find it helpful in determining appropriate therapy if pulmonary edema, oliguria, or blood pressure unresponsive to therapy results.

NURSING PROCESS

PREVENTION

Because the etiology of the disease is unknown, it is difficult to outline a protocol for prevention. Based on scientific studies, some general principles, however, appear to decrease the incidence of this disease.

- **Adequate Nutrition:** All pregnant patients should receive instructions regarding the benefits of eating a nutritious, balanced diet containing at least 60 to 70 g of protein; 1200 mg of calcium; and an adequate intake of magnesium, sodium (salt), other minerals, and vitamins every day. Drinking 6 to 8 glasses of water or fluid per day should be included in the instructions. If the pregnant patient is not including adequate calcium in her diet, a supplement of 2 g of total calcium gluconate per day has been shown by research to reduce the risk of preeclampsia (Sanchez-Ramos and others, 1994).

- **Adequate Rest:** Bed rest facilitates venous return, increasing the circulatory volume, enhancing renal and placental perfusion, and lowering blood pressure. Therefore high risk patients may benefit from 8 to 12 hours of sleep each night with a rest period in the middle of the day. Bed rest also mobilizes edematous fluid back into the intravascular space (Zuspan, 1991a).

- **Water Therapy:** In the presence of severe edema, research has demonstrated that shoulder-deep immersion in water can mobilize extravascular fluid; initiate diuresis; and decrease the renin, angiotensin, aldosterone, and vasopressin levels (Katz and others, 1990). Therefore water therapy may be helpful in the prevention or slowing of the progression of preeclampsia. It has also been shown to help reverse oligohydramnios resulting from uteroplacental insufficiency (Strong, 1993).

- **Early and Appropriate Prenatal Care:** Early, appropriate treatment is effective in preventing the severe form of preeclampsia or eclampsia. Therefore early detection of its development is effective in lowering the high maternal and fetal mortality associated with the disease. Detection should begin on the first prenatal visit early in pregnancy. The nurse practitioner or nurse should obtain an in-depth patient history that includes age and parity; a medical history of such things as diabetes and persistent hypertensive disorders; and familial history of preeclampsia or eclampsia. On each prenatal visit the patient should be weighed, an accurate blood pressure reading obtained, and an early-morning urine specimen checked for protein. If protein is noted in the urine, it should be checked for bacteria and another specimen obtained by clean-catch midstream collection or minicatheterization, because bacteria, vaginal discharge, blood, and amniotic fluid can give a false-positive result.

- **Low-Dose Aspirin:** A number of recent studies but not all have demonstrated that low-dose aspirin therapy (60 to 80 mg/day) may reduce the incidence of preeclampsia in some women at risk for the disease (Hauth, Cunningham, 1995; Royal College of Obstetricians and Gynecologists, 1996; Sibai and others, 1993b; Zuspan, Samuels, 1993). Aspirin selectively inhibits thromboxane production with minimal effect on prostacyclin synthesis. Therefore it restores the prostacyclin/thromboxane balance. This low dose appears to have no harmful effects on the fetus or neonate (CLASP Collaborative Group, 1995; Hauth, Cunningham, 1995; Hauth and others, 1993; Louden and others, 1994). However, some researchers found an increased incidence of abruptio placentae (Hauth and others, 1993; Sibai and others, 1993b). Further studies are needed to approve aspirin for prevention of preeclampsia. Therefore it should be used only in selected high risk patients (Cunningham and others, 1997; Hines, Jones, 1994).

ASSESSMENT

MATERNAL WELL-BEING

When any patient is diagnosed with preeclampsia, the nurse must continually gather in-depth data to detect early indicators that the condition is deteriorating.

- **Assess Cardiovascular System:** Blood pressure and pulse should be checked every 4 hours while the patient is awake or more often if indicated. The blood pressure should be taken

TABLE 20-5 Degree of edema

Physical findings	Score
Minimal edema of lower extremities	+1
Marked edema of lower extremities	+2
Edema of lower extremities, face, hands	+3
Generalized massive edema including abdomen and sacrum	+4

TABLE 20-6 Proteinuria

Dipstick reading	Protein
Trace	—
+1	30 mg/L
+2	100 mg/L
+3	300 mg/L
+4	>2000 mg/L

Multistix package insert, Bayer Corp. Diagnostic Division, Elkhart, Ind, 1995.

on the same arm with the patient in the same position each time. Preferably the patient should be lying on her left side with the cuff on the right arm. The degree of edema should be evaluated every 8 hours and scored as shown in Table 20-5. A daily weight should be obtained before breakfast.

- **Assess Renal System:** The urine should be evaluated for protein, specific gravity, pH, and glucose daily or every 8 hours. The gram equivalent of protein as indicated on the dipstick is outlined in Table 20-6. A 24-hour urine collection for protein may be ordered. The loss of 5 g or more of protein per 24 hours indicates severe preeclampsia. An intake and output record should be kept. If the urinary output is less than 30 ml/hr or 120 ml/4 hr, oliguria is present. This indicates that the condition is deteriorating.
- **Assess Central Nervous System:** Deep tendon reflexes (DTRs) should be checked daily or more often if indicated. The easiest DTR to check is the patellar reflex (knee jerk). The response elicited should be graded as shown in Table 20-7. At the same time it should be determined whether clonus is present. If clonus is present, dorsiflexion of the foot causes spasms of the muscle. This is seen as convulsive movement of the foot and indicates neuromuscular irritability.

TABLE 20-7   Deep tendon reflex (DTR) grading

Physical result	Grade
None elicited	0
Sluggish or dull	+1
Active, normal	+2
Brisk	+3
Brisk with transient clonus	+4
Brisk with sustained clonus	+5

Data from Barkauskas V and others: *Health and physical assessment,* St Louis, 1994, Mosby.

- **Assess Pulmonary System:** The respiration rate should be checked every 4 hours while the patient is awake or more often if indicated. The lung fields should be auscultated for wheezing or crackles, which can indicate pulmonary edema. Signs of dyspnea, tightness of the chest, shallow respiration, or a cough should be noted.
- **Assess for Worsening Signs:** The nurse should assess for subjective signs and symptoms that indicate that the condition is deteriorating. Severe, persistent headache, visual disturbances, epigastric pain, and restlessness are warning signs of impending eclampsia. Epigastric or right upper quadrant pain, nausea, vomiting, malaise, headache, jaundice, and hematuria are signs of possible development of the HELLP syndrome. Signs of bleeding, such as oozing from IV sites, nosebleeds, and petechiae, may indicate DIC development.
- **Assess Reproductive System:** Assess for the presence of uterine contractions because decreased uteroplacental blood flow can initiate labor. Assess for signs of an abruptio placentae, which are dark red vaginal bleeding, sustained abdominal pain, uterine tenderness, tetanic contractions, and increasing fundal height.

FETAL SURVEILLANCE STUDIES

Because of the reduced blood supply to the fetus, constant surveillance is critical.

- **Fetal Heart Rate:** Fetal heart rate (FHR) should be checked every 4 hours with a Doppler FHR device, or a continuous electronic fetal monitor (EFM) should be used if the condition so indicates.
- **Fetal Movement:** Fetal movements should be recorded daily. This has been shown to correlate with fetal well-being. Fetal

movements reduced from the patient's previous pattern may indicate fetal hypoxia. Rayburn (1987) has developed a protocol for interpreting fetal activity. According to his protocol, inactivity is indicated when there are fewer than four fetal movements per hour for 2 consecutive days (Cunningham and others, 1997).

- **Other Fetal Surveillance Studies:** Appropriate fetal surveillance tests, such as nonstress test (NST), contraction stress test (CST), or biophysical profile (BPP) with frequent amniotic fluid assessment, are carried out at appropriate intervals after 28 to 30 weeks of gestation.

NURSING DIAGNOSES AND INTERVENTIONS

- **RISK FOR ALTERED NUTRITION: LESS THAN BODY REQUIREMENTS** related to the increased requirements of pregnancy.

  DESIRED OUTCOMES: The patient's daily diet will include six 1-oz servings of protein (60 to 70 g), four servings from the milk group (1200 mg of calcium), six to eleven servings from the grain group (half are whole grains), three to five servings from the vegetable group, and two to four servings from the fruit group. The patient will gain approximately 1 pound per week during the second and third trimesters of pregnancy.

  INTERVENTIONS
  1. Assess the patient's nutritional status, and obtain a diet profile.
  2. Analyze the patient's diet for adequate calories, protein, calcium, salt, and vitamins.
  3. Based on the analysis, instruct the patient regarding needed changes, keeping in mind the patient's likes and dislikes.
  4. Teach the patient to avoid foods high in sodium, such as processed foods or already prepared foods such as potato chips and salted nuts.
  5. Provide the patient with information regarding the relationship of diet and preeclampsia.

- **RISK FOR INJURY** related to disease progression causing musculoskeletal trauma or aspiration if eclampsia develops.

  DESIRED OUTCOME: The patient will not have seizures, or, if eclampsia develops, the patient will not be injured.

  INTERVENTIONS

  Seizure precautions
  1. Assess for signs of impending eclampsia, such as epigastric or right upper quadrant pain, nausea and vomiting, headache, jaundice, and hematuria.

2. Implement seizure precautions by having oxygen, suction, a padded tongue blade, and supplies to pad side rails at bedside.

3. Provide a quiet, pleasant environment with limited lighting so as not to activate further the already overstimulated CNS.

4. Limit visitors except the patient's family.

5. Administer magnesium sulfate as ordered. Teach patient about the possible side effects of hot flashes, nausea, or vomiting.

6. Assess for signs of magnesium toxicity, such as absence of DTRs, respirations fewer than 12/min, or a significant drop in pulse or blood pressure. Monitor urinary output, since magnesium sulfate is excreted by way of the kidneys. Note serum magnesium levels.

7. Have antidote of calcium gluconate at bedside.

8. Notify attending physician of any worsening signs, including signs of magnesium sulfate toxicity.

During the seizure

1. Remain with the patient. Assess patency of airway.

2. Facilitate insertion of airway when seizure activity permits.

3. Observe seizure activity for time of occurrence, length of seizure, and type of seizure activity.

4. Lower and turn patient's head to one side to keep airway open and decrease risk of aspiration.

5. Call for help by turning on the patient's call light.

6. Protect the patient from injury by having side rails up and padded if possible.

7. Administer oxygen by face mask to increase fetal oxygenation.

8. Notify physician at the first sign of convulsive activity.

After the seizure

1. Assess airway, and suction if needed. Maintain adequate oxygenation by administering oxygen via face mask at 10 L/min.

2. Start an IV line as soon as possible. Monitor IV fluid closely with infusion pump.

3. Administer magnesium sulfate as ordered to prevent another seizure.

4. Check blood pressure to assess for hypertension.

5. Check FHR (bradycardia may result from the hypoxic and acidotic state).

6. Assess urine for protein.

7. Provide a quiet environment.

8. Assess for signs of restlessness or fundal tightening, which may indicate the start of labor.

9. Notify attending physician of signs of labor.

■ **ALTERED MATERNAL TISSUE PERFUSION (RENAL, HEPATIC, AND CEREBRAL)** related to disease progression causing cerebral or renal ischemia and hepatic failure.

DESIRED OUTCOMES: The patient will maintain a stable blood pressure and weight gain on limited activity, with less than +2 proteinuria and +2 reflexes. The patient will manifest no signs of headache, visual changes, epigastric pain, nausea, vomiting, or oliguria.

INTERVENTIONS

1. Take pulse, respirations, and blood pressure every 4 hours or as ordered.

2. Take temperature four times daily or as ordered. (Fever can decrease platelet survival.)

3. Assess fluid retention by monitoring input and output, checking daily weight before breakfast each day, and observing for signs of edema.

4. Check urine for pH, specific gravity, and protein every 8 hours.

5. Observe for signs that indicate condition is deteriorating, such as headache, visual changes, epigastric pain, oliguria, increasing blood pressure, and dyspnea.

6. Check DTRs every shift.

7. Refer to laboratory data that facilitate diagnosis of the HELLP syndrome, such as platelet count, fibrin split products, and liver enzymes such as aspartate aminotransferase (AST), alanine aminotransferase (ALT), and lactic dehydrogenase (LDH).

8. Assess for signs of DIC such as oozing blood from the IV site, easy bruising, bleeding gums, or petechiae.

9. Institute limited activity, and encourage left lateral position when in bed.

10. Teach self-care such as the therapeutic effects of limiting activity and danger signs to report immediately.

11. Teach the patient that exercises are important in keeping the muscles in tone and in increasing blood flow. The patient should be instructed to do leg exercises such as foot circles at least twice each day. She should also be instructed to do the super Kegel and abdominal tightening exercises to keep the perineal and abdominal muscles in tone. If the patient

complains of back pain, the pelvic rock can help relieve this discomfort (see Box 1-1).

12. Notify the attending physician if the blood pressure increases 10 mm Hg or more, DTR is +3 or greater, or proteinuria is +3 or greater and if any subjective signs develop that indicate condition is deteriorating.

- **RISK FOR FLUID VOLUME EXCESS** related to excessive fluid administration causing congestive heart failure or pulmonary or cerebral edema.
  DESIRED OUTCOMES: The patient will exhibit no signs of dyspnea, crackles, headache, and nausea or vomiting. She will have a balanced intake and output, edema will be +1 or less, and her heart rate will be maintained under 100 beats/min.
  INTERVENTIONS
  1. Weigh patient daily before breakfast for pathologic edema signs.
  2. Assess for signs of pulmonary edema such as tightness in the chest, shortness of breath, cough, shallow respirations, wheezing, and diminished breath sounds.
  3. Assess heart rate and rhythm.
  4. Note change in hematocrit level.
  5. Keep an accurate intake and output record.
  6. Administer isotonic crystalloid fluids or colloid-containing fluids to increase colloid osmotic pressure as ordered. Avoid the use of hypotonic fluids in fluid replacement therapy since they may further decrease the serum osmolarity.
  7. Base initial intake of fluid on the need to combat dehydration. (Usual amount for first 24 hours is 1500 to 3000 ml of fluid. Therefore, if patient is not dehydrated, fluid intake equals amount of urinary output of the previous 24 hours plus 1000 ml except in acute renal failure; then intake should not exceed 500 ml.) If oliguria develops, fluid administration is best guided by pulmonary capillary wedge pressure (PCWP).
  8. Notify attending physician if urinary output is less than 120 ml/4 hr or patient exhibits any signs of fluid volume excess.

- **FEAR** related to lack of predictable outcome for self and her fetus.
  DESIRED OUTCOME: The patient and her family will communicate their fears and concerns openly.

INTERVENTIONS
1. Provide time for the patient and her family to express their concerns regarding the possible outcome for the baby and inconvenience to the mother and family during the treatment. Encourage them to vent any feelings, fears, and anger they may experience.
2. Assess family's support system and coping mechanisms.
3. Provide understandable information to the patient and her family regarding the disease process, plan of treatment, and implications for mother and fetus.
4. Explain all treatment modalities and reasons for each.
5. Keep patient informed of health status, results of tests, and fetal well-being.
6. Refer to a spiritual counselor or chaplain on request.

- **RISK FOR ALTERED ROLE PERFORMANCE** related to hospitalization and treatment with limited activity.
  DESIRED OUTCOME: The patient will verbalize a plan that will take care of all her responsibilities.
  INTERVENTIONS
  1. Assess the patient's responsibilities to determine difficulties she will face in implementing prescribed limited activity.
  2. Teach the patient and her family about the importance of limited activity even though she feels reasonably well.
  3. Help the patient and her family in problem solving difficulties in implementing limited activity.
  4. Make needed referrals, for example, to the social worker, if problems are identified.
  5. Encourage participation in her care and decision making as much as possible.

- **DIVERSIONAL ACTIVITY DEFICIT** related to the therapeutic treatment of limited activity.
  DESIRED OUTCOME: The patient will verbalize various activities she would like to do.
  INTERVENTIONS
  1. Assess patient's interest in various diversional activities within the activity limit.
  2. Provide crafts, reading, and puzzles that can be done in bed, or encourage patient to have these things brought in.
  3. Provide classes in preparation for childbirth by way of video, the hospital television, or group classes that can be attended while reclining.

4. Refer to a diversional therapist or volunteer to provide reading materials, handicrafts, or other interesting things.

■ **RISK FOR IMPAIRED FETAL GAS EXCHANGE** related to the possible effect of the disease on uterine blood flow and the development of a complication such as abruptio placentae.

DESIRED OUTCOMES: The fetus will remain active, and its heart rate will remain between 110 and 160 beats/min. The BPPs will continue to be over 6 with a negative, reactive CST and a reactive NST.

INTERVENTIONS

1. Monitor FHR manually or electronically as indicated.
2. Carry out NST, CST, or BPP as ordered.
3. Assess for signs of abruptio placentae, such as dark vaginal bleeding, sustained abdominal pain, uterine tenderness, tetanic contractions, and increasing fundal height.
4. Teach patient to keep a daily fetal movement chart by counting the number of fetal movements felt in 1 hour. If there are fewer than four movements felt in that hour, she should report it, because fetal activity decreases if hypoxia develops (Cunningham and others, 1997; Rayburn, 1987).
5. Explain any ordered test such as a BPP, CST, and amniocentesis for L/S ratio or phosphatidyl glycerol (PG).
6. If the patient smokes, she should be instructed that smoking further decreases the blood flow to the uterus. Make appropriate referrals if she chooses to quit.
7. Notify physician if FHR drops from baseline or patient reports decreased fetal movements.

COLLABORATIVE INTERVENTION FOR ANTICONVULSANT THERAPY

Magnesium sulfate

Magnesium sulfate is the ideal drug in the prevention and treatment of convulsions related to preeclampsia (ACOG, 1996; Roberts, 1994b).

Action

Magnesium sulfate acts by doing the following:

1. Decreasing neuromuscular irritability and blocking the release of acetylcholine at neuromuscular junctions. Acetylcholine is the excitatory substance that transmits nerve messages across the synapse.
2. Depressing the vasomotor center by acting on the peripheral vascular system. This causes slight vasodilation, which increases blood flow to the uterus and can cause a transient

episode of lowered blood pressure for 30 to 45 minutes after administration.

3. Depressing the CNS, thereby decreasing CNS irritability.

Other beneficial actions

Magnesium sulfate has been shown to cause peripheral vasodilation, increase uterine and renal blood flow, increase prostacyclin production by endothelial cells, reduce platelet aggregation, and decrease the action of plasma renin and angiotensin (Eclampsia Trial Collaborative Group, 1995). It is superior to phenytoin (Lucas and others, 1994, 1995; Sibai, 1996a).

Dosage

Therapeutic administration of magnesium sulfate usually consists of an initial loading dose of 4 g by IV push administered over 15 to 20 minutes, followed by a maintenance dose of 2 to 3 g/hr diluted in 5% dextrose and lactated Ringer's solution administered by an infusion pump to maintain hyporeflexia. The maintenance dose can also be administered intramuscularly. The normal dosage is 5 g per buttock or a total of 10 g every 4 hours. Intramuscular injections of magnesium sulfate are seldom used because the rate of absorption cannot be controlled, tissue necrosis can develop, and the injections are painful. If magnesium sulfate is administered intramuscularly, Z-track technique should be used with a 3-inch, 20-gauge dry needle to ensure that the medication is injected deep into the gluteal muscle, and the site should be gently massaged to facilitate absorption. A local anesthetic agent can be added to the magnesium sulfate solution to minimize the discomfort.

Side effects

Frequently experienced side effects are lethargy, sensations of heat or burning, headache, nausea and vomiting, visual blurring, and constipation. The patient should be prepared for these normal side effects. Because magnesium sulfate decreases smooth muscle contractility by moving calcium out of the smooth muscle, it decreases uterine activity and can prolong labor. However, it is ineffective in suppressing uterine activity once labor becomes active. Because magnesium blocks neuromuscular and cardiac transmission of nerve impulses and depresses the CNS, respiratory paralysis and cardiac arrest can result if serum magnesium levels rise too high. Plasma levels of 4 to 7 mEq/L are very effective in preventing convulsions, demonstrated by depressed DTRs. Plasma levels between 8 and 10 mEq/L cause a loss of DTRs, which is the first sign of toxicity. Other early signs are nausea, a feeling of warmth, flushing, somnolence, double vision, slurred speech, and weakness.

Plasma levels above 13 to 15 mEq/L can cause respiratory paralysis, and levels greater than 20 to 25 mEq/L can cause cardiac arrest (Table 20-8). Therefore serum magnesium levels should be assessed daily. Magnesium can have some detrimental effects on the fetus as well. Relatively less FHR variability at therapeutic levels and neonatal neuromuscular and respiratory depression have been seen.

Nursing interventions

Based on the action of the drug, the nurse should assess any patient receiving magnesium sulfate for early signs of magnesium toxicity. The DTR should be checked every hour if the patient is on continuous IV drip and before administering each dose if the patient is on intermittent therapy (see Table 20-7). The respiratory rate, pulse, and blood pressure should be checked initially every 5 minutes and then every 15 to 30 minutes if the patient is receiving a continuous IV drip or before administering each dose if the patient is receiving intermittent therapy.

Magnesium is excreted largely in the urine so the patient with kidney involvement can develop toxicity rapidly. Therefore the patient's intake and output should be monitored closely. If the patient is receiving a continuous IV drip, the urinary output should be at least 30 ml/hr. If the patient is receiving intermittent doses of magnesium, the urinary output should be obtained every 4 hours and should be at least 120 ml/4 hr. To decrease the risk of pulmonary edema, the total fluid intake for 24 hours should not exceed 2000 ml.

Magnesium sulfate should be discontinued or withheld and the

TABLE 20-8 Serum magnesium levels

Magnesium levels (mEq/L)	Magnesium levels (mg/dl)	Interpretation
1.5-2.5	1.7-2.1	Normal
4-7	5-8	Therapeutic
8-10	10-12	Loss of deep tendon reflexes
13-15	16-18	Respiratory paralysis
15-20	18-25	Heart block
20-25	25-30	Cardiac arrest

Data from Heppard M, Garite T: *Acute obstetrics: a practical guide,* St Louis, 1996, Mosby.

attending physician notified if any of the following signs are present:

- No DTR or a sudden change in the DTR
- Respirations fewer than 12/min
- Urinary output less than 30 ml/hr or 120 ml/4 hr
- A significant drop in pulse or blood pressure
- Signs of fetal distress

Serum magnesium levels are also useful in assessing magnesium toxicity. Therapeutic levels are between 4 and 7 mEq/L.

Calcium gluconate is the antidote for magnesium toxicity because calcium stimulates the release of acetylcholine at the nerve synapse. Ten milliliters of a 10% solution (1 g) is the normal dose given by IV push. This should be administered by the physician over 3 minutes to avoid undesirable reactions such as bradycardia, dysrhythmias, and ventricular fibrillation. It can also be administered intravenously at a rate of 1 g/hr if needed.

Phenytoin

Phenytoin (Dilantin) is one of the most commonly used anticonvulsants for the nonpregnant patient. Recently it has been under research investigation and has been found to be a suitable alternative anticonvulsant for preeclampsia, but magnesium sulfate is superior (ACOG, 1996; Eclampsia Trial Collaborative Group, 1995; Lucas and others, 1995; Sibai, 1996b). The possibility of convulsions is increased in the preeclamptic patient being treated with phenytoin because of the latency of onset (Dommisse, 1990; Ryan and others, 1989).

Action

Phenytoin acts by doing the following (Ryan and others, 1989):

- Suppressing the influx of sodium ions across cell membranes during potential repetitive neuronal activity
- Blocking the changes in the concentrations of potassium and calcium ions that occur before seizure activity, thus lowering the neuronal excitation threshold

Dosage

The therapeutic loading dose is usually 10 mg/kg of current weight, diluted in 250 ml of normal saline or lactated Ringer's solution. A dextrose solution should not be used since a precipitation will occur (Lucas, Jordan, 1997). The rate of infusion is between 25 and 40 mg/min. An additional dose of 5 mg/kg is given 2 hours later. Because the half-life of this drug is 12 hours, which is relatively long compared with that of magnesium sulfate, a maintenance dose may not be needed. It is given based on the serum phenytoin levels. The therapeutic range for phenytoin is 10 to 20 μg/ml.

Side effects

Burning at the IV site is the most common side effect and is related to the alkalinity of the dissolver (Ryan and others, 1989). Hypotension occurs if the IV infusion is given too rapidly (Lucas, Jordan, 1997). Other side effects seen are cardiac dysrhythmias, bradycardia, and heart block; ataxia, slurred speech, mental confusion, and decreased coordination; nausea/vomiting; and double or blurred vision (Heppard, Garite, 1996). This drug does not appear to cause decreased FHR variability or decreased neonatal tone (Repke, Chez, 1989). Phenytoin has no effect on suppression of labor. Mothers are more alert, awake, and able to breast-feed compared with mothers who received magnesium (Lucas, Jordan, 1997).

COLLABORATIVE INTERVENTION FOR ANTIHYPERTENSIVE THERAPY: PREECLAMPSIA

Hydralazine

If the diastolic blood pressure is greater than 110 mm Hg or the systolic greater than 180 mm Hg, the mother's risk of a cerebrovascular accident (CVA) is increased. Treatment should be implemented to reduce the blood pressure to a level that will provide a margin of maternal safety without compromising adequate uterine perfusion. Hydralazine (Apresoline) is the antihypertensive drug of choice in the United States because it is more effective in lowering mean arterial pressure to safe levels (Cunningham and others, 1997). Because of production process issues, availability of hydralazine may be questionable for the future (Heppard, Garite, 1996).

Action

Hydralazine acts on the following systems:

- The arterioles, causing them to relax, thereby decreasing arteriolar spasms
- The vasomotor center, thereby decreasing blood pressure
- The heart, stimulating cardiac output

Because of these three actions, peripheral blood flow is increased, which increases renal, cerebral, liver, coronary, and placental blood flow (Wilson and others, 1997).

Dosage

The normal method of administration is 5 to 10 mg by IV push administered over 10 minutes. The dose can be repeated every 20 minutes until the diastolic blood pressure is between 90 and 100 mm Hg. The diastolic blood pressure should not be allowed to fall below 90 mm Hg to prevent further reduction in blood flow to the placenta. Hydralazine is administered whenever the diastolic blood pressure again reaches 110 mm Hg.

Side effects
Side effects the patient can experience are tachycardia, dizziness, faintness, headache, palpitations, numbness, tingling of the extremities, and disorientation.

Nursing interventions
The nurse is responsible for checking the blood pressure every minute for the first 5 minutes following administration and then every 5 minutes for the next 30 minutes. This is best accomplished with an automatic blood pressure cuff if available. The drug is excreted in breast milk so the patient should not start breast-feeding until 48 hours after the last dose of this medication has been given (Brengman, Burns, 1988; Lawrence, 1994).

Labetalol hydrochloride
Labetalol hydrochloride (Normodyne, Trandate) is an antihypertensive agent and is an acceptable alternative for use in the treatment of severe gestational hypertension (ACOG, 1996).

Action
Labetalol hydrochloride is a combined alpha- and beta-blocker that decreases peripheral vascular resistance without changing cardiac output. Therefore labetalol lowers blood pressure while maintaining placental blood flow (Walker, 1991). It may not be effective in patients receiving alpha- or beta-antagonists (Heppard, Garite, 1996).

Dosage
Labetalol may be administered by a bolus IV injection of 50 mg over 10 minutes followed by a continuous infusion of 1 to 2 mg/kg/hr (Heppard, Garite, 1996).

Side effects
Side effects the patient can experience are nausea, vomiting, scalp tingling, hypotension, bronchospasm, and in rare cases, heart block and heart failure (Dildy, Clark, 1993).

Nifedipine
Nifedipine (Procardia) is another hypertensive medication that is used occasionally.

Action
Nifedipine is a calcium channel blocker that causes vasodilation of the coronary arteries, maximizing blood flow to the cardiac muscle, and reduces total peripheral resistance, reducing cardiac afterload (Zatuchni, Slupik, 1996).

Dosage
The normal dose is 10 to 20 mg taken orally every 20 to 30 minutes until BP<140/100. According to Eglinton (1996), in a hypertensive

emergency the patient may bite, chew, and swallow the capsule to achieve therapeutic effect in 3 minutes.

Side effects

Side effects the patient can experience are dizziness, light-headedness, headache, facial flushing, heat sensation, and peripheral edema (Wilson and others, 1997).

COLLABORATIVE INTERVENTION FOR ANTIHYPERTENSIVE THERAPY: CHRONIC HYPERTENSION

Chronic hypertension occurs in approximately 4% to 5% of all pregnancies, with 21% developing superimposed preeclampsia (Zuspan, 1996). According to Zuspan (1996) the best therapy is periodic bed rest of 45 minutes in the middle of the day and 1 hour before the evening meal to promote uterine blood flow. A regimen of tapering and stopping hypertensive medication is usually tried (Cunningham and others, 1997; Rey, Couturier, 1994). When the diastolic blood pressure exceeds 90 to 100 mm Hg or there is left ventricular hypertrophy, drug therapy is usually initiated. The drug of choice continues to be methyldopa (Aldomet) (ACOG, 1996). The usual dose for methyldopa is 750 to 2000 mg/day. The alternative hypertensive drugs used to treat chronic hypertension during pregnancy are either a beta-blocker, such as atenolol (Tenormin), labetalol (Trandate), or pindolol (Visken), or a calcium channel blocker, such as nifedipine. (See Table 20-9 for common dosages of these hypertensive medications.) The new angiotensin-converting enzyme inhibitors are contraindicated during pregnancy since they decrease uterine blood flow and may increase the chance of intrauterine growth restriction or fetal death (Walker, 1991; Zuspan, 1991a). All chronic hypertensive pregnant patients should be monitored carefully for an abruption as well as superimposed preeclampsia. They have a fourfold to eightfold increased risk of an abruption and a 20% chance of developing superimposed preeclampsia (Zuspan, 1996). Antepartum fetal assessment should begin at 28 to 30 weeks of gestation since the fetus is at greater risk of IUGR.

COLLABORATIVE INTERVENTION FOR INVASIVE HEMODYNAMIC MONITORING

Recommended use

Because it is impossible to differentiate clinically among the varying causative factors of severe preeclampsia or eclampsia, invasive hemodynamic monitoring is being recommended for severe preeclampsia or eclampsia complicated with pulmonary edema, persistent oliguria, or severe hypertension unresponsive to hydralazine treatment (ACOG, 1996; Cowles and others, 1994).

TABLE 20-9   Antihypertensive medications for chronic hypertension during pregnancy

Medication	Drug classification	Usual dosages	Maximum dosage
Methyldopa (Drug of choice: Aldomet)	Central acting antiadrenergic agent	250 mg po bid or tid	2000 mg
Atenolol (Tenormin)	Beta-blocker	50-100 mg po qd	100 mg
Labetalol (Trandate)	Beta-blocker	Start at 100 mg po bid Usual dose 200-400 mg bid	
Pindolol (Visken)	Beta-blocker	Start at 5 mg po bid	60 mg/day
Nifedipine (Procardia)	Calcium channel blocker	10 mg po tid or 10-20 mg po q 4-6 h	120 mg/day

Developed from information in Lindsay L, Barbour L: In Queenan J, Hobbins J, editors: *Protocols for high-risk pregnancies,* ed 3, Cambridge, England, 1996, Blackwell Science. *bid,* Twice daily; *tid,* three times daily; *po,* orally; *q,* every.

Hemodynamic monitoring with a pulmonary artery catheter (Swan-Ganz catheter) to measure central venous pressure (CVP) and pulmonary capillary wedge pressure (PCWP) allows precise assessment of the underlying pathophysiology, thus allowing the medical team to specifically tailor and evaluate the therapy. However, its routine use even if pulmonary edema develops is questioned by Cunningham and others (1997) because of the usual quick response to IV furosemide.

Causes of varying hemodynamic patterns

Severe preeclampsia or eclampsia manifests varying hemodynamic patterns related to the disease process. For example, elevated blood pressure may be related to increased vascular resistance or increased cardiac output. Pulmonary edema may result from volume overload and is the result of left ventricular failure from extremely high vascular resistance or excessive fluid infusion during treatment of the disease. Volume overload can also occur during the postpartum period when normal mobilization of the third-space fluid occurs. The two other factors that can cause pulmonary edema are (1) further reduced colloid osmotic pressure and (2) increased pulmonary capillary permeability related to capillary wall damage. Oliguria is related to decreased renal blood flow as the result of intravascular volume depletion or severe vascular resistance, which can cause left ventricular failure. Occasionally specific renal arteriospasms disproportionate to the systemic vasospasms can cause oliguria.

Table 20-10 gives manifestations of preeclampsia that should be evaluated with invasive hemodynamic monitoring.

COLLABORATIVE INTERVENTION FOR HELLP SYNDROME

Signs and symptoms

Epigastric pain or right upper quadrant tenderness

Epigastric pain occurs in 65% of cases of HELLP syndrome and is related to obstructed hepatic blood flow because of fibrin deposition (Usta, Sibai, 1996).

Flulike symptoms

Flulike symptoms, such as malaise, occur 90% of the time with HELLP syndrome (Usta, Sibai, 1996).

Generalized edema

Patients with HELLP syndrome usually present with significant edema (Barton, Sibai, 1991).

Nausea and vomiting

Nausea and vomiting related to hepatic stretching (Usta, Sibai, 1996) occur in 50% of cases of HELLP syndrome.

Severe elevated blood pressure

A severe elevation in blood pressure is not present with HELLP syndrome in 20% of the cases (Usta, Sibai, 1996).

Proteinuria

Protein in the urine is variable and is not always present in HELLP syndrome (Poole, 1988).

Criteria for diagnosis

All three of the following parameters must be present for the diagnosis of HELLP syndrome to be made.

Hemolysis

Hemolysis is indicated by an abnormal peripheral smear and total bilirubin greater than 1.2 mg/dl.

Elevated liver enzymes

Elevated liver enzymes include AST (SGOT) greater than 72 U/L; ALT (SGPT) greater than 50 U/L, and serum LDH greater than 600 IU/L.

Low platelet count

The platelet count is less than 100,000/mm^3.

TABLE 20-10 Manifestations of preeclampsia that should be evaluated with invasive hemodynamic monitoring

Disease manifestation	Causes	Hemodynamic values	Possible treatment
Hypertensive crisis	Increased cardiac output related to increased heart rate and stroke volume	Normal preload High cardiac output	Reduce cardiac preload with beta-blocker agents and vasodilators
	Increased systemic vascular resistance	Increased PCWP ($\geq$18 mm Hg)	Reduce systemic vascular resistance Bed rest in left lateral position Antihypertensive therapy such as hydralazine hydrochloride
Pulmonary edema	Noncardiogenic Decreased colloid osmotic pressure	Normal PCWP (6-10 mm Hg) (AWHONN, 1994)	Administer colloid fluids
	Increased pulmonary capillary permeability	Normal PCWP	Maintain filling pressures in lower-normal range
	Cardiogenic Volume overload related to left ventricular failure resulting from high vascular resistance	Increased PCWP	Decrease afterload with bed rest and antihypertensive therapy

Oliguria	Volume overload related to iatrogenic fluid overload Volume overload related to normal postpartum mobilization of third-space fluid (diuresis)	Increased CVP Normal or increased PCWP	Attempt diuresis with diuretic such as furosemide
	Decreased renal blood flow related to intravascular volume depletion	Decreased CVP (<4 mm Hg)	Administer colloid or crystalloid fluid boluses
	Decreased renal blood flow related to severe vascular resistance causing left ventricular failure	Increased PCWP (>18 mm Hg)	Decrease vascular resistance Bed rest in the left lateral position Antihypertensive drugs such as hydralazine hydrochloride
	Specific renal arteriospasms disproportionate to systemic vasospasms	Normal PCWP Normal CVP (1-7 mm Hg) (AWHONN, 1994)	Treat with low-dose dopamine infusion

PCWP, Pulmonary capillary wedge pressure; *CVP,* central venous pressure.

Nursing interventions

If possible, the patient should be transferred to a tertiary-care center.

Assess maternal status

Assess for signs of the HELLP syndrome, and assist with obtaining ordered diagnostic tests. Observe for signs of renal failure, DIC, hepatic hematoma or rupture, and abruption. Signs of hepatic rupture are shock, oliguria, and fever. Check for the development of hypoglycemia, which may indicate an acute fatty liver. Implement the same monitoring protocol as for the severe preeclamptic patient.

Assess fetal status

Monitor FHR, and carry out ordered fetal surveillance studies such as an NST or BPP. Be prepared to assist with fetal lung maturity studies.

Assist with stabilization

Stabilization management is the same as for a patient with severe preeclampsia.

Prepare for delivery

If the fetus is immature, attempts may be made to stabilize the patient, undelivered, until steroids can be administered. If the fetus is mature and the cervix is ripe, a vaginal delivery may be attempted. Otherwise, a cesarean delivery is usually performed after stabilization (Sibai, 1996a).

Postpartum considerations

The onset of the HELLP syndrome develops 30% of the time during the postpartum period. Clinical manifestations of the syndrome usually occur within the first 48 hours postpartum.

COLLABORATIVE INTERVENTION FOR ECLAMPSIA

Warning signs of impending eclampsia

Severe, persistent headache, visual disturbances, epigastric pain, and restlessness are warning signs of impending eclampsia.

Eclamptic seizure

The convulsive activity begins with facial twitching followed by generalized muscle rigidity (Cunningham and others, 1997). During the convulsion, respiration ceases because of muscle spasms. Coma usually follows the seizure-like activity, and respiration naturally resumes.

Nursing interventions

Reduce the risk of aspiration

Establish the airway patency by lowering and turning the head to one side to keep the airway open and minimize aspiration. Suction any secretions from the mouth.

Prevent maternal injury

If possible, a padded tongue blade should be inserted with care between the teeth to prevent tongue injury and to facilitate the insertion of an airway if needed. Make sure the side rails are up and padded if possible.

Ensure maternal oxygenation after seizure

Assess breathing pattern, and administer oxygen at 10 L/min by tight face mask as needed to increase the maternal oxygen concentration and improve the oxygen supply to the fetus, which is lessened during a convulsion. Assess blood pressure, pulse, and respirations every 5 minutes until stable. Auscultate lung sounds to rule out aspiration.

Ensure fetal oxygenation after seizure

The FHR should be assessed continuously with a fetal monitor since the hypoxic and acidotic state of a seizure may cause fetal distress. The patient's position should be changed from left lateral to right lateral every 30 minutes to increase uterine and renal blood flow.

Establish seizure control with magnesium sulfate

Magnesium sulfate therapy is usually initiated as soon as the seizure stops. An IV line should be started with an 18-gauge intracatheter (if it has not already been inserted). The normal dosage is a 4-g IV loading dose followed by a continuous infusion of 2 g/hr. Delivery of IV fluid should be monitored closely to avoid exceeding 125 ml/hr to decrease risk of pulmonary edema. A Foley catheter should be inserted for hourly output, proteinuria, and specific gravity. Assess frequently for uterine contractions; a seizure frequently stimulates labor. During the coma phase, restlessness may indicate uterine contractions. Assess for abruptio placentae, which occurs in 23% of eclamptic patients (Sibai, 1996a), by checking for fundal height changes, uterine hyperactivity, vaginal bleeding, or fetal bradycardia. Assess for signs of the HELLP syndrome and DIC. There is a high frequency of HELLP syndrome and DIC in eclamptic patients (Miles and others, 1990). Throughout the delivery of care, the environment should be kept as quiet as possible and bright lights should be avoided to decrease CNS stimulation.

Treat severe hypertension

The blood pressure should be checked according to previously stated protocol as soon as possible to determine whether a hypertensive agent will be needed. Be prepared to administer an antihypertensive agent, such as hydralazine, if the diastolic blood pressure is greater than 110 mm Hg.

Correct maternal acidemia

Obtain blood gases following a seizure, and administer sodium bicarbonate only if pH is less than 7.10.

Initiate process of delivery

Once stabilization of mother and fetus has been achieved, delivery is usually initiated. If labor is not already underway, induction by a labor stimulant is usually attempted if there is no fetal malpresentation or distress and if the fetus is at least 33 weeks of gestational age. If the fetus is less than 33 weeks of gestation but the cervix is ripe, labor induction may be attempted. Cesarean birth will be the choice of delivery for all others.

Postpartum considerations

Thirty percent of the cases of eclampsia develop during the postpartum period (Usta, Sibai, 1996).

INTRAPARTUM INTERVENTION

Indications for delivery

Delivery is indicated in the PIH patient for the following reasons:

- Deterioration of fetal well-being
- Treatment ineffective in improving the disease as evidenced by worsening maternal symptoms or laboratory evidence of end-organ dysfunction
- Eclampsia or warning signs of eclampsia

Route of delivery

Vaginal delivery is usually attempted and achieved after induction with oxytocin; cesarean birth is the method of delivery if the following conditions are present:

- Labor does not begin promptly after attempted induction.
- Vaginal delivery is contraindicated for other obstetric reasons.
- The fetus weighs less than 1500 g.

Nursing interventions

The same precise care that was outlined for the antepartum period should be continued throughout the intrapartum period. If oxytocin is used, the contractions must be assessed frequently for hypertonus because the uterus may be more sensitive to oxytocin than usual (Cunningham and others, 1997). The progress of labor should be monitored closely because the patient may not be aware of the strength and frequency of her contractions. The fetus should be monitored very closely because the uteroplacental blood flow is already compromised and the added stress of labor may be too much for the fetus. Magnesium sulfate crosses the placenta readily. It can cause decreased beat-to-beat variability as seen on the fetal monitor strip. However, there is no indication that it adversely affects the fetus as long as the mother's serum magnesium level does not reach toxic levels.

The patient is usually very anxious about the well-being of the fetus and her own condition. Most women with preeclampsia or eclampsia are transferred to a high risk center. This can mean that they are a long way from home without any family members. This adds to the anxiety and stress of the condition. Therefore it is important for nurses who are providing skilled care to attempt to allay anxiety.

Analgesia and anesthesia

Analgesia during labor is limited to small doses and is withheld during the 2 hours before delivery. If the fetus is premature, analgesics should be avoided; they further depress an already compromised fetus. Administering anesthesia to a patient with PIH has added risks. Intrathecal or epidural block may induce hypotension detrimental to the fetus and mother because of the danger of administering large volumes of IV fluids to treat the hypotension. A general anesthesia may further elevate the blood pressure, especially during induction and awakening (Sibai, 1990). If the HELLP syndrome complicates the case, a low platelet count may increase the risk of hemorrhage associated with an epidural or pudendal block. Therefore the administration of any anesthetic should be done judiciously, with careful monitoring, and the most experienced anesthesiologist or nurse anesthetist involved.

POSTPARTUM INTERVENTION

Nursing interventions

If the patient has been receiving magnesium sulfate or another anticonvulsant, it is usually continued for 24 to 48 hours following delivery or longer if the HELLP syndrome coexisted (Martin and others, 1990; Miles and others, 1990). During this time the patient's condition should be monitored as closely as before; her condition can still deteriorate. This risk may be enhanced by normal postpartum diuresis. As diuresis takes place, an increased loss of magnesium leads to a drop in serum magnesium below therapeutic levels, and a convulsion could result. Blood loss is not tolerated as well as in the healthy postpartum patient because of the reduced blood volume caused by the disease process. Therefore the nurse should monitor the blood loss very closely. If the HELLP syndrome coexists, platelets, AST, ALT, and LDH levels are appropriate indicators of severity and progress toward recovery (Martin and others, 1990). There is a direct correlation between severity of the disease and the length of time for recovery (Martin and others, 1990).

Psychologic needs are great during the postpartum period. If the mother was not fully alert for all or part of the labor and delivery, it is important to fill in the gaps of the event for her. Most parents are also very concerned about their neonate's well-being. If the neonate was born prematurely or has IUGR and is in the intensive care nursery (ICN), the mother should be shown pictures of the infant and kept informed regarding the infant's condition. The father should be encouraged to visit the ICN. Then, when the mother's condition becomes stable, arrangements should be made for her to visit the ICN. Even if the neonate is healthy, the mother will need extra support, because she will be separated from her infant for a large portion of the first day or two following delivery. The mother needs limited neuromuscular stimulation and therefore will be kept in a dark, quiet environment with limited visitors.

The parents might be concerned about the effects of magnesium on their neonate. They should be reassured that it has no long-term negative side effects. The neonate may appear hypotonic at first. The parents should be informed that this is a temporary condition and it does not indicate neurologic damage. The mother may also be concerned about breast-feeding and the effects of magnesium. She should be reassured that no negative effect has been implicated and that the levels in breast milk are usually less than even in some formulas (Lawrence, 1994).

The patient who has chronic hypertension and must continue on hypertensive therapy should understand that antihypertensives are excreted in breast milk. The effect on the infant is unknown. If the patient has mild hypertension, the health care provider may withhold the medication during breast-feeding and closely observe the patient's blood pressure. The patient with severe hypertension that can be managed on a reduced antihypertensive drug dosage under close blood pressure observation may breast-feed; otherwise, breast-feeding is contraindicated (Working Group on High Blood Pressure in Pregnancy, 1990).

Long-term effects

In counseling a patient regarding the recurring incidence of preeclampsia and later development of hypertension, the following information should be considered:

1. If the patient developed transient gestational hypertension, she has a high probability of developing chronic hypertension later in life (Working Group on High Blood Pressure in Pregnancy, 1990).

2. The nulliparous patient who developed preeclampsia has a low risk of a subsequent gestational hypertensive disorder and no greater risk of developing chronic hypertension later in life (Working Group on High Blood Pressure in Pregnancy, 1990).

3. The multiparous patient who developed preeclampsia has a high risk of subsequent preeclampsia as well as other pregnancy complications such as abruptio placentae, IUGR, and preterm labor. With severe preeclampsia that develops during the second trimester the risk of recurrence is as high as 65% (Usta, Sibai, 1996; Working Group on High Blood Pressure in Pregnancy, 1990).

CONCLUSION

The ultimate goal of the nurse is to prevent hypertensive disorders of pregnancy or to assist in early diagnosis and appropriate treatment of these disorders to maximize outcome. Preeclampsia is a much studied disease of pregnancy, but the triggering factor remains unknown. This makes prevention difficult; however, because research indicates that several factors, such as early appropriate prenatal care, adequate fluid intake, and optimal nutrition, play important roles, the nurse should include these in the prenatal instructions. When a patient develops preeclampsia during pregnancy, the goal becomes the prevention of eclampsia and uteroplacental insufficiency while attempting to facilitate fetal maturity. Therefore preeclampsia is treated in hopes of stabilizing the condition until fetal maturity is reached. If treatment is effective, diuresis should occur within 18 to 36 hours. Positive signs of stabilization are increased output and a decrease in weight, blood pressure, edema, and proteinuria. If preeclampsia does not respond to treatment, delivery is the treatment of choice to prevent eclampsia and uteroplacental insufficiency.

Other hypertensive disorders of pregnancy are treated to keep the diastolic blood pressure below 100 to prevent maternal cardiovascular complications and uterine insufficiency.

BIBLIOGRAPHY

American College of Obstetricians and Gynecologists (ACOG): Hypertension in pregnancy, *ACOG Techn Bull,* no. 219, 1996.

Association of Women's Health, Obstetric, and Neonatal Nurses (AWHONN): *Invasive hemodynamic monitoring in high-risk intrapartum nursing: clinical commentary,* Washington, DC, 1994, The Author.

Barton J, Sibai B: Care of the pregnancy complicated by HELLP syndrome, *Obstet Gynecol Clin North Am* 18(2):165-179, 1991.

Barton J, Sibai B: Hepatic imaging in HELLP syndrome (hemolysis, elevated liver enzymes, and low platelet count), *Am J Obstet Gynecol* 174:1820, 1996.

Barton J, Stanziano G, Sibai B: Monitored outpatient management of mild gestational hypertension remote from term, *Am J Obstet Gynecol* 170:765, 1994.

Beer A, Need J: Immunological aspects of preeclampsia/eclampsia, *Birth Defects* 21:131-154, 1985.

Belizan J and others: Calcium supplementation to prevent hypertensive disorder of pregnancy, *N Engl J Med* 325:1399, 1991.

Branch D, Dudley D, Michell M: Preliminary evidence for homeostatic mechanism regulating endothelin production in preeclampsia, *Lancet* 337:943, 1991.

Branch D and others: Outcome of treated pregnancies in women with antiphospholipid syndrome: an update of the Utah experience, *Obstet Gynecol* 80:614-620, 1992.

Brengman S, Burns M: Hypertensive crisis in L&D, *Am J Nurs* 88(3):325-332, 1988.

Brown M and others: Sodium excretion in normal and hypertensive pregnancy: a prospective study, *Am J Obstet Gynecol* 159:297-307, 1988.

Brown M and others: Measuring blood pressure in pregnant women: a comparison of direct and indirect methods, *Am J Obstet Gynecol* 171(3):661-667, 1994.

Carroli G, Duley L, Belizan V: Calcium supplementation during pregnancy: a systematic review of randomised controlled trials, *Br J Obstet Gynaecol* 101:753, 1994.

Chang J, Roman C, Heymann M: Effect of endothelium-derived relaxing factor inhibition on the umbilical placental circulation in fetal lambs in utero, *Am J Obstet Gynecol* 166:727-734, 1992.

Chesley L, Cooper D: Genetics of hypertension in pregnancy: possible single gene control of pre-eclampsia and eclampsia in the descendants of eclamptic women, *Br J Obstet Gynaecol* 93:898-908, 1986.

Clark B and others: Plasma endothelin levels in preeclampsia: elevation and correlation with uric acid levels and renal impairment, *Am J Obstet Gynecol* 166:962-968, 1992.

CLASP Collaborative Group: Low dose aspirin in pregnancy and early childhood development: follow up of collaborative low dose aspirin study in pregnancy, *Br J Obstet Gynaecol* 102:861, 1995.

Cowles T, Saleh A, Cotton D: Hypertensive disorders in pregnancy. In James D and others, editors: *High risk pregnancy: management options,* London, 1994, Saunders.

Crawther C, Boumeester A, Ashwist H: Does admission to hospital for bedrest prevent disease progression or improve fetal outcome in pregnancy complicated by nonproteinuric hypertension? *Br J Obstet Gynaecol* 99:13, 1992.

Cunningham F, MacDonald P, Gant N: *Williams' obstetrics,* ed 20, Norwalk, Conn, 1997, Appleton & Lange.

Davey D, MacGillivray I: The classification and definition of the hypertensive disorders of pregnancy, *Am J Obstet Gynecol* 158:892-898, 1988.

Davidge S, Stranko C, Roberts J: Urine but not plasma nitric oxide metabolites are decreased in women with preeclampsia, *Am J Obstet Gynecol* 174:1008-1013, 1996.

De Groot C and others: Plasma from preeclamptic women increases human endothelial cell prostacyclin production without changes in cellular enzyme activity or mass, *Am J Obstet Gynecol* 172:976, 1995.

deJong C, Dekker G, Sibai B: The renin-angiotensin-aldosterone system in preeclampsia, *Clin Perinatol Hypertens Pregnancy* 18:683-711, 1991.

Dekker G, Sibai B: Early detection of preeclampsia, *Am J Obstet Gynecol* 165:160, 1991.

Dildy G, Clark S: Hypertensive crisis, *Contemp OB/GYN* 38(6):11-22, 1993.

Dizon-Townson D and others: Severe preeclampsia is associated with the factor V Leiden mutation, *Am J Obstet Gynecol* 174:343, 1996.

Dommisse J: Phenytoin sodium and magnesium sulphate in the management of eclampsia, *Br J Obstet Gynaecol* 97:104-109, 1990.

Eclampsia Trial Collaborative Group: Which anticonvulsant for women with eclampsia? Evidence from the collaborative eclampsia trial, *Lancet* 345:1455-1463, 1995.

Eglinton G: Medications in labor. In Queenan J, Hobbins J: *Protocols for high-risk pregnancies,* ed 3, Cambridge, England, 1996, Blackwell Science.

Franx A and others: Validation of automated blood pressure recording in pregnancy, *Br J Obstet Gynaecol* 101(1):66-69, 1994.

Friedman S: Pathophysiology of preeclampsia, *Clin Perinatol* 18(4):661-681, 1991.

Friedman S, Taylor R, Roberts J: Pathophysiology of preeclampsia, *Clin Perinatol Hypertens Pregnancy* 18:661-682, 1991.

Friedman S and others: Biochemical corroboration of endothelial involvement in severe preeclampsia, *Am J Obstet Gynecol* 172:202, 1995.

Ghabour M and others: Immunohistochemical characterization of placental nitric oxide synthase expression in preeclampsia, *Am J Obstet Gynecol* 173:687-694, 1995.

Gilstrap L, Gant N: Pathophysiology of preeclampsia, *Semin Perinatol* 14:147-151, 1990.

Green L, Froman R: Blood pressure measurement during pregnancy: auscultatory versus oscillatory methods, *J Obstet Gynecol Neonatal Nurs* 25:155-159, 1996.

Grohar J: Nursing protocols for antepartum home care, *J Obstet Gynecol Neonatal Nurs* 23(8):687-694, 1994.

Guyton A, Hall J: *Textbook of medical physiology,* ed 9, Philadelphia, 1996, Saunders.

Hauth J, Cunningham F: Low-dose aspirin during pregnancy. In *Williams' obstetrics,* ed 19, suppl 14, Norwalk, Conn, 1995, Appleton & Lange.

Hauth J and others: Low-dose aspirin therapy to prevent preeclampsia, *Am J Obstet Gynecol* 168:1083, 1993.

Helewa M and others: Community-based home-care program for the management of pre-eclampsia: an alternative, *Can Med Assoc J* 14:829, 1993.

Heppard M, Garite T: *Acute obstetrics: a practical guide,* St Louis, 1996, Mosby.

Hines T, Jones M: Can aspirin prevent and treat preeclampsia? *MCN Am J Matern Child Nurs* 19(5):258-263, 1994.

Johenning A, Barron W: Indirect blood pressure measurement in pregnancy: Korotkoff phase 4 versus phase 5, *Am J Obstet Gynecol* 167:577-580, 1992.

Katz V and others: A comparison of bed rest and immersion for treating the edema of pregnancy, *Obstet Gynecol* 75:147-151, 1990.

Knuppel R, Drukker J: *High risk pregnancy: a term approach,* ed 2, Philadelphia, 1993, Saunders.

Lawrence R: *Breastfeeding,* ed 4, St Louis, 1994, Mosby.

Leduc L and others: Coagulation profile in severe preeclampsia, *Obstet Gynecol* 79:14-18, 1992.

Lindsay L, Barbour L: Medications cited. In Queenan J, Hobbins J, editors: *Protocols for high-risk pregnancies,* ed 3, Cambridge, England, 1996, Blackwell Science.

Louden K and others: Neonatal platelet reactivity and serum thromboxane B2 production in whole blood: the effect of maternal low dose aspirin, *Br J Obstet Gynaecol* 101:203, 1994.

Lowenstein C, Dinerman J, Snyder S: Nitric oxide: a physiologic messenger, *Ann Intern Med* 120:227-237, 1994.

Lucas L, Jordan E: Phenytoin as an alternative treatment for preeclampsia, *J Obstet Gynecol Neonatal Nurs* 26(3):263-269, 1997.

Lucas M, Leveno K, Cunningham F: A comparison of magnesium sulfate with phenytoin for the prevention of eclampsia, *N Engl J Med* 333:201, 1995.

Lucas M and others: A simplified phenytoin regimen for preeclampsia, *Am J Perinatol* 11(2):153-156, 1994.

Mabie W: Critical care obstetrics. In Gabbe S, Niebyl J, Simpson J: *Obstetrics: normal and problem pregnancies,* ed 3, New York, 1996, Churchill Livingstone.

Maloni J: Bed rest and high-risk pregnancy, *Nurs Clin North Am* 31(2):313-325, 1996.

Martin J, Blake P, Lowry S: Pregnancy complicated by preeclampsia-eclampsia with the syndrome of hemolysis, elevated liver enzymes, and low platelet count: how rapid is postpartum recovery? *Obstet Gynecol* 76:737, 1990.

Martin J and others: The natural history of HELLP syndrome: patterns of disease progression and regression, *Am J Obstet Gynecol* 164:1500-1513, 1991.

McAnulty J, Metcalfe J, Ueland K: Cardiovascular disease. In Burrow G, Ferris T: *Medical complications during pregnancy,* ed 4, Philadelphia, 1995, Saunders.

Miles J and others: Postpartum eclampsia: a recurring perinatal dilemma, *Obstet Gynecol* 76:328, 1990.

Mitchell M, Koening J: Increased production of 15-hydroxy-eiconsatetraenoic acid by placentae from pregnancies complicated by pregnancy-induced hypertension, *Prostaglandins Leukot Essent Fatty Acids* 43:61, 1991.

National Research Council (NRC): *Recommended dietary allowances: report of the Subcommittee on the tenth edition of the RDA's Food and Nutrition Board, Commission on Life Sciences,* ed 10, Washington, DC, 1989, National Academy Press.

Need J, Bell B, Meffin E: Preeclampsia in pregnancies from donor inseminations, *J Reprod Immunol* 5:329-338, 1983.

Newman V, Fullerton J: Role of nutrition in the prevention of preeclampsia: review of the literature, *J Nurse Midwifery* 35(5):282-291, 1990.

Nova A and others: Maternal plasma levels of endothelin are increased in preeclampsia, *Am J Obstet Gynecol* 164:794, 1991.

Perry I and others: Conflicting views on the measurement of blood pressure in pregnancy, *Br J Obstet Gynaecol* 98:214-243, 1991.

Phelan J, Easter T: HELLP syndrome: the great masquerader, *Female Patient* 15(2):79-84, 1990.

Poole J: Getting perspective on HELLP syndrome, *MCN Am J Matern Child Nurs* 13(6):432-437, 1988.

Rayburn W: Monitoring fetal body movements, *Clin Obstet Gynecol* 3:899-911, 1987.

Repke J: Calcium, magnesium, and zinc supplementation and perinatal outcome, *Clin Obstet Gynecol* 34(2):262-267, 1991.

Repke J, Chez R: Treating preeclampsia with phenytoin, *Contemp OB/GYN* 34(6):57-59, 1989.

Rey F, Couturier A: The prognosis of pregnancy in women with chronic hypertension, *Am J Obstet Gynecol* 171:410, 1994.

Roberts J: Current perspectives on preeclampsia, *J Nurse Midwifery* 39(2):70-90, 1994a.

Roberts J: Pregnancy-related hypertension. In Creasy R, Resnik R, editors: *Maternal-fetal medicine: principles and practice,* ed 3, Philadelphia, 1994b, Saunders.

Roberts J, Taylor R, Goldfien A: Endothelial cell activation as a pathogenetic factor in preeclampsia, *Semin Perinatol* 15(1):86-93, 1991.

Robillard P and others: Association of pregnancy-induced hypertension with duration of sexual cohabitation before conception, *Lancet* 344:973, 1994.

Royal College of Obstetricians and Gynecologists: Report of a workshop: where next for prophylaxis against preeclampsia? *Br J Obstet Gynaecol* 103:603, 1996.

Ryan G, Lange I, Naugler M: Clinical experience with phenytoin prophylaxis in severe preeclampsia, *Am J Obstet Gynecol* 161:1297-1304, 1989.

Sanchez-Ramos L and others: Prevention of pregnancy-induced hypertension by calcium supplementation in angiotensin II-sensitive patients, *Obstet Gynecol* 84:349, 1994.

Shennan A and others: Lack of reproducibility in pregnancy of Korotkoff phase IV as measured by mercury sphygmomanometry, *Lancet* 347:139, 1996.

Sibai B: Preeclampsia-eclampsia: maternal and perinatal outcome, *Contemp OB/GYN* 32(6):109-118, 1988.

Sibai B: Eclampsia: maternal perinatal outcome in 254 consecutive cases, *Am J Obstet Gynecol* 163:1049-1055, 1990.

Sibai B: Management of preeclampsia, *Clin Perinatol* 18(4):793-808, 1991.

Sibai B: Hypertension in pregnancy. In Gabbe S, Niebyl J, Simpson J: *Obstetrics: normal and problem pregnancies,* ed 3, New York, 1996a, Churchill Livingstone.

Sibai B: Treatment of hypertension in pregnant women, *N Engl J Med* 335:257, 1996b.

Sibai B, Mabie W: Hemodynamics of preeclampsia, *Clin Perinatol* 18(4):727-747, 1991.

Sibai B, Mercer B, Sarinoglu C: Severe preeclampsia in the second trimester: recurrence risk and long term prognosis, *Am J Obstet Gynecol* 165:1408-1412, 1991.

Sibai B, Sarinoglu C, Mercer B: Eclampsia: pregnancy outcome after eclampsia and long-term prognosis, *Am J Obstet Gynecol* 166:1757-1763, 1992.

Sibai B and others: A comparison of no medication versus methyldopa or labetalol in chronic hypertension during pregnancy, *Am J Obstet Gynecol* 162:920-967, 1990.

Sibai B and others: Maternal morbidity and mortality in 442 pregnancies with hemolysis, elevated liver enzymes, and low platelets (HELLP syndrome), *Am J Obstet Gynecol* 169:1000-1006, 1993a.

Sibai B and others: Prevention of preeclampsia with low-dose aspirin in healthy, nulliparous pregnant women, *N Engl J Med* 329:1213, 1993b.

Sibai B and others: Pregnancies complicated by hemolysis, elevated liver enzymes, and low platelets (HELLP): subsequent pregnancy outcome and long-term prognosis, *Am J Obstet Gynecol* 172:125, 1995.

Silver H: Hypertensive disorders. In Niswander K, Evans A, editors: *Manual of obstetrics,* Boston, 1995, Little, Brown.

Smarson A, Sargent I, Redman C: Endothelial cell proliferation is suppressed by plasma but not serum from women with preeclampsia, *Am J Obstet Gynecol* 174:787, 1996.

Strong T: Reversal of oligohydramnios with subtotal immersion: a report of five cases, *Am J Obstet Gynecol* 169:1595-1597, 1993.

Tuffnell D and others: Randomised controlled trial of day care for hypertension in pregnancy, *Lancet* 339:224-227, 1992.

Twaddle S, Harper V: An economic evaluation of daycare in the management of hypertension in pregnancy, *Br J Obstet Gynaecol* 99:459-463, 1992.

Usta I, Sibai B: Preeclampsia. In Queenan J, Hobbins J: *Protocols for high-risk pregnancies,* ed 3, Cambridge, England, 1996, Blackwell Science.

Walker J: Hypertensive drugs in pregnancy-antihypertensive therapy in pregnancy, preeclampsia, and eclampsia, *Perinatol Hypertens Pregnancy* 18:845-873, 1991.

Wallenburg H: Hemodynamics in hypertensive pregnancy. In Rubin P, editor: *Hypertension in pregnancy,* Amsterdam, 1988, Elsevier Publisher.

Wallenburg H: Detecting hypertensive disorders of pregnancy. In Chalmers I, Enken M, Keirse M, editors: *Effective care in pregnancy and childbirth,* vol 1. *Pregnancy,* Oxford, England, 1989, Oxford University Press.

Wallenburg H, Dekker G, Makovitz J: Effect of low dose aspirin on vascular refractoriness in angiotensin sensitive primigravid women, *Am J Obstet Gynecol* 164:1169-1173, 1991.

Walsh S: Physiology of low dose aspirin therapy for the prevention of preeclampsia, *Semin Perinatol* 14(2):152-170, 1990.

Wang Y and others: The imbalance between thromboxane and prostacy-clin in preeclampsia is associated with an imbalance between lipid peroxides and vitamin E in maternal blood, *Am J Obstet Gynecol* 165:1695-1700, 1991a.

Wang Y and others: Maternal levels of prostacyclin, thromboxane, vitamin E, and lipid peroxides throughout normal pregnancy, *Am J Obstet Gynecol* 165:1690, 1991b.

Ward K and others: A molecular variant of angiotensinogen associated with preeclampsia, *Nat Genet* 4:59, 1993.

Weinstein L: Preeclampsia/eclampsia with hemolysis, elevated liver enzymes, and thrombocytopenia, *Obstet Gynecol* 66:657, 1985.

Wenger N, Speroff L, Packard B: Cardiovascular health and disease in women, *N Engl J Med* 329:247-256, 1993.

Wilson B, Shannon M, Stang C: *Nurses' drug guide 1997,* Stamford, Conn, 1997, Appleton & Lange.

Working Group on High Blood Pressure in Pregnancy: National high blood pressure education program working group report on high blood pressure in pregnancy, *Am J Obstet Gynecol* 163:1689-1712, 1990.

World Health Organization (WHO) Study Group: *The hypertensive disorders of pregnancy. WHO Technical Report Series no. 758,* Geneva, 1987, World Health Organization.

Worthington-Roberts B, Williams S: *Nutrition in pregnancy and lactation,* ed 5, St Louis, 1997, Mosby.

Zatuchni G, Slupik R: *Obstetrics and gynecology drug handbook,* ed 2, St Louis, 1996, Mosby.

Zeeman G, Dekker G: Pathogenesis of preeclampsia: a hypothesis, *Clin Obstet Gynecol* 35:317, 1992.

Zuspan F, Samuels P: Preventing preeclampsia, *N Engl J Med* 329:1265, 1993.

Zuspan F: Chronic hypertension. In Queenan J, Hobbins J: *Protocols for high-risk pregnancies,* ed 3, Cambridge England, 1996, Blackwell Science.

Zuspan F: Dealing with chronic hypertension, *Contemp OB/GYN* 37(1):31-44, 1991a.

Zuspan F: New concepts in the understanding of hypertensive diseases during pregnancy, *Clin Perinatol* 18(4):653-659, 1991b.

CHAPTER

21

Preterm Labor

Preterm labor can be defined as regular uterine contractions that cause progressive dilation of the cervix after 20 weeks of gestation and before 36 completed weeks.

INCIDENCE

Approximately 8% to 10% of all pregnancies end in preterm labor. According to 1989 vital statistics, the rate is increasing despite innovative perinatal technology. Prematurity in the newborn continues to account for 75% to 80% of neonatal morbidity and mortality (Creasy, Merkatz, 1990; Creasy, Resnik, 1994; Freda and others, 1991).

ETIOLOGY

The cause cannot be identified in 50% of patients who experience preterm labor (Papiernik and others, 1989). Factors frequently related to preterm labor can be classified as past history, altered life-style practices, stress, altered uterine factors, and infections (Box 21-1).

Another factor that predisposes a woman to preterm labor is a low socioeconomic status. The deterrent factor is unknown, but altered nutrition, bacterial or viral flora of the reproductive tract caused by inadequate hygiene, lack of education, higher incidence of teenage pregnancies, higher frequency of grand multiparity, and

---

Box 21-1
Predisposing Factors of Preterm Labor

History
Previous preterm labor (single most important factor)
Altered life-style practices
Altered nutrition that leads to low maternal weight gain
Smoking
Illicit drug use, especially cocaine (Hoskins and others, 1991)
Stress
Emotional stress
Long, tiring commutes
Two or more children at home
Heavy work
Altered uterine factors
Decreased blood flow:
   Abruptio placentae
   Placenta previa
   Diabetes
   Renal disease
   Cardiovascular disease
   Preeclampsia
Overdistention of uterus
   Multiple gestation
   Polyhydramnios
Abdominal trauma
Abdominal surgery
Premature rupture of membranes
Diethylstilbestrol (DES) exposure in utero resulting in uterine abnormalities
Incompetent cervix
Uterine anomalies
Infections
Urinary tract
Vagina/uterus/fetus
Febrile illness

---

psychologic and physical stress have all been suggested. Causes that can be identified include the following:

1. Multiple gestation
2. Infection, especially urinary tract infection (UTI)
3. Febrile illness
4. Abdominal surgery

5. Uterine anomalies
6. Placenta previa and/or abruption

Factors that may contribute to the risk of preterm labor include the following (Freston and others, 1997; Iams and others, 1994):

1. Low socioeconomic status
2. Less than high school education
3. Teen pregnancy
4. Substance abuse, legal or illegal
5. Lack of or late prenatal care
6. Poor nutritional status

NORMAL PHYSIOLOGY

To have a physiologic understanding of possible causes and current medical treatments for preterm labor, one must understand the physiology of labor contractions. What actually initiates labor remains unknown. However, several concepts have developed from research efforts, and there is strong scientific evidence that various hormones interplay to influence uterine activity.

Initiation of Labor

Prostaglandins

An unknown alteration in fetal metabolism, related to certain fetal maturational milestones, may interrupt the support of systems that serve to promote uterine quiescence and maintain pregnancy (Huszar, 1994). This unknown fetal signal appears to stimulate macrophage-like decidua, the endometrium of pregnancy, to release interleukin-1-beta. Interleukin-1-beta, an immune hormone, causes hydrolysis of glycerophospholipids found in the decidua, fetal membranes, and myometrium. Esterified arachidonic acid, which is stored in the glycerophospholipids, is released to free arachidonic acid (Casey, MacDonald, 1988; Huszar, 1994). The release of arachidonic acid is accomplished either directly by phospholipase A_2 or indirectly by phospholipase C. Both of these agents hydrolyze the membrane to release arachidonic acid (Creasy, Resnik, 1994).

Free arachidonic acid is then converted into prostaglandins and thus stimulates the platelet-activating factor. Each tissue synthesizes a type of prostaglandin (PG). For example, the decidua produces primarily $PGF_{2\alpha}$ and a small amount of PGE_2. The amnionic and chorionic fetal membranes produce PGE_2, and the myometrium produces prostacyclin (PGI_2) and a small amount of $PGF_{2\alpha}$.

During labor, prostaglandins $PGF_{2\alpha}$ and PGE_2 and platelet-activating factor accumulate in the amniotic fluid. Along with arachidonic acid and interleukin-1-beta, $PGF_{2\alpha}$, PGE_2, and platelet-activating factor remain active for 4 to 6 hours.

Thromboxane, $PGF_{2\alpha}$, and PGE_2 prepare the myometrial muscle for labor by promoting the development of gap junctions, which are cell-to-cell contact areas, and coordinate smooth muscle contractions. These three substances stimulate myometrial contractions by facilitating the movement of calcium into the smooth muscle so that the muscle can contract and promote cervical ripening.

During pregnancy, prostacyclin (PGI_2) quiets the uterus by inhibiting the formation of gap junction and release of phospholipases A_2 and C and by blocking movement of calcium into cells. Production of prostacyclin is suppressed during labor secondary to high levels of maternal and fetal cortisol (MacKenzie and others, 1988).

Estrogen

Estrogen is produced by the corpus luteum for the first 2 to 4 weeks of gestation. Then the placenta takes over the production. Low density lipoprotein (LDL) cholesterol is used by the fetal and maternal adrenals to secrete a precursor for placental estrogen. Near term, the adrenal gland, the largest fetal organ, is the primary source for placental estrogen precursor. Estriol, one form of placental estrogen, stimulates the fetal membranes and decidua to deposit glycerophospholipids.

Estrogen influences the increased number of cells and size of the myometrium, stimulates Braxton Hicks contractions, facilitates the development of gap junctions (Huszar, 1994), and promotes oxytocin receptors. It is for this reason that oxytocin is an ineffective stimulator of myometrial contractions until late in pregnancy when estrogen levels are high (Carsten, Miller, 1987). Estrogen also stimulates prostaglandin biosynthesis and inhibits progesterone synthesis in fetal membranes, thus effecting a local change in the progesterone/estrogen ratio in amniotic fluid at term (Romero and others, 1988).

Progesterone

Progesterone is produced by the corpus luteum for the first 4 to 6 weeks of gestation. Then it is produced by the fetal syncytiotrophoblasts at an increasing rate until 32 to 34 weeks by converting maternal plasma LDL cholesterol into progesterone. Then progesterone is maintained at a constant level, approximately

250 mg/day, until birth (Casey, MacDonald, 1988). Progesterone withdrawal does not cause the initiation of true labor but may stimulate the synthesis of the precursor for interleukin-1-beta. At the same time progesterone prevents the release of interleukin-1-beta and of phospholipase A_2 and blocks the effect of estrogen on the induction of oxytocin receptors. Therefore protesterone appears to influence preparation for labor while maintaining quiescence of the myometrial muscle.

Oxytocin

It was once thought that oxytocin initiated normal labor, but it is now known to maximize uterine contraction of second-stage labor and, after delivery, to stimulate decidual prostaglandin release. Oxytocin is ineffective at stimulating uterine contractions during early pregnancy since the uterus is not yet sensitized by high estrogen levels. Oxytocin is also ineffective at promoting gap junctions and cervical ripening (Cunningham and others, 1989).

• • •

Fig. 21-1 shows the interrelationships among the different endocrine factors that contribute to the control of labor.

Uterine Contractions

Prostaglandins and oxytocin stimulate the uterus to contract related to their capability of increasing intracellular concentrations of calcium, which activates the muscle to contract. First, prostaglandins and oxytocin block calcium from being bound to the sarcoplasmic reticulum where it is stored. Second, they block the beta-adrenergic receptors from stimulating adenyl cyclase. If stimulated, the plasma enzyme adenyl cyclase accelerates the transport of sodium out of the cell in exchange for potassium. This increases the sodium gradient, and sodium is exchanged for calcium, causing an intracellular decrease in calcium (Fig. 21-2). Carsten and Miller (1987) noted that there is little difference in the capability of prostaglandins to inhibit storage of calcium in a pregnant or nonpregnant uterus. However, they noted a marked difference in the capability of oxytocin, which is effective only in late pregnancy when estrogen levels are high.

PATHOPHYSIOLOGY

Preterm labor is usually caused by factors that stimulate uterine irritability or the release of prostaglandins. A genetic trait may be an influencing factor in some cases.

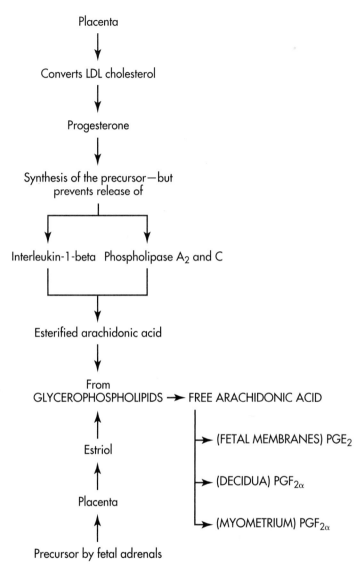

FIG. 21-1 Interrelationships among different endocrine factors that contribute to control of labor. *LDL,* Low density lipoprotein; *PGE,* prostaglandin E; *PGF,* prostaglandin F.

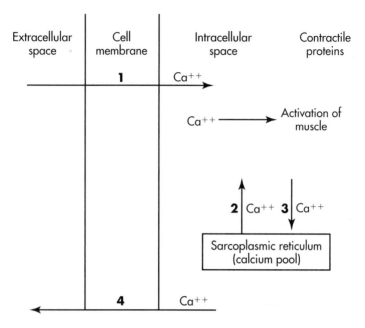

FIG. 21-2 Final steps that lead to contraction and relaxation of myometrium. *1,* Calcium flows in from extracellular space. *2,* Calcium is released from sarcoplasmic reticulum. Steps 1 and 2 increase calcium level inside muscle, which activates muscle to contract. *3,* Calcium returns to sarcoplasmic reticulum. *4,* Calcium returns to extracellular space. Steps 3 and 4 decrease calcium level inside muscle, which causes muscle to relax.

Infection

Bacterial endotoxins can stimulate prostaglandin release directly or indirectly by stimulating the release of interleukin (Romero and others, 1989). In this manner a urinary tract, vaginal, uterine, or fetal infection may stimulate preterm labor.

Altered Uterine Factors

Physical stressors such as myometrial stretch, hyperosmolarity, and fetal membrane or uterine trauma cause lysosomes to release phospholipase A_2. Prostaglandins are then produced, stimulating the myometrium to contract. In this way, premature rupture of membranes (PROM), abdominal trauma, multiple gestations, uterine anomalies causing overdistention of the uterus, and polyhydramnios can stimulate preterm labor.

Factors that decrease blood flow to the uterus may lead to uterine irritability and decreased placental function. These in turn cause the lysosomes to become unstable and release phospholipase A_2. Therefore conditions during pregnancy that interfere with uterine or placental blood flow can trigger preterm labor. Some of these conditions are preeclampsia, poorly controlled diabetes, heart disease, renal disease, abruptio placentae, or placenta previa. Altered nutrition, smoking, or illicit drug use may stimulate preterm labor in this manner as well.

Stress

Emotional or physical stress can stimulate the release of catecholamines, which affect placental function and make the uterus irritable.

Multiple Gestation

Because of the increased likelihood for infertile couples who become pregnant with any one of the fertility methods to have twins or more, we now see many more successful pregnancy outcomes. However, with this success comes an increased incidence of preterm birth of the multiples. Currently, some perinatal programs are reporting equally successful outcomes with quadruple births as with twin births. Although quadruplets are more likely to deliver by 32 weeks than are twins, ultimately their outcome successes rival twins. Preterm labor with multiple gestation is more difficult for the pregnant woman to identify because of confusion with extra aches and pains from rapid stretching and pressure, as well as differentiating kicks and movement of multiple babies from contractile activity of the uterus. In addition, the overdistention of the uterus contributes to increased irritability of the uterus.

Bed rest, except for up to the bathroom and for meals, is still the preferred treatment once signs of preterm cervical changes are identified. Usually larger doses of magnesium sulfate or other tocolytics are needed than with a singleton preterm pregnancy.

Other complications are also more likely with a multiple gestation pregnancy, including pregnancy-induced hypertension (PIH), which may be modified by hydrotherapy by 26 to 28 weeks and thus gain more time in utero. There is no doubt that multiple gestation presents management problems to the provider, as well as self-management challenges for the patient and her family.

Abdominal Surgery

If a surgical emergency presents itself before 36 weeks of gestation, regardless of previous risk, the pregnant patient is at high risk for preterm labor and delivery. It is postulated that the higher production of prostaglandins for the healing process increases the likelihood of preterm contractions. The pregnant woman may find it difficult to impossible to recognize these from abdominal pain at the surgical site. Add to this, pain medication, which masks contraction discomfort as well, and contractions are probably not going to be the identified complaint. After abdominal surgery, it is therefore a good idea to monitor with an electronic monitor the contraction pattern of the uterus. Some providers will treat with subcutaneous terbutaline every 2 to 4 hours, or with intravenous (IV) magnesium sulfate as a preventative, for 24 to 48 hours after abdominal surgery, if the woman is more than 20 weeks pregnant.

• • •

Fig. 21-3 shows the pathophysiologic effects of the causative factors of preterm labor.

MATERNAL EFFECTS

The most common direct effect on the mother is psychologic stress from the threat of a preterm delivery on the health and well-being of the expected baby. Other maternal consequences are related to the side effects of the medical treatment, such as prolonged bed rest and the use of labor suppressant drugs, on the mother's health.

FETAL AND NEONATAL EFFECTS

Preterm labor leads to the birth of an infant whose body processes are immature. Therefore these infants have an increased risk of birth trauma and an increased difficulty adjusting to extrauterine life. Special problems seen in the preterm infant are as follows:

1. Respiratory distress syndrome
2. Intraventricular or pulmonary hemorrhage
3. Hyperbilirubinemia
4. Increased susceptibility to infections
5. Anemia
6. Neurologic disorders
7. Metabolic disturbances
8. Ineffective temperature regulatory mechanism

The severity of each of these problems depends greatly on the gestational age of the infant. The greatest potential problem of the preterm infant is respiratory distress. If it is severe, hypoxia can ensue and cerebral hemorrhage, seizure disorders, and neonatal death can result. In fact, preterm labor accounts for 75% to 85% of all neonatal mortality and morbidity (Morrison, 1990).

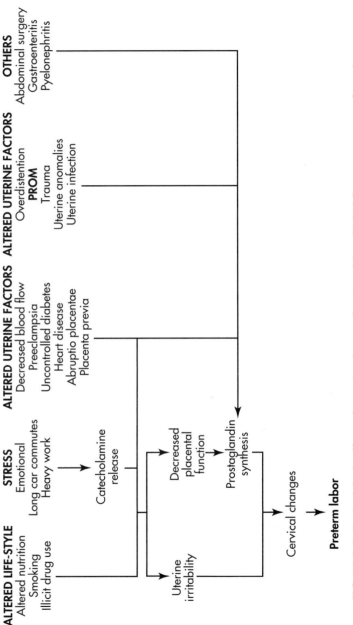

FIG. 21-3 Pathophysiologic effects of causative factors of preterm labor. *PROM,* Premature rupture of membranes.

NATIONAL EFFECTS

Despite technologic and pharmacologic advances in the treatment of preterm labor, the preterm birth rate is higher in the United States than in 18 other industrialized nations. At the same time, the economic importance of preterm births has direct and indirect impacts on us as a nation. Neonatal intensive care, primarily because of premature births, is the most expensive care service in our health care system, with estimated costs of 5 billion dollars annually.

DIAGNOSTIC TESTING

When a patient comes in experiencing regular, rhythmic uterine contractions, the medical team must first determine whether the patient is in true labor. The diagnosis is usually made in the presence of (1) contractions that occur every 7 to 10 minutes, last at least 30 seconds, and have been present for at least 1 hour and (2) a cervix that is beginning to dilate or efface. Cervical dilation may be diagnosed by cervical/vaginal ultrasound (Iams and others, 1994).

USUAL MEDICAL MANAGEMENT AND PROTOCOLS FOR NURSE PRACTITIONERS

When the diagnosis of preterm labor is made, the medical team should attempt to determine the cause and whether further continuation of the pregnancy will be beneficial or harmful to the fetus or harmful to the mother. The choice of treatment depends on the answers to these questions and the age and maturity of the fetus.

Contraindications to Halting Labor

In 20% of the cases that present in preterm labor, delivery will be indicated because of a medical or obstetric reason (ACOG, 1995):

1. Mature fetus as demonstrated by a lecithin/sphingomyelin (L/S) ratio of 2:1 or greater or the presence of phosphatidyl glycerol in the amniotic fluid
2. Fetal death
3. Fetal anomaly incompatible with life
4. Intrauterine growth restriction related to an unfavorable intrauterine environment
5. Fetal compromise
6. Active hemorrhage
7. Intraamniotic infection
8. Severe preeclampsia, heart disease, or significant amount of bleeding from placenta previa or abruptio placentae

Diagnostic Data

Diagnostic data in preterm labor include the following:

1. Blood studies: a complete blood count with differential and platelets
2. Urinalysis for culture and sensitivity to rule out a UTI
3. Cervical cultures for gonorrhea, group B streptococci, *Chlamydia, Bacteroides bivius,* and *Bacteroides fragilis* to rule out an infection (Krohn and others, 1991)
4. Fetal surveillance studies to determine signs of fetal compromise
5. Fetal lung maturity if gestational age is between 32 and 36 weeks
6. Fibronectin evaluation (Clark and others, 1995)

Fibronectins are a family of proteins found in plasma and extracellular matrix. Fetal fibronectins are found in amniotic fluid and extracts of placental tissue. It is postulated that fetal fibronectin may be released into the cervix and the vagina when mechanical- or inflammatory-mediated damage occurs to the membranes. A new immunoassay test to detect fetal fibronectins is being used in research trials to predict women at risk for preterm labor. The test is done by placing a sterile speculum in the vagina and swabbing first the external circle of the cervix and then, with a new swab, the posterior fornix of the vagina. This is done as a test for women who have preterm labor risk factors or signs and symptoms and who are at 24 to 37 weeks of gestation (Lockwood and others, 1991).

Labor Suppression

Modified Activity

Until recently, bed rest at home or in the hospital was the first line of treatment. Recent research on the efficacy and the negative physical and psychosocial effects of complete bed rest has shown that a plan of modified activities, spaced with periods of rest, is as effective, without the negative impact (Goldenberg and others, 1994; Josten and others, 1995; Maloni, 1993, 1994, 1996; Maloni and others, 1993; Schroeder, 1996). Home care for high risk perinatal patients stresses the value of supporting nursing care that assesses more than just the physical symptoms of preterm labor. It is expected that a psychosocial impact on the family as well as the woman is an important consideration when developing a personal program of acceptable activity levels for prevention of preterm labor (Dahlberg, Kolorutis, 1994).

Hydration

It is controversial whether increased hydration measures should be implemented initially. In the event tocolytic drugs are to be used, the complication of pulmonary edema is increased if large amounts of fluids are given (Pircon and others, 1989). However, oral fluid hydration, especially fluids with nutritive calories, such as fruit juices, milk, and gelatin, do help and are not contraindicated for most patients in the initial evaluation period.

Tocolytic Drug Therapy

Tocolytic drugs may be used in an attempt to stop contractions. If these drugs are to be used, the next management dilemma arises regarding which tocolytic drug should be used. Many drugs have been used in an attempt to slow labor, but because none are without serious, undesirable side effects and a statistical history of drug ineffectiveness, the selection is complicated. The drugs currently being used are beta-sympathomimetics such as ritodrine (Yutopar) and terbutaline sulfate (Brethine); magnesium sulfate; a prostaglandin inhibitor, indomethacin; and a calcium channel blocker, nifedipine. Ritodrine is the only drug approved by the U.S. Food and Drug Administration for use in suppressing labor. However, by common practice terbutaline and magnesium sulfate are more frequently used, equally as safe, and less expensive. Prostaglandin inhibitors and calcium channel blockers are currently being researched and are frequently reserved for treatment when the other drugs have failed to be effective in suppressing labor. However, some obstetricians use them as first-line drugs in selected situations (Besinger and others, 1991; Creasy, Resnik, 1994; Eronen and others, 1991; Niebyl, 1988).

Home Uterine Activity Monitoring Program

There are a number of choices for preterm labor home care. Home uterine contraction monitoring may be used with self-palpation only or with the use of a home monitor unit that prints out objectively the contractions a woman is experiencing.

Home Uterine Contraction Monitoring

Home uterine contraction monitoring is done for the following reasons:
- Unless the woman concentrates, she may feel fewer than 50% of her contractions. However, without specific education, many patients who perceive the sensations will not report them or seek care. Research has also demonstrated that

frequent contractions may be reported as many as 3 days before physicians respond to patient-perceived contractions (Freston and others, 1997).

- When patients report the contractions they feel, there are no objective data for evaluation and documentation and therefore physicians may be inclined to postpone response. Thus by the time contractions are reported and diagnosed, advanced cervical dilation may have occurred, precluding prevention of preterm delivery.

- Presumably, home uterine contraction monitoring, with early, objective contraction data, fosters early response to patient-perceived contractions before cervical changes occur. However, much controversy surrounds this assumption. Many studies have concluded that it is the frequency of monitoring that improves the outcomes.

Components of a Uterine Contraction Monitoring Program

Home uterine contraction monitoring may be ordered by physicians when a woman at risk for preterm labor and delivery reports or is treated for signs of preterm labor. The home uterine contraction monitor can be rented from several privately owned perinatal home care companies. The monitor consists of a monitoring device and a battery-operated recording unit. The monitoring device is a large disk with a curved surface and serves as a tocodynamometer. It is designed so that the entire surface, unlike a conventional electronic fetal monitor (EFM) tocodynamometer, is capable of sensing a low-intensity contraction. Daily follow-up is provided by the nursing services of the uterine contraction monitoring company guided by the orders of the attending physician.

Advantages and Disadvantages of Home Uterine Monitoring Devices

Controversy exists regarding the efficacy and cost effectiveness of home uterine monitoring devices for assessment. It has been suggested that the studies promising better outcomes are flawed in that most did not separate the comprehensive nursing care follow-up from the technologies (ACOG, 1995; Creasy, Merkatz, 1990; Freston and others, 1997; Morrison, 1990). Further, most of the studies have been monetarily supported by the companies who own the equipment and stand to gain from increased use. Improved outcomes are seen in groups of patients with multiple gestation when discriminating among fetal movements, abdominal discomforts in general, and contractions is difficult (Garite and others,

1990; Knuppel and others, 1990). Uterine contraction monitoring has been reported to be more beneficial than when the patient self-palpates and has telephone visits from a nurse.

Subcutaneous Terbutaline Pump

The terbutaline pump is a device designed for continuous subcutaneous infusion of small amounts of terbutaline (Fig. 21-4). Frequently, terbutaline pump therapy is offered by the uterine contraction monitoring preterm prevention programs, but it may be used with self-palpation as well.

Reasons for Subcutaneous Terbutaline Pump

Subcutaneous terbutaline pumps are used for the following reasons:

- Contraction breakthrough with oral beta-sympathomimetics frequently occurs, especially after 3 weeks of administration. The myometrial beta-adrenergic receptor sites become desensitized, and a drug tolerance builds up.
- There is a poor patient compliance with scheduling and consistent self-administration when oral maintenance therapy is used.
- Frequently there is a patient intolerance to the unpleasant side effects related to oral therapy.

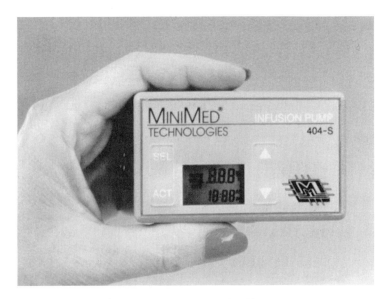

FIG. 21-4 Subcutaneous terbutaline pump.

Function of Pump

The pump delivers a small, continuous basal rate, usually 0.05 to 0.075 mg/hr. It is also present for boluses of 0.25 mg. The bolus schedule is determined from observing and analyzing a pattern of contraction frequencies over a 24-hour monitoring period. Normally, the maximum pump dose delivered in 24 hours is 3 mg compared with an oral 24-hour dose of 15 to 30 mg.

Advantages

Low-dose pump delivery has the following advantages:
- It does not rely on episodic patient administration and therefore improves compliance.
- Unpleasant side effects are reduced.
- Length of time before contraction breakthrough occurs is increased as much as 6 weeks.

Disadvantages

Low-dose pump delivery has the following disadvantages:
- It requires additional learning to operate the pump.
- Risk of infection at the needle site is increased.
- The infusion pump therapy is more expensive than oral tocolytics (Romeo, Jones, 1994).

NURSING PROCESS

PREVENTION

Prematurity is the most frequent cause of infant mortality and is on the rise in the United States despite advanced pharmacologic agents and technologic improvements. No treatment is consistently effective for prevention of preterm birth. At the same time, the economic importance of preterm births has direct and indirect impacts. Neonatal intensive care, primarily caused by premature births, is the most expensive care service in our health care system, with estimated costs of 5 billion dollars annually. In addition, many newborns become permanently functionally affected, families are temporarily or permanently disrupted, and associated medicolegal claims increase in numbers and awards. Therefore the best approach to lowering infant mortality is to prevent preterm labor.

Preventive measures must center around counteracting or improving the conditions that predispose to preterm labor. According to Morrison (1990), although preterm birth prevention remains a puzzle for the 1990s, a comprehensive team approach shows promise in reducing the preterm birth rate. Physicians, nurses, social workers, health care policymakers, and patients must make a concerted effort to orchestrate and provide a model of preventive prenatal care. Nurses play a very significant role in any comprehensive preterm birth prevention program. Studies suggest that the key factor in preterm birth prevention is frequent contact by caring, involved, and educated nurses who empower the patient with knowledge (Dyson and others, 1991; Hill and others, 1990; Iams and others, 1994; Maloni, 1993, 1994; Maloni and others, 1993; Ross and others, 1994).

NURSING DIAGNOSES/COLLABORATIVE PROBLEMS AND INTERVENTIONS

■ **RISK FOR ALTERED HEALTH MAINTENANCE** related to insufficient knowledge of risks of preterm labor, subtle symptoms, and self-care measures to prevent preterm labor.

DESIRED OUTCOME: The patient's pregnancy will continue for 37 weeks of gestation or longer without the development of preterm labor. If preterm labor develops, it will be detected before the cervix dilates 2 cm and effaces 50%.

INTERVENTIONS

1. Because patients who receive prenatal care have a decreased risk of preterm labor, nurses should be actively involved in the legislative process that would enhance access to prenatal care for all. This means that prenatal care is conveniently located, culturally and ethnically acceptable, and universally available regardless of pay status.

2. All patients should be screened for risks of preterm labor on their first and every prenatal visit. A screening assessment tool should be used to ensure consistency. Several scoring systems to predict a pregnant woman at risk for preterm labor have been developed and tested and can be adapted for the specific subpopulations and locality being served (Freston and others, 1997).

3. Analyze all pregnant patients' nutritional status as to dietary intake and meal patterns. Provide education based on the analysis. Inadequate weight gain and preterm labor are correlated (Abrams, Parker, 1990; Scholl and others, 1990). Meal patterns should be assessed also. If the patient goes for long periods without eating, this can provoke prostaglandin release. Motivational strategies appropriate to the patient are important in a successful teaching plan. An ongoing assessment of weight gain and nutritional habits should be obtained at each prenatal visit. Appropriate refer-

rals for nutritional counseling or nutritional supplement programs should be made as indicated.

4. Encourage the patient to drink at least one 8-oz glass of water or fruit juice at least every waking hour. Caffeine drinks should be avoided. Adequate hydration decreases the release of antidiuretic hormone and oxytocin from the posterior pituitary gland and increases uterine blood flow, thereby stabilizing the decidual lysosomes so arachidonic acid will not be freed to be converted into prostaglandins. It can also decrease the risk of UTIs.

5. Because of the stimulating effect of bacterial endotoxins in prostaglandin production, infection prevention should be taught. Prevention of urinary tract and vaginal infections is most important. Adequate fluid, perineal hygiene, the wearing of cotton-lined underwear, the avoidance of scented bath salts, and the limiting of sexual contacts to only one person are beneficial in lowering the risk of these infections. The patient should understand the signs of an infection and the need to report any signs immediately.

6. Evaluate the patient's employment and home responsibility as to stress, level of heavy work, and amount of commute time. Instruct to decrease activities that cause fatigue and plan daily rest periods to increase blood flow to the uterus, which decreases the risk of prostaglandin release. If work responsibilities involve strenuous activities, problem solve with the patient and her family as to ways to avoid or lessen this type of activities.

7. Emphasize that appropriate exercise, such as walking or swimming, can be beneficial in decreasing fatigue and stress.

8. Educate the patient as to the importance of emptying her bladder every 2 hours while awake. A full bladder can stimulate the uterus to contract and increase the risk of UTIs.

9. Assess level of anxiety, and assess for the presence of economic or family stressors. Teach relaxation techniques to decrease the effects of stress. Encourage problem solving to reduce stress by avoiding or altering stressful situations. Make appropriate referrals as needed.

10. An assessment for substance abuse, especially for smoking and cocaine, should be included in the initial prenatal assessment. If substance abuse is determined, refer to Chapter 25 for interventions.

Additional education for patients at risk for preterm labor

1. Empower the patient with knowledge about the subtle nature of preterm labor symptoms and the importance of immediate reporting of any symptoms. Before establishing an education program for preterm prevention, determine the local population's basic knowledge of the subject so the program can emphasize the most critical areas (Freda and others, 1991).

2. Educate the patient about what a contraction feels like. It is a tightening sensation that does not have to be painful.

3. Empower the patient with the importance of self-palpating for uterine contractions twice each day for 1 hour between 20 and 36 weeks of gestation. This should be done by lying down, placing her fingertips on the fundus, and consciously determining if the uterus is tightening.

4. Emphasize the warning signs of preterm labor. These include menstrual-like or abdominal cramps; low, dull, back-ache; pelvic pressure; a change in vaginal discharge; or diarrhea (Iams and others, 1990a, 1990b; Katz and others, 1990).

5. If the patient experiences any of the warning signs just mentioned, instruct her to empty her bladder, lie down on her side, drink 2 to 3 cups of fluid, and check for contractions.

6. Impress on the patient the importance of calling her health care provider if she is experiencing more than four contractions in 1 hour or if the warning signs do not go away after the hour of rest and hydration. (It has been determined that patients who do not go into preterm labor have three or fewer uterine contractions per hour throughout their pregnancy [Nageotte and others, 1988]. There is always a surge of uterine activity before the onset of labor [Bentley and others, 1990].)

7. Encourage abstinence or condom use during sexual relations since prostaglandins are in semen. Manipulation of the cervix can cause prostaglandin release as well.

8. Prepare the patient for vaginal examinations during her prenatal visits after 16 to 20 weeks of gestation to detect early cervical change. (There is a correlation between early cervical dilation and preterm labor [Main, Gabbe, 1987].)

9. Avoid prenatal preparation such as nipple rolling or brushing. (Breast stimulation causes the release of oxytocin.)

10. Build a rapport with the patient so she feels free to call at any time she perceives a problem.
11. Refer to a high risk pregnancy support group such as Confinement Connection, Confinement Line, or High Risk Moms.
12. Refer to a preterm labor prevention nurse and a home uterine activity monitoring program if at very high risk for preterm labor or after an initial preterm labor episode (Jones, Collins, 1996; Rhoads and others, 1991).

- ■ **POTENTIAL COMPLICATIONS OF PRETERM LABOR: PRETERM BIRTH, INTRAUTERINE INFECTION**
  DESIRED OUTCOME: The pregnancy will continue for 36 or more weeks of gestation without signs of infection.
  INTERVENTIONS
    1. Place the EFM to assess fetal heart rate (FHR), fetal well-being, and uterine contraction pattern.
    2. Assess for vaginal discharge; assess presence and character of bleeding to begin to rule out abruptio placentae or placenta previa; and assess fluid discharge to rule out rupture of membranes before a digital vaginal examination is done.
    3. If there is no bleeding or signs of leakage of amniotic fluid, assess amount of cervical changes for parity and gestational appropriateness.
    4. Collect a clean-catch or catheterized specimen of urine for culture analysis and sensitivity.
    5. Assess for signs of maternal infection by evaluating maternal temperature and referring to the white blood count.
    6. Determine estimated date of delivery.
    7. Prepare to assist with amniocentesis to assess for an intraamniotic infection or fetal lung maturity and an ultrasound for fetal growth and gestational age assessment.
    8. Evaluate patient's level and source of anxiety, fear, and anticipatory grief.
    9. Obtain medical orders for treatment of preterm labor contractions within 30 minutes of initial hospital evaluation if the patient reports symptoms.
    10. Treat preterm contractions by having the patient void and placing her in a lateral recumbent position. If tocolytic drugs are ordered, start an IV infusion and administer the tocolytic drug as outlined in this chapter under collaborative interventions for the respective tocolytic drug.
    11. Carry out fetal surveillance tests as ordered.

Preparation for discharge home

1. Discuss and verbally contract with patient for modifications of activities so that bed rest is possible for as much of the day as possible or at least activities are modified and altered with increased periods of rest.
2. Include supportive family members in all instructions.
3. Teach about self-administration of medications.
4. Teach or reinforce the prevention and early detection program of further preterm labor events as outlined under the previous nursing diagnosis.

- **RISK FOR ALTERED ROLE PERFORMANCE** related to impaired ability to perform role responsibilities while on bed rest or limited activity.

    DESIRED OUTCOME: The patient will verbalize a plan that will take care of all her responsibilities.

    INTERVENTIONS *(Maloni, 1993; Maloni and others, 1993; Schroeder, 1996)*

    1. Assess the patient's responsibilities to determine difficulties she will face in implementing prescribed bed rest or limited activity.
    2. Teach the patient and her family about the importance of limited activity even though she feels reasonably well.
    3. Facilitate the patient and her family in problem solving difficulties in implementing limited activity.
    4. Make needed referrals, for example, to the social worker, if problems are identified.
    5. Encourage participation in her care and decision making as much as possible.
    6. If there are other children that the mother must continue to care for, refer to Box 21-2 for ways to entertain children while the mother is on bed rest.

- **DIVERSIONAL ACTIVITY DEFICIT** related to limited activity.

    DESIRED OUTCOME: The patient will verbalize various activities she would like to do and can do within the activity limit.

    INTERVENTIONS

    1. Assess patient's interest in various diversional activities within the activity limit.
    2. Explore interests for acceptable alternatives.
    3. Provide ideas. Refer to Box 21-3 for helpful hints for bed rest preterm labor patients.

Box 21-2

Entertaining Children While Mother is on Bed Rest

Keep supplies in a laundry basket near your bed.

Keep a roll of paper towels near your bed for spills.

Use an old sheet or blanket as a playtime cover to spare your bedspread.

Keep activities brief.

Have a remote-control television.

Don't feel guilty about "neglecting your children." They live through it, and it is a small portion out of their lives in comparison with the rest of your unborn baby's life.

Let your child play under the covers.

Play "bed bowling" with paper cups and a small ball.

Play "bed basketball" with rolled-up socks and an empty laundry basket.

Direct bedspread traffic using small cars to follow the design on the bedspread.

Use a mirror to make faces. This would be a good time to express feelings and show them on your faces in the mirror.

Make hand shadows on the wall with a flashlight.

Build with blocks.

Play board games.

Go bed fishing using magnets and paper fish.

Play red light–green light, with mom as the traffic cop.

Cut up magazines and paste them on cardboard.

Make an alphabet book by cutting up magazines and pasting in a photograph album using a separate page for each letter.

Get children's books from the library, and read to your child!

Color in coloring books.

Play with Colorforms sets.

Play "I see something"; find something in the room, say its color, and then ask your child to guess what you are "seeing."

Play with Play-doh.

Trace letters or numbers on your child's back and have him or her guess what you wrote.

Use this time constructively. Once the baby gets here you will never have this opportunity to spend this "special" time with this child again!

Modified from Maurer L: *Confinement Connection: a home support program,* Phoenix, 1992.

Box 21-3

Helpful Hints for Bed Rest Preterm Labor Patients

Wear clothes during the day if possible.

Be neat and clean; keep up personal hygiene.

Have as much contact and involvement with children as possible.

Set goals, and keep them in mind.

Shop by phone using the yellow pages and catalogs.

Plan your menus, and organize the grocery list.

Do long put-off projects, such as pictures in albums, letters, stitchery, or Christmas cards.

Keep a journal of your pregnancy.

Do things with your children: television, reading, games, video games, special "just talking" time, making a paper chain and having child take one off for every day, puzzles.

Have visitors when you feel up to it, but keep this under control.

If you do not have child care, make your bedroom into a giant playpen. Put everything out of reach, and shut the door so you don't have to worry about where your child is.

Have a small ice chest next to your bed packed with the day's supplies of drinks and snacks.

Do something special to pick you up when you are down, such as a manicure, facial, or favorite show.

Keep a calendar close by to chart your progress. Focus on how far you have come, not how far you have to go!

Get books on tape if you tire of reading.

Make a list of things that people can do for you, so when they ask you can easily come up with something and you can even give them a choice! And do take them up on their offer; people mean it, or they would not offer in the first place.

Obtain a childbirth class in the home if this is available in your area.

Have a "date" with your partner: have him pick up take-out food and bring out the candles.

Do craft projects such as cross-stitch, needlepoint, or knitting. Make something special for the baby or maybe someone else!

Do passive bed rest exercises with prior approval from your physician.

Read books available on high risk pregnancy and premature babies. Be informed, and become involved as a partner with your physician in your care.

Focus on *why* you are doing this, not *what* you are doing.

Utilize your local support group for empathy and understanding when you need to talk to someone who can understand your feelings and fears.

Box 21-3
Helpful Hints for Bed Rest Preterm Labor Patients—cont'd

Pay the bills.
Compile tax data.
Reorganize files.
Update your address book.
Do mending.
Learn a new language with tapes from the library.
Order and address birth announcements.
Call a friend, relative, or support person each day.
Do crossword, word search, or jigsaw puzzles.

Modified from Maloni J: *J Obstet Gynecol Neonatal Nurs* 23(8):696-706, 1994; Mauer L: *Confinement Connection: a home support program,* Phoenix, 1992.

4. Refer to self-support programs where childbirth preparation classes are modified to meet special needs and socialization opportunities are available with couples experiencing a similar high risk pregnancy.

- **RISK FOR FEAR** related to the real threat of a preterm delivery on the health and well-being of the expected baby.
  DESIRED OUTCOMES: The patient and her family will communicate their fears and concerns openly. They will establish a trusting relationship between themselves and the health care professionals.
  INTERVENTIONS
  1. Provide time for the patient and her family to express their concerns regarding the possible outcome for the baby and inconvenience to the mother and family during treatment. Encourage them to vent any feelings, fears, and anger they may experience.
  2. Assess family's support system and coping mechanisms.
  3. Provide patient and her family with honest appraisal of the situation and plan of treatment.
  4. Give adequate information for decisions about alternatives of care.
  5. Refer to support groups with home care programs.
  6. Refer to a spiritual counselor or chaplain on request.

COLLABORATIVE INTERVENTION FOR TOCOLYTIC DRUG THERAPY

Tocolytic agents are currently divided into four classes: (1) beta-sympathomimetics, (2) magnesium sulfate, (3) calcium antagonists, and (4) prostaglandin inhibitors.

Beta-sympathomimetics

Action

Sympathomimetic drugs supplement or mimic the effects of norepinephrine and epinephrine on the body's organs innervated by the adrenergic nerve fibers. There are two types of adrenergic receptors: alpha and beta. Alpha-receptors primarily cause contractions of smooth muscle; beta-receptors primarily cause relaxation of smooth muscle, except in the heart, where they cause cardiac stimulation. There are two types of beta-receptors: $beta_1$ and $beta_2$. $Beta_1$-receptors are more predominant in the heart, and their stimulation results in tachycardia and increased myocardial contractility. $Beta_2$-receptors are more predominant in the uterus, blood vessels, bronchioles, and diaphragm. The contractility of the smooth muscle is decreased, which results in uterine and bronchial relaxation and peripheral vasodilation. Contractility of smooth muscle is decreased by binding calcium to the sarcoplasmic reticulum and activating adenyl cyclase, thereby decreasing intracellular concentration of calcium (Kosasa and others, 1994).

Dosage for ritodrine

When IV ritodrine is ordered, 150 mg is usually diluted in 500 ml of IV fluid such as normal saline or lactated Ringer's solution, yielding a 0.3 mg/ml or 300 µg/ml concentration. It is usually started at 50 to 100 µg/min (0.05 to 0.1 mg/min) and increased 50 µg/min (0.05 mg/min) every 10 minutes until one of the following events occurs:

1. Uterine contractions stop.
2. Intolerable side effects develop.
3. A maximum dose of 350 µg/min (0.35 mg/min) is reached.

The patient is usually maintained on the dose that is effective for her for 12 to 24 hours after uterine contractions cease. Then the IV medication is usually tapered off, and the patient is placed on oral therapy 30 minutes before stopping the IV infusion. The initial oral dosage is 10 mg every 2 to 4 hours for 24 hours and then 10 to 20 mg every 4 to 6 hours. The maximum oral dose during a 24-hour period is 120 mg.

Dosage for terbutaline

When IV terbutaline is ordered, 5 mg is usually diluted in 500 ml of lactated Ringer's solution or normal saline. It is usually started at 2.5 to 20 µg/min and increased 5 µg/min every 10 minutes until one of the following occurs (Clark and others, 1987):

1. Uterine contractions cease.
2. Intolerable side effects develop.
3. A maximum dose of 80 mg/min is reached.

The patient is usually maintained on a dose that is effective for her for 12 to 24 hours after uterine contractions cease. The medication is then tapered off, and the patient is started on subcutaneous injections of 0.25 mg every 4 hours or oral therapy of 5 mg every 6 to 8 hours or 2.5 mg every 4 hours.

Side effects

Side effects that frequently occur with ritodrine or terbutaline include the following:

- Slight hypotension or a widening of maternal pulse pressure related to a slight increase in systolic and a slight decrease in diastolic pressure, thereby decreasing coronary perfusion
- Light-headedness, tremors, and a flushed feeling related to relaxation of vascular smooth muscle
- Restlessness, emotional upset, and anxiety related to epinephrine release
- Maternal and fetal tachycardia, heart palpitations, and frequent skipping of a heartbeat related to cardiac stimulation
- Transient maternal hyperglycemia related to drug stimulation of the liver and muscle, causing glycogenolysis, gluconeogenesis, and decreased uptake of glucose by peripheral tissue
- Elevated lactate and free fatty acids related to hyperglycemia
- Increased insulin and glucagon secretion related to drug stimulation of the pancreas
- Decreased serum potassium caused by an intracellular shift from the extracellular space
- Decreased hematocrit by 20% to 25% related to plasma volume expansion
- Nausea or vomiting related to decreased intestinal motility
- Bronchial relaxation

Intolerable side effects

- Maternal tachycardia greater than 140 beats/min
- Drop in blood pressure to less than 90/60
- Chest pain or tightness
- Cardiac dysrhythmias

Potential life-threatening complications

Potential life-threatening complications that have resulted from the IV administration of ritodrine or terbutaline are listed below:

- Pulmonary edema, which may result from myocardial failure and fluid overload

- Subendocardial myocardial ischemia
- Cardiac dysrhythmias, such as premature ventricular contractions, premature nodal contractions, and atrial fibrillation
- Cerebral vasospasm in patients who have a history of migraine headaches

Nursing interventions for IV therapy

1. Obtain a patient history that includes a medical history of cardiovascular disease, cardiac dysrhythmias, hypertension, uncontrolled maternal hyperthyroidism, or migraine headaches. If the patient has a severe cardiac disease, she is not a candidate for this type of labor suppressant therapy. If she has any of the other disorders listed, it should be used only with extreme caution.

2. Assess for signs of bleeding. Because beta-sympathomimetics antagonize the body's normal compensatory mechanism for blood loss by their effects on heart rate and systolic and diastolic pressure, these drugs should not be used if there are any indications that bleeding is present.

3. Assess for signs of an intraamniotic infection. Refer to Chapter 22. Suppression of labor is contraindicated in the presence of an intraamniotic infection, but especially with beta-sympathomimetics, because of the increased risk of developing maternal pulmonary edema.

4. Assess for signs of a UTI. Obtain a clean-catch midstream or catheterized urine specimen for urinalysis and urine culture.

5. Obtain such baseline data as FHR, uterine activity, maternal vital signs, weight, electrocardiogram, and laboratory studies that include a complete blood count with differential, blood glucose, urea nitrogen, and serum electrolytes.

6. Start an IV infusion of normal saline with an 18-gauge needle to piggyback the IV administration of ritodrine or terbutaline. Because incremental titration is essential, an infusion pump should be used.

7. Encourage the patient to maintain a left lateral position to minimize the risk of hypotension during IV administration.

8. An external monitor should be used to record FHR and uterine activity continuously.

9. Blood pressure, pulse rate and rhythm, and temperature should be monitored closely.

10. To avoid fluid overload and pulmonary edema, the total fluid intake for 24 hours should not exceed 2.5 L.

11. Accurately measure and record intake and output and a daily weight.

12. If intolerable side effects develop, the drug should be discontinued, oxygen administered via face mask, the attending physician notified, and preparation made to obtain an electrocardiogram.

13. Have available cardiopulmonary resuscitation (CPR) equipment and an appropriate beta-blocking antidote such as propranolol (Inderal), 0.25 mg, or verapamil.

14. Be prepared to reverse pulmonary edema with IV furosemide (Lasix).

15. Be prepared to obtain diagnostic data, such as serum potassium, hemoglobin, hematocrit, and renal function studies periodically during the IV treatment. Although hypokalemia can develop as the result of potassium moving from the extracellular space to the intracellular space, there is no change in the total body potassium level. Therefore supplemental potassium is usually not necessary. The potassium level will return to normal within 24 hours after the IV therapy is discontinued.

16. Measure blood glucose twice daily with B-G Chemstrips or the Dextrometer. Diabetic patients can become hyperglycemic if treated with either terbutaline or ritodrine. Therefore they require careful monitoring of plasma glucose and usually require IV insulin administration.

17. Anticipate that glucocorticoids may be administered to stimulate a more mature fetal surfactant production. In this event, refer to the collaborative interventions for stimulation of fetal lung maturity outlined in this chapter.

Nursing interventions for oral therapy

Every patient to be discharged and continued on oral therapy at home should be instructed in medication administration with the following self-assessments:

1. Check pulse before taking the medicine. If pulse is greater than 120 beats/min, contact physician before taking medication.

2. Report any medication side effects such as heart palpitations, tremors, or nervousness.

3. Check temperature daily.

4. Report the development of any early signs of preterm labor, such as four or more uterine contractions in 1 hour, or any warning signs, such as intermittent backache or change in amount or character of vaginal discharge.

5. Report signs of rupture of membranes, vaginal bleeding, and signs of infection, such as an elevated temperature.
6. Return for weekly prenatal visits, fetal surveillance studies, and glucose monitoring.

Long-term effects

The only major side effect to the fetus is tachycardia, but no adverse physical or neurologic effects have been noted. In contrast, beneficial effects have been demonstrated even when delivery is postponed for only 24 to 72 hours. A beneficial effect is acceleration of the phospholipid synthesis caused by stress on the fetus. Therefore the incidence of neonatal respiratory distress syndrome is decreased. The only side effect noted in the neonate has been mild, transient hypoglycemia or hyperglycemia during the first 24 hours.

Magnesium sulfate

Delineative reports of the efficacy of magnesium sulfate as a tocolytic were reviewed by Elliott (1984). Subsequent reports support this original work (Hollander and others, 1987; Wilkins and others, 1988). In the past, magnesium sulfate has been used in obstetrics primarily to treat preeclampsia. It is now being used more often in the treatment of preterm labor (Kosasa and others, 1994).

Action

Magnesium relaxes the smooth muscle of the uterus by substituting itself in place of calcium. Magnesium acts not only at the cellular level to decrease uterine activity but also at a nerve transmission level. Magnesium blocks the release of acetylcholine at the nerve synapse by displacing calcium, thus blocking nerve transmission to the muscle. Secondary effects of magnesium, such as decreasing arteriole pressure and increasing uterine blood flow, can also be therapeutic in suppressing preterm labor.

Dosage

A loading IV dose of 6 to 8 g is usually recommended in the treatment of preterm labor, followed by a maintenance dose of 2 to 4 g/hr until uterine contractions cease or signs of toxicity develop. The patient being treated for preterm labor can tolerate a much higher dose of magnesium than the preeclamptic patient. Kidney function is usually not compromised in the preterm labor patient as it can be in the preeclamptic patient.

Signs of toxicity

- Respirations fewer than 12/min

- Absence of deep tendon reflexes
- Severe hypotension
- Extreme muscle relaxation

Side effects

During the loading dose, the patient frequently complains of hot flashes, nausea, vomiting, drowsiness, and blurred vision. These side effects usually subside when the loading dose is completed.

Nursing interventions

1. Monitor vital signs frequently, especially blood pressure and respiration. (Because magnesium relaxes skeletal as well as smooth muscle, respiratory and circulatory failure can occur if toxic levels are allowed to develop.)
2. Check the deep tendon reflex every hour. (The reflexes are frequently suppressed before significant respiratory suppression.)
3. Keep an hourly intake and output record. Because magnesium is rapidly secreted from the mother's body by way of the kidneys, urinary output should be at least 30 ml/hr or magnesium will accumulate in the body and toxicity will develop.
4. Refer to serum magnesium levels daily. Therapeutic serum levels of 4 to 7.5 mEq/L are effective in reducing uterine contractions. Toxicity can develop with levels of 10 mEq/L or greater.
5. Do not administer concurrently with a narcotic or sedative. (Concurrent administration potentiates the effect of respiratory depression.)
6. Have CPR equipment and the antidote, calcium gluconate (1 to 2 g), available.
7. Restrict total fluids to 2500 ml/24 hr.

Nursing intervention for oral therapy

Oral magnesium oxide or magnesium gluconate may be used for maintenance tocolysis. The normal dose for magnesium gluconate is 1 g every 2 to 4 hours. Research has indicated that either drug is as effective as an oral beta-sympathomimetic in suppressing preterm labor with fewer side effects (Martin and others, 1988; Ridgway and others, 1990). The most common side effects experienced by patients are nausea/vomiting and diarrhea.

Long-term effect on neonate

Neonatal side effects are rare as long as the mother's serum level is maintained below 8 mEq/L. Infants born to mothers who received magnesium sulfate intravenously demonstrate no negative long-term effects. Only slight muscle flaccidity and hypocalcemia may be noted. Both symptoms are treatable.

Calcium channel blockers

Action

Calcium channel blockers do not allow the movement of calcium into the smooth muscle of the uterus. Contraction of smooth muscle depends on the availability of calcium.

Dosage

Dosage is 10 to 20 mg of nifedipine orally or sublingually every 3 to 8 hours.

Side effects

The following side effects are uncommon, but if they occur they are related to peripheral vasodilation:

- Headache
- Fatigue
- Hypotension
- Dizziness
- Peripheral edema

Prostaglandin inhibitors

Action

Prostaglandin inhibitors, such as indomethacin or ibuprofen (Motrin), act by inhibiting prostaglandin synthesis.

Contraindications

Prostaglandin inhibitors are contraindicated in patients who have a peptic ulcer or a drug sensitivity to salicylates.

Dosage

The initial loading dose of indomethacin is 50 mg orally or by rectal suppository followed by a maintenance oral dose of 25 mg every 4 hours for 24 to 48 hours (Heppard, Garite, 1996; Niebyl, Chez, 1988). If contractions recur, a second course of indomethacin may be given (Heppard, Garite, 1996). Others have treated patients for 1 month or more with the drug (Besinger and others, 1991; Eronen and others, 1991; Niebyl, Chez, 1988). Ibuprofen, 600 mg every 6 hours, may be used instead.

Side effects

Oligohydramnios, premature closure of the ductus arteriosus, and neonatal pulmonary hypertension have been noted if a prostaglandin inhibitor is used longer than 48 hours (Besinger and others, 1991; Eronen and others, 1991). The risk of transient obstruction of the ductus arteriosus increases with increasing gestational age (Eronen and others, 1991).

Nursing interventions

1. Because of the potential seriousness of the side effects, prostaglandin inhibitors are currently used only with very immature gestations in which other tocolysis has failed. They should not be used after 35 weeks of gestation.
2. Be prepared to assist with fetal surveillance studies such as an echocardiogram and amniotic fluid index.

COLLABORATIVE INTERVENTIONS FOR STIMULATION OF FETAL LUNG MATURITY

Betamethasone or dexamethasone

Action

Steroid therapy stimulates the production of a more stable lecithin, which is a surface-active phospholipid mainly responsible for facilitating normal alveolar function. Steroid therapy is thought to decrease the risk of neonatal respiratory distress in the fetus born between 28 and 34 weeks of gestation.

Side effects

The effects on the mother include increased risk of infection and delayed wound healing. If she has diabetes or hypertension of pregnancy, steroids can aggravate these disorders. There is an increased risk of maternal endometritis if steroids are administered in the presence of premature rupture of membranes.

Dosage

Betamethasone and dexamethasone are the two drugs of choice because they cross the placenta unchanged whereas other steroids do not. Betamethasone (Celestone) has short- and long-term activities and is usually favored. The routine dose is two doses of 12 mg 24 hours apart. At 48 hours following the first dose, the steroid window is reached. This means that the full effect on maturing the surfactant has been obtained. Steroid therapy has a transient effect on lecithin. Therefore if the patient does not deliver within 1 week, the treatment should be repeated if the fetus is less than 34 weeks of gestation (Mazor and others, 1994).

Nursing interventions

1. Ensure that the patient has been informed, understands the advantages and the risk involved with steroid therapy, and has been provided an opportunity to give an informed consent.
2. Monitor the fetus closely for signs of compromise.
3. Notify the neonatal intensive care team or neonatologist of the delivery when imminent.
4. If steroids are used in the diabetic patient, she should receive IV insulin and have her blood sugar levels evalu-

ated frequently for hyperglycemia because of the effect of steroids on blood sugar.

COLLABORATIVE INTERVENTIONS FOR HOME UTERINE ACTIVITY MONITORING

The benefits of home uterine activity monitoring, with electronic monitoring equipment or self-palpation, have been comparatively studied. These programs were initiated because early signs and symptoms of preterm labor were often difficult to detect and many times the diagnosis of preterm labor was not made until after advanced cervical dilation had occurred, when tocolysis is ineffective. Presumably, home uterine contraction monitoring facilitates early detection of uterine contractions, thereby fostering early treatment before cervical changes occur.

Components of uterine activity monitoring program

Program initiation

The physician may order home uterine contraction monitoring when a woman who is at risk for preterm labor reports or is treated for signs of preterm labor. In the event home uterine contraction monitoring is ordered, the patient monitors for uterine contractions either by self-palpation or with a home uterine contraction monitor. Self-palpation is done by teaching the woman to spread her fingers across all four quadrants of her abdomen, pressing in just enough to feel the uterine wall through the abdominal muscle (Fig. 21-5). If a home uterine contraction monitor is to be used, the patient must be referred to one of the uterine contraction monitoring companies to rent the monitor. She is taught how to place the ambulatory tocodynamometer, which is connected to a battery-operated recording unit, just below the umbilicus and comfortably secure it with a belt. When the device for home uterine activity monitoring is used, self-palpation must also be taught to the patient.

Uterine monitoring

Whether using the device for monitoring or self-palpation alone, uterine activity is recorded for 1 full hour twice each day. With the monitoring equipment, contraction data are stored for later transmission via the telephone. With self-palpation alone, the woman is instructed to record the period of cramping or the numbers of contractions and whether they were palpated only or also perceived as a specific sensation, such as backache, tightening, tingling, or discomfort.

Daily nursing contact

Once each day a preterm birth prevention nurse contacts the patient at home, discusses with her any home management problems, and

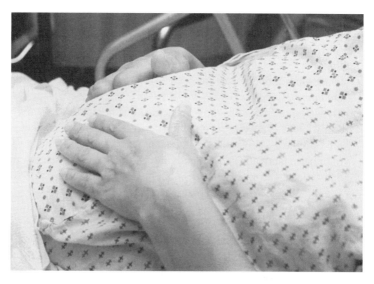

FIG. 21-5 Self-palpation for uterine contractions.

encourages her to share her perception of how the past 24 hours have been.

Transmission of data

After the nurse contact, the patient, using the monitoring equipment, is instructed to transmit both of the stored hours of contraction information. This is done by connecting the home telephone receiver into the recorder and pressing a button on the recorder to send. Within a matter of minutes, the 2 hours worth of contraction monitoring is received on the receiving center's equipment. If self-palpation is used, the woman describes times and type of uterine activity noted to the nurse.

Analysis of data

The received data are analyzed by the nurse.

Nursing interventions

The information from contraction monitoring is relayed verbally to the patient, and instructions for further monitoring, continuing care, or reporting to the hospital for treatment are given. The instructions are based on a tolerable baseline of no more than four contractions (or other number determined by the attending physician) per hour or patient's report of symptoms. Standing physician orders or immediate referral to the attending physician guides the nurse's instructions to the patient.

Expense

The patient's third-party reimbursement is charged a separate daily fee for the rental of the equipment and for the nursing care follow-up. The cost/benefit ratio for indiscriminate use of the uterine contraction monitor has not been firmly established by research.

Outcome

To date, most research studies conclude that home uterine activity monitoring, used in concert with perinatal nursing, can reduce preterm births. The results of these studies show earlier diagnosis of preterm labor and subsequently more effective tocolysis (Dyson and others, 1991; Grimes, Schulz, 1992; Hill and others, 1990; Koehl, Wheeler, 1989; Merkatz, Merkatz, 1991).

However, the nurse contact, along with uterine self-palpation, may be the key element in the success of the home uterine monitoring program. Four prospectively randomized studies (Dyson and others, 1991; Iams and others, 1988; Porto and others, 1987; Scioscia and others, 1988) have compared the two methods, that is, nurse contact along with daily home uterine monitoring with a device versus daily nurse contact with uterine self-palpation. In all the studies, both groups had a significant reduction in preterm birth when compared with a control group. However, there were no differences between the two groups who received daily nurse contact with or without the uterine contraction monitoring device. According to the ACOG (1989), home uterine activity devices are not recommended for clinical use, but for research only, until further research answers this question.

COLLABORATIVE INTERVENTION FOR SUBCUTANEOUS TERBUTALINE PUMP

The terbutaline pump delivers a small, continuous basal rate, usually 0.05 to 0.075 mg/hr. It is also preset for boluses of 0.25 mg. The bolus schedule is determined from observing and analyzing a pattern of contraction frequencies over a 24-hour monitoring period.

Nursing interventions before discharge

1. The patient's contraction pattern is stabilized with magnesium sulfate for at least 24 hours before starting the terbutaline pump therapy. This allows the myometrial receptor sites for beta-sympathomimetics to recover their sensitivity to terbutaline.
2. Be prepared to assist with baseline screening for electrolyte imbalance; carbohydrate intolerance; anemia; and vaginal infections such as gonorrhea, *Chlamydia,* group B streptococci, *Bacteroides fragilis,* and *Bacteroides bivius.*

3. Be prepared to obtain an electrocardiogram as part of the baseline data.

4. Obtain a 24-hour uterine contraction pattern to be used by the physician in ordering the basal rate and setting the bolus schedule.

5. Develop a consistent patient education program that includes the following:
   a. Physiologic basis of pump therapy
   b. Mechanics of pump operation
   c. Mechanism of loading prefilled syringes into pump
   d. Subcutaneous needle insertion in lower abdomen and upper thighs
   e. Side effects to be monitored and reported, such as pulse rate greater than 120 beats/min, chest pains or tightness, heart palpitations, and signs of infection at injection site
   f. Importance of daily uterine activity evaluation either with a uterine monitor or uterine self-palpation
   g. Daily fetal activity recording
   h. Reinforce or educate as to ways to decrease risk of preterm labor recurrence as outlined in the altered health maintenance nursing diagnosis.

• • •

WEEKLY NURSING ASSESSMENT IN HOME

Refer to Boxes 21-4 and 21-5 for a guide to the nursing assessment in the home.

Box 21-4
Home Visit Physical Assessment

Vital signs, including blood pressure, respiratory rate, and temperature
Breath sounds
Fetal heart rate
Fetal activity
Cervical status
Fasting blood glucose because of possible drug-induced alteration in glucose metabolism
Weight
Fundal height
Urine for ketones, protein, leukocyte esterase
Signs of pathologic edema

Box 21-5

Functional Health Pattern Assessment for Home Visit

Health perception/health management assessment

Which prenatal health care resources have you used or do you plan to use, such as childbirth education classes, support groups, social service, and community agencies?

Nutritional assessment

What is a typical daily food and fluid intake?

Appetite?

Elimination assessment

Urinary elimination pattern: changes or problems perceived, such as odor or burning pain on urination?

Bowel elimination pattern: changes or problems perceived, such as flatulence or constipation?

Activity/exercise assessment

What activity level are you maintaining? What kinds of limited activity exercises are you doing?

Sleep/rest assessment

How do you feel after a night's sleep?

Cognitive/perceptual assessment

Describe your uterine activity pattern. How many contractions do you palpate during the assessment hour? What activities seem to stimulate contractions?

What kind of management problems have you experienced with the pump, home bed rest, or other recommendations?

Self-perception/self-concept assessment

Describe how you and your family feel everything is going.

Role-relationship assessment

How are all your role responsibilities being managed while you are maintaining limited activity?

How are you dealing with boredom?

Sexuality/reproductive assessment

Have you experienced any warning signs of preterm labor? How are you and your partner dealing with the restricted sexual activity?

Coping/stress tolerance assessment

What are you most concerned or worried about at this time?

How are other family members dealing with their concerns, anxiety, or fear?

CONCLUSION

The ultimate goal of prevention and treatment of preterm labor is delivery of a healthy term infant. It is a fact that neonatal outcomes are greatly improved when intrauterine life can be extended until fetal lungs mature. It is therefore suggested that delaying labor for even days can be beneficial. Screening and education for self-monitoring and home care are the key factors to preventing preterm labor and delivery. Early diagnosis and frequent health care contact can have a positive effect on early treatment of preterm labor before advanced cervical changes take place. Perinatal nurses can have a positive impact on neonatal morbidity by doing what nurses do so uniquely well. Screening, motivating, providing health care education, and frequent caring and sensitive contact with at-risk pregnant women can make a significant contribution to lowering neonatal morbidity and mortality from preterm delivery.

BIBLIOGRAPHY

Abrams B, Parker J: Maternal weight gain in women with good pregnancy outcome, *Obstet Gynecol* 76(1):1-7, 1990.

Alexander G and others: Preterm birth prevention: an evaluation of programs in the United States, *Birth* 18(3):160-169, 1991.

American College of Obstetricians and Gynecologists (ACOG): *ACOG committee opinion: strategies to prevent prematurity: home uterine contraction monitoring,* no. 74, Washington, DC, 1989, The College.

American College of Obstetricians and Gynecologists (ACOG): *Preterm ACOG Techn Bull,* no. 206, 1995.

Bentley D and others: Relationship of uterine contractility to preterm labor, *Obstet Gynecol* 76:36S-38S, 1990.

Besinger R and others: Randomized comparative trial of indomethacin and ritodrine for the long-term treatment of preterm labor, *Am J Obstet Gynecol* 164:981-988, 1991.

Caritis S and others: Pharmacokinetics of orally administered ritodrine, *Am J Obstet Gynecol* 161(1):32-34, 1989.

Carsten M, Miller J: A new look at urine muscle contraction, *Am J Obstet Gynecol* 157:1303-1305, 1987.

Casey M, MacDonald P: Bimolecular processes in the initiation of parturition: decidual activation, *Clin Obstet Gynecol* 31(3):533-552, 1988.

Clark I and others: Tissue inhibitor of metalloproteinases: serum levels during pregnancy and labor, term and preterm, *Obstet Gynecol* 83(4):532-542, 1995.

Clark S and others: *Critical care obstetrics,* ed 2, Boston, 1987, Blackwell Scientific Publications.

Creasy R, Merkatz I: Prevention of preterm birth: clinical opinion, *Obstet Gynecol* 76:2S-4S, 1990.

Creasy R, Resnik R, editors: *Maternal-fetal medicine: principles and practice,* ed 3, Philadelphia, 1994, Saunders.

Cunningham R, MacDonald P, Gant N: *Williams' obstetrics,* ed 20, Norwalk, Conn, 1997, Appleton & Lange.

Dahlberg N, Kolorutis M: Hospital based perinatal home care program, *J Obstet Gynecol Neonatal Nurs* 23(8):682-686, 1994.

Dyson D and others: Prevention and preterm birth in high risk patients: the role of education and provider contact versus home uterine monitoring, *Am J Obstet Gynecol* 164(3):756-762, 1991.

Eganhouse D: A nursing model for a community hospital preterm birth prevention program, *J Obstet Gynecol Neonatal Nurs* 23(9):756-766, 1994.

Elliott J: Magnesium sulfate as a tocolytic agent, *Am J Obstet Gynecol* 147:277, 1984.

Eronen M and others: The effects of indomethacin and a B-sympathomimetic agent on the fetal ductus arteriosus during treatment of premature labor: a randomized double-blind study, *Am J Obstet Gynecol* 164:141-146, 1991.

Ferguson J and others: A comparison of tocolysis with nifedipine or ritodrine: analysis of efficacy and maternal, fetal, and neonatal outcome, *Am J Obstet Gynecol* 163:105-111, 1990.

Freda M, Damus K, Merkatz I: What do pregnant women know about preventing preterm birth? *J Obstet Gynecol Neonatal Nurs* 20(2):140-145, 1991.

Freston M and others: Responses of pregnant women to potential preterm labor symptoms, *J Obstet Gynecol Neonatal Nurs* 26(1):35-41, 1997.

Garite T and others: Uterine activity characteristics in multiple gestations, *Obstet Gynecol* 76:56S-59S, 1990.

Gill P, Smith M, McGregor C: Terbutaline by pump to prevent recurrent preterm labor, *MCN Am J Matern Child Nurs* 14(3):163-167, 1989.

Goldenberg R and others: Bedrest in pregnancy, *Obstet Gynecol* 84(1):131-136, 1994.

Grimes D, Schulz K: Randomized controlled trials of home uterine activity monitoring: a review and critique, *Obstet Gynecol* 79(1):137-142, 1992.

Heppard M, Garite T: *Acute obstetrics: a practical guide,* ed 2, St Louis, 1996, Mosby.

Hill W and others: Home uterine activity monitoring is associated with a reduction in preterm birth, *Obstet Gynecol* 76:13S-17S, 1990.

Hollander D, Nagey D, Pupkin M: Magnesium sulfate and ritodrine hydrochloride: a randomized comparison, *Am J Obstet Gynecol* 156:631, 1987.

Hoskins I and others: Relationship between antepartum cocaine abuse, abnormal umbilical artery Doppler velocimetry, and placental abruption, *Obstet Gynecol* 78(2):279-282, 1991.

Huszar G: Physiology of the myometrium. In Creasy R, Resnik R, editors: *Maternal-fetal medicine: principles and practice,* ed 3, Philadelphia, 1994, Saunders.

Iams J, Johnson F, Hamer C: Uterine activity and symptoms as predictors of preterm labor, *Obstet Gynecol* 76:42S-45S, 1990a.

Iams J, Johnson F, O'Shaughnessy R: A prospective random trial of home uterine activity monitoring in pregnancies at increased risk of preterm labor. II, *Am J Obstet Gynecol* 159:595-603, 1988.

Iams J and others: Symptoms that precede preterm labor and preterm premature rupture of the membranes, *Am J Obstet Gynecol* 162:486-490, 1990b.

Iams J and others: A prospective evaluation of the signs and symptoms of preterm labor, *Obstet Gynecol* 84(2):227-230, 1994.

Katz M, Goodyear K, Creasy R: Early signs and symptoms of preterm labor, *Am J Obstet Gynecol* 162:1150-1153, 1990.

Jones D, Collins B: The nursing management of women experiencing preterm labor: clinical guidelines and why they are needed, *J Obstet Gynecol Neonatal Nurs* 25(7):569-592, 1996.

Josten L and others: Bedrest compliance for women with pregnancy problems, *Birth* 22(1):1-12, 1995.

Knuppel R and others: Preventing preterm birth in twin gestation: home uterine activity monitoring and perinatal nursing support, *Obstet Gynecol* 76(1):24S-27S, 1990.

Koehl L, Wheeler D: Monitoring uterine activity at home, *Am J Nurs* 89(2):200-203, 1989.

Kosasa T and others: Long-term tocolysis with combined intravenous terbutaline and magnesium sulfate: a 10 year study of 1000 patients, *Obstet Gynecol* 84(3):369-376, 1994.

Kristensen J and others: Idiopathic preterm deliveries in Denmark, *Obstet Gynecol* 85(4):549-557, 1995.

Krohn M and others: Vaginal *Bacteroides* species are associated with an increased rate of preterm delivery among women in preterm labor, *J Infect Dis* 164(1):88-93, 1991.

Lam F: Miniature pump infusion of terbutaline: an option in preterm labor, *Contemp OB/GYN* 33(1):58-70, 1989.

Lockwood C and others: Fetal fibronectin in cervical and vaginal secretions as a predictor of preterm delivery, *N Engl J Med* 325(10):672-674, 1991.

MacKenzie L and others: Prostacyclin biosynthesis by cultured human myometrial smooth muscle cells: dependency on arachidonic acid in the culture medium, *Am J Obstet Gynecol* 159:1365-1372, 1988.

Main D, Gabbe S: Risk scoring for preterm labor: where do we go from here? *Am J Obstet Gynecol* 157:789-793, 1987.

Maloni J: Bedrest during pregnancy: implications for nursing, *J Obstet Gynecol Neonatal Nurs* 22(5):422-426, 1993.

Maloni J: Home care of the high risk pregnant woman requiring bed rest, *J Obstet Gynecol Neonatal Nurs* 23(8):696-706, 1994.

Maloni J: Bedrest and the high risk pregnancy, *Matern Fetal Nurs* 31(2):313-325, 1996.

Maloni J and others: Physical and psychosocial side effects of antepartum hospital bedrest, *Nurs Res* 42(4):197-203, 1993.

Martin R and others: Comparison of oral ritodrine and magnesium gluconate for ambulatory tocolysis, *Am J Obstet Gynecol* 158:1440-1445, 1988.

Martin R and others: Uterine activity compared with symptomatology in the detection of preterm labor, *Obstet Gynecol* 76(1):19S-23S, 1990.

Maurer L: *Confinement Connection: a home support program,* Phoenix, 1992.

Mazor M and others: Association between preterm birth and increased maternal plasma cortisol concentrations, *Obstet Gynecol* 84(4):521-528, 1994.

Merkatz R, Merkatz I: The contributions of the nurse and the machine in home uterine activity monitoring systems, *Am J Obstet Gynecol* 164(5):1159-1162, 1991.

Mitchell M: Pathways of arachidonic acid metabolism with specific application to the fetus and mother, *Semin Perinatol* 10(4):242-254, 1986.

Morrison J: Preterm birth: a puzzle worth solving, *Obstet Gynecol* 76:5S-11S, 1990.

Morrison J and others: Cost/health effectiveness of home uterine activity monitoring in a medicaid population, *Obstet Gynecol* 76(1):76S-81S, 1990.

Nageotte M and others: Quantitation of uterine activity preceding preterm, term, and postterm labor, *Am J Obstet Gynecol* 158:1254-1259, 1988.

Nagey D and others: Randomized comparison of home uterine activity monitoring and routine care in patients discharged after treatment for preterm labor, *Obstet Gynecol* 82(3):319-323, 1993.

Niebyl J: Averting preterm labor with first-line tocolytics, *Contemp OB/GYN* 32(6):65-78, 1988.

Niebyl J, Chez R: Indomethacin for preterm labor, *Contemp OB/GYN* 31(4):69-72, 1988.

Papiernik E and others: *Effective prevention of preterm birth: the French experience measured at Haguenau,* New York, 1989, March of Dimes.

Pircon R and others: Controlled trial of hydration and bed rest versus bed rest alone in the evaluation of preterm uterine contractions, *Am J Obstet Gynecol* 161:775-779, 1989.

Porto M: Home uterine activity monitoring: essential tool or expensive accessory? *Contemp OB/GYN* 35(1):112S-119S, 1990.

Porto M and others: *The role of home uterine activity monitoring in the prevention of preterm birth.* Presented at the Society of Perinatal Obstetricians, Orlando, Feb 5-7, 1987.

Rhoads G, McNellis D, Kessel S: Home monitoring of uterine contractility, *Am J Obstet Gynecol* 165:2-6, 1991.

Ridgway L and others: A prospective randomized comparison of oral terbutaline and magnesium oxide for the maintenance of tocolysis, *Am J Obstet Gynecol* 163:879-882, 1990.

Romeo C, Jones P: Home infusion therapies for obstetric patients, *JOGNN* 23(8):675-681, 1994.

Romero C, Jones P: Home infusion therapies for obstetric patients, *J Obstet Gynecol Neonatal Nurs* 23(8):675-681, 1994.

Romero R, Mazor M, Tarkakovsky B: Systemic administration of interleukin induces preterm parturition, *Am J Obstet Gynecol* 165(4):969-972, 1991.

Romero R, Oyarzun E, Mazor M: Mechanisms at work when infection triggers preterm labor, *Contemp OB/GYN* 33(1):133-150, 1989.

Romero R and others: Evidence for a local change in the progesterone/estrogen ratio in human parturition at term, *Am J Obstet Gynecol* 159:657-660, 1988.

Ross M and others: The West Los Angeles preterm birth prevention project II: cost effectiveness analysis of high risk pregnancy interventions, *Obstet Gynecol* 83(4):506-511, 1994.

Sala D, Moise K: The treatment of preterm labor using a portable subcutaneous terbutaline pump, *J Obstet Gynecol Neonatal Nurs* 19(2):108-115, 1990.

Scholl T and others: Weight gain during pregnancy in adolescence: predictive ability of early weight gain, *Obstet Gynecol* 75:948-953, 1990.

Schroeder C: Women's experience of bedrest in high risk pregnancy, *IMAGE* 28(3):253-258, 1996.

Scioscia A and others: *A randomized clinical trial of outpatient monitoring of uterine contractions in women at risk for preterm delivery: self palpation versus tocodynamometer.* Eighth Annual Meeting of Society of Perinatal Obstetricians, Las Vegas, 1988.

Stanton R: Comanagement of the patient on subcutaneous terbutaline pump therapy, *J Nurs Midwifery* 36(3):204-208, 1991.

Watson D and others: Management of preterm labor patients at home: does daily uterine activity monitoring and nursing support make a difference? *Obstet Gynecol* 76(1):32S-35S, 1990.

Wilkins I and others: Efficacy and side effects of magnesium sulfate and ritodrine as tocolytic agents, *Am J Obstet Gynecol* 159:685-689, 1988.

CHAPTER

22

Premature Rupture
of Membranes

Premature rupture of membranes (PROM) is defined as
rupture of the amniotic sac surrounding the fetus before the
onset of labor. *Preterm PROM* is commonly used to refer to the
rupture of the membranes when it occurs before term.

INCIDENCE

PROM occurs in 2% to 18% of all pregnancies, and approximately
20% of these cases occur before 36 weeks of gestation (Allen,
1991; Creasy, Resnik, 1994; Vintzileos and others, 1991).

ETIOLOGY

The cause of PROM is unknown in most cases. Increased intrauterine pressure with multiple gestation and polyhydramnios, inflammatory processes such as cervicitis and amnionitis, placenta previa, abruptio placentae, abnormalities of the internal cervical os,
multiple amniocenteses, and therapeutic abortions are factors that
are at times associated with PROM. It was once believed that an
inherently weak fetal membrane might be a cause of PROM.
However, when fetal membranes were tested after premature rupture, they were found to be just as strong as membranes from
normal term deliveries (Gibbs, Sweet, 1994). Current information

reveals that a bacterial invasion can often precede and may possibly be the cause of PROM in 30% to 40% of the cases (Greenberg, Hankins, 1991; Kilbride and others, 1989; Schoonmaker and others, 1989). However, this does not mean the patient has an intraamniotic infection.

The most common risk factor for PROM is a positive history in a prior pregnancy (Allen, 1991; Asrat and others, 1991). The risk of PROM is increased in socioeconomically disadvantaged patients, sexually promiscuous teenagers, patients who have inadequate nutrition especially in zinc (Sikorski and others, 1990), patients who smoke (Harger and others, 1990), and patients with decreased immunity.

NORMAL PHYSIOLOGY

The developing fetus is protected from the outside world by two fetal membranes, the amnion and the chorion, which form a sac around the fetus. These membranes are thin but tough. They contain no blood vessels or nerve endings. However, they are rich in collagen, which gives them their strength and elasticity. Regulatory inhibitors control collagenolytic enzymes such as trypsin and collagenase from breaking down the collagen throughout pregnancy. As the pregnancy nears term, a normal decrease in regulatory inhibitors and an increase in collagenolytic enzyme activity occur. At the same time, phospholipase enzymes are activated that convert phospholipids to arachidonic acid, the precursor of prostaglandins. These prostaglandins initiate labor. The decrease in phospholipids creates a rubbing force between the chorion and amnion. During labor this increase in collagenolytic enzymes and the decrease in phospholipids are what normally cause the membranes to rupture (Polzin, Brady, 1991).

Amniotic fluid is produced within the amniotic sac, allowing the developing fetus to float freely. The fluid is slightly alkaline (pH 7.0 to 7.5). In early pregnancy the primary source of the fluid appears to be the amnion. The amnion produces the amniotic fluid by actively transporting solute and passively transporting water from maternal serum to the amniotic fluid space throughout pregnancy. As pregnancy advances, fetal urine significantly contributes. By way of fetal swallowing and breathing, amniotic fluid is reabsorbed. Thus the fluid is constantly being formed and reabsorbed with replacement about every 3 hours. At 12 weeks the average volume is 50 ml; at 20 weeks the average volume is 400 ml. The maximum volume of 1000 ml is reached between 36 and 38 weeks.

Amniotic fluid serves many functions. It provides a medium in which the fetus can move, grow, and develop symmetrically without pressure on its delicate tissue. Blood flow is also unrestricted as blood is transported through the umbilical cord. The fluid also helps to maintain an even environmental temperature for the fetus.

Normal amniotic fluid contains an antibacterial substance, which gradually increases with gestational age until term and then decreases (Blanco and others, 1982). The level of this antibacterial substance varies with individuals. A diet deficient in protein and zinc may decrease the antibacterial and antiviral activity of the amniotic fluid (Sikorski and others, 1990).

PATHOPHYSIOLOGY

Premature rupture of the fetal membranes occurs when there is focal weakening as the result of extensive changes in collagen metabolism or the intraamniotic pressure is increased (Vadillo-Ortega and others, 1990). In the presence of many bacteria, bacterial protease(s) and collagenases are produced. These enzymes plus the inflammatory response of neutrophils act together to decrease the collagen content of the membranes, thus focally weakening the strength and elasticity of the membranes (McGregor and others, 1990; Vadillo-Ortega and others, 1990). Bacterial proteases also activate the prostaglandin cascade (Polzin, Brady, 1991). After prolonged rupture of membranes an intraamniotic infection often develops as the result of ascending vaginal organisms such as *Ureaplasma urealyticum, Mycoplasma hominis, Bacteroides bivius,* group B streptococci, and *Gardnerella vaginalis. Neisseria gonorrhoeae,* herpes simplex virus, cytomegalovirus, and *Candida albicans* have been implicated as well. There are two possible mechanisms that cause an intraamniotic infection. Some patients have normal inhibitory activity of the amniotic fluid, but when large volumes of bacteria enter the amniotic cavity, they are unable to overpower the inhibitors. In other patients, inhibitory activity in the amniotic fluid may be lacking. These patients are susceptible to an intraamniotic infection if any bacteria enter the amniotic fluid.

MATERNAL EFFECTS

If an intraamniotic infection develops as a result of rupture of membranes, it can very quickly cause a serious maternal infection. This can lead to septicemia and death if not treated promptly. If this occurs, it usually develops during the postpartum period as endometritis (Greenberg, Hankins, 1991) and is more prevalent after a cesarean delivery (Veille, 1988).

FETAL AND NEONATAL EFFECTS

Approximately 10% of all perinatal deaths are associated with PROM (Veille, 1988).

Prematurity

Preterm PROM causes one third of all preterm births (Asrat, Garite, 1991; Harger and others, 1990; McGregor and others, 1990). Before 36 weeks of gestation, respiratory distress syndrome is the main cause of morbidity and mortality of the neonate resulting from a preterm PROM (Iams, 1991; Moretti, Sibai, 1988).

Fetal/Neonatal Infection

Infection appears to play a very minor role in morbidity and mortality if the rupture occurs before 35 or 36 weeks of gestation. Infection does not appear to correlate directly with the length of time the membranes are ruptured before 35 or 36 weeks (Goldstein and others, 1989; Kilbride and others, 1989; Vintzileos and others, 1991). However, if an intraamniotic infection develops, the fetus has a 10% to 20% risk of developing septicemia, meningitis, or pneumonia (Blanco, 1991). After 36 weeks of gestation, infection is the major risk factor to the fetus, but the risk is relatively low. At this gestational age the risk of infection increases with the duration of the rupture (Kilbride and others, 1989).

Fetal Compromise

PROM can cause fetal compromise as the result of a prolapsed cord or decreased amniotic fluid. The cord can prolapse if the presenting part is not well engaged. If the amniotic fluid volume is affected to a large degree, pressure can be applied on the cord as the fetus moves about, thereby causing fetal compromise. Seventy-five percent of patients with PROM will experience variable decelerations related to cord compression (Kilbride and others, 1989). If fetal compromise is allowed to persist for any length of time, fetal hypoxia can result, causing the anal sphincter to relax and release meconium into the amniotic fluid. Deep, gasping respiratory movements are triggered, which moves the meconium-stained amniotic fluid deep into the alveoli. Then the neonate is at risk of developing aspiration pneumonia.

Developmental Abnormalities

If the membranes rupture before 26 to 28 weeks of gestation and marked oligohydramnios results, the fetus is at an increased risk

(12% to 46%) for skeletal compression deformities and pulmonary hypoplasia (Kilbride and others, 1989; Ohlsson, 1989; Richards, 1991; Rotschild and others, 1990). Pulmonary hypoplasia is more common with PROM because lung development depends more on extrinsic factors such as amniotic fluid than other fetal organs.

DIAGNOSTIC TESTING
Sterile Speculum Examination

When PROM is suspected, a sterile speculum examination is done. If amniotic fluid is observed leaking from the cervix and collecting in the posterior fornix of the vagina, an accurate diagnosis of PROM can be made. A digital vaginal examination should *never* be done if any attempt is to be made in delaying the labor. Vaginal bacteria could be transported into the cervical canal from the vaginal examination, thereby increasing the risk of an intraamniotic infection.

Nitrazine Test

If there is no visual sign of loss of amniotic fluid from the cervix, the secretions of the posterior fornix of the vagina should be tested with Nitrazine paper for pH determination. Because amniotic fluid is alkaline and vaginal secretions are acidic, the Nitrazine paper will turn blue in the presence of amniotic fluid. Blood, cervical mucus, and povidone-iodine (Betadine) should not be allowed to contaminate the specimen; they are alkaline also.

Microscopic Examination

A small amount of the fluid should then be spread on a slide and allowed to dry. Microscopic examination of dried amniotic fluid shows a fernlike pattern because of the fluid's concentration of salt.

USUAL MEDICAL MANAGEMENT AND PROTOCOLS FOR NURSE PRACTITIONERS

The treatment of PROM is one of the most controversial subjects in obstetrics today because of conflicting scientific research. Therefore only general principles will be presented.

Expectant Management

If the fetus is not mature, there are no signs of infection, and no fetal compromise is identified, many physicians use expectant management consisting of bed rest with bathroom privileges and observation for signs of infection and fetal compromise. This is done in the hope that, by lengthening the pregnancy, fetal lungs may mature and decrease the risk of respiratory distress in the neonate. It is postulated by some that PROM also accelerates fetal lung maturity by stimulating the production of glucocorticoids by the fetal adrenals and that this stimulates an increased production of lecithin by the fetal lungs (Eriksen, Blanco, 1991; Kilbride and others, 1989). However, the question of whether rupture of membranes accelerates fetal lung maturity is still undergoing much debate (Iams, 1991). Rarely, fibrin can be laid down to form a clot that may close the tear (Johnson and others; 1990; Kilbride and others, 1989).

Documentation of Fetal Age

Gestational age is usually verified with ultrasound. If the biparietal diameter (BPD) cannot accurately be determined because the head is low in the pelvis, femur length or abdominal circumference is used. Most patients whose membranes rupture after 34 to 36 weeks of gestation are prepared for delivery. In the presence of an unripe cervix, with no signs of infection or fetal compromise, a 24-hour or longer delay is recommended before initiating an induction. This protocol decreases the incidence of cesarean delivery for failure to progress without increasing the risk of an infection (Cammu and others, 1990; Clark, 1989; Duff, 1991). In fact, it may actually decrease the risk of a maternal infection since there is a 10 times greater risk of an infection after cesarean delivery in patients with PROM (Veille, 1988).

Between 26 and 35 weeks of gestation, expectant management is usually the preferred choice of treatment if no signs of infection or fetal compromise are present. Before 26 weeks of gestation, care must be individualized because of the risk of maternal infection and fetal developmental abnormalities. Most obstetricians involve the parents in the decision-making process (Asrat, Garite, 1991; Clark, 1989).

Ruling Out Intraamniotic Infection

Maternal fever is one of the best indicators of an intraamniotic infection (Asrat, Garite, 1991). Maternal and fetal tachycardia, uterine tenderness, and an elevated maternal white blood cell count are earlier indicators; however, they are not as reliable. Some obstetricians will take a culture of the amniotic fluid by way of an amniocentesis. The amniotic fluid is then tested for bacteria by doing a Gram stain (Asrat, Garite, 1991; Morales, 1991). Other obstetricians use daily biophysical profiles to assess for a subclinical infection. A score of 2 for fetal breathing pattern is 100%

accurate in predicting the absence of an intraamniotic infection. The absence of fetal breathing associated with decreased fetal movement indicates an intraamniotic infection (Goldstein and others, 1988; Vintzileos and others, 1991). If signs indicate an intraamniotic infection, some obstetricians recommend antibiotic therapy and expedient delivery (Blanco, 1991; Gibbs, Duff, 1991; Johnston and others, 1990). Other obstetricians favor delaying antibiotic therapy until delivery so cultures of the neonate may be obtained first (Ohlsson, 1989; Veille, 1988). Still other obstetricians use antibiotic prophylaxis, especially if beta-streptococci are cultured from the vagina (Greenberg, Hankins, 1991; Heppard, Garite, 1992).

Fetal Maturity Assessment

Fetal lung maturity can be determined in one of two ways. First, amniotic fluid from the vaginal pool can be tested for phosphatidyl glycerol (PG); if PG is present, fetal lung maturity is probable (Asrat, Garite, 1991; Kilbride and others, 1989). Second, fetal lung maturity can be determined by collecting amniotic fluid by way of an amniocentesis and evaluating it for lecithin/sphingomyelin (L/S) ratio. An L/S ratio from 1.8:1 to 2:1 indicates fetal lung maturity. It may be difficult, however, for the physician to obtain enough amniotic fluid by an amniocentesis if the leak is large. If there is only a small amount of amniotic fluid, the procedure can be facilitated by encouraging the patient to drink fluids and placing the patient in a Trendelenburg position for 1 hour before the procedure. Then, with the aid of ultrasound, a pocket of amniotic fluid can often be found. The L/S ratio may be elevated if the amniotic fluid is contaminated by blood. Because amniotic fluid in the vagina is frequently contaminated with blood from the mucous plug, the L/S ratio is rarely done on vaginal pool amniotic fluid. Should blood contaminate the specimen during amniocentesis, fetal lung maturity should be determined by the presence of PG; it is not affected by blood. In the presence of a mature surfactant, delivery is usually the choice of treatment.

Assessment for Fetal Stressors

Fetal heart rate (FHR) monitoring, fetal movement monitoring, nonstress tests (NSTs), biophysical profiles, and amniotic fluid index are used to determine fetal compromise in the presence of PROM. Fetal compromise may result from cord compression caused by oligohydramnios. This would manifest itself as variable decelerations of the FHR. Decreased fetal movements may indicate an infected fetus since an infected fetus is usually lethargic. A reactive NST indicates an uninfected fetus. In the presence of a nonreactive NST, further testing should be done because of the high false-positive rate of this test (Goldstein and others, 1989). Recently the fetal biophysical profile and amniotic fluid index have been used to detect early signs of an intraamniotic infection after PROM. An intraamniotic infection develops in approximately 50% of the patients with no pocket of amniotic fluid greater than 1×1 cm (Vintzileos and others, 1991).

Assessment for Signs of Preterm Labor

When fetal membranes rupture, there is also a potential risk of preterm labor. At term, 80% of patients with PROM will go into labor within 24 hours (Goldstein and others, 1989; Iams, 1991). The more premature the fetus, the longer the time period before spontaneous labor is usually initiated (Gibbs, Sweet, 1994; Goldstein and others, 1989; Vintzileos and others, 1991). However, 50% of all patients with a gestational age of less than 36 weeks at the time of the rupture of membranes will deliver within 1 week (Richards, 1991).

Tocolysis

The use of tocolysis in the presence of PROM is very controversial. Tocolytic agents are less effective when membranes are ruptured, and they may increase the risk of or mask the signs of an intrauterine infection (Iams, 1991; Olofsson and others, 1988). However, according to Garite and others (1987) tocolytics may be more effective when initiated within 2 hours of rupture.

Corticosteroids

The use of corticosteroids to accelerate fetal pulmonary maturation in the presence of ruptured membranes lacks consensus. Many studies have shown no benefit in reducing the incidence of respiratory distress, and incidence of neonatal infection is increased because of the suppressive effect on the immunologic response (Eriksen, Blanco, 1991; Iams, 1991).

NURSING PROCESS

PREVENTION

Because the actual cause of PROM is unknown, prevention is difficult. However, it may be helpful to look at the risk factors and guard against these during pregnancy. Statistics indicate that socioeconomically disadvantaged patients and teenagers have an increased risk of PROM. The reason for this is unknown, but nutrition probably plays an important role. Therefore these patients should be instructed early in pregnancy regarding a healthful diet for pregnancy and should be provided with reasons to follow this diet. They may also need referral to financial assistance and food supplement programs, as well as instruction in how to prepare nutritious foods.

Cleanliness can also be a factor in decreasing the risk of PROM; vaginal bacterial flora should be kept to a minimum. Daily bathing and wiping the perineum from front to back are important prenatal instructions. Multiple sexual relationships also increase the vaginal bacterial count and should be avoided.

Any attempt to facilitate increased immunity against infection is beneficial. Therefore drinking 6 to 8 ounces of fluid per waking hour, daily exercise with adequate rest to avoid fatigue, an adequate diet high in protein and zinc, and cleanliness are all beneficial in guarding against PROM.

Harger and others (1990) demonstrated in their study a relationship between smoking and PROM. Therefore prenatal patients who smoke should be instructed regarding its effect on pregnancy and should be supported in their attempt to stop smoking.

All pregnant women should be instructed regarding the danger signs in pregnancy, and PROM should be pointed out as one of these signs. The signs of membrane rupture and the necessity of prompt notification if these signs occur should be explained early in prenatal care.

NURSING DIAGNOSES/COLLABORATIVE PROBLEMS AND INTERVENTIONS

- **RISK FOR INFECTION**   related to loss of the membrane barrier.
  DESIRED OUTCOMES: The patient's temperature will remain normal, vaginal discharge will be without odor, and white blood cell count will remain less than $18,000/mm^3$. The fetus will remain active, and its heart rate will remain at its normal baseline between 110 and 160 beats/min.
  INTERVENTIONS
    1. Assess temperature every 4 hours or as indicated. (A fever is the most reliable indicator, but it is a late indicator of an intraamniotic infection [Lee, Thomason, 1988].)
    2. Assess maternal pulse and blood pressure as indicated. (Tachycardia is one of the earlier signs of an intraamniotic infection [Lee, Thomason, 1988].)

3. Assess FHR as indicated. (Fetal tachycardia is one of the earlier signs of an intraamniotic infection [Goldstein and others, 1989].)

4. Assess vaginal discharge for odor or color change.

5. Assess for uterine tenderness.

6. Refer to such diagnostic data as white blood cell count and C-reactive protein (CRP). (A white blood cell count above 18,000/mm^3 is a significant sign of an infection during pregnancy. A normal CRP level is a valuable predictor of no intraamniotic infection [Lee and Thomason, 1988].)

7. Be prepared to assist in obtaining vaginal and urethral cultures for group B streptococci, chlamydia, and gonococcus. If any of these organisms is present, be prepared to start antibiotic therapy to decrease neonatal infection risk. (Group B streptococcus is the most common cause of neonatal sepsis [Clark, 1989].)

8. Be prepared to assist with an amniocentesis to measure for gram-positive bacteria.

9. Assess for signs of a urinary tract infection.

10. Determine nutritional habits.

11. Determine activities since PROM.

12. Teach the benefits of bed rest with bathroom privileges only.

13. Teach the importance of perineal care after each voiding and stool.

14. Perform no vaginal examinations until the patient is in active labor.

15. If patient is discharged home, instruct regarding no intercourse or douching, taking temperature twice daily, showers only, notifying the physician if temperature is more than 38° C or if amniotic fluid loss increases or becomes foul smelling, and returning to the clinical laboratory for a white blood cell count twice weekly.

16. Notify the physician if temperature is greater than 38° C, fetal or maternal tachycardia develops, foul-smelling amniotic fluid develops, or amniotic fluid changes from straw color.

17. If signs of an intraamniotic infection are manifested, be prepared to begin broad-spectrum antibiotic therapy, such as penicillin G and gentamicin; ampicillin and gentamicin; or cephalosporin. If the patient has a cesarean delivery, clindamycin may be administered in addition (Blanco, 1991).

■ **RISK FOR IMPAIRED FETAL GAS EXCHANGE** related to cord compressions resulting from oligohydramnios or prolapsed cord.
   DESIRED OUTCOMES: The fetus will remain active, and its heart rate will be maintained at a baseline between 120 and 160 with normal variability, normal reactivity, and no decelerations. The biophysical profile will continue to be more than 6.
   INTERVENTIONS
   Prenatal
   1. Continuously monitor FHR initially for a prescribed period of time after membrane rupture to rule out fetal stressors.
   2. During expectant management, periodically monitor FHR for variable decelerations and fetal activity.
   3. Observe amount of amniotic fluid that is being lost.
   4. Reposition mother, and administer oxygen by mask if variable decelerations occur.
   5. Instruct patient to report any decrease in fetal activity.
   6. Prepare the patient for ordered fetal well-being and maturity studies. Biophysical profiles, ultrasound, NSTs, amniotic fluid index, and amniocentesis are usually ordered on a frequent basis in an attempt to determine the optimal time for delivery.
   7. Notify physician if a baseline or periodic FHR change is noted, an NST is nonreactive, or a biophysical profile is 6 or less.

   Intrapartum
   1. Use continuous fetal monitoring for early detection of nonreassuring FHR changes.
   2. Assess amniotic fluid for meconium.
   3. Reposition patient, administer oxygen by mask at 8 to 10 L, and increase the intravenous (IV) fluid rate if variable decelerations occur.
   4. Be prepared to manage a saline amnioinfusion if multiple variable decelerations occur related to decreased amniotic fluid (Haubrich; 1990; Owen and others, 1990; Strong and others, 1990).
   5. Notify the physician at the first signs of a nonreassuring FHR change.
   6. Once delivery is imminent, notify the intensive care nursery of a possible high risk infant.

■ **POTENTIAL COMPLICATION OF AMNIOINFUSION: ABRUPTIO PLACENTAE AND AMNIOTIC FLUID EMBOLISM** related to overdistention of the uterus with saline; fetal bradycardia related to infusing cold saline or a rising uterine resting tone; umbilical cord prolapse related to a gush of amniotic fluid.

DESIRED OUTCOME: The severe variable decelerations will be minimized as measured by a significant decline of severity of variable FHR decelerations with FHR baseline variability present.

INTERVENTIONS

1. Rule out cord prolapse.
2. Assess patient's understanding of the procedure.
3. Educate patient as to the reasons for the procedure.
4. Obtain an informed consent.
5. Obtain baseline maternal vital signs, FHR, and uterine activity.
6. Obtain a 1000-ml bag of normal saline that has been stored in a heating unit or warmed in a microwave oven to 37° C.
7. Connect the warmed normal saline to the intrauterine pressure catheter by way of IV tubing.
8. Infuse at a rate of 15 to 20 ml/min. This rate can be accomplished without an infusion pump by hanging the saline bag 3 to 4 feet above the uterus.
9. Continue infusion until (a) the variable decelerations resolve plus 250 ml has been given; (b) 800 ml of normal saline has been infused; or (c) intolerable side effects develop such as an increasing uterine resting tone, signs of fetal compromise, or uterine tenderness.
10. Monitor FHR and uterine activity continuously with a separate or double-lumen intrauterine pressure catheter.
11. Document the amount and character of vaginal discharge.
12. Keep the patient as dry as possible by changing the pads often.
13. Notify the physician if severe variable decelerations are not resolved with 800 ml of warmed saline or signs of maternal or fetal compromise are manifested.
14. For a further nursing update on amnioinfusion refer to Haubrich (1990), Knorr (1989), and Strong and Phelan (1991).

- **FEAR** related to effect on own health status and threat to fetal/ neonatal well-being.

  DESIRED OUTCOME: The patient and her family will be able to communicate their fears and concerns openly.

  INTERVENTIONS

  1. Assess family's anxiety over maternal, fetal/neonatal well-being.

2. Assess family's coping strategies and resources.
3. Encourage expectant parents to communicate openly about their feelings and concerns.
4. Clarify any misconceptions.
5. Provide information to the patient and her family regarding the pregnancy complication, plan of treatment, and implications for mother and fetus in understandable terms.
6. Arrange a tour of the intensive care nursery in the event of a possible preterm delivery.
7. Refer to the social worker if inadequate coping is noted.
8. Refer to pastor, priest, or chaplain per parents' request.

■ **RISK FOR ALTERED ROLE PERFORMANCE** related to prolonged hospitalization and treatment with bed rest.

   DESIRED OUTCOME: The patient will verbalize a plan that will take care of all her work- and family-related responsibilities during her absence.

   INTERVENTIONS
   1. Assess the patient's responsibilities to determine difficulties she will have in implementing prescribed bed rest.
   2. Teach the patient and her family about the importance of bed rest in the lateral position.
   3. Facilitate the family in problem solving if difficulties arise in implementing bed rest.
   4. Make needed referrals, for example, to the social worker, if problems are identified.
   5. Encourage participation in her care and decision making as much as possible.

■ **DIVERSIONAL ACTIVITY DEFICIT** related to the therapeutic treatment of bed rest.

   DESIRED OUTCOME: The patient will verbalize various appropriate activities she would like to do while maintaining bed rest.

   INTERVENTIONS
   1. Assess patient's interest in various diversional activities within the activity limit.
   2. Provide crafts, reading materials, music, and puzzles that can be done in bed or encourage patient to have these things brought in.
   3. Provide classes in preparation for childbirth by way of video, the hospital television, or group classes that can be attended while reclining.
   4. Refer to a diversional therapist or volunteer to provide reading materials, handicrafts, or other interesting things.

CONCLUSION

Because infections and lower amniotic fluid immunity play a significant role in PROM, the ultimate goal of the nurse should be education. Prenatal education should cover the need for adequate fluids and nutrition, appropriate hygiene, and the significance of reporting any signs of an infection immediately. This would decrease the risk of PROM. Once the membranes rupture, the goal of treatment is to maintain the pregnancy to allow for fetal maturity as long as the uterine environment is healthy. If the uterine environment becomes infected or causes fetal compromise, the fetal outcome may be improved by premature delivery.

BIBLIOGRAPHY

Allen S: Epidemiology of premature rupture of the fetal membranes, *Clin Obstet Gynecol* 34(4):685-693, 1991.

American College of Obstetricians and Gynecologists (ACOG): Premature rupture of membranes, *ACOG Techn Bull,* no. 115, 1988.

Asrat T, Garite T: Management of preterm premature rupture of membranes, *Clin Obstet Gynecol* 34(4):730-741, 1991.

Asrat T and others: Rate of recurrence of preterm premature rupture of membranes in consecutive pregnancies, *Am J Obstet Gynecol* 165:1111-1115, 1991.

Blanco J: Recognizing and responding to intra-amniotic infection, *Contemp OB/GYN* 36(9):61-64, 1991.

Blanco J and others: The association between the absence of amniotic fluid bacterial inhibitory activity and intraamniotic infection, *Am J Obstet Gynecol* 143:749-756, 1982.

Cammu H, Verlaenen H, Derde M: Premature rupture of membranes at term in nulliparous women: a hazard? *Obstet Gynecol* 76:671-674, 1990.

Clark S: Managing PROM: a continuing controversy, *Contemp OB/GYN* 33(6):49-55, 1989.

Creasy R, Resnik R, editors: *Maternal-fetal medicine: principles and practice,* ed 3, Philadelphia, 1994, Saunders.

Duff P: Management of premature rupture of membranes in term patients, *Clin Obstet Gynecol* 34(4):723-729, 1991.

Eriksen N, Blanco J: The role of corticosteroids in the management of patients with preterm premature rupture of the membranes, *Clin Obstet Gynecol* 34(4):694-701, 1991.

Garite T and others: A randomized trial of ritodrine tocolysis versus expectant management in patients with premature rupture of membranes at 25 to 30 weeks of gestation, *Am J Obstet Gynecol* 157:388-393, 1987.

Gibbs R, Duff P: Progress in pathogenesis and management of clinical intraamniotic infection, *Am J Obstet Gynecol* 164:1317-1326, 1991.

Gibbs R, Sweet R: Clinical disorders. In Creasy R, Resnik R, editors: *Maternal-fetal medicine: principles and practice,* ed 3, Philadelphia, 1994, Saunders.

Goldstein I, Copel J, Hobbins J: Fetal behavior in preterm premature rupture of the membranes, *Clin Perinatol* 6(3):735-755, 1989.

Goldstein I and others: Fetal body and breathing movements as predictors of intraamniotic infection in preterm premature rupture of membranes, *Am J Obstet Gynecol* 159:363, 1988.

Greenberg R, Hankins G: Antibiotic therapy in preterm premature rupture of membranes, *Clin Obstet Gynecol* 34(4):742-750, 1991.

Harger J and others: Risk factors for preterm premature rupture of fetal membranes: a multicenter case-control study, *Am J Obstet Gynecol* 163:130, 1990.

Haubrich K: Amnioinfusion: a technique for the relief of variable deceleration, *J Obstet Gynecol Neonatal Nurs* 9(4):299-303, 1990.

Heppard M, Garite T: *Acute obstetrics: a practical guide,* St Louis, 1992, Mosby.

Iams J: Tocolytics and steroids for PROM: no reason to use them, *Contemp OB/GYN* 36(8):85-95, 1991.

Johnson J, Egerman R, Moorhead J: Cases with ruptured membranes that "reseal," *Am J Obstet Gynecol* 163:1024-1032, 1990.

Johnston M and others: Antibiotic therapy in preterm premature rupture of membranes: a randomized, prospective, double-blind trial, *Am J Obstet Gynecol* 163:743-747, 1990.

Kilbride H, Yeast J, Thibeault D: Intrapartum and delivery room management of premature rupture of membranes complicated by oligohydramnios, *Clin Perinatol* 16(4):863-888, 1989.

Knorr L: Relieving fetal distress with amnioinfusion, *MCN Am J Matern Child Nurs* 4(5):346-350, 1989.

Lee G, Thomason J: Marshaling evidence for chorioamnionitis, *Contemp OB/GYN* 32(1):47-54, 1988.

McGregor J and others: Antibiotic inhibition of bacterially induced fetal membrane weakening, *Obstet Gynecol* 76:124-128, 1990.

Morales W: Why tocolysis and steroids have a place in PROM management, *Contemp OB/GYN* 36(8):73-82, 1991.

Moretti M, Sibai B: Maternal and perinatal outcome of expectant management of premature rupture of membranes in the midtrimester, *Am J Obstet Gynecol* 159:390-396, 1988.

Ohlsson A: Treatments of preterm premature rupture of the membranes: a meta-analysis, *Am J Obstet Gynecol* 160:890-906, 1989.

Olofsson P, Rydhstrom H, Sjoberg N: How Swedish obstetricians manage premature rupture of membranes in preterm gestations, *Am J Obstet Gynecol* 159:1028-1034, 1988.

Owen J, Henson B, Hauth J: A prospective randomized study of saline solution amnioinfusion, *Am J Obstet Gynecol* 162:1146-1149, 1990.

Polzin W, Brady K: Mechanical factors in the etiology of premature rupture of the membranes, *Clin Obstet Gynecol* 34(4):702-714, 1991.

Richards D: Complications of prolonged PROM and oligohydramnios, *Clin Obstet Gynecol* 34(4):759-768, 1991.

Rotschild A and others: Neonatal outcome after prolonged preterm rupture of the membranes, *Am J Obstet Gynecol* 162:46-52, 1990.

Schoonmaker J and others: Bacteria and inflammatory cells reduce chorioamniotic membrane integrity and tensile strength, *Obstet Gynecol* 74:590-596, 1989.

Sikorski R, Juszkiewicz T, Paszkowski T: Zinc status in women with premature rupture of membranes at term, *Obstet Gynecol* 76:675-677, 1990.

Strong T, Phelan J: Amnioinfusion for intrapartum management, *Contemp OB/GYN* 37(5):15-24, 1991.

Strong T and others: Prophylactic intrapartum amnioinfusion: a randomized clinical trial, *Am J Obstet Gynecol* 162:1370-1375, 1990.

Vadillo-Ortega F and others: Collagen metabolism in premature rupture of amniotic membranes, *Obstet Gynecol* 75:84-88, 1990.

Veille J: Management of preterm premature rupture of membranes, *Clin Perinatol* 15(4):851-862, 1988.

Vintzileos A, Campbell W, Rodis J: Antepartum surveillance in patients with preterm premature rupture of the membranes, *Clin Obstet Gynecol* 34(4):779-793, 1991.

23

Trauma

Trauma is the leading cause of death in women of childbearing years.* An estimated 7% of all pregnant women will suffer some type of trauma during their pregnancy, with 75% of those in motor vehicle crashes (Arneson and others, 1986; Pearlman and others, 1990a; Williams and others, 1990). Nonobstetric injury is the second leading cause of maternal mortality (Rochat and others, 1988). The frequency of injury increases with each trimester, so the highest risk of injury is in the third trimester. Trauma causes death of the fetus more often than death of the mother (Pearlman and others, 1990a; Stafford and others, 1988). Major and minor traumas during pregnancy are associated with an increased risk of spontaneous abortion, preterm labor, placental abruption, fetomaternal transfusion, and stillbirth (ACOG, 1989; Pearlman and others, 1990b).

Because it is not uncommon for pregnant women to continue to participate in a wide variety of activities, they are exposed to the risk of accidental injury. Several factors have been identified that contribute to the risk of injury during pregnancy (Daddario, 1989; Hutzel, Remsburg-Bell, 1996):

1. Active employment and increasing numbers of women in occupations previously held by men

---

*Arneson and others, 1986; Daddario, 1989; Gonik, 1994; Neufield and others, 1987; Pearlman and others, 1990a, 1990b; Williams and others, 1990.

2. Increased societal mobility
3. Increased exposure to violent behavior
4. Participation in sports and recreational activities

When pregnancy is complicated by trauma, emergency care may be delivered in a variety of settings outside trauma units and by providers who are not routinely accustomed to problems associated with trauma. Such settings may be obstetric units and outpatient settings. In addition, trauma teams in emergency centers, although familiar with trauma care, are often unfamiliar with some of the physiologic considerations for pregnancy and with caring for a second, invisible patient, the fetus.

INCIDENCE

Statistics support recognition of trauma as a significant complication in pregnancy. Some of these statistics are as follows:

- Seven percent of pregnant women seek medical care for accidental injury.
- Of the injuries, 10% occur in the first trimester, 40% during the second trimester, and 50% during the third trimester.
- Of all injuries during pregnancy, 54% are from motor vehicle crashes; 70% of the major, life-threatening injuries are from motor vehicle crashes (Daddario, 1989; Stafford and others, 1988).
- Approximately 8% of pregnant women are battered (Helton and others, 1987).

ETIOLOGY

The leading causes of maternal trauma are motor vehicle crashes, falls, burns, and penetrating injuries, such as stabbing and gunshot wounds (Johnson, Oakley, 1991; Neufield and others, 1987; Pearlman and others, 1990a, 1990b; Williams and others, 1990). Battering is also reported as a source of serious injury during pregnancy, but it is difficult to get specific statistics because of underreporting of this type of crime. Studies of battered women in shelters (Bullock and others, 1989; Campbell, 1989; Helton and others, 1987; Hillard, 1985; Parker, McFarlane, 1991) state that 40% to 60% of the women report that they were battered during a pregnancy.

Violent assaults and suicide are the second leading cause of maternal death from trauma. Most of the maternal deaths from trauma of this type are the result of head trauma or intraabdominal hemorrhage.

NORMAL PHYSIOLOGY

A thorough review of maternal physiologic adaptations is provided in Chapter 1.

PATHOPHYSIOLOGY

The pathophysiology to be considered obviously depends on the type of injury, the source of the injury, and the system or part of the body affected. Because head injury and abdominal hemorrhage are the most common lethal maternal effects, discussion of pathophysiology focuses on both. The adverse fetal effects of preterm labor, delivery, abruption, preterm rupture of membranes, and intrauterine death are conditions dealt with in Chapters 14 to 17, 21, and 22.

Hemorrhage

Because of the total blood volume increase during pregnancy, trauma involving abdominal hemorrhage has profound hemodynamic consequences that place the pregnant woman at much greater risk than a nonpregnant counterpart. These consequences include the following:

1. By 32 to 34 weeks of gestation, there is an average of 50% to 70% blood volume increase. Because clinical signs of shock usually present as a function of percentage of total blood loss, the pregnant patient has a greater absolute amount of blood loss than a nonpregnant person in a similar state. Thus a larger amount of blood replacement is needed in resuscitative efforts.

2. Because of the increased volume available to her, the pregnant woman may be able to more readily, although temporarily, maintain hemodynamic stability at the expense of the fetus. Reflex, compensatory, vasoconstrictive responses can significantly decrease uteroplacental perfusion, compromising the fetal compartment.

3. Although cardiac output is increased by 30% to 40% near term, supine positioning is likely to confuse the general picture of potential shock by enhancing hypotension. Supine positioning will decrease cardiac output secondary to decreased cardiac return from mechanical obstruction of the inferior vena cava by the gravid uterus.

4. Because the pregnant woman's heart rate is already increased by approximately 10 to 15 beats/min and blood pressure falls in the second trimester, these two parameters may confuse the clinical picture for the provider who is

unfamiliar with normal, physiologic, hemodynamic alterations in pregnancy.

5. When the gravid abdomen sustains trauma, both the uterus, with its increased circulating volume, and the bladder are more anatomically prone to injury. Abdominal injury adds an additional risk of significant maternal hemorrhage secondary to placental abruption.

6. The kidneys and ureters are relatively protected from injury by the uterus. However, normal dilation of the ureters may be misinterpreted on radiologic examination of the abdomen following injury.

7. Anatomically, the bowel is pushed upward and is more prominent during pregnancy. As a result, the small and large intestines are at greater risk of injury with blunt or penetrating trauma.

8. Because pregnancy is a hypercoagulable state, risks of thrombosis after injury are increased.

9. Disseminated intravascular coagulopathy (DIC), a frequent complication of severe abdominal trauma, also may evidence an atypical presentation. Normal fibrinogen level in pregnancy is four to five times the nonpregnant level. As a result the lower nonpregnant levels when applied to pregnant women may signify early DIC. (See Chapters 17 and 18 for signs and symptoms of shock, DIC, and placental abruption.)

Neurologic Injury

Head injury is often severe enough to result in maternal death. No significant neurophysiologic adaptations in pregnancy alter presentation of the clinical picture. However, if maternal brain death occurs, the fetus may remain a prime, viable consideration. Therefore the concept of brain death needs to be considered from an ethical perspective (Field and others, 1988).

Brain death is the unequivocal and irreversible loss of total brain function. It is a concept used to determine when death has occurred even though cardiopulmonary resuscitation (CPR) and life support technology obscure the conventional criteria for diagnosis of life or death. Once the diagnosis of brain death is made, cardiopulmonary collapse may be expected within 72 hours. In any situation where brain death has occurred, it would generally be considered unethical to squander costly medical resources to continue to support life with artificial means. However, even if the woman has given an advance directive for removal of life support in such a situation, maternal brain death presents a case for continued artificial support for the sake of the fetus. The new, advance directive law (see Chapter 7) does not change this.

Spinal cord injury is another type of neurologic injury that can have pathophysiologic consequences in the pregnant woman. When spinal cord injury occurs during the course of an established pregnancy, the following complications may occur (Creasy, Resnik, 1994; Westgren and others, 1993):

- Spontaneous abortion or stillbirth may occur (see Chapters 14 and 17).
- With lesions above the tenth thoracic segment, the woman will not note onset of abdominal pain or discomfort. Because of the caudal entrance of the afferent uterine nerves, the nerve supply to the uterus is interrupted. Thus the uterus can contract normally, but there is an absence of associated pain sensation with onset of labor contractions.
- Complete cord lesions above the fifth or sixth thoracic segment, above the splanchnic outflow, may cause the development of the syndrome of hyperreflexia with the onset of contractions.

Signs and symptoms of hyperreflexia are caused by the sudden release of catecholamines. These include throbbing headache, hypertension, reflex bradycardia, sweating, nasal congestion, and vasodilation (Baker and others, 1992).

Chest Injury

Physiologic adaptations in respiratory functions may confuse the understanding of the pathophysiology of chest injury and confound resuscitative efforts. During pregnancy there is increased oxygen (O_2) consumption, increased tidal volume, decreased arterial carbon dioxide partial pressure (pCO_2), and decreased serum bicarbonate. Chronic, compensatory respiratory alkalosis may mislead the resuscitation team in evaluation of blood gases. Blood buffering capabilities decrease during pregnancy, and therefore reestablishing acid/base homeostasis is more difficult.

Pelvic Fractures

The major complications of pelvic fractures include retroperitoneal bleeding and placental abruption in the pregnant woman. The pelvis usually fractures in two places in the bony ring. If the fetal head is engaged, fetal skull fracture may occur.

Thermal (Burn) Trauma

Classification of thermal injury is according to the percent of the body burned, the depth involved, and gestational age. If more than 60% of the body is affected, there is significant risk of maternal death. Because of the normally hypervolemic state in pregnancy, fluid resuscitation must be vigorous with prompt evaluation and correction of electrolyte imbalance. Maternal sepsis secondary to burns can lead to intrauterine death or fetal compromise.

SIGNS AND SYMPTOMS

Signs and symptoms of complications of trauma are given in Chapters 11, 12, 14, 17, 18, 21, and 22.

MATERNAL EFFECTS

The following effects may be seen after maternal trauma:
- Hemorrhage and shock
- DIC
- Placental abruption
- Respiratory distress
- Syndrome of hyperreflexia with spinal cord injury
- Brain death
- Maternal death
- Electrolyte imbalance, hypovolemia

FETAL EFFECTS

The fetus is extremely vulnerable to the effects of maternal trauma, especially blunt or penetrating trauma to the abdomen (Bullock, McFarlane, 1989; Pearlman and others, 1990b). Common fetal effects include the following:
- Preterm rupture of membranes
- Premature labor and delivery
- Occult placental abruption with fetomaternal bleed
- Stillbirth
- Fetal skull injuries, especially when the fetal head is engaged and there is a maternal pelvic fracture
- Hypoxic compromise secondary to maternal respiratory embarrassment, shock, DIC, thermal injury, or maternal cardiopulmonary arrest

MEDICAL DIAGNOSIS AND USUAL CRITICAL MANAGEMENT
Resuscitation

The standard CPR procedure should be followed with a pregnant woman. There is increased likelihood that artificial ventilation will be needed because of the anatomic shift of the diaphragm. The patient should be tilted or positioned laterally to prevent supine hypotension. Certain modifications to the conventional CPR procedures should be considered.

Vasopressor Drugs

Avoid use of vasopressor drugs such as epinephrine, dopamine, or norepinephrine bitartrate; these cause vasoconstriction of the placental bed. Epinephrine is a better choice when fetal outcome is also a high priority because it enhances placental blood flow.

Antidysrhythmics

Lidocaine hydrochloride does not appear to cross the placenta and may be helpful in treating some dysrhythmias. Other antidysrhythmics may be toxic to the fetus.

Open Heart Massage

If circulatory function is not restored after 5 to 10 minutes, open heart massage may be needed with an emergency cesarean performed once fetal viability is established by ultrasound.

Defibrillation

If defibrillation is necessary and a fetal spiral electrode is being used to monitor the fetal heart rate (FHR), the wires should be disconnected from the leg plate to reduce the risk of conducting through the fetal spiral electrode to the fetus.

Fluid Replacement

Give vigorous and aggressive fluid replacement.

Perimortem

If maternal resuscitation efforts are not successful after 15 minutes, a perimortem (agonal or postmortem) cesarean delivery should be done unless the fetus is no longer viable or less than 23 weeks.

Minor Injury Management

After a minor injury the initial assessment usually takes place in the trauma or emergency center. Here a history as to the mechanism of injury and circumstances surrounding the incident is obtained. Diagnostic tests and procedures are carried out as dictated by the physical injury. The patient is often then transferred to labor and delivery for fetal assessment and follow-up monitoring for the development of complications.

Major Injury Management

Immediately after major trauma, diagnosis and treatment occur almost simultaneously in three phases.

Initial Care Phase

The initial response to a major trauma usually involves two teams, each with members assigned to very specific and limited components of care. The A team, or first team, focuses on the mother and responds immediately, begins an assessment, and sets priorities for stabilization management. Their focus is on identification of immediate life-threatening injuries and is directed at assessment of airway, breathing, and circulation for the mother. Neurologic injuries, especially head injuries, should next be evaluated as appropriate depending on the type of injury.

As soon as the initial assessment is done, the A team moves out of the way and the B team moves in to focus on the fetus and pregnancy-related issues. Finally, the A team reevaluates the effects of resuscitation efforts for the mother; last, the B team reevaluates resuscitation of the mother as it affects the fetus. The specific efforts of each team are directed toward immediate stabilization and basic life support resuscitation. (See Table 23-1 for a summary of management of the pregnant patient after major trauma. The acronym *TRAUMA* will be used to summarize priorities for immediate management and stabilization.)

Continued Care Phase

Although initial emergency assessment and stabilization may be carried out in any level trauma center or emergency room and surgical service, continued maternal care for serious trauma commonly will be delivered in critical care units.

If the mother is pronounced dead and the fetus is older than 24 weeks and alive, a cesarean delivery will be performed. If the mother is brain-dead, she may be kept on life support until the fetus has an opportunity to grow to maturity.

Recovery and Rehabilitation Phase

During the recovery and rehabilitation phase, assessments are directed at identification of potential long-term complications and sequelae. Interventions during this phase are focused on restoration of optimal functional capabilities.

TABLE 23-1 Priorities for perinatal TRAUMA management

Activity	Team A (mother)	Team B (fetus)

T = Triage*	Assess ABCs
	  Airway
	  Breathing
	  Circulation
		Assess fetus
		  Cardiac activity
		  Gestational age
		  Assess placenta for abruption
		Position mother in left lateral tilt

R = Resuscitation	Perform CPR Infuse crystalloid fluids Administer oxygen at 8-10 L/min by mask Administer blood as indicated (in emergency situation, O-negative blood can be used)	
A = Assessment	Assess for maternal injuries (similar to in nonpregnant patient) Assess vital signs; level of consciousness; respiratory status as to depth, irregularity, and breath sounds	Assess FHR and uterine contractions with EFM Assess for vaginal bleeding and rupture of membranes Kleihauer-Betke test may be done to rule out fetal hemorrhage

U = Ultrasound/uterine evaluation	Evaluate uterine cavity for hemorrhage	Evaluate fundal height Palpate for uterine tenderness, contractions, or irritability Ultrasound may be done to determine placental or fetal injury and placental location Amniocentesis may be done to assess fetal lung maturity or intrauterine bleeding
M = Management/monitor	Decide initial management and needed continual monitoring	Decide to monitor or deliver depending on status of mother and fetus and risk of prematurity
A = Activate transport/transfer	After stabilization, transport/transfer to critical care, operating suite, or level III perinatal unit	Activate neonatal team for consultation, transfer, or transport as necessary

CPR, Cardiopulmonary resuscitation; *FHR,* fetal heart rate; *EFM,* electronic fetal monitor.
*Mother is first priority, then fetus.

NURSING PROCESS

PREVENTION

- **MOTOR VEHICLE CRASHES**

  Because the risk for major trauma during pregnancy is the greatest with motor vehicle crashes, prevention of that source of injury should be targeted. Efforts to teach and demonstrate the safe and consistent use of car safety belts can have a major impact on the degree of injury, especially blunt trauma to the abdomen. Every pregnant patient should be taught that the seat belt harness should be used no matter how short the trip. The current recommendation for seat belt use during pregnancy is for the shoulder strap to cross between the breasts and over the upper abdomen above the uterus. The lap belt should cross over the pelvis below the uterus (ACOG, 1991). A discussion of the pregnant woman's vulnerability should include facts such as avoiding fatigue, late departures, and distractions, for example, loud music and arguing children.

- **OTHER ACCIDENTAL CAUSES**

  Pregnant women should be made aware of sources of injury, such as falls resulting from the displaced center of gravity or increased joint flexibility. Other causes may be burns and domestic or other violence. The topic of potential maternal trauma from any of these sources should be included in early childbirth preparation classes and in the routine anticipatory education presented during prenatal visits.

- **BATTERING**

  Routine prenatal care should include an assessment for physical or sexual abuse (U.S. Department of Health and Human Services, 1986). Observation for families at risk and preventive intervention, such as referral for stress reduction, emotional support, improving communication, and improving interpersonal relationships, should be provided as needed.

  Because battering during pregnancy is a significant health care problem, all pregnant women should be screened. The National Coalition Against Domestic Violence (1993) has estimated that between 15% and 25% of pregnant women are battered (Christian, 1995). Risk factors include the following:
  1. Unmarried adult or teen
  2. Poor support system
  3. Below the poverty level socioeconomically
  4. Poor weight gain
  5. Smoking; alcohol or drug use

6. Poor obstetric history
7. Preterm labor
8. Anemia

Pregnancy provides a window of opportunity for assessment as well as intervention. In most studies reviewed, a specific assessment directed at obtaining information about abuse or battering was more likely to get more accurate responses than a generalized physical assessment and a superficial psychosocial assessment (Hutzel, Remsburg, 1996; Norton and others, 1995; Parker and others, 1994). Responses were more likely to be elicited accurately depicting events when the abuse assessment was done by the prenatal nurse rather than by the physician (Norton and others, 1995) or social worker.

An abuse assessment screen that can be reproduced was developed by the Nursing Research Consortium on Violence and Abuse (Christian, 1995; Norton and others, 1995; Parker and others, 1994). The assessment screen includes four basic questions and a scoring system for the degree of threat pertaining to specific types of abuse. It includes the following questions:

1. Have you ever been emotionally or physically abused by your partner or someone important to you? **Yes** or **No**
2. Within the last year, have you been hit, slapped, kicked, or otherwise physically hurt by someone? **Yes** or **No**
   a. If yes, by whom?
   b. Total number of times?
3. Since you have been pregnant, were you hit, slapped, kicked, or otherwise physically hurt by someone? **Yes** or **No**
   a. If yes, by whom?
   b. Total number of times?
4. Are you afraid of your partner or anyone you listed above? **Yes** or **No**

Perinatal nurses should screen all pregnant women at the earliest opportunity and again at intervals during the pregnancy follow-up for any risks that may present later. Pregnant women who are battered need education, support, and intervention to break out of the cycle of abuse (Christian, 1995).

NURSING DIAGNOSES/COLLABORATIVE PROBLEMS AND INTERVENTIONS

- **PSYCHOSOCIAL DIAGNOSES RELATED TO BATTERING ABUSE**
  - Self-esteem disturbance related to verbal abuse
  - Anxiety and fear related to the ongoing threat of abuse
  - Depression related to verbal abuse from partner

- Fear related to potential physical harm to self and/or fetus from her partner
- Knowledge deficit related to the cycle of violence
- Physical injury, actual
- Ineffective coping, individual and family
- Hopelessness related to ongoing abuse

DESIRED OUTCOMES: The pregnant woman will demonstrate trust in her provider and/or perinatal nurse by accurately portraying her potential for actual abuse. The pregnant woman who is experiencing battering or abuse will be able to verbalize options and resources for assistance and support. The pregnant woman who is experiencing battering or abuse will verbalize trust in and support from her provider and her perinatal nurse in exploring strategies and exercising options for self-care that will reduce or eliminate the threats to self and fetus.

INTERVENTIONS *(Christian, 1995)*

1. Assess and screen specifically for battering and abuse (physical, emotional, and sexual).
2. Assess social support outside the partnership if abuse or battering is occurring.
3. Assess for strengths and deficits.
4. Provide education about battering.
5. Provide information about community resources and how to use them.
6. Assist in planning strategies for safety crisis intervention.
7. Support and advocate for the pregnant woman when she is unable to advocate for herself.

- **RISK FOR ALTERED HEALTH MAINTENANCE** related to domestic violence.

   DESIRED OUTCOMES: The abused woman will verbalize her abuse to the nurse. She will choose from her options, implement a plan of action, and obtain long-term support in her decisions from her provider.

   INTERVENTIONS

   1. Develop and carry out an assessment for physical or sexual abuse as part of the routine prenatal assessment. Questions that might facilitate this type of assessment may include the abuse assessment screen described on p. 609.
   2. Encourage a problem-solving approach with the woman so she is able to look at and evaluate various options. Support her choices whenever possible.
   3. The nurse should become aware of the local laws regarding

reporting procedures and assist the woman if she wishes to file a report.

4. Be prepared to make appropriate referrals to available resources for the family. If the woman or children are in danger of harm, refer immediately to a battered women's shelter. Refer the woman's partner to a resource for abusers if the opportunity presents and it does not violate issues of trust for the woman.

- **POTENTIAL COMPLICATIONS OF TRAUMA: HEMORRHAGE, NEUROLOGIC INJURY, RESPIRATORY DISTRESS, RH SENSITIZA-TION, DECREASED GASTRIC MOTILITY/ASPIRATION, AND MATERNAL DEATH**

DESIRED OUTCOME: The complications of trauma will be minimized and managed as measured by stable vital signs, urinary output of 30 ml/hr or more, absence of signs of shock, hematocrit maintained between 30% and 45%, breath sounds clear, bowel sounds active, and abdomen soft.

INTERVENTIONS

Initial care

1. Keep airway patent.
2. Maintain breathing and circulation.
3. Control bleeding.
4. Administer oxygen at 8 to 10 L/min as indicated.
5. Assess level of consciousness.
6. Assess and document respiratory status for rate, depth, regularity, and breath sounds.
7. Assess and document peripheral pulses, skin color, and capillary bed refill.
8. Monitor blood pressure frequently.
9. Infuse crystalloid fluids and blood as indicated.
10. If the patient remains hypotensive, a suit of medical antishock trousers (MAST) can be applied without using the abdominal flap.
11. Auscultate more laterally for bowel sounds.
12. Intermittent nasogastric suctioning may be ordered because of the increased risk for regurgitation and aspiration related to trauma further decreasing gastrointestinal motility.
13. Monitor urinary output. A Foley catheter may be ordered to monitor urine output and evaluate urologic injuries after some types of trauma.
14. Refer to diagnostic data, such as complete blood count, blood type, antibody screen, Kleihauer-Betke test to deter-

mine a fetomaternal hemorrhage, platelet count, arterial blood gases, or coagulation studies, in case signs of DIC develop.

15. Administer prophylactic tetanus as ordered.
16. If x-ray films are ordered, shield the fetus if at all possible.
17. If the patient is D (Rh) negative, administer D immune globulin as ordered.

Continued care

1. The perinatal nurse should work with the critical care nurse unless the patient is in a tertiary care center with a critical care obstetrics unit.
2. Provide consultation, such as physiologic changes related to pregnancy, fetal monitoring, and signs and treatment of pregnancy complications, such as abruptio placentae, preterm labor, and premature rupture of membranes.

Recovery and rehabilitation care

1. Educate patient in self-care or self-assessment after discharge.
2. If the mother is left physically disabled because of the trauma, physical and occupational therapy may be needed to teach skills for caring for other children and a new baby.

■ **RISK FOR INFECTION** related to tissue injury and blood being an ideal medium for bacterial growth.

DESIRED OUTCOME: The patient's temperature will remain normal, injured tissue will show signs of healing, and white blood cell count will remain less than 16,000/mm^3.

INTERVENTIONS

1. Check temperature every 4 hours.
2. Refer to laboratory work such as white blood cell count.
3. Check injury areas for redness, swelling, and drainage every shift.
4. On discharge, instruct the patient as to the importance of reporting any signs of infection.
5. Notify the physician if signs of an infection develop.

■ **RISK FOR IMPAIRED FETAL GAS EXCHANGE** related to development of complications, such as abruptio placentae, premature labor, or maternal death.

DESIRED OUTCOMES: The fetus will remain active, and its heart rate will remain between 110 and 160 beats/min. The biophysical profiles will continue to be more than 6 with a reactive nonstress test (NST). On delivery the cord pH will be 7.0 or higher.

INTERVENTIONS

1. If the mother needs to be positioned supine, place a small wedge under right hip if no spinal cord injury below thoracic region is suspected. This displaces the uterus off the inferior vena cava.
2. Initially determine FHR.
3. Assist physician with a quick abdominal ultrasound to evaluate fetal status and general gestational age.
4. After stabilization, assess FHR and uterine contractions with electronic fetal monitor (EFM) for 4 to 24 hours after a motor vehicle crash or abdominal injury for early detection of abruptio placentae and preterm labor (Pearlman, Tintinalli, 1991).
5. Assess for signs of abruptio placentae, such as dark vaginal bleeding, sustained abdominal pain, uterine tenderness, or increasing fundal height.
6. Assess for uterine contractions, warning signs of preterm labor, and premature rupture of membranes.
7. If placental abruption, maternal injury resulting in persistent fetal compromise, intrauterine infection, or maternal death occurs and the fetus is more than 24 weeks and alive, prepare for a cesarean birth.
8. Instruct patient as to the importance of reporting the development of these signs of an abruption or preterm labor immediately.
9. In the event of discharge, teach patient to keep a daily fetal movement chart.
10. Explain any ordered test such as biophysical profile or NST for fetal surveillance and amniocentesis for fetal lung maturity or intrauterine bleeding.

■ **POTENTIAL COMPLICATION: FETAL COMPROMISE** related to blunt or penetrating maternal trauma.
   DESIRED OUTCOMES: The fetus will remain active, and its heart rate will remain between 110 and 160 beats/min. The biophysical profiles will continue to be more than 6 with a reactive NST. On delivery the cord pH will be 7.0 or higher.
   INTERVENTIONS
   1. B team assesses as previously outlined.
   2. If signs of fetal compromise develop, prepare for emergent or postmortem cesarean birth.
   3. Prepare for transfer of premature or injured infant to an intensive care nursery.

   4. If not delivered in the initial phase or early continued care phase, assess for spontaneous abortion, preterm labor, preterm rupture of membranes, or intrauterine fetal compromise.

- **RISK FOR ALTERED PARENTING** related to maternal separation from newborn, lack of early contact, separation from rest of family, or maternal or newborn death.

  DESIRED OUTCOMES: The mother and family members will demonstrate attachment behaviors such as calling the infant by name, making positive comments regarding the infant, seeking contact, wanting to touch, showing interest in caretaking, or learning any special caretaking skills that might be necessary. If contact is not possible, the various family members will seek appropriate alternatives, such as verbal reports and photographs.

  INTERVENTIONS
   1. Keep the mother and family informed of the status of the mother and fetus or newborn.
   2. Encourage parent contact with infant using creative methods depending on the individual situation.
   3. Allow older children in the family to visit mother and infant.
   4. Make appropriate referrals based on the family's needs.

- **RISK FOR ANTICIPATORY GRIEVING** related to loss of the pregnancy, death of the newborn or mother, and loss of the expected experiences of parenting. Refer to Chapters 5 and 6.

CONCLUSION

Maternal trauma as the leading cause of maternal death is a serious consequence of the increase in societal violence, lack of protection of pregnant women, and a general apathy to the need for maternal protection from injury. Life-threatening injuries to mother and fetus resulting from motor vehicle crashes could be prevented by safe and consistent use of car seat belts. Other injuries related to falls, burns, and acts of individual violence might be prevented by education. Pregnant women, family members, employers, and society in general need to be made more aware of the incidence of, risks for, and potential dangers of exposure of pregnant women to possible physical injury and trauma.

BIBLIOGRAPHY

Amato P, Quercia R: A historical perspective and review of the safety of fat emulsion in pregnancy, *NCP* 6(5):189-192, 1991.

American College of Obstetricians and Gynecologists (ACOG): *ACOG Techn Bull,* no. 124, 1989.

American College of Obstetricians and Gynecologists (ACOG): Automobile passenger restraints for children and pregnant women, *ACOG Techn Bull,* no. 151, 1991.

Arneson S and others: Automobile seat belt practices of pregnant women, *J Obstet Gynecol Neonatal Nurs* 15(4):339-344, 1986.

Baker E and others: Risks associated with pregnancy in spinal cord injured women, *Obstet Gynecol* 80(3):425-428, 1992.

Bohn D: Domestic violence and pregnancy: implications for practice, *J Nurse Midwifery* 35(2):86-98, 1990.

Bullock L, McFarlane J: The birth weight/battering connection, *Am J Nurs* 89(9):1153-1155, 1989.

Bullock L and others: The prevalence and characteristics of battered women in a primary care setting, *Nurse Practitioner* 14(6):49-54, 1989.

Campbell J: A test of two explanatory models of women's response to battering, *Nurs Res* 38(1):18-24, 1989.

Christian A: Home care of the battered pregnant woman: one woman's battered pregnancy, *J Obstet Gynecol Neonatal Nurs* 24(9):836-842, 1995.

Creasy R, Resnik R, editors: *Maternal-fetal medicine: principles and practice,* ed 3, Philadelphia, 1994, Saunders.

Daddario J: Trauma in pregnancy, *J Perinatal Neonatal Nurs* 3(2):14-22, 1989.

Dunn P and others: Assessing a pregnant woman after trauma, *Nurs 90* 20(2):52-57, 1990.

Field D and others: Maternal brain death during pregnancy: medical and ethical issues, *JAMA* 260(6):816, 1988.

Gonik B: Intensive care monitoring of the critically ill pregnant patient. In Creasy R, Resnik R, editors: *Maternal-fetal medicine: principles and practice,* ed 3, Philadelphia, 1994, Saunders.

Hutzel P, Remsburg-Bell E: Fetal complications related to minor maternal trauma, *J Obstet Gynecol Neonatal Nurs* 25(2):121-124, 1996.

Helton A, McFarlane J, Anderson E: Battered and pregnant: a prevalence study, *Am J Public Health* 77(10):1337-1339, 1987.

Hillard P: Physical abuse in pregnancy, *Obstet Gynecol* 66(2):185-189, 1985.

Howard J, Nyari D: Traumatic fetal death, *Dimensions Crit Nurs* 8(4):217, 1989.

Johnson J, Oakley L: Managing minor trauma during pregnancy, *J Obstet Gynecol Neonatal Nurs* 20(5):379-384, 1991.

Kettel L, Branch W, Scott J: Occult placental abruption after maternal trauma, *Obstet Gynecol* 71(3, pt 2):449-453, 1988.

National Coalition Against Domestic Violence: 1993.

Neufield J and others: Trauma in pregnancy, *Emerg Med Clin North Am* 5(3):623-640, 1987.

Norton L and others: Battering in pregnancy: an assessment of tool screening methods, *Obstet Gynecol* 85(3):321-325, 1995.

Parker B, McFarlane J: Identifying and helping battered pregnant women, *MCN Am J Matern Child Nurs* 16:161-164, 1991.

Parker B and others: Abuse during pregnancy: effects on maternal complications and birth weight in adult and teenage women, *Obstet Gynecol* 84(3):323-328, 1994.

Pearlman M, Tintinalli J: Evaluation and treatment of the gravida and the fetus following trauma during pregnancy, *Obstet Gynecol Clin North Am* 18(2):371-376, 1991.

Pearlman M and others: Blunt trauma during pregnancy, *N Engl J Med* 123(23):1609-1613, 1990a.

Pearlman M and others: A prospective controlled study of outcome after trauma during pregnancy, *Am J Obstet Gynecol* 162(6):1502-1507, 1990b.

Rochat R and others: Maternal mortality in U.S.: report from maternal mortality collaborative study, *Obstet Gynecol* 72:91-97, 1988.

Rodgers B and others: Criminal prosecution for prenatal injury, *Obstet Gynecol* 80(3):522-523, 1992.

Scott J and others, editors: *Danforth's obstetrics and gynecology,* Philadelphia, 1990, Lippincott.

Stafford P and others: Lethal intrauterine fetal trauma, *Am J Obstet Gynecol* 159(2):485-489, 1988.

U.S. Department of Health and Human Services: *Surgeon general's workshop on violence and public health,* Washington, DC, 1986, Public Health Service.

Westgren N and others: Pregnancy and delivery in women with a traumatic spinal cord injury in Sweden, 1980-1981, *Obstet Gynecol* 81(6):926-930, 1993.

Williams J and others: Evaluation of blunt abdominal trauma in the third trimester of pregnancy: maternal and fetal considerations, *Obstet Gynecol* 75(1):33-37, 1990.

U N I T

VI

Teratogens and Social Issues Complicating Pregnancy

The rise in the incidence of sexually and nonsexually transmitted infections and substance abuse during pregnancy has posed increased threats to fetal and maternal well-being. Because cell-mediated immunity is normally suppressed during pregnancy, women are more prone to infections during pregnancy (Moss, Kreiss, 1990). Chapter 24 describes the implications of the most common sexually and nonsexually transmitted infections on pregnancy and discusses nursing care responsibilities. Knowledgeable and involved perinatal nurses and nurse practitioners can significantly decrease the risk to the pregnant woman and her fetus.

Abuse of substances known to be teratogenic during pregnancy has increased dramatically in the past decade. Any pattern of habitual use and some isolated uses of substances, such as alcohol, cocaine, heroin, marijuana, and tobacco, can have adverse teratogenic effects on the development and growth of the fetus. Nurse practitioners and nurses have a unique opportunity during preconceptual and early prenatal care to educate and empower patients to abstain from contact with all substances that might potentially threaten the well-being of the fetus. Chapter 25 focuses on the six most commonly abused substances (alcohol, amphetamines, cocaine, heroin, marijuana, and tobacco) and describes in-depth nursing assessment techniques and interventions.

CHAPTER

24

Sexually and Nonsexually Transmitted Genitourinary Infections

currently more than 50 sexually transmitted diseases and numerous other genitourinary infections are recognized that impact the outcome of the pregnancy (Youngkin, 1995). Because of the continuing rise in incidence of sexually and nonsexually transmitted diseases in the United States, the development of microbial resistance to antibiotics, the emergence of incurable and fatal disease types, and the risk that they pose to the fetus and expectant mother, it is imperative that nurse practitioners and nurses caring for families during their childbearing years have an in-depth understanding of these diseases. This chapter focuses on the seven most common sexually transmitted diseases and the five most common nonsexually transmitted diseases and how each can affect pregnancy.

BACTERIAL VAGINOSIS
Organism

The organisms responsible for bacterial vaginosis (BV) are anaerobic bacteria, such as *Gardnerella vaginalis;* anaerobes, such as *Mobiluncus, Prevotella, Porphyromonas, Bacteroides, Fusobacterium,* and *Peptostreptococcus;* and general mycoplasmas (Duff, 1996; Hillier, Arko, 1996).

Transmission

BV is not considered a sexually transmitted disease. It usually results from a disturbance in normal vaginal flora initiated by sexual intercourse, hormonal changes, pregnancy, antibiotic administration, or use of nonoxynol-9 spermicidal products because they have a bactericidal effect on lactobacilli (Freeman, 1995; LeVasseur, 1992).

Signs and Symptoms

Signs and symptoms of BV are as follows:
- 50% asymptomatic (Ament, Whalen, 1996)
- Thin, gray, watery vaginal discharge
- Increased vaginal discharge odor (fishy) after intercourse
- Alkaline pH (greater than 4.5)

BV does not cause vaginal itching or dysuria.

Screening

Patients should be screened for BV if they are symptomatic. Clinical diagnosis is made if three of the following five characteristics are present:
- Saline wet mount: shows clue cells that are characterized by 1 in 5 epithelial cell margins obscured by bacteria
- Whiff test (fishy odor prevalent when vaginal fluid is mixed with 10% potassium hydroxide [KOH])
- Vaginal pH more than 4.5
- Homogeneous white to gray discharge that adheres to the vaginal wall
- No cervical or vaginal inflammation

Treatment in Pregnancy

After the first trimester treat with either metronidazole (Flagyl), 500 mg orally twice daily for 7 days, or clindamycin, 300 mg orally twice daily for 7 days. During the first trimester treat with topical clindamycin vaginal cream (2%), one applicatorful per day for 7 days. Then follow up with metronidazole after 12 weeks of gestation (CDC, 1993). During breast-feeding the woman should be treated with one dose of metronidazole, 2 g orally, and instructed to pump and discard breast milk for 24 hours (Ament, Whalen, 1996; Lawrence, 1994).

Current treatment of the woman's sexual partner or partners is not necessary and does not improve outcome.

Effect on Pregnancy Outcome

BV has the following effects on pregnancy:
1. Increases the risk of premature rupture of membranes (PROM) and preterm labor (Hillier and others, 1995)

2. Increases the risk of vaginosis and postpartum endometritis (Thomason, 1991)
3. May cause neonatal septicemia

Pregnancy Considerations

Bacterial vaginosis affects 15% to 20% of all pregnancies (Ament, Whalen, 1996). It changes the normal vaginal flora to (1) a small amount of lactobacilli that normally produce lactic acid and protect against vaginal pathogens by maintaining an acid pH and (2) a high concentration of anaerobes.

CANDIDIASIS
Organism

Candida albicans is the most common cause (90% of cases) of candidiasis. *Candida tropicalis* and *Candida glabrate* are two other possible causes of candidiasis, a fungal (yeast) infection.

Transmission

Candidiasis is not considered a sexually transmitted disease. It usually results from a disturbance in normal vaginal flora and conditions that cause vaginal pH to be more alkaline, such as pregnancy, antibiotic administration, large amounts of simple sugars in the diet, douching, wearing tight clothing, uncontrolled diabetes, or use of estrogen oral contraceptives (Eschenbach, Mead, 1992).

Signs and Symptoms

Signs and symptoms of candidiasis are as follows:
- Vaginal and vulvar irritation (erythematous and edematous)
- Pruritic, white, curdlike vaginal discharge
- Yeasty odor
- Dysuria
- Dyspareunia

Screening

Screening for candidiasis is as follows:
- Saline or KOH wet mount microscopically examined: shows hyphae, pseudohyphae, and budding yeast
- Culture with Saboraud medium reserved for cases when clinical signs are present but the wet mount is negative (Hillier, Arko, 1996)

Treatment in Pregnancy

Only symptomatic women should be treated for candidiasis. Use an antifungal agent, such as clotrimazole (e.g., Gyne-Lotrimin and Mycelex) or miconazole (e.g., Monistat). These drugs come in a vaginal tablet or cream form. Duration of treatment is usually 7 days (Youngkin, 1995).

Sitz baths twice daily may decrease the external irritation. Instruct to abstain from intercourse and use of tampons, avoid bubble baths, use cotton undergarments, and practice good perineal hygiene.

Pregnancy Considerations

Candidiasis is the second most common vaginal infection (Freeman, 1995). The risk of getting candidiasis during pregnancy is two to ten times greater than when a woman is not pregnant (Wang, Smaill, 1989), with the highest risk in patients with diabetes and patients receiving antibiotic therapy, because of the decrease in lactobacilli.

Candidiasis may be more resistant to treatment during pregnancy. Treat all symptomatic pregnant patients vigorously to avoid neonatal thrush.

CHLAMYDIA
Organism

Chlamydia trachomatis, an intracellular, bacteria-like parasite, is the organism responsible for chlamydia.

Transmission

Chlamydia is transmitted by close sexual contact.

Signs and Symptoms

The pregnant woman with chlamydia will be asymptomatic or exhibit some or all of the following symptoms:
- Increased, clear, white to yellowish mucous vaginal discharge
- Painful, frequent urination
- Dyspareunia
- Bleeding between periods

Objective Findings

- Bartholin, urethral, and skene glands (BUS): swelling and abnormal discharge may be present

- External genitalia: erythema, edema, excoriation may be present
- Vagina: abnormal discharge
- Cervix: mucopurulent cervicitis; edematous, erythematous, and friable; CMT (cervical motion tenderness) may be present

Screening

Routine screening for chlamydia is the standard of practice. All pregnant women should be screened on the first prenatal visit, and high risk patients should be screened again during the third trimester, since the disease is asymptomatic in 20% of cases (ACOG, 1994). Screening is as follows:

- Culture is the most commonly used screening method. Use a plastic- or metal-shafted, fiber-tipped swab to obtain many epithelial cells, place directly into the transport medium, and refrigerate. A cotton-tipped swab should be used first to remove mucus and debris from the cervical os. Obtain a Papanicolaou (Pap) smear first before collecting this culture.
- Antigen detection tests: direct fluorescent antibody (DFA) or enzyme-linked immunosorbent assay (ELISA).
- Pap smear shows inflammation that suggests additional testing needed (Schachter, Barnes, 1996).

Treatment in Pregnancy

Treatment for the pregnant woman with chlamydia is with erythromycin base, 500 mg orally four times daily for 7 days (CDC, 1993). If gastrointestinal side effects occur, erythromycin base, 250 mg four times daily for 14 days (CDC, 1993), is given. Erythromycin should be taken with 8 ounces of water 1 to 2 hours after a meal. For patients who cannot tolerate erythromycin, azithromycin, 1 g orally for one dose, or amoxicillin, 500 mg orally three times daily for 7 to 10 days, is an acceptable alternative (CDC, 1993).

Avoid tetracycline, doxycycline, and ofloxacin during pregnancy because of their harmful effect on fetal teeth and cartilage.

All sexual partners within 30 days should be tested and treated as well.

Effect on Pregnancy Outcome

Chlamydia is an ascending infection that can cause 25% to 50% of all pelvic inflammatory diseases (PIDs), which can later lead to infertility and ectopic pregnancies (Kottmann, 1995; Schachter, Barnes, 1996). However, PID is very unlikely during pregnancy.

Chlamydia's effect on pregnancy progression (Faro, 1991) is very controversial. It modestly increases the risk of PROM, prematurity, low birth weight, and perinatal mortality related to placental transfer of the organism (McGregor, French, 1991; Paavonen, 1991; Ryan and others, 1990).

Pregnancy Considerations

Chlamydia is the most common sexually transmitted disease in the United States and most developed countries (CDC, 1993; Duff, 1996; Schachter, Barnes, 1996), occurring in approximately 26% of all pregnancies (ACOG, 1994). If the infection is present at the time of vaginal birth, the neonate has a 50% risk of conjunctivitis and an 18% risk of pneumonitis (CDC, 1993; Crombleholme, 1992; Duff, 1996); therefore all neonates' eyes should be treated with either 0.5% erythromycin or 1% tetracycline ophthalmic ointment. Any neonate who develops conjunctivitis should be screened for chlamydia. Chlamydia may cause a delayed endometritis (Paavonen, 1991).

GENITAL HERPES

Organism

The organism responsible for herpes is herpes simplex virus (HSV-2), a double-stranded deoxyribonucleic acid (DNA) virus.

Transmission

Transmission occurs through direct, intimate contact.

Signs and Symptoms

Signs and symptoms of primary infection are as follows:
- Prodrome: lasts 2 to 10 days
    - Neuralgia
    - Paresthesia
    - Hypesthesias
- Vesicle pustule: lasts approximately 6 days
    - Painful vesicular lesions
    - Dysuria
    - Fever
    - Malaise
    - Cervicitis
- Wet ulcer: lasts approximately 6 days
- Dry crust: lasts approximately 8 days

Recurrent infections are usually less severe and of shorter duration.

Objective Findings With Lesions

- Papules, vesicles, ulcerations, pustules, or crusts on the vulva, vagina, or perianal area
- Cervical lesions resembling mucous patches, with central necrosis and elevated borders
- General cervicitis

Screening

The first prenatal assessment should include questions regarding a history of HSV infection. If the history is positive, screen for other sexually transmitted diseases (STDs), such as gonorrhea, chlamydia, syphilis, hepatitis B, and human immunodeficiency virus (HIV). At the time of delivery the health care provider should ask about prodromal symptoms and examine for cervical, vaginal, and vulvar lesions. Pregnant women who have a negative history for HSV but have a suspicious lesion should be screened to determine HSV by the following methods:

- Visualization of classic lesions
- Viral culture (most accurate screening method)
- Cytology: multinucleated, giant cells with intranuclear inclusion bodies on a Pap smear

Treatment in Pregnancy

No therapy can eradicate HSV. Symptomatic relief is the treatment of choice during pregnancy. This could include keeping the lesions dry and clean, the use of topical Campho-Phenique lotion on external lesions, and compresses of cold milk, colloidal oatmeal, or aluminum sulfate–calcium acetate (Domeboro solution) applied every 2 to 4 hours.

Acyclovir, 200 mg five times per day for 10 days, is the treatment of choice for HSV-2 to lessen symptoms and decrease viral shedding. However, it has not been approved by the U.S. Food and Drug Administration (FDA) for use during pregnancy. Therefore the drug is not usually used except in the presence of a disseminated infection (Duff, 1996). However, in one research study several hundred patients were given acyclovir with no toxic fetal effect. Therefore ongoing research is occurring to determine if there are adverse effects in infants exposed in utero to this antiviral drug (CDC, 1993). Patients who receive acyclovir during pregnancy should be registered into the International Acyclovir in Pregnancy Registry by calling 1-800-722-9292, ext. 8465.

Natural remedies such as boric acid Sitz baths can also be used, and instructions should be given so the patient will abstain from intercourse while lesions are present to decrease the spread of infection.

The use of acyclovir is contraindicated during breast-feeding.

Effect on Pregnancy Outcome

Intrauterine infection is the result of a primary maternal infection during pregnancy and is rare. If infection occurs, it may cause a spontaneous abortion, intrauterine growth restriction (IUGR), or preterm labor (Cook, Gall, 1994; Hatcher and others, 1994; Swanson and others, 1995).

Pregnancy Considerations

Contact at the time of delivery is the most common mode of transmission to the baby. Primary HSV-2 infection has a 40% to 50% risk of perinatal transmission, and a recurrent HSV-2 infection has only a 1% to 5% risk (Duff, 1996; Mann, Grossman, 1996), which suggests that maternal antibodies provide some protection. However, 50% to 60% of neonatal HSV infections occur without a positive maternal history of genital herpes (Moreland and others, 1996).

Prevention is the goal. If active lesions are present at the time of labor or rupture of membranes, cesarean birth is the method of delivery; otherwise, a vaginal birth should be expected. Weekly cultures are ineffective at predicting live HSV-2 at the time of birth (Roberts and others, 1995).

An infected mother should be counseled regarding the importance of good hand washing and hygiene in preventing transmission to her infant.

If the neonate develops HSV-2 infection, it is disseminated, involving multiple organs; localized, involving the skin, eyes, and mucosa; or localized, involving the central nervous system (CNS) (Moreland and others, 1996). Without antiviral therapy, disseminated infections are associated with a 90% mortality, and of those who survive, 90% will be mentally retarded (Radetsky, 1990).

Any skin lesions present at birth should be cultured for HSV-2. The currently accepted antiviral therapy for the neonate is either vidarabine or acyclovir (Schachter, Barnes, 1996).

GONORRHEA
Organism

The organism responsible for gonorrhea is *Neisseria gonorrhoeae,* a bacterium that is a gram-negative intracellular diplococcus.

Transmission

Gonorrhea is transmitted by close sexual contact. The risk of transmission from an infected man to an uninfected woman is 50% to 60%, and there is a 20% risk from an infected woman to an uninfected man (Whittington and others, 1996).

Signs and Symptoms

Gonorrhea is asymptomatic in 50% of cases (ACOG, 1994; Whittington and others, 1996). Signs and symptoms of gonorrhea are as follows:

- Vaginal discharge: may be profuse, purulent, yellow-green
- Anal discharge
- Itching or swelling of vulva
- Dysuria
- Dyspareunia
- Joint and tendon pain

Objective Findings

- Inguinal or cervical adenopathy
- BUS: Skene and Bartholin glands tender to palpation
- External genitalia: erythematous, edematous; excoriation may be present
- Vagina: abnormal discharge, blood or pus may be visualized
- Cervix: Cervicitis indicated by erythema; friable, cervical os with CMT
- Rectal examination: assess for discharge, bleeding, or tenderness

Screening

Routine screening for gonorrhea is the standard of practice. All pregnant women should be screened on the first prenatal visit, and high risk patients should be screened again during the third trimester since the disease is asymptomatic in 50% of cases. Screening should also be done before such procedures as dilation and curettage (D & C) and chorionic villus sampling. The test for gonorrhea is an endocervical culture. To collect, insert a cotton, polyester, or calcium alginate swab moistened with warm water 2 to 3 cm into the cervical canal and move it in and out with a rotary motion for 10 seconds to allow absorption of exudate. If a Pap smear is to be taken during the same examination, it should be obtained first.

Treatment in Pregnancy

For the pregnant woman with gonorrhea the drug of choice is ceftriaxone, 125 mg intramuscularly (IM) for one dose, followed by erythromycin base, 500 mg four times daily for 7 days, because of the increased risk of coinfection of chlamydia (CDC, 1993). If the patient is allergic to cephalosporins, spectinomycin, 2 g IM for one dose, can be given, followed by erythromycin base, 500 mg four times daily for 7 days (ACOG, 1994).

Avoid tetracyclines and quinolones during pregnancy because of their injurious effect on fetal teeth and cartilage (CDC, 1993).

Sexual partners within the preceding 30 days should be identified, examined, cultured, and treated.

Effect on Pregnancy Outcome

Gonorrhea can affect pregnancy outcome in any trimester, causing spontaneous abortion, preterm delivery, or PROM (Ament, Whalen, 1996). If the organism is present at the time of delivery, the greatest neonatal risk is an eye infection called *gonococcal ophthalmia,* which can cause blindness. This is one of the reasons all newborns' eyes should be treated with either 0.5% erythromycin or 1% tetracycline ophthalmic ointment within 1 hour of birth (CDC, 1993). If the organism is known to be present in the birth canal at delivery, the infant should be treated with a single injection of ceftriaxone, 50 mg/kg intravenously (IV) or IM for a maximum dose of 125 mg.

Pregnancy Considerations

Gonorrhea is an ascending infection that causes 8% to 70% of all pelvic inflammatory infections, depending on geographic location (Whittington and others, 1996). PID can cause infertility. Untreated gonorrhea is an important cause of postpartum endometritis. The risk of coexisting chlamydia infection is 45% (Kottmann, 1995; Whittington and others, 1996).

GROUP B STREPTOCOCCAL INFECTION (GBS)
Organism

Streptococcus agalactiae is a gram-positive encapsulated coccus, a two–cell wall polysaccharide.

Pregnancy Considerations

Streptococcus agalactiae is present in the lower genital tract or rectum of 10% to 30% of all healthy pregnant women. These women are asymptomatic carriers of GBS, which causes a 1% to 2% risk of GBS disease in the newborn (CDC, 1996). Approximately 80% of these neonatal cases will develop the early-onset invasive GBS disease that occurs in the first 7 days of the neonate's life. In the event a newborn contracts early-onset invasive GBS, mortality is 5% to 20% and morbidity for permanent neurologic sequelae is 15% to 30% if the newborn survives the meningeal infection (ACOG, 1996).

GBS has maternal morbidity implications as well. In pregnancy there is an increased risk of abnormal vaginal discharge, urinary tract infections, chorioamnionitis, and endocarditis (Clay, 1996). There is a 2% to 22% risk of developing a puerperal infection (Katz, 1993).

Risk Factors

The following risk factors increase the likelihood of early-onset neonatal GBS infection:
- Positive prenatal culture for GBS this pregnancy
- Preterm birth of less than 37 weeks of gestation
- PROM for longer than 18 hours
- Intrapartum maternal fever greater than 38° C
- Positive history for early-onset neonatal GBS

Screening

Identification of a GBS carrier during pregnancy is difficult because of the variable duration of carrier status. Prenatal screening cultures may not identify the woman who will be a GBS carrier at the time of labor. Cultures obtained between 35 and 37 weeks of gestation appropriately identify intrapartum carrier status; however, that is not helpful in the case of preterm labor. The current recommendations are that cultures should be obtained from the anorectal area and vagina and not from the cervix in the following situations:
- Prenatal symptomatic cervicitis
- Premature or prolonged rupture of membranes
- Preterm labor
- Intrapartum maternal fever
- Prenatal urinary tract infection (UTI)

The culture should be obtained without use of a speculum. The swabs should be placed in transport broth immediately (CDC, 1996).

Recommendations for Intrapartum Prophylaxis and Appropriate Therapy

The CDC (1996) recommendation to decrease the risk of neonatal GBS infection involves two alternative treatment plans. One approach recommends intrapartum treatment of all women who develop risk factors for GBS during the antepartum or intrapartum period. The other approach includes GBS screening protocols at 36 weeks of gestation in addition to treating all high risk women. The antibiotic of choice for either treatment plan is penicillin G, 5 million units by IV load and then 2.5 million units IV every 4 hours during labor. Ampicillin, 2-g loading dose and then 1 g IV every 4 hours during labor, is an alternative therapy. If the patient is penicillin allergic, clindamycin, 900 mg IV every 8 hours, or erythromycin, 500 mg IV every 6 hours, can be administered during labor (CDC, 1996). Antibiotic therapy is not recommended if there are no clinical risk factors or if reliable tests for GBS are negative (Larsen, 1996). Refer to Figs. 24-1 and 24-2 for two algorithms for prevention of early-onset GBS disease according to the 1996 CDC recommendations.

Other Considerations

Treat all symptomatic or asymptomatic pregnant patients who have a positive urine culture for group B streptococcus with a 10-day course of antibiotics.

Notify the pediatrician of any group B streptococcal infection during pregnancy.

HEPATITIS B
Organism

Hepatitis B virus (HBV), a hepadnavirus, is a partially double-stranded DNA virus consisting of a core antigen (HBcAg) carried in a lipoprotein envelope that contains the surface antigen (HBsAg). It carries a third antigen, the e antigen (HBeAg), that is highly infectious (Crawford, Pruss, 1993).

Transmission

Hepatitis B is transmitted by blood and body fluids, such as semen, vaginal secretions, and saliva. The organism is extremely hardy and can survive outside the body in dried blood or body secretions for 1 week or more. Therefore the two major modes of HBV transmission are contact with contaminated blood or blood products and participation in sexual intercourse.

Signs and Symptoms

Acute HBV infection usually resolves as the body develops protective antibodies, but a chronic infection (the carrier state) may result. The risk of becoming a carrier is inversely associated with the age at which the infection is acquired. Young children have the greatest risk (Shapiro, Alter, 1996). The pregnant woman with

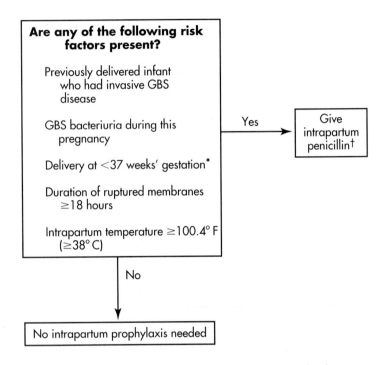

* If membranes ruptured at <37 weeks' gestation and the mother has not begun labor, collect group B streptococcal culture and either (1) administer antibiotics until cultures are completed and the results are negative or (2) begin antibiotics only when positive cultures are available.
† Broader spectrum antibiotics may be considered at the physician's discretion, based on clinical indications.

FIG. 24-1 Algorithm for prevention of early-onset group B streptococcal (GBS) disease in neonates, using prenatal screening at 35 to 37 weeks of gestation.
From Centers for Disease Control and Prevention: *MMWR Morb Mortal Wkly Rep* 45(RR-7):1-24, 1996.

acute hepatitis B may be asymptomatic, or she may exhibit some or all of the following signs and symptoms:
- Chronic low grade fever
- Anorexia
- Nausea and vomiting
- Fatigue
- Skin rashes
- Arthralgia

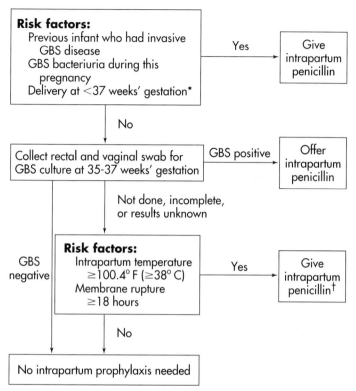

*If membranes ruptured at <37 weeks' gestation and the mother has not begun labor, collect group B streptococcal culture and either (1) administer antibiotics until cultures are completed and the results are negative or (2) begin antibiotics only when positive cultures are available. No prophylaxis is needed if culture obtained at 35-37 weeks' gestation was negative.

†Broader spectrum antibiotics may be considered at the physician's discretion, based on clinical indications.

FIG. 24-2 Algorithm for prevention of early-onset group B streptococcal (GBS) disease in neonates, using risk factors.
From Centers for Disease Control and Prevention: *MMWR Morb Mortal Wkly Rep* 45(RR-7):1-24, 1996.

Screening

The Centers for Disease Control and Prevention (CDC) and the American College of Obstetricians and Gynecologists (ACOG) recommend routine prenatal screening of all pregnant women at the initial visit and rescreening of all high risk women during the third trimester. Women who were not screened prenatally should be screened on admission to labor and delivery (ACOG, 1990; CDC, 1993). High risk individuals for HBV infection are the following (Duff, 1996):

- Persons of Central African, Southeast Asian, Middle Eastern, Pacific Islands, and Alaskan descent
- IV drug users
- Persons with multiple sexual partners
- Health care workers with blood and needle stick exposure
- Recipients of multiple blood transfusions

Screening for the presence of HBV is easily done by drawing blood and testing it for HBsAg. If HBsAg is positive, order HBeAg, anti-HBe, anti-HBc, aspartate transaminase (AST), alkaline phosphatase, and liver profile studies per consult. In the presence of an acute HBV infection, HBsAg, HBeAg, and immunoglobulin M (IgM) anti-HBe are all elevated. In chronic HBV infection (the carrier state), HBsAg remains elevated as does the IgG antiHBc but IgM antiHBe is absent (Shapiro, Alter, 1996).

Treatment in Pregnancy

If exposure occurs during pregnancy and the patient is HBsAg negative, hepatitis B immune globulin (HBIG), 0.06 mg/kg IM, should be given; the HBIG dose is repeated 1 month later, followed by the hepatitis B vaccination series (ACOG, 1990; Duff, 1996; Zatuchni, Slupik, 1996). If an expectant mother contracts the disease during pregnancy, symptomatic treatment only is given. This usually includes increased bed rest; a high-protein, low-fat diet; adequate hydration; and avoidance of medications that are metabolized in the liver.

Pregnancy Considerations

HBV does not usually affect the course of pregnancy, except that if the severe acute phase occurs during the third trimester, it can increase the risk of preterm delivery (Pastorek, 1993).

Newborn Care if the Mother is HBsAg Negative

The CDC recommends routine HBV vaccination of all newborns. Vaccine for these infants is Recombivax HB, 2.5 μg, or Engerix-B, 10 μg, IM in the anterolateral thigh. If option 1 is used, the series should be started soon after birth, the second injection given at 2 months of age, and the third at 6 to 18 months (CDC, 1991). If option 2 is followed, the first dose is given between 1 and 2 months, the second dose at 4 months, and the third between 6 and 18 months.

Newborn Care if the Mother is HBsAg Positive

If the mother is HBsAg and HBeAg positive, the child has a 90% risk of becoming infected or if only HBsAg positive, a 10% to 20% risk (CDC, 1991; Duff, 1996). Transmission can occur in the following ways (Crawford, Puss, 1993; Margolis and others, 1991; Sweet, 1990):

1. Intrapartum as the result of exposure to blood and vaginal secretions
2. Transplacental after 28 weeks of gestation
3. Postpartum related to blood contact or through breast milk

The infant rarely develops signs and symptoms, but 90% become chronic carriers if not treated (Margolis and others, 1991; Sweet, 1990). Chronic carriers have a 25% risk of developing liver cancer or cirrhosis by 50 years of age (CDC, 1991).

If the mother has a positive HBsAg test, the newborn should be treated with HBIG, 0.5 ml by 12 hours postdelivery, and an initial dose of hepatitis B vaccine (Recombivax HB), 5 μg or Engerix-B 10 μg IM. Follow-up care should include a subsequent hepatitis B vaccination at 1 and 6 months of age and diagnostic studies between 12 and 15 months to determine the infant's carrier status. If anti-HB antibodies are present, the prophylactic program was effective. However, if HBsAg is detected, the prophylactic program was ineffective and the infant is a carrier of HBV (Sweet, 1990).

The prophylactic program just described is 85% to 95% effective in preventing exposed infants from becoming chronic carriers (CDC, 1991). It is ineffective in 5% to 15% of all infants and may be related to a transplacental exposure.

Advise that breast-feeding is not contraindicated if the infant was immunized.

HUMAN IMMUNODEFICIENCY VIRUS
Organism

The organism human immunodeficiency virus (HIV) is a cyto-pathic retrovirus.

Transmission

Transmission occurs from exposure to infected blood or body secretions of semen or vaginal fluid. The most common means is unprotected sexual activity or the sharing of contaminated needles.

Normal Physiology of Immune System of Pregnancy

In HIV the helper T cells (T4) are suppressed and the suppressor T cells (T8) are not affected. Therefore there is a normal reduction of the T4/T8 ratio (Spach, Keen, 1996). The polymorphonuclear leukocyte function is decreased. Antibody formation is not affected. The net result is the pregnant woman is not more susceptible to an infection but, once she contracts an infection, it is harder to eradicate.

Pathophysiology

HIV is an envelope virus consisting of a p24 protein capsule (p24 antigen) containing two short strands of genetic material (ribonucleic acid [RNA]) and a unique reverse transcriptase enzyme encapsulated in a lipid envelope.

A virus can reproduce only inside a cell. To get into the cell, there must be an attachment molecule on its wall for the virus to attach to and then enter the cell. HIV attaches to the glycoprotein antigen (CD4) receptors on the helper T-lymphocytes (T4 cells), B-lymphocytes, macrophages, and monocytes, as well as other cells in the immune and central nervous systems, and enters these cells.

The virus reproduces inside the CD4 cells, such as the helper T-lymphocytes, and eventually destroys them. The helper T-lymphocytes (T4 cells) are the master immune cells. They send out alerting messages, by way of hormones, to the rest of the immune system. This activates the killer T-lymphocytes that hunt down and destroy microbes, monocytes that engulf microbes, and B cells that produce antibodies (Barrick, 1990; Grady, 1989). Therefore HIV weakens the immune system, causing the patient to be very susceptible to opportunistic infections that can lead to death.

Severity of the disease can be determined by measuring the CD4 (T4-lymphocytes) helper cell level. Decreasing the CD4 helper cells by one half will cause a low-grade chronic infection in the lymph glands. If the level is below 200 T4 cells/ml, opportunistic infections develop.

HIV Disease Continuum

Initial infection with HIV may manifest with mononucleosis-like symptoms, such as fever, fatigue, lymphadenopathy, and a skin rash. In the asymptomatic phase the patient is infectious without any signs or symptoms. Next is persistent generalized lymphadenopathy that lasts at least 3 months.

Acquired immune deficiency syndrome (AIDS) is the final phase. In this phase the immune system is suppressed and the patient (1) develops the wasting syndrome, manifested by an involuntary weight loss of more than 10% or persistent diarrhea, (2) contracts various opportunistic infections, or (3) develops an unusual malignancy.

Screening

The CDC (1995) recommends that all pregnant women be offered HIV antibody screening.

Screening Methods Currently Used

The screening methods currently used for HIV are viral antibody detection and viral culture.

Viral antibody detection. Viral antibody detection is with ELISA or the Western blot test. ELISA is currently the most commonly used screening test. The Western blot is a confirmatory test if the ELISA is positive.

HIV culture. Viral culture for HIV is a difficult, time-consuming, and expensive test that is of low sensitivity (Spach, Keen, 1996).

Other Screening Methods

Viral antigen detection. Viral antigen detection is for quantitative p24 (p24 is the major HIV core protein). This screening method is currently used to diagnose an acute HIV infection during the "window period" when antibodies are not yet developed.

Polymerase chain reaction. Polymerase chain reaction (PCR) is an amplification of DNA/RNA test used when other tests are undeterminate in the diagnosis.

Risk Factors

Risk factors for HIV are as follows (Radetsky, 1990):

1. Exhibits signs of HIV
2. Has used illicit IV drugs
3. Is an emigrant from an endemic area such as Haiti or Africa
4. Has been or is employed in sexual activities (prostitution)
5. Received a blood transfusion between 1977 and 1985
6. Is the sex partner of an IV drug abuser, a bisexual, a hemophiliac, a transfusion recipient between 1977 and 1985, or an emigrant from an endemic area

Signs and Symptoms

Signs and symptoms of HIV depend on the stage of the disease. They are as follows:

- Persistent fatigue
- Fever, chills
- Night sweats
- Diarrhea
- Unexpected weight loss
- Skin rashes or lesions
- Floaters in the eyes
- Oral ulcers
- Generalized lymphadenopathy
- Dry cough
- Persistent yeast infections
- Opportunistic infections

Diagnoses of Disease Progression

- Early stage is indicated by a CD4 cell count more than 500 cells/mm^3
- Middle stage is indicated by a CD4 cell count between 200 and 500 cells/mm^3
- Late stage is indicated by a CD4 cell count less than 200 cells/mm^3

Treatment in Pregnancy

At 14 weeks of gestation, patients who test positive for HIV should be offered the option of zidovudine (ZDV), 100 mg five times per day orally antepartum, 2 mg/kg IV over a 1-hour period and then a maintenance infusion of 1 mg/kg per hour intrapartum, followed by 2 mg/kg orally every 6 hours for 6 weeks to the newborn for the purpose of decreasing perinatal transmission. According to research done by Connor and others (1994) the perinatal transmission risk is decreased to 8% with this regimen. The benefits of this regimen are unstudied in pregnant individuals who have previously received ZDV or have a CD4 count less than 200/μl. Because of the risk of hematologic changes, the patient who chooses this treatment option must be checked with the following:

1. Complete blood count (CBC) every 2 weeks for two times and then every month
2. Liver profile each month
3. Creatinine every month

The treatment plan should be discontinued if any of the following develop:

1. Hemoglobin less than 8 g/dl
2. Platelet count less than 100,000/mm^3
3. Granulocytes less than 750/mm^3
4. AST and alanine transaminase (ALT) five times normal

Pregnancy Outcome

According to MacGregor (1991) and Minkoff and others (1990), HIV has minimal effect on causing pregnancy complications and a negative birth outcome if the patient does not drink, smoke, or use IV drugs.

The risk of transmission to the fetus or neonate is approximately 30% to 40% (Minkoff, 1996). Transmission appears to occur transplacentally at any gestational age, during vaginal or cesarean delivery, and through breast milk (CDC, 1993). Research has recently indicated that zidovudine (ZDV) administered during pregnancy can reduce the transmission rate to 8% (Connor and others, 1994). Vitamin A deficiency has been shown to increase the risk of perinatal transmission (Semba and others, 1994).

Infants who acquire HIV before birth will show clinical manifestations faster since the incubation time is shorter; 50% will manifest symptoms in the first year of life.

Pregnancy may mask the symptoms of HIV infection since such clinical manifestations of HIV as fatigue, nausea, and weight loss can be common discomforts of pregnancy. However, pregnancy does not appear to accentuate the course of HIV infection (Lindberg, 1995).

Pregnancy Considerations

Antepartum

If HIV infection is diagnosed during a pregnancy, the woman needs education as to potential consequences of pregnancy on HIV disease progression, referrals for appropriate crisis counseling such as WARN (Women and AIDS Resource Network; 718-596-6007), and adequate psychosocial support services to help her cope with what the diagnosis means to her, as well as risk of transmission and consequences to her child (Jones, 1991).

To facilitate health promotion, the woman needs adequate instructions in ways to enhance the immune system, such as (1) adequate sleep; (2) decreasing stress; (3) adequate protein since a deficiency can cause depression of cell-mediated immunity, complement, and phagocytes; (4) a balanced intake of polyun-saturated fatty acids and vitamin E since a high intake can depress the humoral- and cell-mediated immunity; (5) adequate zinc and vitamin A for overall growth and development of immune cells; (6) adequate pyridoxine, pantothenic acid, and folic acid for general cell synthesis (a deficiency in any of these nutrients can impair both humoral- and cell-mediated immunity); and (7) avoidance of infections. Screen for other sexually transmitted diseases. Assist in the notification plan of all sexual partners.

Intrapartum

Decrease risk of inoculation of the virus into the neonate during labor by not using a scalp electrode for fetal monitoring or doing a scalp blood sampling for fetal pH (Minkoff, 1996). Delay am-niotomy to possibly decrease the transmission rate of HIV. If the woman gives birth within 4 hours of rupture of membranes, there is a 50% less likelihood of transmitting HIV to her neonate (Mandelbrot and others, 1996). Avoid such invasive procedures as forceps- or vacuum-assisted delivery (Benson, 1994; Shannon, 1994). An episiotomy or cesarean delivery does not appear to have an obvious effect on the infection rate (Mandelbrot and others, 1996).

Postpartum

Because the actual risk of contracting an HIV infection through breast milk is unknown, the CDC (1993) recommends that HIV-infected mothers in the United States avoid breast-feeding (Cutting, 1994).

Neonate

Because it appears that length of exposure is important, bathe the infant as soon as possible after delivery (Mandelbrot and others, 1996). Percutaneous needle sticks should be done only after the initial bath and with thorough cleansing of the skin just before the injection (Benson, 1994). Antibody screening is not reliable during infancy since maternally produced immunoglobulin G (IgG) antibodies to HIV are present in all infants born to HIV-infected mothers and can continue to be present in the blood up to 6 to 15 months of age (Lindberg, 1995). Infants who do not serorevert by 18 months are considered infected with HIV (Rogers and others, 1991). The new immune complex–dissociated HIV p24 antigen test detects the presence of the p24 antigen in fetal blood after separating out the passively acquired maternal antibodies. The test has been shown to be very sensitive if two or more neonatal blood samples are tested and may become more commonly used in the near future (Spach, Keen, 1996).

In summary, it is very difficult to determine early if the infant has acquired an HIV infection because of the presence of passive acquired maternal antibodies until 12 to 18 months (CDC, 1993).

Health Care Workers

Use Standard Precautions when caring for all pregnant women during labor, during delivery, and postpartum and for infants until they have had their first bath (CDC, 1996). This should include wearing gloves, protective eyewear, and water-repellent gowns and, when doing neonatal suctioning, using a DeLee catheter to wall suction using less than 140 mm Hg pressure or a bulb suction (Minkoff, 1996).

HUMAN PAPILLOMAVIRUS
Organism

The organisms responsible for human papillomaviruses (HPVs) are human wart viruses. Currently 70 HPV types are identified (Moreland and others, 1996). Ninety percent of cases of condylomata acuminata, known as genital warts, are caused by HPV types 6 and 11 and have a low oncogenic potential (Carson, 1997). HPV types 16, 18, 31, and 33 are found to be strongly associated with genital dysplasia and invasive cancer.

Transmission

Sexual contact is the most common form of transmission, with a higher transmission rate in young adolescents (ACOG, 1994; Richart, Wright, 1993).

Signs and Symptoms

Signs and symptoms of HPVs are as follows:
- Warty growths: soft, fleshy colored, generally painless, flat or papular clusters that appear within 3 to 6 months of exposure (ACOG, 1994)
- Itching
- Vulvar pain
- Vaginal discharge

Eighty percent of women have a coexisting candidiasis infection (Deitch, Smith, 1990).

Screening

Screening for HPV includes the following:
- Visualization
- Application of acetic acid to wart to magnify its presence
- Cytology: Pap smear is the most important screening tool
- Dot hybridization technique (VirPap or Viratype kit)

Treatment in Pregnancy

No treatment has been shown to eradicate HPV. Therefore the goal is to remove the lesions and ameliorate the signs and symptoms only but not to eliminate the virus (Heppard, Garite, 1996; Youngkin, 1995). Then one must wait for the immune response to control replication of the virus. A number of treatments are used to do this. TCA (trichloroacetic acid), 80% to 90%, can be topically applied only to the warts weekly or up to three times per week (ACOG, 1994; Carson, 1997). Xylocaine jelly can be applied to the surrounding skin to decrease the burning sensation of TCA. Cryotherapy with liquid nitrogen can be used safely during the second and third trimesters. CO_2 laser can be safely used throughout pregnancy.

Electrocautery is effective on small lesions throughout pregnancy. Surgical removal during pregnancy has an increased risk of hemorrhage related to the increased vascularity. Podophyllin, interferon, and 5-fluorouracil are not safe treatment modalities during pregnancy because of their teratogenic potential.

If the patient smokes, instruct her regarding the effect that smoking has on the immune system, which can decrease the effectiveness of any HPV treatment.

All sexual partners should be examined for any evidence of warts and instructed to use condoms to decrease transmission.

Effect on Pregnancy Outcome

Condylomata acuminata have an insignificant adverse effect on pregnancy.

Pregnancy Considerations

HPV is the most common viral sexually transmitted disease currently in North America (Carson, 1997). Warts tend to proliferate and become friable during pregnancy (Heppard, Garite, 1996). During delivery, condylomata can cause pelvic outlet obstruction and severe hemorrhage related to lacerations of the friable condylomatous tissue.

HPV, especially types 6 and 11, can cause laryngeal papillomas in infants and children exposed during delivery through an infected birth canal; however, the incidence is low (0.04% risk) (Carson, 1997). These laryngeal papillomas usually appear between 2 and 5 years of age, causing such symptoms as an abnormal cry, voice changes, stridor, or evidence of airway obstruction (Wood, 1991).

There is an increased risk of poor episiotomy healing in the presence of condylomata. This risk is increased if the woman smokes (Snyder and others, 1990).

Cesarean delivery is indicated only when warts are so large at the time of delivery that the risk of dystocia and hemorrhage is great (CDC, 1993).

There is a 25% to 33% risk of coexisting sexually transmitted diseases such as trichomoniasis, BV, and chlamydia.

HPV types 16 and 18 and related viruses, such as 31 and 33, carry a high risk of causing dysplasia and squamous cell genital carcinoma (ACOG, 1994). Types 6 and 11 have a lower but increased risk of dysplasia (Moreland and others, 1996). Therefore all patients with HPV should be instructed regarding the risk and impressed with the importance of a yearly Pap smear.

Smoking and vitamin A, vitamin C, and folic acid deficiency can increase the risk of progressive development of invasive carcinoma in the presence of HPV (Carson, 1997; Kelley and others, 1992).

SYPHILIS
Organism

The organism responsible for syphilis is *Treponema pallidum,* a spirochete bacterium.

Transmission

Transmission is by way of sexual contact during the primary and secondary stages.

Signs and Symptoms

Primary syphilis is evidenced by a chancre, which is a painless sore that does not get better fast. It may last 10 days to 3 months.

Secondary syphilis is evidenced by a rash and a low-grade fever, which usually manifest from 6 weeks to 6 months after the infection. This is because the spirochete enters the bloodstream and resides in the small arteries that lead to every organ, eventually causing infection of every organ and skin manifestations.

Latent syphilis is usually asymptomatic when the spirochete goes into hiding for 5 to 20 years. This phase is subdivided into two phases: early and late. Early latency encompasses the first year after the secondary infection. Relapses of a secondary infection can occur during this phase. Many years later, manifestations of late latency syphilis are cardiovascular, granulomatous, and meningovascular (neural) (Larsen and others, 1996).

Tertiary syphilis is a remanifestation of the disease itself as it slowly destroys the heart, brain, central nervous system (CNS), and occasionally the liver, bones, and skin.

Screening

Routine screening is considered a standard of practice to be done on the first prenatal visit and repeated during the third trimester if the patient is at high risk (CDC, 1993). All cord blood should be tested as well. Common screening tests for syphilis are one of the nontreponemal tests, that is, either the Venereal Disease Research Laboratory (VDRL) test or the rapid plasma reagin (RPR) test. Common tests used to confirm the diagnosis are the treponemal antibody titer tests, either the microhemagglutination assay for antibodies to *T. pallidum* (MHA-TP) or the fluorescent treponemal antibody absorption test (FTA-ABS).

Treatment in Pregnancy

If the patient had the disease for less than 1 year, she is given benzathine penicillin G, 2.4 million units IM for one dose. If the patient had the disease for more than 1 year, she is given benzathine penicillin G, 2.4 million units IM for three doses 1 week apart for 3 consecutive weeks for a total of 7.2 million units (CDC, 1993).

The above therapy will cure a maternal infection and prevent congenital syphilis 98% of the time (CDC, 1993; Heppard, Garite, 1996). Sixty percent will experience a Jarisch-Herxheimer reaction, that is, a fever, myalgia, headache, mild hypotension, tachycardia, decreased fetal activity, and uterine contractions (Crane, 1992). These side effects are related to prostaglandin production stimulated by the endotoxin released from the spirochete (Gilstrap, Wendel, 1996).

If the patient is allergic to penicillin, the CDC (1993) guidelines suggest skin testing and referral for penicillin desensitization. This is indicated because tetracycline and doxycycline are contraindicated during pregnancy and nonpenicillin drugs such as erythromycin fail to prevent congenital syphilis (CDC, 1993).

Monthly quantitative nontreponemal serologic tests for the remainder of the pregnancy should be drawn. If the titers show a fourfold rise, the pregnant woman should be retreated.

Effect on Pregnancy Outcome

The spirochete can cross the placenta at any time. However, treatment is very effective before 16 weeks of gestation related to fetal immune competence before that gestational age (Gilstrap, Wendel, 1996).

Untreated syphilis can profoundly affect the fetus, depending on the stage of maternal infection and the length of exposure to the organism.

During the active phases of the disease the organism load is the highest and will have the gravest effect on the fetus. Almost 100% of infants will have congenital syphilis if the mother has untreated primary or secondary syphilis. If the mother has untreated early latent syphilis, infection of the fetus is possible but there is significantly less risk (Larsen and others, 1996).

Exposure during the second trimester can cause the following:
- Spontaneous abortion
- Preterm labor
- Stillbirth
- Congenital effects such as multisystem failure of the lungs, spleen, liver, and pancreas; and structural bone damage as well as nervous system involvement

If exposure occurs during the third trimester, the neonate will most likely be asymptomatically infected. Signs of asymptomatic infections are the following:
- Enlarged liver (100%)
- Enlarged spleen (100%)
- Skin rash (50%)
- Jaundice

Placental estriol is decreased if the fetus contracts congenital syphilis. This is believed to be related to decreased secretion of the precursor for estriol by the fetal adrenal glands (Parker, Wendel, 1988).

TRICHOMONIASIS
Organism

The organism responsible for trichomoniasis is *Trichomonas vaginalis,* a flagellated protozoan that is sexually transmitted.

Transmission

Trichomoniasis generally is caused by sexual activity. However, it may be contracted by swimming in contaminated water, using contaminated towels, or sitting in hot tubs.

Signs and Symptoms

The pregnant woman with trichomoniasis may be asymptomatic, or she may exhibit some or all of the following signs and symptoms:

- Frothy, yellow-green, foul discharge
- Constant perineal itching
- Erythema (strawberry spots)
- Vaginal pH alkaline (greater than 4.5)
- Vaginal mucosa erythematous
- Cervix with punctate hemorrhages

Screening

If the pregnant woman is symptomatic for trichomoniasis, a saline wet mount will show motile trichomonads with an increased number of white blood cells. The routine Pap smear may detect trichomonads.

Treatment in Pregnancy

Avoid treatment until after the first trimester (Ament, Whalen, 1996) and while the patient is breast-feeding. If the patient is undergoing a chorionic villus sampling, treat preprocedurally. Bacteria can adhere to trichomonads; thus trichomonads can serve as a vector for a chorionic infection (Hammill, 1989).

Treatment of choice for trichomoniasis is metronidazole (Flagyl), 250 mg three times daily for 7 days or a single oral dose of 2 g.

No alcoholic beverages or vinegar products are allowed for 48 hours after therapy to avoid nausea, vomiting, cramping, and headaches (Ament, Whalen, 1996). No intercourse is allowed for 2 weeks for pelvic and cervical rest.

During the first trimester and if the woman is breast-feeding, symptomatic relief with clotrimazole is the treatment of choice. During breast-feeding the woman could be treated with metronidazole, 2 g orally for one dose, and instructed to pump and discard breast milk for 24 hours (Lawrence, 1994). All sexual partners should be treated also.

Effect on Pregnancy Outcome

Trichomonas vaginalis is diagnosed in 20% of all pregnancies. For the woman with trichomoniasis, no known fetal risk exists; thus it is believed best to avoid treating unless necessary during the first trimester. Metronidazole does cross the placenta, but there is no known teratogenic effect (Wendel, Wendel, 1993). However, trichomoniasis has been implicated in premature rupture of membranes and postpartum endometritis (Freeman, 1995).

URINARY TRACT INFECTION

UTI is manifested by the following three clinical types:
- Asymptomatic bacteriuria
- Cystitis
- Pyelonephritis

Organism

The most common causative organisms are coliforms, particularly *Escherichia coli* gram-negative pathogenic bacteria. They account for approximately 85% of all UTIs. Other gram-negative pathogenic bacteria (*Klebsiella pneumoniae, Proteus* species) are important pathogens, especially in recurrent UTIs. Less frequent causative organisms involved in UTIs are gram-positive organisms: group B streptococci, enterococci, and staphylococci. They account for approximately 3% to 7% of the infections (Duff, 1996). Two other causative organisms are *N. gonorrhoeae* and *C. trachomatis* (sexually transmitted pathogens).

Transmission

Coliform organisms are a normal part of the perineal flora and may be introduced into the urethra during intercourse or improper wiping after defecation. *N. gonorrhoeae* and *C. trachomatis* are transmitted by sexual contact.

Signs and Symptoms

Signs and symptoms of a UTI depend on the location of the infection. In 5% to 10% of the cases they are asymptomatic. In cystitis or lower UTI the following symptoms are common:
- Urinary frequency
- Urinary urgency
- Dysuria
- Hesitancy or dribbling
- Suprapubic tenderness
- Gross hematuria

Accompanying symptoms with pyelonephritis (upper UTI) are usually chills, fever, and back pain with costovertebral angle (CVA) tenderness. Signs of a lower UTI may be present as well.

Screening

Routine screening for UTI is the standard of practice at the first prenatal visit and is repeated at 32 to 34 weeks of gestation. It should also be performed if there are complaints of any signs or symptoms.

- Microscopic examination shows white blood cells; bacteria may or may not be present
- Dip urine may be positive for nitrites and leukocyte esterase
- Clean-catch midstream specimen for culture and sensitivity

Treatment in Pregnancy for Asymptomatic or Acute Cystitis

Refer to Table 24-1 for the most common antibiotics used in treatment of asymptomatic or acute cystitis. In the initial infection, a 3-day course of treatment is usually as effective as 7 to 10 days (Duff, 1996). However, with a recurrent infection a 7- to 10-day course of treatment is necessary. To facilitate antibacterial action, acidify urine with cranberry juice, ascorbic acid, prunes, or plums (Zatuchni, Slupik, 1996). Teach the patient to drink at least one glass of water per waking hour and to void before and after intercourse to decrease the risk of recurrent UTIs. At all remaining prenatal visits, screen the urine for nitrites and leukocyte esterase. If either of these tests is positive, repeat urine culture and re-treat as culture indicates.

Treatment in Pregnancy for Pyelonephritis

The patient may be treated as an outpatient if the disease manifestations are mild and the patient is hemodynamically stable and without evidence of preterm labor. The usual treatment is amoxicillin and clavulanate potassium (Augmentin), 500 mg three times daily for 7 to 10 days, or trimethoprim and sulfamethoxazole (Bactrim DS), twice daily for 7 to 10 days. If the patient is hemodynamically unstable; disease manifestations are severe, such as high fever, chills, and tachycardia; or the patient is experiencing uterine contractions, she must be hospitalized for treatment. Obtain a catheterized urine sample, and send immediately for culture and sensitivity. Initiate antibiotic therapy immediately. If the patient is hemodynamically stable, common IV antibiotic therapy is a first-generation cephalosporin, such as Cefadyl, 2 g IV piggyback every 6 hours, or a third-generation penicillin, such as ampicillin, 2 g IV piggyback every 4 hours (Heppard, Garite, 1996). If the patient has a high fever, chills, and tachycardia, alternate ampicillin and gentamicin. The usual dose of

TABLE 24-1 Antibiotics for asymptomatic bacteriuria or cystitis

Antibiotics	Organism sensitivity	Oral dose	Administration considerations
Penicillin (amoxicillin)	70%-80% of *Escherichia coli*, most *Proteus* species, group B streptococci, enterococci, some staphylococci	250 mg three times daily	Do not use this drug unless sensitivity tests indicate sensitivity Side effects: diarrhea and candidiasis
Penicillin (Augmentin)	Most gram-negative aerobic bacilli Most gram-positive cocci	250 mg three times daily	Best to use if suspect drug-resistant *Escherichia coli* Side effects: diarrhea and candidiasis
Cephalosporin (Keflex)	Most *Escherichia coli* *Klebsiella* *Proteus* species Group B streptococci Staphylococci	250 mg four times daily	
Sulfonamides (Bactrim DS)	Most gram-negative aerobic bacilli	1 tab twice daily	Do not use near delivery because of its possible effect on protein binding of bilirubin
Nitrofurantoin (Macrobid)	Most gram-negative aerobic bacilli	100 mg twice daily	Best to use if suspect drug-resistant *Escherichia coli*

Modified from Duff P: In Gabbe S, Niebyl J, Simpson J, editors: *Obstetrics: normal and problem pregnancies*, ed 3, New York, 1996, Churchill Livingstone.

gentamicin is 1 mg/kg every 8 hours. If the patient is at high risk for a resistant organism, aztreonam, 500 mg to 1 g every 8 to 12 hours, may be administered until susceptibility test results are available. Consider changing the IV antibiotic therapy if the culture and sensitivity indicate or the patient has not responded to therapy within 48 hours. Obtain blood cultures if the patient has an unexplained heart murmur or signs of subacute bacterial endocarditis (Twickler and others, 1991).

Discontinue the IV antibiotics when the patient is afebrile for 48 hours, and continue on oral antibiotics to complete a 10-day course of therapy. Commonly used oral antibiotics are listed in Table 24-1. Repeat a urine culture and sensitivity before discharge.

Effect on Pregnancy Outcome

The endotoxins released from gram-negative bacteria may stimulate the production of prostaglandins and thus cause preterm labor.

Pregnancy Considerations

Five to ten percent of all pregnancies are complicated with a UTI. Approximately 1% to 2% of these cases will be pyelonephritis, usually as a consequence of undiagnosed asymptomatic bacteriuria or inadequately treated cystitis.

NURSING PROCESS

NURSING DIAGNOSES AND INTERVENTIONS

■ **ALTERED HEALTH MAINTENANCE** related to lack of knowledge, type of life-style, and sexual contacts.
   DESIRED OUTCOMES: The patient will choose to implement safe sex practices and will describe correctly signs of sexually transmitted disease that should be reported.
   INTERVENTIONS
   Prevention of STDs
   1. Nurses should be actively involved in accurate, timely education programs that teach about the symptoms of sexually transmitted diseases, method of transmission, and preventive measures.
      a. Absolutely safe sexual practice is abstinence until one establishes a mutually monogamous relationship.
      b. Safe sexual practice if one chooses to have sex out of a mutually monogamous relationship is use of a barrier method of contraception, such as a latex condom with a nonoxynol-9 spermicide.

    c. Abstaining from illegal drug use, especially the sharing of needles and syringes with anyone, is important.

    d. Periodic examinations for sexually transmitted diseases if in the at-risk group are beneficial.

    e. Expression of values and beliefs that might not permit following this type of suggested life-style should be allowed.

2. Conduct motivation seminars to increase one's reason to delay sex, for example:

    a. Job training

    b. Importance of staying in school

    c. Building self-esteem

    d. Life planning and counseling

    e. Recreational activities available

Prevention of vaginal infections related to nonsexually transmitted diseases

1. Teach behaviors to promote normal vaginal flora.

    a. Wear cotton undergarments.

    b. Maintain good perineal hygiene.

    c. Reduce simple sugars in the diet.

    d. Refrain from douching for hygienic reasons.

    e. Eat yogurt or drink milk with acidophilus when taking an antibiotic.

Prevention of urinary tract infection

1. Drink one glass of water every waking hour except for the 2 hours before bedtime.

2. To facilitate antibacterial action, keep the urine acid with cranberry juice, ascorbic acid (chewable vitamin C tablets), prunes, or plums (Lutz, Przytulski, 1997; Zatuchni, Slupik, 1996).

3. Void before and after intercourse.

Early recognition

1. When women of childbearing age seek health care, a thorough history should be taken and include the following:

    a. Cultural background

    b. Sexual practices

    c. Drug use

2. Further investigate manifested signs such as the following:

    a. Perineal, vaginal, or cervical lesions or "sores"

    b. Increased, abnormal, or malodorous vaginal discharge

    c. Dysuria

3. Educate at-risk patients regarding significant signs and symptoms to report to health care workers so effective

treatment can be initiated early and risk reduction behavior can be taught.

Prevention of further spread

1. Inform the patient of the requirement to report certain sexually transmitted diseases, such as syphilis, gonorrhea, and HIV, to community health officials, and explain local follow-up procedures in this event.
2. Educate as to the importance of notifying all sexual partners who could have been infected when a sexually transmitted disease is diagnosed.
3. Encourage abstinence from sex until follow-up cultures are negative.
4. Educate as to the importance of using condoms lubricated with a spermicide containing nonoxynol-9 to prevent reinfection.
5. Educate as to the importance of seeking immediate medical treatment if any symptoms reappear or if a sexual partner is diagnosed with a sexually transmitted disease.
6. Inform the patient that cigarette smoking may accelerate the pathogenic course of many STDs, especially HPV.

Possible herbal treatments for candidiasis, bacterial vaginosis, or trichomoniasis (Lichtman, Papera, 1990)

1. Acidification of the vagina with vinegar and water douches (1 to 2 tablespoons of plain vinegar in 1 quart of water)
2. Acidophilus vaginal tablet at bedtime for 1 to 2 weeks to restore *Lactobacillus acidophilus* in the vagina
3. Garlic suppository twice daily for 10 days (does not cause an unpleasant odor)
4. Yogurt (plain) douches with active culture twice daily for 1 week

- **PAIN** related to vaginal itching, lesions, and increased discharge as well as dysuria.

  DESIRED OUTCOME: The patient will express increasing relief with appropriate prescribed treatment.

  INTERVENTIONS

  1. Identify level of discomfort.
  2. Provide information that warm sitz baths, cornstarch, and use of a hair dryer on genital area may decrease vulvar burning, itching, or dysuria.
  3. Educate regarding hygienic measures such as use of cotton underwear and frequent bathing.
  4. Instruct on correct procedure for taking prescribed medications.

- **SELF-ESTEEM DISTURBANCE** related to difficulty accepting the fact that the condition is sexually transmitted and may be incurable.
  DESIRED OUTCOME: The individual will be able to verbalize a positive self-image.
  INTERVENTIONS
  1. Provide opportunities to discuss feelings in a nonjudgmental environment.
  2. Provide referrals to support groups if indicated.
  3. Assist the patient in planning for her future with regard to sexual activity.

- **ALTERED FAMILY PROCESSES** related to the effects of a diagnosis of sexually transmitted disease on a family's relationship.
  DESIRED OUTCOME: The family will demonstrate effective coping strategies.
  INTERVENTIONS
  1. Provide assistance with notification of sexual partners if applicable.
  2. Provide opportunities for family members to discuss feelings in a nonjudgmental environment.
  3. Provide appropriate referrals as needed.
  4. Suggest alternative methods of sexual gratification for couples who have an active sexually transmitted disease.

- **RISK FOR FETAL INJURY** related to the teratogenic effect of the disease or the necessary treatment.
  DESIRED OUTCOME: The neonate will be free of any teratogenic effect.
  INTERVENTIONS
  1. Monitor fetal growth and well-being.
  2. Educate regarding implications for pregnancy and type of delivery.
  3. Inform regarding possible fetal effects of necessary treatment.
  4. Educate regarding appropriate newborn care and follow-up.

CONCLUSION

Most sexually transmitted diseases pose a risk not only to the pregnant woman but also to the fetus she carries. It is particularly important that childbearing women be free of a sexually transmitted disease. Nurses who provide health care to childbearing families can participate in primary prevention by conducting education programs and consistently providing ongoing education about the risk and prevention of these diseases. Nurses should also be involved in secondary prevention, which includes early diagnosis and appropriate intervention if the problem arises. Only by addressing these diseases at every level will progress be made in diminishing their prevalence and devastating effects.

BIBLIOGRAPHY

General

Moss G, Kreiss J: The interrelationship between human immunodeficiency virus infection and other sexually transmitted diseases, *Med Clin North Am* 74:1647-1660, 1990.

Youngkin E: Sexually transmitted diseases: current and emerging concerns, *J Obstet Gynecol Neonatal Nurs* 24(8):743-758, 1995.

Bacterial Vaginosis

Ament L, Whalen E: Sexually transmitted diseases in pregnancy: diagnosis, impact and intervention, *J Obstet Gynecol Neonatal Nurs* 25(8):657-666, 1996.

Centers for Disease Control and Prevention (CDC): Sexually transmitted diseases treatment guidelines. U.S. Department of Health and Human Services, Public Health Service, *MMWR Morb Mortal Wkly Rep* 42:RR-14, 1993.

Duff P: Maternal and perinatal infection. In Gabbe S, Niebyl J, Simpson J, editors: *Obstetrics: normal and problem pregnancies,* ed 3, New York, 1996, Churchill Livingstone.

Freeman S: Common genitourinary infections, *J Obstet Gynecol Neonatal Nurs* 24(8):735-742, 1995.

Hillier S, Arko R: Vaginal infections. In Morse S, Moreland A, Holmes K, editors: *Atlas of sexually transmitted diseases and AIDS,* ed 2, Baltimore, 1996, Mosby-Wolfe.

Hillier S and others: Association between bacterial vaginosis and preterm delivery of a low-birth-weight infant, *N Engl J Med* 333:1737-1742, 1995.

Lawrence R: *Breastfeeding: a guide for the medical profession,* St Louis, 1994, Mosby.

LeVasseur J: Vulvovaginitis: promotion of condom use to prevent sexually transmitted disease, *Nurse Practitioner Forum* 3(3):177-180, 1992.

Thomason J: Bacterial vaginosis: current review with indications for asymptomatic therapy, *Am J Obstet Gynecol* 165(4):1210-1215, 1991.

Thomason J, Gelbart S, Scaglione N: Bacterial vaginosis: current review with indications for asymptomatic therapy, *Am J Obstet Gynecol* 165:1210-1217, 1991.

Candidiasis

Eschenbach D, Mead P: Managing problem vaginitis, *Patient Care* 26(14):137-152, 1992.

Freeman S: Common genitourinary infections, *J Obstet Gynecol Neonatal Nurs* 24(8):735-742, 1995.

Hillier S, Arko R: Vaginal infections. In Morse S, Moreland A, Holmes K, editors: *Atlas of sexually transmitted diseases and AIDS,* ed 2, Baltimore, 1996, Mosby-Wolfe.

Wang E, Smaill F: Infection in pregnancy. In Chalmers I, Enkin M, Keirse M, editors: *Effective care in pregnancy and childbirth,* Oxford, England, 1989, Oxford University Press.

Youngkin E: Sexually transmitted diseases: current and emerging concerns, *J Obstet Gynecol Neonatal Nurs* 24(8):743-758, 1995.

Chlamydia

American College of Obstetricians and Gynecologists (ACOG): Gonorrhea and chlamydial infections, *ACOG Techn Bull,* no. 190, 1994.

Cates W, Wasserheit J: Genital chlamydial infections: epidemiology and reproductive sequelae, *Am J Obstet Gynecol* 164:1771-1781, 1991.

Centers for Disease Control and Prevention (CDC): Sexually transmitted diseases treatment guidelines. U.S. Department of Health and Human Services, Public Health Service, *MMWR Morb Mortal Wkly Rep* 42:RR-14, 1993.

Crombleholme W: Neonatal chlamydial infections. In Mead P, Hager W, editors: *Infection protocols for obstetrics and gynecology,* Montvale, NJ, 1992, Medical Economics Publishing.

Duff P: Maternal and perinatal infection. In Gabbe S, Niebyl J, Simpson J, editors: *Obstetrics: normal and problem pregnancies,* ed 3, New York, 1996, Churchill Livingstone.

Faro S: *Chlamydia trachomatis:* female pelvic infection, *Am J Obstet Gynecol* 164:1767-1770, 1991.

Hatcher R and others: *Contraceptive technology,* ed 16, New York, 1994, Irvington Publishers.

Kottmann L: Pelvic inflammatory disease: clinical overview, *J Obstet Gynecol Neonatal Nurs* 24(8):759-767, 1995.

McGregor J, French J: *Chlamydia trachomatis* infection during pregnancy, *Am J Obstet Gynecol* 164:1782-1789, 1991.

Paavonen J: Chlamydial disease during pregnancy, *Contemp OB/GYN* 37(3):91-96, 1991.

Radetsky M: *Sexually transmitted diseases.* Presented at the Hocus Pocus Perinatal Focus conference, Scottsdale, Ariz, Nov 16, 1990.

Ryan G and others: *Chlamydia trachomatis* infection in pregnancy and effect of treatment on outcome, *Am J Obstet Gynecol* 162:34-39, 1990.

Schachter J, Barnes R: Chlamydia. In Morse S, Moreland A, Holmes K, editors: *Atlas of sexually transmitted diseases and AIDS,* ed 2, Baltimore, 1996, Mosby-Wolfe.

Swanson J, Dibble S, Chenitz C: Clinical features and psychosocial factors in young adults with genital herpes, *Image J Nurs Sch* 27(1):16-22, 1995.

Genital Herpes

American College of Obstetricians and Gynecologists (ACOG): Perinatal herpes simplex virus infections, *ACOG Techn Bull,* no. 122, 1988.

American College of Obstetricians and Gynecologists (ACOG): *Committee opinion: prevention of early-onset group B streptococcal disease in newborns,* Washington, DC, 1996, The Author.

Centers for Disease Control and Prevention (CDC): Hepatitis B virus: a comprehensive strategy for eliminating transmission in the United States through universal vaccination: recommendations of the Immunization Practices Advisory Committee (ACIP), *MMWR Morb Mortal Wkly Rep* 40:1, 1991.

Centers for Disease Control and Prevention (CDC): Pregnancy outcomes following systemic prenatal acyclovir exposure, June 1, 1984–June 30, 1993, *MMWR Morb Mortal Wkly Rep* 42:806, 1993.

Cook C, Gall S: Herpes in pregnancy, *Infect Dis Obstet Gynecol* 1:298, 1994.

Duff P: Maternal and perinatal infection. In Gabbe S, Niebyl J, Simpson J, editors: *Obstetrics: normal and problem pregnancies,* ed 3, New York, 1996, Churchill Livingstone.

Freij B, Sever J: Herpesvirus infections in pregnancy: risks to embryo, fetus, and neonate, *Clin Perinatol* 15(2):203-231, 1988.

Hatcher R and others: *Contraceptive technology,* ed 6, New York, 1994, Irvington.

Mann M, Grossman III J: Herpes simplex. In Queenan J, Hobbins J, editors: *Protocols for high-risk pregnancies,* ed 3, Cambridge, England, 1996, Blackwell Science.

Moreland A and others: Genital herpes. In Morse S, Moreland A, Holmes K, editors: *Atlas of sexually transmitted diseases and AIDS,* ed 2, Baltimore, 1996, Mosby-Wolfe.

Radetsky M: *Sexually transmitted diseases.* Presented at the Hocus Pocus Perinatal Focus conference, Scottsdale, Ariz, Nov 16, 1990.

Roberts S and others: Genital herpes during pregnancy: no lesions, no cesarean, *Obstet Gynecol* 85:261-264, 1995.

Swanson J and others: Clinical features and psychosocial factors in young adults with genital herpes, *Image: Journal of Nursing Scholarship* 27(1):16-22, 1995.

Whitley R, Gramm J: Acyclovir: a decade later, *N Engl J Med* 327:782, 1992.

Gonorrhea

Ament L, Whalen E: Sexually transmitted diseases in pregnancy: diagnosis, impact and intervention, *J Obstet Gynecol Neonatal Nurs* 25(8):657-666, 1996.

American College of Obstetricians and Gynecologists (ACOG): Gonorrhea and chlamydial infections, *ACOG Techn Bull,* no. 190, 1994.

Cates W, Hinman A: Sexual transmitted diseases in the 1990s, *N Engl J Med* 325(19):1368-1370, 1991.

Centers for Disease Control and Prevention (CDC): Sexually transmitted diseases treatment guidelines. U.S. Department of Health and Human Services, Public Health Service, *MMWR Morb Mortal Wkly Rep* 42:RR-14, 1993.

Kottmann L: Pelvic inflammatory disease: clinical overview, *J Obstet Gynecol Neonatal Nurs* 24(8):759-767, 1995.

Wendel G: Sexually transmitted diseases in pregnancy, *Semin Perinatol* 14(2):171-178, 1990.

Whittington W, Ison C, Thompson S: Gonorrhea. In Morse S, Moreland A, Holmes K, editors: *Atlas of sexually transmitted diseases and AIDS,* ed 2, Baltimore, 1996, Mosby-Wolfe.

Group B Streptococcal Infection

American College of Obstetricians and Gynecologists (ACOG): *Committee opinion: prevention of early-onset group B streptococcal disease in newborns,* Washington, DC, 1996, The Author.

Centers for Disease Control and Prevention (CDC): Sexually transmitted diseases treatment guidelines. U.S. Department of Health and Human Services, Public Health Service, *MMWR Morb Mortal Wkly Rep* 42:RR-14, 1993.

Centers for Disease Control and Prevention (CDC): Prevention of perinatal group B streptococcal disease: a public health perspective, *MMWR Morb Mortal Wkly Rep* 45(RR-7):1-24, 1996.

Clay L: Group B streptococcus in the perinatal period: a review, *J Nurse Midwifery* 41(5):355-363, 1996.

Katz V: Management of group B streptococcal disease in pregnancy, *Clin Obstet Gynecol* 36:832-842, 1993.

Larsen J: Group B streptococcus. In Queenan J, Hobbins J, editors: *Protocols for high-risk pregnancies,* ed 3, Cambridge, England, 1996, Blackwell Science.

Larwon J: Group B streptococcus. In Patorek J, editor: *Obstetric and gynecologic infectious diseases,* New York, 1994, Raven Press.

Zangwill K, Schuchat A, Wenger J: Group B streptococcal disease in the United States, 1990: report from a multistate active surveillance system (CDC surveillance summaries), *MMWR Morb Mortal Wkly Rep* 41(SS-6):25-32, 1992.

Hepatitis B

American College of Obstetricians and Gynecologists (ACOG): *Guidelines for hepatitis B virus screening and vaccination during pregnancy: ACOG committee opinion.* No. 78, Washington, DC, 1990, The College.

Centers for Disease Control and Prevention (CDC): Hepatitis B virus: A comprehensive strategy for eliminating transmission in the United States through universal childhood vaccination, *MMWR* 40:1-24, 1991.

Centers for Disease Control and Prevention (CDC): *Sexually transmitted diseases treatment guidelines.* U.S. Department of Health and Human Services, Public Health Service, *MMWR Morb Mortal Wkly Rep* 42:RR-14, 1993.

Crawford N, Pruss A: Preventing neonatal hepatitis B infection during the perinatal period, *J Obstet Gynecol Neonatal Nurs* 22(6):491-497, 1993.

Duff P: Hepatitis B infection: managing the risk in health care workers, *Obstet Gynecol Rep* 2:153-154, 1990.

Duff P: Maternal and perinatal infection. In Gabbe S, Niebyl J, Simpson J, editors: *Obstetrics: normal and problem pregnancies,* ed 3, New York, 1996, Churchill Livingstone.

Immunization Practices Advisory Committee: Prevention of perinatal transmission of hepatitis B virus: prenatal screening of all pregnant women for hepatitis B surface antigen, *MMWR Morb Mortal Wkly Rep* 37:341-346, 1988.

Margolis H, Alter M, Hadler S: Hepatitis B: evolving epidemiology and implications for control, *Semin Liver Dis* 11(2):84-91, 1991.

Pastorek J: The ABCs of hepatitis in pregnancy, *Clin Obstet Gynecol* 36(4):843-854, 1993.

Shapiro C, Alter M: Hepatitis. In Morse S, Moreland A, Holmes K, editors: *Atlas of sexually transmitted diseases and AIDS,* ed 2, Baltimore, 1996, Mosby-Wolfe.

Sweet R: Hepatitis B infection in pregnancy, *Obstet Gynecol Rep* 2:128-139, 1990.

Zatuchni G, Slupik R: *Obstetrics and gynecology drug handbook,* ed 2, St Louis, 1996, Mosby.

Human Immunodeficiency Virus

American College of Obstetricians and Gynecologists (ACOG): *Voluntary testing for human immunodeficiency virus: ACOG committee opinion.* No. 97, Washington, DC, 1991, The College.

Barrick B: Light at the end of a decade, *Am J Nurs* 90(11):36-40, 1990.

Benson M: Management of infants born to women infected with human immunodeficiency virus, *J Perinatal Neonatal Nurs* 7(4):79-87, 1994.

Centers for Disease Control and Prevention (CDC): Sexually transmitted diseases treatment guidelines. U.S. Department of Health and Human Services, Public Health Service, *MMWR Morb Mortal Wkly Rep* 42:RR-14, 1993.

Centers for Disease Control and Prevention (CDC): U.S. Public Health Service recommendations for human immunodeficiency virus counseling and voluntary testing for pregnant women, *MMWR Morb Mortal Wkly Rep* 44:RR-17, 1995.

Centers for Disease Control and Prevention (CDC): Update: Mortality attributable to HIV infection among persons age 25-44 years—United States, *MMWR* 45:1, 1996.

Connor E and others: Reduction of maternal-infant transmission of human immunodeficiency virus type I with zidovudine treatment, *N Engl J Med* 331(18):1173-1180, 1994.

Cutting W: Breastfeeding and HIV: a balance of risks, *J Tropical Pediatr* 40:6-11, 1994.

Grady C: The immune system and AIDS/HIV infection. In Flaskerud J, editor: *AIDS/HIV infection,* Philadelphia, 1989, Saunders.

Jones D: HIV-seropositive childbearing women: nursing management, *J Obstet Gynecol Neonatal Nurs* 20(6):446-452, 1991.

Lindberg C: Perinatal transmission of HIV: How to counsel women, *MCN* 20(4):207-212, 1995.

MacGregor S: Human immunodeficiency virus infection in pregnancy, *Clin Perinatol* 8(1):33-50, 1991.

Mandelbrot L and others: Obstetric factors and mother-to-child transmission of human immunodeficiency virus Type I: the French perinatal cohorts, *Am J Obstet Gynecol* 175:661-667, 1996.

Minkoff H: Human immunodeficiency virus infection. In Queenan J, Hobbins J, editors: *Protocols for high-risk pregnancies,* ed 3, Cambridge, England, 1996, Blackwell Science.

Minkoff H and others: Pregnancy outcomes among mothers infected with human immunodeficiency virus and uninfected control subjects, *Am J Obstet Gynecol* 163:1598-1604, 1990.

Radetsky M: *Sexually transmitted diseases.* Presented at the Hocus Pocus Perinatal Focus conference, Scottsdale, Ariz, Nov 16, 1990.

Rogers M and others: Advances and problems in the diagnosis of human immunodeficiency virus infection in infants, *Pediatr Infect Dis J* 10(7):523-531, 1991.

Semba R and others: Maternal vitamin A deficiency and mother-to-child transmission of HIV-1, *Lancet* 343:1593-1597, 1994.

Shannon M: Clinical issues and therapeutic interventions in the care of pregnant women infected with the human immunodeficiency virus, *J Perinatal Neonatal Nurs* 7(4):13-27, 1994.

Sipes C: Guidelines for assessing HIV in women, *MCN Am J Matern Child Nurs* 20(1):29-33, 1995.

Spach D, Keen P: HIV and AIDS. In Morse S, Moreland A, Holmes K, editors: *Atlas of sexually transmitted diseases and AIDS,* ed 2, Baltimore, 1996, Mosby-Wolfe.

Human Papillomavirus

American College of Obstetricians and Gynecologists (ACOG): Genital human papillomavirus infections, *ACOG Techn Bull,* no. 193, 1994.

Carson S: Human papillomatous virus infection update: impact on women's health, *Nurse Practitioner* 22(4):24-37, 1997.

Centers for Disease Control and Prevention (CDC): Sexually transmitted diseases treatment guidelines. U.S. Department of Health and Human Services, Public Health Service, *MMWR Morb Mortal Wkly Rep* 42:RR-14, 1993.

Deitch K, Smith J: Symptoms of chronic vaginal infection and microscopic condyloma in women, *J Obstet Gynecol Neonatal Nurs* 19(2):133-138, 1990.

Heppard M, Garite T: *Acute obstetrics: a practical guide,* ed 2, St Louis, 1996, Mosby.

Kelley K, Galbraith M, Vermund S: Genital human papillomavirus infection in women, *J Obstet Gynecol Neonatal Nurs* 21(6):503-515, 1992.

Moreland A, Majmudar B, Vernon S: Genital human papillomavirus infections. In Morse S, Moreland A, Holmes K, editors: *Atlas of sexually transmitted diseases and AIDS,* ed 2, Baltimore, 1996, Mosby-Wolfe.

Richart R, Wright J: Controversies in the management of low-grade cervical intraepithelial neoplasia, *Cancer* 15:1413-1421, 1993.

Snyder R, Hammond T, Hankins G: Human papillomavirus associated with poor healing of episiotomy repairs, *Obstet Gynecol* 76:664-667, 1990.

Wood C: Laryngeal papillomas in infants and children: relationship to maternal venereal warts, *J Nurse Midwifery* 36(5):297-302, 1991.

Youngkin E: Sexually transmitted diseases: current and emerging concerns, *J Obstet Gynecol Neonatal Nurs* 24(8):743-758, 1995.

Syphilis

Centers for Disease Control and Prevention (CDC): Sexually transmitted diseases treatment guidelines. U.S. Department of Health and Human Services, Public Health Service, *MMWR Morb Mortal Wkly Rep* 42:RR-14, 1993.

Crane M: The diagnosis and management of maternal and congenital syphilis, *J Nurse Midwifery* 37(1):4-15, 1992.

Gilstrap L, Wendel G: Syphilis. In Queenan J, Hobbins J, editors: *Protocols for high-risk pregnancies,* ed 3, Cambridge, England, 1996, Blackwell Science.

Heppard M, Garite T: *Acute obstetrics: a practical guide,* ed 2, St Louis, 1996, Mosby.

Larsen S, Thompson S, Moreland A: Syphilis. In Morse S, Moreland A, Holmes K, editors: *Atlas of sexually transmitted diseases and AIDS,* ed 2, Baltimore, 1996, Mosby-Wolfe.

Parker C, Wendel G: The effect of syphilis on endocrine function of the fetoplacental unit, *Am J Obstet Gynecol* 159:1327-1331, 1988.

Trichomoniasis

Ament L, Whalen E: Sexually transmitted diseases in pregnancy: diagnosis, impact and intervention, *J Obstet Gynecol Neonatal Nurs* 25(8):657-666, 1996.

Freeman S: Common genitourinary infections, *J Obstet Gynecol Neonatal Nurs* 24(8):735-742, 1995.

Hammill H: Trichomonas vaginalis, *Obstet Gynecol Clin North Am* 16(3):531-539, 1989.

Hillier S, Arko R: Vaginal infections. In Morse S, Moreland A, Holmes K, editors: *Atlas of sexually transmitted diseases and AIDS,* ed 2, Baltimore, 1996, Mosby-Wolfe.

Hughes V, Hillier S: Microbiologic characteristics of lactobacillus products used for colonization of the vagina, *Obstet Gynecol* 75:244-248, 1990.

Lawrence R: *Breastfeeding: a guide for the medical profession,* St Louis, 1994, Mosby.

Wendel P, Wendel G: Sexually transmitted diseases in pregnancy, *Semin Perinatol* 17(6):443-451, 1993.

Urinary Tract Infection

Duff P: Maternal and perinatal infection. In Gabbe S, Niebyl J, Simpson J, editors: *Obstetrics: normal and problem pregnancies,* ed 3, New York, 1996, Churchill Livingstone.

Heppard M, Garite T: *Acute obstetrics: a practical guide,* ed 2, St Louis, 1996, Mosby.

Spellacy W: Urinary tract infections. In Queenan J, Hobbins J, editors: *Protocols for high-risk pregnancies,* ed 3, Cambridge, England, 1996, Blackwell Science.

Twickler D and others: Renal pelvicalyceal dilation in antepartum pyelonephritis: ultrasonographic findings. 1, *Am J Obstet Gynecol* 165(4):1115-1119, 1991.

Zatuchni G, Slupik R: *Obstetrics and gynecology drug handbook,* ed 2, St Louis, 1996, Mosby.

Nursing Interventions

Lichtman R, Papera S: *Gynecology: well-woman care,* Norwalk, Conn, 1990, Appleton & Lange.

Lutz C, Przytulski K: *Nutrition and diet therapy,* ed 2, Philadelphia, 1997, Davis.

Zatuchni G, Slupik R: *Obstetrics and gynecology drug handbook,* ed 2, St Louis, 1996, Mosby.

CHAPTER

25

Substance Abuse

Substance abuse among childbearing women continues to increase dramatically. According to ACOG (1994), 10% of all pregnant women have a substance abuse problem. Practicing any kind of substance abuse increases the risk of pregnancy complications in the childbearing woman and the risk of adverse physical and mental outcomes in her fetus. It is imperative that nurse practitioners and nurses caring for families during their childbearing years understand substance abuse. This chapter focuses on six of the most commonly abused substances and provides insight into the management of care of pregnant women who are using these six substances.

ALCOHOL
Incidence

Currently alcohol is the most common teratogen. Approximately 7% to 15% of childbearing women are heavy drinkers, consuming five or six drinks on occasion and at least 45 drinks per month (Jannke, 1994). In the United States 70% of embryos and fetuses are exposed to alcohol (Sokol, Martier, 1996).

Pathophysiologic Effects

Alcohol use during pregnancy can have varied pathophysiologic effects, including the following:

1. Interferes with the absorption of many nutrients (Wardlaw and others, 1997)

2. Interferes with overall cell growth and cell division (Armant, Saunders, 1996)
3. Impairs neuronal differentiation (Armant, Saunders, 1996)
4. Inhibits deoxyribonucleic acid (DNA) synthesis and interferes with amino acid availability to the fetus (Pietrantoni, Knuppel, 1991)

Maternal Complications

Maternal complications with alcohol use during pregnancy include increased risk for the following problems (Armant, Saunders, 1996; Grodstein and others, 1994; Pietrantoni, Knuppel, 1991):
1. Infertility
2. Spontaneous abortion
3. Abruptio placentae

Fetal Complications

Alcohol can have varying adverse effects on the fetus, depending on such factors as genetic sensitivity, time of exposure, and dose (Armant, Saunders, 1996). The continuum for adverse fetal outcome can range from no effect to a fetal alcohol syndrome (FAS) with alcohol-related birth defects (ARBDs) spread out in varying degrees in the middle of the continuum.

FAS is a pattern of defects that are the result of prenatal exposure to alcohol characterized by three clinical features. To make the diagnosis of FAS, one manifestation from each of the three deficits must be present. Other deficits are seen with increasing frequency but are not required for the diagnosis.
1. Prenatal or postnatal growth restriction characterized by growth deficiency in length, weight, and head circumference below the tenth percentile
2. Craniofacial anomalies
   a. Flattened midface
   b. Sunken, narrow nasal bridge
   c. Flattened and elongated philtrum (the groove between the nose and upper lip)
   d. Short, upturned nose
3. Neurologic disorders
   a. Microcephaly
   b. Mental retardation
   c. Poor motor coordination
   d. Attention deficit disorder
   e. Hyperactivity
   f. Poor short-term memory

4. Other major organ system malformations
   a. Congenital heart defects 30% to 40% of the time
   b. Skeletal abnormalities such as a congenital hip dislocation

ARBDs present with lesser and varying degrees of mental, physical, and behavior defects but lack the full set of characteristics that define FAS. These may include major malformations, decreased immune function, hearing impairment, and developmental delays (Armant, Saunders, 1996).

Childhood Effects

These children continue to demonstrate growth deficiency, the dysmorphic characteristics, performance deficits, and varying degrees of learning difficulties. Their social and emotional development depends somewhat on their environment. FAS is the most common cause of mental retardation (ACOG, 1994; Hankin, Sokol, 1995). Recurrent otitis media is commonly related to eustachian tube dysfunction.

Screening

The best screening method for alcohol abuse is a self-administered questionnaire given to all pregnant women on their first prenatal visit. The questions should be worded in a manner that assumes alcohol use in order to lessen defensive responses and increase honesty. Two different ways of wording the questions have been found to facilitate disclosure. The first way is a simple question such as "How many times per week do you drink beer, wine, or liquor?" (Mason, Lee, 1995; Rosett and others, 1981). A second way is to use a multiple-choice question such as "Choose the response that best matches your drinking pattern": "I drink regularly now"; "I drink regularly, but I've cut down since becoming pregnant"; "I drink occasionally"; "I have quit drinking"; or "I wasn't drinking at the time I got pregnant" (Mullen and others, 1991). If it is determined that the pregnant woman drinks, administer a questionnaire to determine at-risk levels of drinking. The T-ACE and the CAGE are two such instruments. Refer to Table 25-1 for the T-ACE and Table 25-2 for the CAGE.

Screen, very carefully, women who are particularly at risk, including the following groups:

1. Single pregnant women
2. Women of American Indian descent
3. Smokers
4. Women with alcoholic husbands

TABLE 25-1   T-ACE questionnaire for at-risk drinking patterns

	Questions	Score
T	How many drinks does it take to make you feel high (**T**olerance)?	6 or more drinks = 2 Less than 6 drinks = 1
A	Have people **A**nnoyed you by criticizing your drinking?	Yes = 2 No = 1
C	Have you felt you ought to **C**ut down on your drinking?	Yes = 2 No = 1
E	Have you ever had a drink first thing in the morning to steady your nerves or get rid of a hangover (**E**ye opener)?	Yes = 2 No = 1

Modified from American College of Obstetricians and Gynecologists (ACOG): *ACOG Techn Bull,* no. 195, 1994.
A score of two on any question indicates a high probability of being a "risk drinker."

TABLE 25-2   CAGE questionnaire for at-risk drinking patterns

	Questions
C	Have you ever felt you ought to **C**ut down on drinking?
A	Have people **A**nnoyed you by criticizing your drinking?
G	Have you ever felt bad or **G**uilty about your drinking?
E	Have you ever had a drink first thing in the morning to steady your nerves or get rid of a hangover (**E**ye opener)?

Modified from Lowdermilk D, Perry S, Bobak I: *Maternity and Women's Health Care,* ed 6, St Louis, 1997, Mosby.
More than one positive response suggests an alcohol "at-risk" problem.

Pregnancy Considerations

No level of alcohol has been proven safe for the fetus, and alcohol should be completely avoided when planning for conception and during pregnancy (ACOG, 1994). Because alcohol readily passes to the infant through breast milk and research has shown that infants consume significantly less breast milk when it contains alcohol (Mennella, Beauchamp, 1991), drinking is not recommended during breast-feeding as well.

The teratogenic effect of alcohol is dose related, and "risk drinking" is of the greatest concern. This is defined as maternal drinking that produces blood alcohol levels high enough and for long enough to produce fetal damage (Hankin, Sokol, 1995). However, the precise level of alcohol varies with each individual. Therefore no safe drinking level has been established.

Maternal nutrition is usually affected if the pregnant woman drinks. Ethanol is a source of energy; therefore a person with alcoholism usually has a low intake of nutrients. Ethanol can also interfere with intestinal absorption of such nutrients as calcium, amino acids, and some vitamins, such as thiamin, folate, and vitamin K (Institute of Medicine, 1990). Affected liver function compounds the vitamin deficiencies of vitamin A, thiamin, vitamin C, and vitamin D (Wardlaw and others, 1997).

Women are frequently more receptive to making life-style changes during pregnancy than at any other time during their lives. Offering advice that can be easily remembered versus mass media education is more effective in motivating a woman to choose to stop drinking (Hankin, Sokol, 1995). Examples are as follows:

1. You have a whole life to drink but only 9 months to grow a healthy baby.
2. Although only 1 in 10 heavy drinkers has a baby with fetal alcohol syndrome, you cannot predict that you will not be the one.
3. The most important thing you can do to influence the health of your baby is to cut your drinking or quit altogether.

If the woman comes into labor intoxicated, the fetal heart rate (FHR) variability will be decreased and FHR acceleration response to fetal movement will be suppressed related to the effects of the alcohol (Barbour, 1990).

Treatment During Pregnancy

The risk of FAS decreases if an alcohol-abusing pregnant woman stops her alcohol use during the third trimester. Therefore when a pregnant woman identifies that she does use alcohol to some degree, classify her drinking pattern according to (1) social drinking, (2) symptom-relief drinking (drinking to relieve depression or to elevate mood), or (3) syndrome drinking (physiologic and psychologic dependence on alcohol). Then implement nursing interventions based on the woman's drinking pattern to facilitate her quitting or at least decreasing her drinking.

The social drinker just needs complete information as to the effects of alcohol on her unborn child, and she will most likely quit. However, in a qualitative study Barbour (1990) found that 60% of pregnant women received information that occasional drinking was not likely to be harmful. Nevertheless, to decrease undue anxiety, a woman who has had a few social drinks before the pregnancy was recognized should be reassured of a relatively low risk of fetal damage but instructed as to the importance of avoiding alcohol for the remainder of the pregnancy. The symptom-relief drinker will need the same education as to the effects of alcohol but will need supportive counseling as well. This can be provided effectively in the prenatal office setting by trained health care workers. The woman with alcoholism will require referral to an appropriate detoxification program as well as support programs. However, the nurse practitioner and the prenatal nurse need to remain actively involved after making the appropriate referrals.

AMPHETAMINES

Amphetamines and methamphetamines, known as *ice* or *blue ice,* have vasoconstrictive properties like cocaine and are used in a similar manner.

Maternal Complications

The following complications are known to occur with amphetamine use:

- Abruptio placentae (ACOG, 1994)
- Hyperactivity
- Insomnia
- Loss of appetite
- Cardiac dysrrhythmias

Perinatal Effects

- Strongest correlation: intrauterine growth restriction (IUGR) and reduced brain growth (ACOG, 1994)
- Congenital anomalies and fetal stress have been reported (Evans, 1995)
- May cause neonatal withdrawal

Treatment

Ideal treatment is as follows:

- Cessation of use
- Optimal nutrition
- Ongoing prenatal care

COCAINE

Cocaine comes in two forms: powder and crystals. Cocaine hydrochloride, cocaine sulfate, and cocaine base come in the form of a powder and are inhaled ("snorted" or "sniffed"); therefore they are readily absorbed through the mucous membranes or dissolved and taken intravenously. Cocaine powders are only 15% to 25% pure and have many street names, such as *lady, snow, coke, white girl, nose candy, Cadillac,* and *gold dust.* Crack, which is 90% pure cocaine, comes in the form of crystals called *rocks* and is smoked ("free based"); therefore it is absorbed through the lung tissue.

Sniffing cocaine produces a high after several minutes, and the effect lasts for more than 1 hour. Intravenous cocaine and smoking cocaine produce a high in seconds that causes rapid euphoria that lasts only about 30 minutes. Thus they are usually repeated more often and are therefore highly addicting. Most people are hooked after their first experience with it.

Incidence

The use of cocaine during pregnancy has continued to dramatically increase in the past few years. It is estimated that 8% to 30% of pregnant women use cocaine (Chazotte and others, 1995).

Pathophysiologic Effects

Cocaine interferes with the reuptake of dopamine and norepinephrine at the nerve synapses, resulting in increased circulating levels of these two neurotransmitters. Cocaine also alters the metabolism of serotonin and acetylcholine. The resulting neurotransmitter imbalance overactivates certain receptors that regulate (1) mood, causing euphoria (a feeling of confidence and sexual arousal); (2) sleep, causing a hyperaroused state; (3) motor function, causing excitation and restlessness; and (4) sympathetic nervous system stimulation, causing tachycardia, tachypnea, hyperthermia (38.8° to 46° C[102° to 106° F]), hypertension (increased mean arterial pressure approximately 50%), and intense, generalized vasoconstriction (Buehler and others, 1996; Chasnoff, 1991; Dolkart and others, 1990). After depletion of the neurotransmitters, depression, malaise, and an extreme craving for the drug ensue.

Resulting complications that can occur from cocaine use are as follows:

- Decreased blood flow to the heart muscle, which predisposes to dysrhythmias, a myocardial infarction, and platelet aggregation (Chao, 1996)
- Decreased blood flow to the brain, which predisposes to seizures, stroke, and cerebral infarction (Burkett and others, 1990)

- Decreased blood flow to the intestines, which can cause peristaltic stimulation but can lead to tissue death
- Decreased uterine blood flow by 50% and increased uterine vascular resistance by 190% (Chao, 1996)
- Increased levels of fetal neurotransmitters (The resulting consequences are the same as for the adult, such as increased fetal mean arterial pressure by 24%, increased FHR by 50%, and decreased fetal oxygen partial pressure [pO_2] by 30%, which may cause various teratogenic effects [Buehler and others, 1996; Dolkart and others, 1990].)
- Damage to the fetal brain neurotransmitters, causing permanent neurobehavioral abnormalities (Burkett and others, 1990; Landry, Whitney, 1996)

Cocaine is metabolized by plasma and liver cholinesterase to water-soluble substances called *metabolites* that are excreted in the urine. Because the plasma cholinesterase is decreased during pregnancy and is much less in the fetus and neonate, cocaine is more toxic during pregnancy and to the fetus (Chao, 1996; Dombrowski, Sokol, 1990).

Maternal Complications

Cocaine can stimulate uterine contractions. Therefore its use in the first trimester of pregnancy increases the risk of a spontaneous abortion (Lindenberg and others, 1991). Its use in the second and third trimesters can increase the risk of preterm labor and premature rupture of membranes (Hurd and others, 1991; Monga, 1996).

Cocaine decreases blood flow to the heart, brain, and uterus to a greater extent during pregnancy (Chao, 1996). Because of this vasoconstrictor effect of the drug, cardiovascular failure, intracerebral hemorrhage, respiratory failure, seizures, and hypertensive crisis that may mimic pregnancy-induced hypertension (PIH) occur significantly more frequently (Rosenak and others, 1990; Woods, Plessinger, 1990).

Abruptio placentae and stillbirth are recognized complications of cocaine usage (Dombrowski, Sokol, 1990; Hoskins and others, 1991; Jones, 1991) that can occur immediately after taking the drug or as the result of placental damage done during early gestational development (Chasnoff and others, 1989). Cocaine-using expectant mothers are in real need of adequate prenatal care but are very unlikely to obtain appropriate care (McCalla and others, 1991).

Fetal and Neonatal Complications

Because of the dramatic decrease in uterine blood flow with resultant fetal hypoxia and the blocking reuptake of the neurotransmitters that occur with maternal cocaine use, complications are prevalent. Prematurity caused by a preterm delivery is related to cocaine-induced uterine contractions (Smith and others, 1995).

Small for gestational age including small head circumference, even when controlled for weight gain and smoking and alcohol use, has consistently been observed in cocaine-exposed infants (Chazotte and others, 1995; McCalla and others, 1991).

Congenital malformations have been reported in the literature and include cardiac anomalies, urinary tract defects, segmental intestinal atresia, and central nervous system (CNS) abnormalities (ACOG, 1994). However, available research data do not provide unequivocal proof. The strongest association is between intrauterine exposure to cocaine and an increased incidence of genitourinary tract malformations (Buehler and others, 1996).

Cases of cerebral infarctions and seizure activity in the fetus when exposed to large quantities of cocaine or in the neonate when the mother used cocaine just before delivery have been reported (Heier and others, 1991).

Infants exposed to cocaine during pregnancy do not exhibit physiologic withdrawal symptoms as seen when other types of substances are abused but frequently manifest neurobehavioral abnormalities (Lindenberg and others, 1991; Peters, Theorell, 1991), such as the following (Cherukuri and others, 1988):

- Hyperreflexia, which can be seen as an exaggerated startle response and tremulousness
- Abnormal state patterns such as difficulty sleeping and maintaining an alert, inactive state, thus spending prolonged time in the crying and alert active state
- Inappropriate interactive behaviors and inability to respond appropriately to parents, affecting parent-infant attachment
- Difficulty in habituating and therefore extreme sensitivity to environmental stimuli
- Extremely short attention to a stimulus before showing signs of agitation, such as color changes, rapid respirations, and agitated motor activity
- Deficient self-consoling abilities and poor response to comforting by care providers
- Difficulty in eating because of an ineffective suck

The preceding neurobehavioral abnormalities may partially correct but frequently lead to learning difficulties caused by attention deficits and behavioral problems, such as a flat, apathetic mood later in life (Rosenak and others, 1990).

Gastrointestinal dysfunction in the neonate may be seen as diarrhea or prolonged time between stools.

The risk of sudden infant death syndrome (SIDS) appears to be increased from 0.05% in the general population to 15% in the cocaine-exposed infant (ACOG, 1994; Durand and others, 1990).

Birth complications, such as meconium-stained amniotic fluid and fetal distress, are observed more frequently (ACOG, 1994; Burkett and others, 1990; Mastrogiannis and others, 1990).

Effect of Paternal Cocaine Use

If the male is exposed to cocaine before mating, the offspring has an increased risk of abnormalities. Research has demonstrated that cocaine binds to the human spermatozoa (Yazigi and others, 1991).

Screening

During the initial prenatal assessment, all pregnant women should be asked about cocaine use. About 80% of health care providers (Gillogley and others, 1990; Matera and others, 1990) screen prenatally for cocaine use if the history is positive, as shown by one of the following:

- No or inadequate prenatal care
- Inadequate prenatal weight gain
- Previous induced abortion
- Preterm labor
- Abruptio placentae
- History of substance abuse, such as cigarettes, alcohol, or cocaine
- A sexually transmitted disease diagnosed
- An inconsistent support system
- Chronic nasal congestion

Other health care providers recommend urine toxicology screening to be done on all pregnant women because drug use is missed significantly if one screens only those with an indicating history (Matera and others, 1990; McCalla and others, 1991).

ACOG (1994) states it may be desirable to do periodic screening on pregnant women who have admitted to prior cocaine use.

Toxicology urine screen detects cocaine use by the pregnant woman during the last week because of its slow metabolism during pregnancy. Meconium can be analyzed by radioimmunoassay (RIA) for drug metabolites (Rosengren and others, 1993), and analysis of hair is being used as well (Mason, Lee, 1995).

Treatment During Pregnancy

Be able to recognize the signs of possible cocaine use, such as sweatiness, tachycardia, flushed skin, tremulousness, irritability, difficulty sitting still, and being "high" or sleepy. Dispel myths, such as that recreational use is not harmful and cocaine will bring about a shorter, easier labor. Educate as to the harmful effects of cocaine since many feel it is harmless.

When it is determined that the pregnant woman is taking cocaine, she should be told the best thing to do is to stop immediately. Then provide supportive services so she can stop, such as drug rehabilitation programs that address women's needs, individual and family counseling, support groups such as Narcotics Anonymous, financial assistance, and home nurse visitation. A cocaine addict usually will resist treatment. Therefore the health care provider must persist in all avenues appropriate for the patient, such as patient support systems and multidisciplinary resources, in attempting to get her to admit that cocaine is harmful to her and her fetus and that she should stop using the drug.

Compose a list of available community and state resources. A helpful national treatment referral and information service resource is 1-800-COCAINE. This resource can give health care providers names of local perinatal cocaine treatment centers. This same number serves as a cocaine hotline that is available for a cocaine addict or family.

Assess for multiple risk factors, such as cigarette smoking, alcohol use, use of other drugs, and inadequate prenatal care.

Become familiar with the legislative issues related to drug testing, reporting drug use, and fetal rights for your state, and become involved, in cooperation with the risk management department of your institution, in policy development to legally manage the care of pregnant women who use cocaine.

Care of the laboring patient who has recently used cocaine should include close observations for signs of complications, oxygen by mask at 7 to 10 L/min to enhance fetal oxygenation, and notification of the intensive care nursery of a potential high risk neonate. Cocaine may induce fetal tachycardia and increase beat-to-beat variability (Lynch, McKeon, 1990). These patients experience labor pains as much as any other patient, and withholding pain medication is not beneficial. If epidural anesthesia is necessary, the nurse should monitor very closely for hypotension since it appears to occur more frequently in the cocaine-positive laboring woman (Birnbach and others, 1991).

If there is a chance that the mother will use cocaine after the birth of her infant, she should be counseled not to breast-feed since cocaine readily passes to the infant by way of breast milk (Lawrence, 1994).

HEROIN

Heroin is most commonly injected intravenously, referred to as "mainlining." Smoking or inhaling the drug is becoming more popular because of the fear of human immunodeficiency virus (HIV) from needles. The drug taken by any route is extremely addicting. Street names for this drug are *snow, stuff, junk, smack, horse,* and *joy powder.*

Maternal Complications

Infertility is common since heroin frequently inhibits ovulation. A woman usually becomes pregnant when heroin levels drop.

It is difficult to ascribe specific maternal effects to heroin since 75% of women who use heroin report using more than one drug (Little and others, 1990b). A pregnant heroin addict has a threefold to sevenfold increased risk of preterm labor (ACOG, 1994). Infections such as hepatitis, tuberculosis, and HIV are common complications of heroin because the route of administration is likely intravenous.

Fetal and Neonatal Complications

Fetal and neonatal complications of heroin use include the following:
- Preterm birth and prematurity (Lee, 1995)
- IUGR, which is compounded by maternal abuse of other substances and malnutrition (Little and others, 1990a)
- Appears to accelerate fetal lung maturity but increases the risk of meconium-stained amniotic fluid, and the risk of sudden infant death syndrome is higher (Kendig, 1996)
- Signs of withdrawal manifested by 60% to 80% of the infants exposed to prenatal heroin; withdrawal usually occurs within the first 24 to 72 hours but may be delayed up to 10 days of life (ACOG, 1994) (Box 25-1 gives signs of withdrawal.)
- Postnatal growth deficiency, mild developmental delays, and

---

Box 25-1

Signs of Drug Withdrawal

W   Wakefulness
I   Irritability
T   Tremulousness, Temperature variation, and Tachypnea
H   Hyperactivity and High-pitched or continuous cry
D   Diarrhea, Diaphoresis, and Disorganized suck
R   Rub marks, Restless sleeping, and Respiratory difficulty
A   Apneic attacks
W   Weight loss or failure to gain weight
A   Alkalosis (respiratory)
L   Lacrimation (runny eye syndrome)

Modified from American Academy of Pediatrics Committee on Drugs: Neonatal drug withdrawal, *Pediatrics* 72(6):895-902, 1983; Torrence C, Horns K: *Neonatal Network* 8(3):49-59, 1989.

---

behavior problems observed in follow-up studies of children exposed to perinatal heroin; however, these problems are felt to be more related to poor maternal nutrition and inappropriate postnatal environment than to the direct effect of the perinatal heroin (Robins, Mills, 1993)

Treatment During Pregnancy

Sudden withdrawal from heroin can be harmful and is not recommended during pregnancy because of heroin's high physical and psychologic addictive properties. Methadone treatment is frequently used to get the pregnant mother off heroin. Because methadone can cause detrimental fetal effects and neonatal withdrawal, a pregnant woman should be withdrawn from heroin with a small dose of methadone to control symptoms of withdrawal before delivery (Mason, Lee, 1995).

MARIJUANA

Street names for marijuana are *grass, pot, joint, reefer,* and *weed.*

Incidence

It is estimated that approximately 20% to 30% of pregnant women are using marijuana (MacGregor and others, 1990). It is the most commonly used illicit drug among childbearing women (Day, Richardson, 1991).

Pathophysiologic Effects

One of the active ingredients of marijuana is delta-9-tetrahydrocannabinol, which crosses the placenta and is fat soluble. Therefore it may take 30 days for the drug to be excreted from the fetal body (Mason, Lee, 1995).

Marijuana interferes with the production of follicle-stimulating hormone, luteinizing hormone, and prolactin, thereby inhibiting ovulation.

Marijuana increases the carbon monoxide levels in blood five times more than tobacco smoke and therefore decreases fetal oxygenation.

Maternal Complications

Marijuana can cause infertility problems, especially in the male.

Marijuana does not cause physical addiction, but it can cause psychologic addiction.

Marijuana smoke contains more cancer-causing properties than tobacco smoke. One joint affects the lungs as much as smoking 16 cigarettes (Wu and others, 1988).

Fetal Complications

Little is still known about the effects of marijuana on the development and well-being of the fetus. Research results are equivocal as to its effect on fetal growth, neurobehavioral activities, and length of gestation (Day, Richardson, 1991). In a very controlled study of Jamaican women, insignificant problems were noted (Hayes and others, 1988). However, marijuana is not harmless since smoking marijuana has similar effects to smoking tobacco (Wu and others, 1988). A dose-related risk of IUGR has been reported, but it is not known whether it is directly related to marijuana or to malnutrition and other substances the woman may be using (Robins, Mills, 1993). Maternal marijuana use appears to have no teratogenic effect (Cyr, Moulton, 1990). However, significantly lower scores in childhood verbal and memory abilities have been associated with maternal marijuana use (Fried, Watkinson, 1990). The neonate is at more risk for jitteriness, which can lead to an infant who is difficult to console when crying and therefore can impact parent-infant attachment (Parker and others, 1990).

Screening

Many marijuana users, as well as substance users of most illegal drugs, will go undetected if a drug toxicity screen is not done on all pregnant patients. A commonly used toxicity urine screen is the enzyme multiplied immunoassay. It is effective in detecting marijuana use for the past 3 to 30 days (Mason, Lee, 1995).

Meconium is a useful sample for drug screening in newborns (Maynard and others, 1991).

Treatment During Pregnancy

Because no drug has been proven safe for the unborn child, neither has marijuana. Therefore a woman should be encouraged to stop its use. She should be closely evaluated for the use of other substances as well.

TOBACCO
Incidence

Approximately 20% to 30% of all pregnant women smoke (ACOG, 1993; USDHHS NIDA Center for Substance Abuse Research, 1994).

Pathophysiologic Effects

A cigarette contains more than 2500 poisonous compounds (ACOG, 1993). One of them, carbon monoxide, readily crosses the placenta and decreases the oxygen-carrying capacity of the hemoglobin. Nicotine, another substance, stimulates adrenergic release, which causes generalized vasoconstriction, leading to decreased uterine perfusion and narrowing of the umbilical arteries. Compensatory signs are manifested, such as increased maternal and fetal heart rate and decreased fetal movement. Another harmful compound is cadmium, which interferes with placental transfer of zinc (Bottoms, 1996).

Research indicates that smokers have a poorer diet than nonsmokers (Bottoms, 1996; Haste and others, 1990). Cigarette smoking also interferes with the assimilation of various essential vitamins and minerals, resulting in an increased loss of calcium caused by mobilization from bones, decreased intestinal synthesis of vitamin B_{12}, and increased usage of vitamin C (Institute of Medicine, 1990).

Maternal Complications

The risk of the following complications is increased in the pregnant woman who smokes:

- Infertility related to ovulatory dysfunction and alteration in sperm (ACOG, 1993)

- Ectopic pregnancy related to altered tubal motility (ACOG, 1993)
- Spontaneous abortion (Brown, 1996; Lambers, Clark, 1996)
- Placenta previa (Andres, 1996)
- Abruptio placentae (Andres, 1996)
- Premature rupture of membranes (Andres, 1996)
- Preterm delivery (Brown, 1996; Lambers, Clark, 1996; Wisborg and others, 1996)

Fetal and Neonatal Complications

The risk of the following complications is increased in the fetus, neonate, and infant when exposed to cigarette smoke.

Low birth weight (175 to 300 g smaller) is a consistently documented effect of smoking (Brown, 1996; Walsh, 1994). The severity of low birth weight is in direct proportion to the number of cigarettes smoked per day or the amount of exposure to passive ("side stream") smoke (Lambers, Clark, 1996; Vik and others, 1996). Perinatal and neonatal mortality is increased 33% when the fetus is exposed to cigarette smoke (Walsh, 1994). This is associated with an increased risk of prematurity (Economides, Braithwaite, 1994).

Research has been inconsistent in showing an increased teratogenic effect of cigarette smoking. However, according to Li and others (1996), there appears to be a causal association between maternal smoking and the risk of congenital urinary tract anomalies.

An increased risk of childhood cancer related to prenatal exposure to cigarette smoking is inconsistent (Floyd and others, 1991).

Lower IQ and behavioral abnormalities such as attention deficit hyperactivity disorder (ADHD) that result in later learning difficulties have been observed in follow-up studies (Lambers, Clark, 1996; Milberger and others, 1996).

Smoking can reduce breast milk and expose the infant to its harmful compounds since they pass freely into breast milk (Lambers, Clark, 1996).

Children of mothers who smoke run a twofold risk of developing asthma. Prenatal exposure to cigarette smoke is as great, if not greater, an influence on the later development of asthma (Barber and others, 1996; Stick and others, 1996).

Postnatal exposure to passive smoke can increase the infant's risk of SIDS (Floyd and others, 1991; Haglund, Chattingius, 1990) and childhood respiratory illnesses such as pneumonia, bronchitis, and inner ear infections (Floyd and others, 1991; Taylor, 1990).

Treatment During Pregnancy

The goal of treatment for smokers during pregnancy is to get all pregnant women and those around them to stop smoking. Quitting before 16 weeks significantly decreases the adverse risks (Li and others, 1993). This is very challenging, and the counseling must be individualized. According to Devonport (1996), health professionals must motivate their patients to choose to stop smoking and then empower them to be successful. Some guidelines are provided in the following list:

1. Set the right example as a health care provider by not smoking or at least not smoking in the presence of patients. Make the health care facility a smoke-free environment.

2. Assess the woman's smoking habits on the initial prenatal visit. Determine in a nonthreatening manner whether the woman smokes, how long she has smoked, approximately how many cigarettes she smokes daily, and for what reasons (O'Campo and others, 1995).

3. Improve disclosure by using multiple-choice questions, such as "Choose the answer that best describes your pattern of cigarette smoking": "I smoke regularly now—about the same amount as before I was pregnant"; "I smoke regularly now but I have cut down since finding out I was pregnant"; "I quit after finding out I was pregnant"; or "I do not currently smoke and was not smoking at the time I got pregnant" (Mullen and others, 1991).

4. Determine the woman's reasons for smoking by using, for example, a self-test for smokers produced by the U.S. Department of Health and Human Services, no. (CDC) 75-8716.

5. Present a clear, brief message on the need to quit, keeping it positive and nonjudgmental. Relate the effects of smoking to the fetus; for example, during an ultrasound or when taking the FHR have the mother smoke so she can see the direct effects. This has been shown to increase one's motivation to want to stop (Li and others, 1993). Include personal health benefits in the counseling as well.

6. Assess the woman's motivation to quit.

7. Emphasize how to quit smoking by tailoring it to the woman personally as to her reasons for smoking.

8. If the woman verbalizes a desire to quit, together develop a quitting plan tailored to her needs. Include ways to change smoking behaviors, social and family support, a referral to an appropriate cessation program, appropriate self-help educational materials (Table 25-3), and a follow-up mechanism that provides ongoing encouragement.

9. If the woman is reluctant to quit, assess her reasons. For example, she may be afraid of gaining too much weight, fear withdrawal symptoms, need smoking as a psychologic support, believe it really will not hurt her baby because it did not hurt someone else's baby, believe smoking cannot be harmful since her health care provider smokes, or have tried and failed in the past.

10. If the woman chooses to keep smoking, encourage her to reduce the amount she smokes since the fetal effects are dose related (Li and others, 1993) and counsel her to increase her intake of calcium, vitamins B_{12} and C, and folic acid to compensate for the smoking-induced loss of these vitamins and minerals.

11. Also, give family members a clear, brief message on the need to quit or at least never smoke in the presence of the expectant mother or young child since passive smoke is harmful prenatally as well as postnatally (Lambers, Clark, 1996).

12. Take an active part in legislative and legal strategies to reduce cigarette smoking, such as increasing cigarette taxes, banning cigarette advertisement, or enforcing provisions to make public places smoke free. Short-term use of nicotine gum or the patch delivers less nicotine than usual cigarette smoking and can be used if other methods fail (Oncken and others, 1996).

NURSING PROCESS

NURSING DIAGNOSES AND INTERVENTIONS

- **ALTERED HEALTH MAINTENANCE** related to lack of knowledge and life situations and stressors.

  DESIRED OUTCOME: The woman will stop abusing any substance during pregnancy and lactation or if she continues to use them will reduce the amount consumed.

  INTERVENTIONS

  1. Nurse practitioners and nurses should be actively involved in accurate, timely education programs that teach about the

TABLE 25-3 Self-help educational materials to stop smoking

Titles	Resource
Smart Move! (stop-smoking guide)	American Cancer Society
Fresh Start (group guide)	1599 Clifton Road NE
Quitter's Guide: 7 Day Plan to Help You Stop Smoking Cigarettes	Atlanta, GA 30329
	1-800-227-2345 or call local chapter
Special Delivery: Smoke Free (stop-smoking book)	
Calling It Quits	American Heart Association
	7320 Greenville Ave
	Dallas, TX 75231
	214-373-6300 or call local chapter
Freedom from Smoking: For You and Your Baby (10 day quit-smoking program for pregnant women)	American Lung Association
	1740 Broadway
	New York, NY 10017
	212-315-8700 or call local chapter
Quit Kit	
A Healthy Beginning: the Smoke-Free Family Guide for New Parents (kit)	
Nurses: Help Your Patients Stop Smoking (pub. no. 92-2962)	National Heart, Lung and Blood Institute
	4733 Bethesda Ave, Suite 530
	Bethesda, MD 20814
	301-951-3260
How to Help Your Patient Stop Smoking: Physician's Manual (pub. no. 95-3064)	National Cancer Institute
	Building 31
	Room 10A24
	Bethesda, MD 20892
	1-800-4 CANCER
12-Step Program	Nicotine Anonymous World Service: 1-415-750-0328 or call the local chapter
Breathe Free Plan Clinic	Seventh-day Adventists: call the local church
Group clinic and audiocassette	SmokEnders: 1-800-828-HELP

effects of practicing substance abuse on one's personal health and the potential teratogenic effects on the growing fetus. These programs should be available in grade school, in high school, during contraceptive counseling, and on gynecologic visits.

2. Develop and consistently use a self-administered, matter-of-fact, nonjudgmental questionnaire to obtain a substance abuse assessment on the first prenatal visit.

3. Assess for barriers such as peer pressure, socioeconomic status, psychologic stress, or other environmental factors.

4. Analyze the responses for potential risk.

5. In a positive, nonjudgmental manner motivate the child-bearing woman-to-be or childbearing woman to want to make life-style changes to improve health-related behavior by providing her with information about health risks and the effects of substance abuse on her fetus.

6. Consistently assess for risk factors indicative of substance abuse, such as the following (Mason, Lee, 1995):
   a. Noncompliance
   b. Inadequate support system, especially an unsupportive father of the baby
   c. History of abuse by spouse
   d. History of sporadic employment
   e. Inadequate housing
   f. History of poor parenting by her own mother or father, psychiatric illness, or physical or sexual abuse
   g. Involvement with the legal system
   h. Lack of self-esteem with feelings of insecurity
   i. Abnormal affect, such as lethargy or agitation

7. Assess the family's need for detoxification and, if so, determine whether outpatient, inpatient, or family treatment would be most effective.

8. Negotiate a plan with the patient.

9. Provide supportive counseling to aid the patient in making changes and help her to build self-esteem and overcome feelings of inadequacy. Avoid using threatening statements that make her feel like a bad mother for practicing substance abuse. If possible, have the patient commit to an appropriate, workable treatment plan for her (Kaufman, 1996).

10. Make appropriate community referrals to resources that enable implementation, such as exercise, counseling, and

other methods of stress reduction as well as supportive group referrals.

11. If efforts fail in total abstinence, provide a message of potential benefits from reduction.

12. Become active in legislative issues to block punitive legislation dealing with childbearing women practicing substance abuse since this will drive women away and interfere with their seeking help when they need it the most (Starn and others, 1993).

- **ALTERED NUTRITION: LESS THAN BODY REQUIREMENTS** related to the appetite suppressant effect of substance abuse.

  DESIRED OUTCOME: The patient will follow a nutritionally sound pregnancy diet and gain adequate prenatal weight.

  INTERVENTIONS

  1. Assess dietary intake.
  2. Determine pregnancy weight, and compare with height and gestational age.
  3. Counsel about benefits of adequate nutrition for fetal well-being and one's own health and well-being.
  4. Use effective teaching strategies to teach an appropriate prenatal diet.
  5. Make appropriate referral to WIC (women, infants, and children) program if finances make it difficult for the patient to obtain nutritious foods.
  6. Implement a follow-up program by setting realistic goals with the patient and closely monitoring her progress. Provide encouragement if she reaches her goals, and provide more counseling if she is unable to reach her goals.

- **INEFFECTIVE INDIVIDUAL COPING** related to lack of a support system, low self-esteem, and personal abuse.

  DESIRED OUTCOMES: The woman will voluntarily become involved in a drug therapy program and seek appropriate counseling.

  INTERVENTIONS

  1. Make appropriate referrals to self-help groups such as the following:
     a. Alcoholics Anonymous
     b. Women for Sobriety
     c. Al-Anon for the family of an alcoholic
     d. A stop-smoking clinic

      e. Cocaine hotline: 1-800-COCAINE

      f. Narcotics Anonymous

      g. Local clinics dealing specifically with pregnant substance abusers

  2. Provide ongoing encouragement and support

■ **RISK FOR IMPAIRED FETAL GAS EXCHANGE** related to decreased placental blood flow caused by substance abuse.

  DESIRED OUTCOMES: The fetus will remain active, and its heart rate will remain between 110 and 160 beats/min. The biophysical profile will continue to be more than 6 with a negative contraction stress test (CST) and a reactive nonstress test (NST).

  INTERVENTIONS

    1. Monitor FHR manually or electronically as indicated.

    2. Carry out NST or CST as ordered.

    3. Explain any ordered test such as a biophysical profile or CST.

    4. Emphasize the importance of consistent prenatal care.

    5. Notify physician if FHR drops from baseline or patient reports decreased fetal movement.

■ **RISK FOR FETAL/INFANT INJURY** related to the teratogenic effect of substance abuse and malnutrition.

  DESIRED OUTCOMES: The fetus or infant will show a continuous normal growth pattern without structural defects. The infant will not experience respiratory distress.

  INTERVENTIONS

    1. Assess uterine growth and fundal height each prenatal visit.

    2. Assess fetal growth and structural development with ultrasound examinations.

    3. Carry out a toxicology drug screen as indicated.

    4. Provide counseling regarding possible adverse fetal outcome from practicing substance abuse.

    5. Mothers who use drugs may benefit from cardiopulmonary resuscitation (CPR) training since their infants are at increased risk for SIDS.

CONCLUSION

Health care providers have a unique opportunity to help prevent birth defects by providing education about the effects of substance abuse on the fetus and by early identification of childbearing women who are abusing substances such as alcohol, cigarettes, and illicit drugs. Women who practice substance abuse are at greater risk of spontaneous abortion, preterm labor, low birth weight infants, and abruptio placentae (Robins, Mills, 1993).

Nurses who provide health care to childbearing families can participate in primary prevention by conducting education programs and consistently providing ongoing education about the risks of practicing substance abuse. Nurses should also be involved in secondary prevention, which includes early diagnosis and appropriate intervention if the problem exists. Obtaining an accurate assessment can be exceptionally complex related to the varying symptoms manifested and the need of the patient to conceal her habit. Planning appropriate nursing care is very challenging for these patients.

BIBLIOGRAPHY
Alcohol

American College of Obstetricians and Gynecologists (ACOG): Substance abuse in pregnancy, *ACOG Techn Bull,* no. 195, 1994.

Armant D, Saunders D: Exposure of embryonic cells to alcohol: contrasting effects during preimplantation and postimplantation development, *Semin Perinatol* 20(2):127-139, 1996.

Barbour B: Alcohol and pregnancy, *J Nurse Midwifery* 35(2):78-85, 1990.

Blessed W and others: The prenatal effects of alcohol. In Studd J, editor: *Progress in obstetrics and gynaecology,* vol 11, London, 1994, Churchill Livingstone.

Ewing J: Detecting alcoholism: the CAGE questionnaire, *JAMA* 252:1905-1907, 1984.

Grodstein F, Goldman M, Cramer D: Infertility in women and moderate alcohol use, *Am J Public Health* 84:1429, 1994.

Hankin J, Sokol R: Identification and care of problems associated with alcohol ingestion in pregnancy, *Semin Perinatol* 19(4):286-292, 1995.

Institute of Medicine, Food and Nutrition Board, Subcommittee on Nutritional Status and Weight Gain During Pregnancy: *Nutrition during pregnancy: weight gain,* Washington, DC, 1990, National Academy Press.

Jannke S: When the mother-to-be drinks, *Childbirth Instructor Magazine* 4(1):28-31, 1994.

Mason E, Lee R: Drug abuse. In Barron W, Lindheimer M: *Medical disorders during pregnancy,* ed 2, St Louis, 1995, Mosby.

Mennella J, Beauchamp G: The transfer of alcohol to human milk: effects on flavor and the infant's behavior, *N Engl J Med* 325(14):981-985, 1991.

Mullen P, Carbonari J, Glenday M: Identifying pregnant women who drink alcoholic beverages, *Am J Obstet Gynecol* 165:1429-1430, 1991.

Pietrantoni M, Knuppel R: Alcohol use in pregnancy, *Clin Perinatol* 18(1):93-111, 1991.

Rosett H, Weiner L, Edelin K: Strategies for prevention of fetal alcohol effects, *Obstet Gynecol* 57:1-7, 1981.

Sodol R and others: The T-ACE questions: practical prenatal detection of risk drinking, *Am J Obstet Gynecol* 163:864-875, 1990.

Sokol R, Martier S: Alcohol. In Queenan J, Hobbins J, editors: *Protocols for high-risk pregnancies,* ed 3, Cambridge, Mass, 1996, Blackwell Science.

Wardlaw G, Insel P, Seyler M: *Contemporary nutrition: issues and insights,* ed 2, St Louis, 1997, Mosby.

Weiner L, Rosett H, Mason E: Training professionals to identify and treat pregnant women who drink heavily, *Alcohol Health Res World* 10(1):32, 1985.

Worthington-Roberts B, Williams S: *Nutrition in pregnancy and lactation,* ed. 6, Madison, Wis, 1997, Brown & Benchmark.

Amphetamines

American College of Obstetricians and Gynecologists (ACOG): Substance abuse in pregnancy, *ACOG Techn Bull,* no. 195, 1994.

Evans A: Perinatal substance abuse. In Niswander K, Evans A, editors: *Manual of obstetrics,* ed 5, Boston, 1995, Little, Brown.

Cocaine

American College of Obstetricians and Gynecologists (ACOG): Substance abuse in pregnancy, *ACOG Techn Bull,* no. 195, 1994.

Birnbach D and others: The effect of cocaine on epidural anesthesia, *Am J Obstet Gynecol* 164(1, pt 2):400, 1991.

Buehler B, Conover B, Andres R: Teratogenic potential of cocaine, *Semin Perinatol* 20(2):93-98, 1996.

Burkett G, Yasin S, Palow D: Perinatal implications of cocaine exposure, *J Reprod Med* 35(1):35-42, 1990.

Chao C: Cardiovascular effects of cocaine during pregnancy, *Semin Perinatol* 20(2):107-114, 1996.

Chasnoff I: Cocaine and pregnancy: clinical and methodologic issues, *Clin Perinatol* 18(1):113-123, 1991.

Chasnoff I and others: Temporal patterns of cocaine use in pregnancy: perinatal outcome, *JAMA* 261:1741-1744, 1989.

Chazotte C, Youchah J, Freda M: Cocaine use during pregnancy and low birth weight: the impact of prenatal care and drug treatment, *Semin Perinatol* 19(4):293-300, 1995.

Cherukuri R and others: A cohort study of alkaloidal cocaine ("crack") in pregnancy, *Obstet Gynecol* 72(2):147-151, 1988.

Dolkart L, Plessinger M, Woods J: Effect of alpha receptor blockade upon maternal and fetal cardiovascular responses to cocaine, *Obstet Gynecol* 75:745, 1990.

Dombrowski M, Sokol R: Cocaine and abruption, *Contemp OB/GYN* 35(4):13-19, 1990.

Durand D, Espinoza A, Nickerson B: Association between prenatal cocaine exposure and sudden infant death syndrome, *J Pediatr* 117:909-911, 1990.

Gillogley K and others: The perinatal impact of cocaine, amphetamine, and opiate use detected by universal intrapartum screening, *Am J Obstet Gynecol* 163:1535-1542, 1990.

Heier L and others: Maternal cocaine abuse: the spectrum of radiologic abnormalities in the neonatal CNS, *Am J Neuroradiol* 12:951-956, 1991.

Hoskins I and others: Relationship between antepartum cocaine abuse, abnormal umbilical artery Doppler velocimetry, and placental abruption, *Obstet Gynecol* 78(2):279-282, 1991.

Hurd W and others: Cocaine directly augments the α-adrenergic contractile response of the pregnant rabbit uterus, *Am J Obstet Gynecol* 164:182-187, 1991.

Jones K: Developmental pathogenesis of defects associated with prenatal cocaine exposure: fetal vascular disruption, *Clin Perinatol* 18(1): 139-145, 1991.

Landry S, Whitney J: The impact of prenatal cocaine exposure: studies of the developing infant, *Semin Perinatol* 20(2):99-106, 1996.

Lawrence R: *Breastfeeding: a guide for the medical profession,* ed 4, St Louis, 1994, Mosby.

Lindenberg C and others: A review of the literature on cocaine abuse in pregnancy, *Nurs Res* 40(2):69-75, 1991.

Lynch M, McKeon V: Cocaine use during pregnancy: research findings and clinical implications, *J Obstet Gynecol Neonatal Nurs* 19(4):285-292, 1990.

Mason E, Lee R: Drug abuse. In Barron W, Lindheimer M: *Medical disorders during pregnancy,* ed 2, St Louis, 1995, Mosby.

Mastrogiannis D and others: Perinatal outcome after recent cocaine usage, *Obstet Gynecol* 76:8-11, 1990.

Matera C and others: Prevalence of use of cocaine and other substances in an obstetric population, *Am J Obstet Gynecol* 163:797-801, 1990.

McCalla S and others: The biologic and social consequences of perinatal cocaine use in an inner-city population: results of an anonymous cross-sectional study, *Am J Obstet Gynecol* 164:625-630, 1991.

Mercado A and others: Cocaine, pregnancy and postpartum intracerebral hemorrhage, *Obstet Gynecol* 73:467-468, 1989.

Monga M: The effect of cocaine on myometrial contractile activity: basic mechanisms, *Semin Perinatol* 20(2):140-146, 1996.

Peters H, Theorell C: Fetal and neonatal effects of maternal cocaine use, *J Obstet Gynecol Neonatal Nurs* 20(2):122-126, 1991.

Rosenak D and others: Cocaine: maternal use during pregnancy and its effect on the mother, the fetus, and the infant, *Obstet Gynecol Surv* 45(6):348-359, 1990.

Rosengren S and others: Meconium testing for cocaine metabolite: prevalence, perceptions, and pitfalls, *Am J Obstet Gynecol* 168:1449-1456, 1993.

Smith Y and others: Decrease in myometrial beta-adrenergic receptors with prenatal cocaine use, *Obstet Gynecol* 85:357-360, 1995.

Spence M and others: The relationship between recent cocaine use and pregnancy outcome, *Obstet Gynecol* 78:326-329, 1991.

Woods J, Plessinger M: Pregnancy increases cardiovascular toxicity to cocaine, *Am J Obstet Gynecol* 162:529-533, 1990.

Yazigi R, Odem R, Polakoski K: Demonstration of specific binding of cocaine to human spermatozoa, *JAMA* 266:1956-1959, 1991.

Heroin

American College of Obstetricians and Gynecologists (ACOG): *Substance abuse in pregnancy, ACOG Techn Bull,* no. 195, 1994.

Kendig S: Substance abuse in pregnancy, *Childbirth Instructor Magazine* 6(3):18-24, 1996.

Lee R: Drug abuse. In Burrow G, Ferris T, editors: *Medical complications during pregnancy,* ed 4, Philadelphia, 1995, Saunders.

Little B and others: Maternal and fetal effects of heroin addiction during pregnancy, *J Reprod Med* 35(2):159-162, 1990a.

Little B and others: Patterns of multiple substance abuse during pregnancy: implications for mother and fetus, *South Med J* 83(5):507-509, 1990b.

Mason E, Lee R: Drug abuse. In Barron W, Lindheimer M: *Medical disorders during pregnancy,* ed 2, St Louis, 1995, Mosby.

Robins L, Mills J: Effects of in utero exposure to street drugs, *Am J Public Health* 83(suppl 32), 1993.

Nursing Interventions

Kaufman E: Diagnosis and treatment of drug and alcohol abuse in women, *Am J Obstet Gynecol* 174:21-27, 1996.

Mason E, Lee R: Drug abuse. In Barron W, Lindheimer M: *Medical disorders during pregnancy,* ed 2, St Louis, 1995, Mosby.

Robins L, Mills J: Effects of in utero exposure to street drugs, *Am J Public Health* 83(suppl 32), 1993.

Starn J and others: Can we encourage pregnant substance abusers to seek prenatal care? *MCN Am J Matern Child Nurs* 18:147-152, 1993.

Marijuana

Cyr M, Moulton A: Substance abuse in women, *Obstet Gynecol Clin North Am* 17(4):905-925, 1990.

Day N, Richardson G: Prenatal marijuana use: epidemiology, methodologic issues, and infant outcome, *Clin Perinatol* 18(1):77-91, 1991.

Fried P, Watkinson B: 36- to 46-month neurobehavioral follow-up of children prenatally exposed to marijuana, cigarettes, and alcohol, *J Dev Behav Pediatr* 11(2):49-58, 1990.

Hayes J, Dreher M, Nugent J: Newborn outcomes with maternal marijuana use in Jamaican women, *Pediatr Nurs* 14(2):107-110, 1988.

MacGregor S and others: Prevalence of marijuana use during pregnancy: a pilot study, *J Reprod Med* 35(12):1147-1149, 1990.

Mason E, Lee R: Drug abuse. In Barron W, Lindheimer M: *Medical disorders during pregnancy,* ed 2, St Louis, 1995, Mosby.

Maynard E, Amoruso L, Oh W: Meconium for drug testing, *Am J Dis Child* 145(6):650-652, 1991.

Parker S and others: Jitteriness in full-term neonates: prevalence and correlates, *Pediatrics* 85(1):17-23, 1990.

Robins L, Mills J: Effects of in utero exposure to street drugs, *Am J Public Health* 83(suppl 32), 1993.

Wu T and others: Pulmonary hazards of smoking marijuana as compared with tobacco, *N Engl J Med* 318:347-351, 1988.

Zuckerman B and others: Effects of maternal marijuana and cocaine use on fetal growth, *N Engl J Med* 320:762-768, 1989.

Smoking

American College of Obstetricians and Gynecologists (ACOG): Smoking and reproductive health, *ACOG Techn Bull,* no. 180, 1993.

Andres R: The association of cigarette smoking with placenta previa and abruptio placentae, *Semin Perinatol* 20(2):154-159, 1996.

Barber K, Mussin E, Taylor D: Fetal exposure to involuntary maternal smoking and childhood respiratory disease, *Ann Allergy Asthma Immunol* 76(5):427-430, 1996.

Bottoms S: Smoking. In Queenan J, Hobbins J, editors: *Protocols of high risk pregnancies,* ed 3, Cambridge, Mass, 1996, Blackwell Science.

Brown D: Smoking cessation in pregnancy, *Can Fam Physician* 42(1):102-105, 1996.

Centers for Disease Control and Prevention (CDC): Cigarette smoking among reproductive-aged women. U.S. Department of Health and Human Services, Public Health Service, *MMWR Morb Mortal Wkly Rep* 40:719-723, 1991.

Devonport C: Support for pregnant women who wish to stop smoking, *Nurs Times* 92(10):36-37, 1996.

Economides D, Braithwaite J: Smoking, pregnancy and the fetus, *J R Soc Health* 114:198-201, 1994.

Floyd R and others: Smoking during pregnancy: prevalence, effects, and intervention strategies, *Birth* 18(1):48-53, 1991.

Haglund B, Chattingius S: Cigarette smoking as a risk factor for sudden infant death syndrome: a population based study, *Am J Public Health* 80:29-32, 1990.

Haste F and others: Nutrient intakes during pregnancy: observations on the influence of smoking and social class, *Am J Clin Nutr* 51:29-36, 1990.

Institute of Medicine, Food and Nutrition Board, Subcommittee on Nutritional Status and Weight Gain During Pregnancy: *Nutrition during pregnancy: weight gain,* Washington, DC, 1990, National Academy Press.

Lambers D, Clark K: The maternal and fetal physiologic effects of nicotine, *Semin Perinatol* 20(2):115-126, 1996.

Li C and others: The impact on infant birth weight and gestational age of continue-validated smoking reduction during pregnancy, *JAMA* 269: 1519-1524, 1993.

Li D and others: Maternal smoking during pregnancy and the risk of congenital urinary tract anomalies, *Am J Public Health* 86:249-253, 1996.

Milberger S and others: Is maternal smoking during pregnancy a risk factor for attention deficit hyperactivity disorder in children? *Am J Psychol* 153: 1138-1142, 1996.

Mullen P and others: Improving disclosure of smoking by pregnant women, *Am J Obstet Gynecol* 165:409-413, 1991.

O'Campo P, Davis M, Gielen A: Smoking cessation interventions for pregnant women: review and future directions, *Semin Perinatol* 19(4):279-285, 1995.

Oncken C and others: Effects of short-term use of nicotine gum in pregnant smokers, *Clin Pharmacol Ther* 59(6):654-661, 1996.

Robins L, Mills J: Effects of in utero exposure to street drugs, *Am J Public Health* 83(suppl 32), 1993.

Stick S and others: Effects of maternal smoking during pregnancy and a family history of asthma on respiratory function in newborn infants, *Lancet* 348(9034):1060-1064, 1996.

Taylor B: Prevention of pediatric pulmonary problems: the importance of maternal smoking, *Lung* 168(suppl):327-332, 1990.

USDHHS NIDA Center for Substance Abuse Research: Press briefing, Sept. 12, 1994.

Vik T and others: Pre- and post-natal growth in children of women who smoked in pregnancy, *Early Hum Dev* 45(3):245-255, 1996.

Walsh R: Effects of maternal smoking on adverse pregnancy outcomes: examination of the criteria of causation, *Hum Biol* 66:1059-1092, 1994.

Wisborg K and others: Smoking during pregnancy and preterm birth, *Br J Obstet Gynaecol* 103(8):800-805, 1996.

U N I T

VII

Alterations in the Mechanism of Labor

Successful termination of pregnancy heralded by labor requires the harmonious interplay of the uterus, placenta, fetus, and pelvis. Disruptions can result if labor is not stimulated on time, the uterus contracts ineffectively, the fetus is larger than the pelvis, or the fetus is in a presentation that makes it impossible to accommodate to the pelvis. When a disruption in the mechanism of labor develops, early detection, active medical management, and nursing interventions are important to facilitate the best maternal and fetal outcome. A variety of nursing measures to facilitate progress in labor, if employed, can significantly reduce the need for obstetric and surgical interventions.

26

Labor Stimulation

Induction of labor is any attempt to initiate uterine contractions before their spontaneous onset to facilitate a vaginal delivery. Augmentation of labor is any attempt to stimulate uterine contractions during the course of labor to facilitate a vaginal delivery. It is frequently used for certain types of uterine dysfunction. A labor should not be augmented until noninvasive interventions have been tried, such as the following:

- Making sure the bladder is empty
- Encouraging ambulation if possible or changing positions
- Allaying anxiety, since epinephrine decreases uterine efficiency
- Making sure the patient is properly nourished and hydrated

Labor stimulant methods considered in this chapter are pharmacologic means, including oxytocin and prostaglandins; physiologic means, including breast stimulation, amniotomy, and stripping of fetal membranes; and dilators and mechanical means, including natural and synthetic dilators.

INCIDENCE

Use of a labor stimulant for either inducing or augmenting labor varies among countries, cities, and hospitals. According to the National Center for Health Statistics, approximately 27% of all labors in the United States are stimulated (Ventura and others, 1995).

CRITERIA

Criteria for an induction of labor are listed below:
- An engaged presenting part
- No previous classical uterine incision
- No fetopelvic disproportion
- No nonreassuring fetal heart rate (FHR) patterns
- No major bleeding from an abruptio placentae
- No placenta previa

Cervical ripening, induction of labor, and augmentation of labor are considered safe for the vaginal birth after previous cesarean (VBAC) if no other contraindication is present (Chez, 1995).

Criteria for augmentation of labor are the same as for an induction. There should also be definite signs that the progress of labor is slowing down.

Labor is seldom induced or augmented (1) on a grand multipara more than five parity, (2) on a multiple pregnancy, or (3) in the presence of polyhydramnios because of the increased risk of uterine rupture related to uterine overdistention.

The success of the induction or augmentation usually depends on a ripe cervix. A cervix is considered ripe when it is soft, anterior, effaced more than 50%, and dilated 2 cm or more. Bishop (1964) developed a 13-point scoring system to predict the responsiveness of a patient to an induction. He found that an induction is usually successful when the pelvic score totals 9 or more for a nullipara or 5 or more for a multipara (Table 26-1).

A newly developed test to determine the presence of fetal fibronectin is being examined for use in determining successful induction. Blanch and others (1996) compared Bishop scores of term

TABLE 26-1 Bishop prelabor scoring system

	Score			
	0	**1**	**2**	**3**
Dilation (cm)	0	1-2	3-4	5-6
Effacement (%)	0-30	40-50	60-70	80
Station	−3	−2	−1/0	+1/+2
Consistency of cervix	Firm	Medium	Soft	
Cervical position	Posterior	Median	Anterior	

Reprinted with permission from the American College of Obstetricians and Gynecologists (*Obstet Gynecol* 24:266, 1964).

patients with the presence of fetal fibronectin with those in which it was absent. They discovered that the presence of fetal fibronectin positively correlated to the changes in the cervix and vaginal secretions that occur close to the onset of labor. They concluded that fetal fibronectin values may provide a quantitative predictor of labor. They may have a place in determining readiness for induction in the near future. However, at present the Bishop cervical scoring system remains the standard used for predicting inducibility (Fuentes, Williams, 1995).

PHYSIOLOGY OF UTEROTROPINS AND UTEROTONINS

Many substances interplay to prepare for and promote labor. Prostaglandins are formed enzymatically from phospholipids and arachidonic acid in most tissues of the body. They act as a local hormone by exerting their action primarily at the site of production. The biosynthesis of reproductive tissue prostaglandins varies among tissue. The myometrium is the primary source of prostacyclin ($PGI_2$2 (PGE_2); and the decidua is the primary source of prostaglandin $F_{2\alpha}$ ($PGF_{2\alpha}$).

During pregnancy, PGI_2 facilitates a quiet uterus by inhibiting the formation of gap junctions and the release of phospholipase A and it blocks calcium movement into cells. Progesterone further regulates the myometrial activity throughout pregnancy by inhibiting the formation of oxytocin receptors and gap junctions (Huszar, Walsh, 1991). Estrogen promotes this process.

During the prelabor phase or preparation phase just before true labor, production of PGE_2 by the amnion increases; this increase is normally induced by the fetus (Casey, MacDonald, 1988). During this phase the body is prepared for labor by the following occurrences:

1. Decreasing myometrial receptors for both progesterone and estrogen (Goff, 1993)
2. Softening and ripening of the cervix caused by enzymatic rearrangement of the collagen fibers into smaller, more flexible fibers and increasing synthesis of hyaluronic acid, thereby facilitating water absorption by the cervix (Leppert, 1995); leads to a softer, more stretchable cervix
3. Increasing elastin in the cervix, which gives the cervix its ability to recoil and regain its shape after birth
4. Increasing the frequency of Braxton Hicks contractions
5. Developing gap junctions in the myometrium that are cell-to-cell contact areas to coordinated myometrium contractions

6. Increasing the number of oxytocin receptors in the myometrium

As true labor is initiated, $PGF_{2\alpha}$ production increases significantly by the decidua, which continues to promote the responses that PGE_2 initiated as well as increasing the contractile responsiveness of the myometrium by moving calcium into the cells. Production of prostacyclin is suppressed during labor because of high levels of cortisol (MacKenzie and others, 1988).

Oxytocin levels in the plasma may not increase significantly until second-stage labor, when oxytocin appears to maximize uterine contractions, and after delivery (Blakemore, Petrie, 1988; Goff, 1993). Oxytocin is ineffective in promoting myometrial contractions until oxytocin receptors are present in the myometrium. These receptors are stimulated by high levels of estrogen, $PGF_{2\alpha}$, and PGE_2 (Carsten, Miller, 1987).

OXYTOCIN

Oxytocin, a normal body hormone secreted from the posterior pituitary gland, is chemically related to vasopressin/antidiuretic hormone (ADH). It promotes smooth muscle contractions of the uterus by activating the myometrium. The effect of oxytocin is enhanced in the presence of high levels of estrogen. This is why oxytocin has very little effect on the pregnant uterus until near term when estrogen levels are high so adequate oxytocin receptors are present in the myometrium.

Oxytocin is administered in synthetic form, such as Pitocin or Syntocinon. It is available in solution form for intravenous (IV) or intramuscular (IM) injections, in a nasal spray, or in buccal tablets for sublingual use. It cannot be administered orally because the digestive enzyme *trypsin* inactivates it. IV administration of dilute oxytocin is the preferred route of administration because the absorption rate is predictable and the absorption of the drug can be stopped at any time by discontinuing the IV infusion. Its effect on the body usually ceases very quickly after the drug is discontinued; the pregnant woman's plasma, near term, contains a high concentration of the enzyme *pitocinase*.

Physiology

If labor must be initiated by oxytocin, the preparation for labor that normally takes place during the prelabor phase may not have occurred. Therefore the initial oxytocin-induced uterine contractions must promote these activities by causing a myometrial cell inflammatory response that frees arachidonic acid so it is converted to prostaglandins. Once enough prostaglandins have been synthesized and myometrial gap junctions formed so the uterus can respond in a coordinated manner, the active phase of labor will begin.

By the middle of the active phase of labor, adequate oxytocin receptors will be formed so the dosage of oxytocin may be decreased. It can frequently be discontinued when 7 to 8 cm of dilation is reached because of adequate endogenous prostaglandins and oxytocin production.

Pharmacologic Characteristics

Individualized Uterine Response to Oxytocin

The uterine response to oxytocin is individualized (Perry and others, 1996).

Sensitivity to Oxytocin Changes During Various Phases of Labor

Sensitivity to oxytocin increases as labor advances related to the development of gap junctions and oxytocin receptors (Dawood, 1989), peaking during the second stage of labor (Shyken, Petrie, 1995).

Oxytocin Secretion in Pulses

During normal labor, oxytocin has been found to be secreted in pulses or spurts (Shyken, Petrie, 1995).

Maximum Uterine Contractile Effect of Oxytocin

A uterine response occurs to oxytocin in 3 to 5 minutes with a half-life of approximately 10 minutes. It takes approximately 40 minutes for a serum plasma state to be reached after oxytocin administration (Brodsky, Pelzar, 1991; Seitchik and others, 1984). However, according to Perry and others (1996), serum plasma levels of oxytocin may not be important in determining dosing of the drug.

Uterine Response to Oxytocin

A triphasic uterine response to oxytocin occurs. During the incremental phase, the uterine response increases evenly as oxytocin dose increases. In the stable phase, the uterine response is unchanged even when oxytocin doses are increased. During the third phase, uterine contractions increase in frequency but intensity decreases, leading to an ineffective uterine contraction pattern. This change in uterine response may be gradual or abrupt (Brindley, Sokol, 1988).

Dosage

There is a wide discrepancy among health care providers as to the most effective protocol for administering oxytocin. Currently there are three schools of thought.

Low-Dose Management

Low-dose management in oxytocin administration is based on research by Seitchik and others (1982; 1985), who recommend starting oxytocin at 1 mU/min and increasing the dosage by 1 mU/min every 40 minutes. The effect that conservative management has on outcome variables of labor has been studied by Blakemore and others (1990), Chua and others (1991), Mercer and others (1991), and Muller and others (1992). The findings of these four studies include decreased hyperstimulation, decreased fetal compromise, and significantly less oxytocin needed without affecting the duration of labor or cesarean rate. Refer to Table 26-2 for examples of current low-dose oxytocin management.

High-Dose (Active) Management

Current high-dose oxytocin protocols are based on the active management by O'Driscoll and others (1984; 1993), who recommend starting oxytocin at 6 mU/min and increasing the dosage by 6 mU/min every 15 minutes. The goal is strong uterine contractions leading to shortened labor and delivery. The effect that active

TABLE 26-2 Examples of low-dose and high-dose oxytocin management for labor stimulation

Oxytocin	Starting dose (mU/min)	Incremental increase (mU/min)	Dosage interval (in minutes)	Maximum dose (mU/min)
Low dose	0.5	1	30-60	20
	1-2	2	30	
	1-2	2	15	40
High dose	6	6	20-40	42
	6	6	15	40
	4	4	15	

Modified from American College of Obstetricians and Gynecologists (ACOG): *ACOG Techn Bull,* no. 218, 1995; American College of Obstetricians and Gynecologists (ACOG): *ACOG Techn Bull,* no. 217, 1995; Cunningham F and others: *Williams' obstetrics,* ed 20, Stamford, Conn, 1997, Appleton & Lange.

management has on outcome variables of labor has been studied by Lopez-Zeno and others (1992), Peaceman and Socol (1996), Satin and others (1991; 1992), and Xenakis and others (1995). The findings of these studies include decreased length of labor, rate of forceps delivery, and rate of cesarean birth for dystocia, with an increase in hyperstimulation and cesarean birth for fetal stress. However, Frigoletto and others (1995) found active management to shorten labor to some degree and decrease risk of maternal fever but not to decrease cesarean delivery rate.

According to O'Driscoll and others (1993), there are other components to the active management protocol than just high-dose oxytocin. Most American obstetricians emphasize the high-dose oxytocin and fail to incorporate all other components (ACOG, 1995a).

Components of active management in Dublin

1. *Childbirth education.* The patient is taught what to expect in labor and that it will not last more than 12 hours.

2. *Criterion for diagnosis of labor.* The Dublin criterion is complete effacement. The healthy primigravida is not admitted until this criterion is met.

3. *Amniotomy.* On admission the membranes are artificially ruptured if still intact. If the amniotic fluid is clear, FHR is auscultated. If the amniotic fluid is meconium stained, a continuous electronic monitor is used.

4. *Criterion for early diagnosis and treatment of dystocia.* The Dublin criterion is 1 cm of progress per hour. If the patient's progress is slower than the standard, high-dose oxytocin (6 mU) is started immediately. It is increased every 15 minutes by 6 mU until the patient dilates 1 cm/hr. Only 12% of the patients are induced (O'Driscoll and others, 1993). If the patient's contraction pattern cannot be stimulated to accomplish a dilation rate of 1 cm/hr in a reasonable time, a cesarean delivery is done. The Dublin cesarean birth rate is 8% (O'Driscoll and others, 1993).

5. *The continual presence of a personal nurse.* One nurse is assigned to one patient, and the nurse remains with the patient until her delivery. According to Thornton and Lilford's review and meta-analysis (1994) of published studies on active labor management, the personal nurse who provides constant emotional and physical support is the only component that is associated with shorter labors and lower cesarean rates.

Refer to Table 26-2 for examples of current high-dose oxytocin management.

Pulsatile Oxytocin Management

Oxytocin is administered by some health care providers in 10-minute pulsed infusions as opposed to a continuous IV infusion. According to Willcourt and others (1994), significantly less oxytocin and infusion fluid is used without loss of effectiveness.

Maternal Side Effects

Uterine Hyperstimulation

Uterine hyperstimulation can cause strong tetanic contractions that occur more often than four in a 10-minute period, last longer than 90 seconds without a period of relaxation, or have an increased uterine resting tone above 20 mm Hg pressure.

Uncoordinated, Unproductive Uterine Activity

Unproductive uterine activity may be seen as an increase in frequency with a decrease in intensity of the contractions. This type of activity is related to the cessation of uterine blood flow during a contraction, causing accumulation of metabolites and hypoxia, which renders the muscle ineffective.

Antidiuretic Effect

Because oxytocin has a weak antidiuretic property, large doses can cause the kidneys to increase the reabsorption of water, decreasing urinary output. Antidiuretic effect is seen more frequently when the oxytocin infusion rate is 20 mU/min or more. This condition is enhanced if large amounts of electrolyte-free dextrose solution are used to administer the oxytocin (Cunningham and others, 1997). Possible signs are decreased urine output, hypotension, tachycardia, headache, and nausea and vomiting.

Cardiovascular Effects

Rapid IV injections can have a generalized relaxing effect on vascular smooth muscle, which can lead to hypotension and tachycardia. With prolonged use, oxytocin may increase blood pressure (ACOG, 1995b; Brodsky, Pelzar, 1991).

Pulmonary Edema

Oxytocin in combination with large IV loads can lead to pulmonary edema.

Fetal and Neonatal Effects

Prematurity

Any time labor is induced, there is a risk of prematurity. Therefore fetal maturity should always be assessed before an induction unless it is being performed because of medical indications when the benefits of delivery outweigh the risks of prematurity.

Fetal Stressors

Labor contractions normally impede uterine blood flow. A healthy fetus who has an adequate oxygen reserve can withstand this stress. However, if the frequency, intensity, duration, or resting tone of the contractions is increased by a labor stimulant, this can further impede the uterine blood flow and can cause fetal compromise, resulting in a nonreassuring FHR pattern.

Hyperbilirubinemia

In the neonate, hyperbilirubinemia is seen more frequently after oxytocin induction if fetal hypoxia develops because of excessive uterine stimulation (Wein, 1989).

Documentation of Fetal Lung Maturity

According to the ACOG (1995b), one of the following criteria must be met to assume fetal maturity:

- FHR correct for 30 weeks of gestation by Doppler or 20 weeks by fetoscope
- Length of time from a positive pregnancy test is 36 weeks
- Gestational age greater than 37 weeks by fetal ultrasound crown-rump length obtained between 6 and 11 weeks
- Gestational age greater than 37 weeks by fetal ultrasound biparietal diameter, head circumference, abdominal circumference, and femur length obtained between 15 and 20 weeks
- Mature fetal lung surfactant levels

Nursing Interventions

Because of the individualized response to oxytocin, the variations of practice philosophy supported by research, and variable resources unique to each institution, the following oxytocin protocol is generic:

1. Initiate oxytocin induction or augmentation only after a physician who can perform a cesarean delivery has evaluated the patient, determined a medical indication, provided documentation of fetal maturity, and ordered oxytocin.
2. A unit- or hospital-based validation program for the

registered labor nurse should be established to prepare the nurse to safely administer and monitor labor stimulants (AWHONN, 1993).

3. Explain the procedure to the patient and her coach.

4. Assess the response of the patient and her coach to labor stimulation. Many times parents feel as if they have failed when such an intervention is needed. An explanation as to the reason can help to alleviate these feelings.

5. Assess the patient's level of fear associated with labor-induced contractions. Many patients have heard alarming reports about oxytocin. The nurse should inform the patient and her coach that stimulated contractions are usually very similar to normal, active labor contraction. An induced labor usually has a shorter latent phase, with contractions that may be more uncomfortable than those occurring with a spontaneous latent phase, but the active phase is not usually altered.

6. Apply an external fetal monitor or assist with the placement of an internal fetal monitor and determine a baseline for maternal vital signs, FHR, and uterine activity for 10 to 20 minutes before initiation.

7. Perform a vaginal examination to determine cervical effacement and dilation, fetal presentation, and station.

8. Prepare the oxytocin solution according to hospital policy, and label properly. (Usually 10 U of oxytocin is mixed with 1000 ml of an IV isotonic electrolyte solution.)

9. Have the patient positioned on her side or sitting up to avoid the vena cava syndrome.

10. Administer the solution by way of a continuous infusion device to ensure precise control over the amount of medication administered.

11. Piggyback the oxytocin solution into a well-functioning infusion line next to the infusion site so that oxytocin can be discontinued and restarted as necessary while maintaining an open vein for any emergency.

12. The pump should usually be started at a low setting per hospital protocol or physician's order.

13. The dose is gradually increased per hospital protocol or physician's orders until a desired contraction pattern is established.

14. When labor has progressed to 5 to 6 cm of dilation, oxytocin may be reduced by 1 to 2 mU/min every 30 to 60 minutes.

15. The goal of oxytocin is to establish an adequate uterine contraction pattern that will promote cervical dilation. Usually a contraction pattern of three contractions every 10 minutes, each lasting 40 to 60 seconds with an intensity of 25 to 75 mm Hg intrauterine pressure that produce between 150 and 350 Montevideo units, in which the uterus returns to baseline (resting tone, which does not exceed 20 mm Hg) for at least 1 minute between each contraction, is effective.

16. Check the patency of the IV infusion frequently so that backup of the oxytocin solution into the IV tubing does not result in a bolus of oxytocin.

17. Assess the FHR and uterine contractions for resting tone, intensity, frequency, and duration according to the institution's policy. According to the Association of Women's Health, Obstetric, and Neonatal Nurses (AWHONN, 1993), the minimum standard is to assess FHR and uterine contractions before every dose increase. However, the American College of Obstetricians and Gynecologists (ACOG, 1995b) recommends continuous monitoring similar to that for any high risk pregnancy.

18. Assess vital signs per institution's policy.

19. Periodic vaginal examinations should be performed to determine cervical dilation and fetal descent. To evaluate the progress of labor, cervical dilation and descent of the presenting part (station) are checked. A 1 cm/hr cervical dilation indicates sufficient progress and adequate oxytocin.

20. Drug doses, times of increase, maternal vital signs, and FHR should be charted on a flow sheet and the fetal monitor strip.

21. Assess the patient's level of pain frequently. The effectiveness of distraction tools should also be determined. If the distraction tools are ineffective for her level of discomfort, the physician should be notified. An analgesic may decrease the pain so that distraction tools are effective and the patient can stay in control. Allow the patient a choice in this regard.

22. The nurse can encourage the patient and her coach by giving them frequent positive reinforcement. This can help alleviate some of the negative feelings associated with a stimulated labor.

23. Ensure adequate hydration to enhance effective contractions and avoid dehydration and exhaustion. A fluid bolus

may be requested before initiating oxytocin, and fluid should usually infuse at a minimum of 125 ml/hr.

24. Keep an accurate intake and output record. Note any decreased urine output.

25. Discontinue oxytocin if a hyperstimulation contraction pattern is noted, and notify the attending physician. Hyperstimulation contractions (a) occur more often than four every 10 minutes, (b) last 90 seconds or more without a period of relaxation, and (c) have an increased uterine resting tone above 20 mm Hg pressure.

26. Discontinue oxytocin, administer oxygen, position patient on her side, and notify the attending physician if a nonreassuring FHR pattern is noted, such as late or variable decelerations, loss of long- or short-term variability, tachycardia, or bradycardia. The oxytocin infusion may be restarted after careful assessment by the attending physician of the uterine contraction pattern and the FHR (ACOG, 1995b).

27. The attending physician must be close to the labor and delivery area to manage any complication that might arise in order for the nurse to carry out the induction.

28. The induction should be discontinued if labor has not started or no progress is made within 2 to 3 hours.

29. If high-dose oxytocin (active management) is used, work to develop and implement all the components of this plan, including continuous emotional support.

PROSTAGLANDINS

Vaginal or cervical application of prostaglandins is widely used for cervical ripening. It causes dissolution of the cervical collagen bundles and increases its submucosal water content (Rayburn and others, 1994). In the past few years, several PGE_2 preparations have been marketed after U.S. Food and Drug Administration (FDA) approval for labor stimulation was granted.

Route of Administration

The two most common routes of prostaglandin administration are intracervical and intravaginal in a gel base. However, the extra-amniotic route has been used. The intracervical route appears to directly affect cervical softening and ripening as well as stimulate uterine contractions, whereas the intravaginal route is thought to affect cervical ripening indirectly by stimulating uterine contractions (Husslein, 1991; Miller, Lorkovic, 1993).

Dosage

$PGF_{2\alpha}$ and PGE_2 have both been used; however, PE_2 is currently used most frequently. The dosage is not standardized yet. Refer to Table 26-3 for a comparison of the most commonly used forms of PGE_2.

Advantages

The advantages of prostaglandin-initiated cervical ripening as demonstrated by research (Bernstein, 1991; Chatterjee and others, 1991; Keirse, 1993; Pollnow, Broekhuizen, 1996; Rayburn, 1989) are as follows:

1. Enhanced cervical ripening
2. Decreased need for oxytocin for induction
3. Decreased oxytocin induction time, when used
4. Reduced amount of oxytocin needed for a successful induction
5. Decreased cesarean birth rate related to failed induction (demonstrated by some research studies)

The effectiveness of cervical ripening before labor induction with prostaglandins has been compared with low-dose oxytocin. According to Pollnow and Broekhuizen (1996), prostaglandin was superior to low-dose oxytocin. This was demonstrated by the incidence of higher Bishop scores, higher rate of successful inductions, and shorter labors. Morbidity and cesarean delivery rates were similar in both groups.

Risks

Uterine Hyperstimulation

Uterine hyperstimulation is seen in approximately 1% to 5% of the patients, with the greatest risk following the intravaginal route (ACOG, 1995; Cunningham and others, 1997). It is defined as six or more contractions in 10 minutes or a single contraction lasting more than 2 minutes. When uterine hyperstimulation occurs, it is effectively reversed with the use of $beta_2$-adrenergic tocolytic therapy, such as IV or subcutaneous terbutaline, 250 µg (ACOG, 1995).

Nonreassuring FHR Pattern Changes

A nonreassuring pattern, such as severe variable decelerations or bradycardia, is seen in less than 1% of patients during prostaglandin labor stimulation (Miller, Lorkovic, 1993). When associated FHR changes occur because of uterine hyperstimulation, they are very responsive to the standard treatment protocol, such as posi-

TABLE 26-3 Comparison of commonly used prostaglandin E$_2$ cervical ripening products

Drug	Route	Dosage	Considerations
Cervidil: vaginal insert—a chip in a polyester mesh net with attached cord	Insert into posterior fornix of vagina transversely	Insert contains 10 mg of dino-prostone, which is released slowly (approximately 0.3 mg/hr for maximum of 12 hr)	Single-dose administration Oxytocin can be administered 30 min after removal of insert Can be removed if labor starts or if hyperstimulation occurs FDA approved Not messy
Individual hospital pharmacy preparations	Insert gel into posterior vaginal fornix	3-mg dosage of PGE$_2$ in K-Y jelly (0.5 mg/ml) May repeat every 6 hr for a maximum of three doses in 24 hr	Lack of standardization (Iriye, Freeman, 1996)
Misoprostol (Cytotec): a synthetic PGE$_1$ analog tablet	Intravaginal	25-µg tablet placed in vagina (Wing, Paul, 1996) May repeat in 3-6 hr for a maximum of 24 hr 50- to 100-µg tablets have been used (Chuck, Huffaker, 1995)	Is FDA approved for prevention and treatment of gastric and duodenal ulcers, not for cervical ripening Inexpensive Stable at room temperature Effective in presence of rupture of membranes (Mundle, Young, 1996)

PGE$_1$, Prostaglandin E$_1$; *PGE$_2$*, prostaglandin E$_2$; *FDA*, U.S. Food and Drug Administration.

Continued

TABLE 26-3 Comparison of commonly used prostaglandin E_2 cervical ripening products—cont'd

Drug	Route	Dosage	Considerations
Pessary: wax-based hydrogel containing 10 mg of timed-release prostaglandin	Intravaginal	Time-released dose of 0.8 mg/hr Medication released up to 12 hr	Not messy More costly Must monitor patient for more than 12 hr Can be removed if labor starts or hyperstimulation develops (Miller, Lorkovic, 1993; Rayburn and others, 1992)
Prepidil gel: prefilled syringe applicator	Intracervical	One syringe application inserted into cervical canal 2.5 ml of gel with 0.5 mg of dinoprostone May repeat every 6 hr Maximum of three doses per 24 hr	FDA approved Requires refrigeration Prompts minimal uterine activity Increased product reliability Quite expensive Efficiency decreased with rupture of membranes Must wait 6-12 hr to start oxyto-cin induction per package insert

PGE₁, Prostaglandin E_1; *PGE₂,* prostaglandin E_2; *FDA,* U.S. Food and Drug Administration.

tion change, increasing IV fluids, and administering oxygen at 10 L/min.

Other Side Effects

Gastrointestinal side effects such as nausea, vomiting, and diarrhea are negligible for patients being treated with low-dose prostaglandins (Cunningham and others, 1997). Rarely a fever or headache occurs. Neonatal adverse effects are not increased with the use of PGE_2 (Keirse, 1993).

Nursing Interventions

Preadministration

1. Obtain an informed consent following an informative discussion as to the procedure, reasons for, what it means to the patient, and potential side effects and risks.
2. Determine the cervical Bishop score (refer to Table 26-1), which is a standard of predicting inducibility. A score of 4 or less indicates an unfavorable cervix that could benefit from prostaglandin softening.
3. Assess for any contraindications of prostaglandin use such as an active pelvic infection, asthma, vaginal bleeding, active cardiopulmonary disease, known hepatic or renal disease, or an allergy to the drug (Zatuchni, Slupik, 1996).
4. Assess amniotic membrane status since the intravaginal route is usually used after rupture of membranes.
5. Obtain a baseline FHR tracing per protocol.
6. Analyze the baseline tracing for any nonreassuring signs, such as bradycardia or late decelerations.
7. Obtain baseline readings of blood pressure, temperature, pulse, and respiration rate.

Administration

1. Assess blood pressure, temperature, pulse, and respiratory rate before each PGE_2 gel application.
2. Prepare medication and equipment for insertion.
3. Instill gel per protocol with patient in a dorsal lithotomy position.
4. Provide ongoing emotional support, and encourage relaxation.
5. Have patient turn on her side and rest in bed for 30 to 60 minutes after each PGE_2 gel application.
6. Monitor for uterine activity and nonreassuring FHR changes per protocol by palpation and auscultation or

continuous electronic FHR monitoring (ACOG, 1995; AWHONN, 1993).

7. Be prepared to treat uterine hyperstimulation and any nonreassuring FHR change by the standard treatment protocol, such as position change, increasing IV fluids, and administering oxygen at 10 L/min. Have a beta$_2$-adrenergic tocolytic drug readily available to give on physician's order. The dosage is usually 250 µg of terbutaline administered subcutaneously or intravenously (ACOG, 1995).

8. Assess for the development of any side effects, such as diarrhea, nausea, or vomiting, that occur most often during the first 30 minutes after administration.

9. Ambulation is usually permitted after the assessment phase until the next dose.

10. Reassess the Bishop score after completion of the prostaglandin protocol.

BREAST STIMULATION

Breast stimulation is a physiologic labor stimulant method that offers an alternative method to pharmacologic induction or augmentation. It has been demonstrated through research to initiate or enhance labor (Salmon and others, 1986) and to shorten, especially the latent phase of, labor (Chayen and others, 1986; Mastrogiannis, Knuppel, 1995).

Physiology

Nipple stimulation does cause the spontaneous release of oxytocin by the posterior pituitary gland.

Procedure

Manual Breast Stimulation

1. The patient gently rolls or brushes one nipple through her clothes for 10 minutes. She then gently rolls or brushes the other nipple for 10 minutes.

2. Discontinue stimulation during a contraction and for 10 minutes of rest following one cycle of stimulation (Moenning, Hill, 1987).

Breast Pump Stimulation

1. Patient stimulates one breast at a time for 10 minutes with the electric breast pump on moderate suction.

2. Patient stops pumping for 10 minutes following one cycle of stimulation.

3. The cycle just described may be repeated up to five times (Young, Poppe, 1987).

Risks

Uterine Hyperstimulation

Research has documented the risk of hyperstimulation from breast stimulation as rare (Young, Poppe, 1987) but supports gentle, gradual stimulation to prevent hyperstimulation.

Nipple Soreness and Engorgement

Nipple soreness and engorgement occur in approximately 25% to 30% of cases of breast stimulation (Young, Poppe, 1987).

Fetal Compromise

Research has documented the risk of fetal compromise from breast stimulation as rare (Salmon and others, 1986; Young, Poppe, 1987).

Nursing Interventions

1. Discuss the benefits of breast stimulation such as increased patient control, early milk production for the breast-feeding mother, and avoidance of invasive measures. Discuss the possible adverse side effects as listed above.
2. Explain the appropriate technique to the patient and her coach.
3. Assess the response of the patient and her family to the procedure.
4. Determine a baseline for maternal vital signs, FHR, and uterine activity for 10 to 20 minutes before having the patient begin the procedure.
5. Perform a vaginal examination to determine cervical effacement and dilation, fetal presentation, and station.
6. Have the patient lie on her side or sit to avoid supine hypotension from obstruction of the vena cava.
7. Evaluate uterine contractions for quality, frequency, duration, and resting tone every 15 to 30 minutes.
8. Assess FHR response to uterine contractions every 15 to 30 minutes.
9. During periods of no stimulation, encourage patient to void, ambulate, and drink fluid unless contraindicated.
10. Have the patient discontinue stimulation if a hyperstimulation contraction pattern occurs. Notify the attending physician, and be prepared to administer a tocolytic. Hyperstimulation contractions are contractions that (a)

occur more often than four every 10 minutes, (b) last 90 seconds or more without a period of relaxation, or (c) have a suspected increased uterine resting tone above 20 mm Hg pressure.

11. Have the patient discontinue stimulation, administer oxygen, position patient on her side, and notify the attending physician if a nonreassuring FHR pattern is noted, such as late or nonreassuring variable decelerations, loss of long- or short-term variability, tachycardia, or bradycardia.

12. Have the patient discontinue stimulation, and notify the physician if labor has not started after five cycles of stimulation.

AMNIOTOMY

An amniotomy is artificial rupture of the fetal membranes with an amniohook. It is used for inducing or augmenting labor.

Physiology

Arachidonic acid release increases with its conversion into prostaglandins following amniotomy (Busowski, Parsons, 1995). Before 4-cm dilation, amniotomy may modestly shorten labor if the cervix is ripe. There is an increased risk of chorioamnionitis and cord compression (Mercer and others, 1995; UK Amniotomy Group, 1994). After 4 cm, amniotomy may improve an uncoordinated uterine contraction pattern related to increased prostaglandin release or enhance a normal uterine contraction pattern because of the dilating wedge of the fetal head on the cervix with no adverse fetal or neonatal effect (Fraser and others, 1993; Garite and others, 1993; Rouse and others, 1994; UK Amniotomy Group, 1994).

Advantages

Amniotomy has two advantages. First, it decreases the length of some labors. Second, it allows for amniotic fluid assessment for meconium and permits internal fetal and uterine contraction monitoring.

Risks

One risk of amniotomy is that once the fetal membranes are ruptured, delivery is expected within a reasonable and safe period of time. Unresolved variable decelerations may progress to a nonreassuring pattern, are more likely to occur at an early stage of labor, and are more likely to be unresponsive to position change. This is the most common risk and can be treated with amnioinfusion.

After 35 weeks the risk of an intraamniotic infection increases with the duration of the rupture (Mercer and others, 1995). Umbilical cord prolapse and change in fetal presentation are two additional risks that can occur with amniotomy.

Fetal stressors can be related to decreased amniotic fluid that results from the rupture in amniotomy or from a prolapsed cord.

If the fetal vessels transfuse through the membranes that lie over the cervix, these may rupture when the membranes are ruptured. If there is an undiagnosed placenta previa, membrane rupture can also cause bleeding.

Caput succedaneum related to direct pressure on the presenting part as it acts as a dilating wedge may occur with amniotomy.

Nursing Interventions

1. Amniotomy should be done only near where an emergency delivery can be performed.
2. Assess for engagement of the presenting part before amniotomy (rupture of membranes [ROM]). (The presenting part must be engaged for an amniotomy to be done.) The health care provider who is rupturing the membranes should assess for fetal blood vessels under fetal membranes before rupture is carried out.
3. Check FHR before ROM.
4. Assist health care provider with rupture. According to AWHONN, an amniotomy is to be performed by an appropriately credentialed health care provider (AWHONN, 1993).
5. During the amniotomy, gentle fundal and suprapubic pressure may be applied, if needed, to decrease risk of cord prolapse.
6. Check FHR immediately following ROM. If an FHR change or nonreassuring pattern occurs, rule out cord prolapse, cord obstruction, or fetal bleeding.
7. Assess the amniotic fluid as to amount, color (clear or meconium stained), and odor.
8. Monitor the uterine contraction pattern following rupture. Oxytocin may be ordered if normal labor does not ensue after rupture.
9. Assess maternal temperature after rupture every 4 hours or more frequently if signs and symptoms of infection occur.

STRIPPING OF FETAL MEMBRANES

During membrane stripping, the chorionic fetal membrane is separated from the decidua of the lower uterine segment.

Physiology

When the membrane is stripped from the decidua, a local decid-uitis results, causing the release of prostaglandins in the area (Busowski, Parsons, 1995; McColgin and others, 1993). It has been shown to decrease the incidence of postdate gestations with-out increasing complications (El Torkey, Grant, 1992; Krammer, O'Brien, 1995; McColgin and others, 1990).

Risks

Risks with stripping the fetal membranes include (1) intrauterine infection, (2) premature rupture of the membranes (PROM) at the time they are stripped, and (3) bleeding if there is an undiagnosed placenta previa.

Interventions

1. Firm documentation must be made that the fetus is at 37 weeks of gestation or older.
2. No medical contraindications such as an abnormal fetal presentation or a low-lying placenta may exist.
3. During the procedure the health care provider will digitally separate 1 to 2 cm of the chorionic membrane from the decidua of the lower uterine segment.

LAMINARIA OR SYNTHETIC DILATORS

Laminaria tents, such as *Laminaria digitata* or *Laminaria japonica,* are natural cervical dilators made from seaweed. Syn-thetic alternatives are currently being used more frequently. Two common synthetic dilators are Dilapan, a hygroscopic cervical dilator, and Lamicel, an alcohol polymer sponge impregnated with 450 mg of magnesium sulfate and compressed into a tent.

Physiology

The dilators are inserted into the full length of the cervical canal, where they absorb cervical fluids and swell, dilating the cervix slowly (Trofatter, 1992).

Advantages

Several research studies have found that the synthetic dilators are effective in ripening the cervix before oxytocin induction (Berkus and others, 1990; Blumenthal, Ramanauskas, 1990; Sanchez-Ramos and others, 1992). It is unclear if the postripening cervical state following dilation is as effective as when the cervix dilates naturally (Krammer, O'Brien, 1995).

Risks

Chorioamnionitis

An infection is caused primarily by beta-hemolytic streptococci. Because of the faster expansion time (4 hours as compared with 12 to 16 hours), the synthetic dilators pose less of a risk of an infection than the *Laminaria* dilators, but the presence of any foreign body may allow vaginal flora to ascend into the uterus (Krammer and others, 1995).

Premature Rupture of Membranes

Because the tents must be placed into the full length of the cervical canal, including the internal os, there is a risk of PROM if the cervix is short.

Cervical Trauma

Cervical trauma is related to insertion technique.

Nursing Interventions

1. Prepare the patient, and assist the physician with the pre-insertion assessment, which includes ruling out ruptured membranes; inspecting the cervix and vagina for an infection, especially for beta-streptococcus or *Neisseria gonorrhoeae;* assessing fetal size, position, amniotic fluid volume, and placental position with ultrasound; and assessing for fetal well-being with a biophysical profile or a contraction stress test.
2. Prepare the patient, and assist the physician with the insertion procedure, which includes a vaginal examination to assess cervical anatomy and cervical status; insertion of a sterile speculum so the cervix can be visualized, stabilized with a ring forcep, and painted with povidone-iodine (Betadine); insertion of four to nine tents to fill the cervix; and packing of the upper vagina with 4×4-inch sponges to hold the tents in place.
3. Instruct the patient that she might experience mild cramping during the insertion.
4. Document the number of dilators and sponges placed.
5. Continue to assess urinary output following insertion since pressure on the bladder may cause urinary retention.
6. Continually assess for ROM, uterine tenderness, or uterine bleeding. If any of these signs occur, assess for signs of fetal compromise and notify the physician so tents can be removed.

SELF-HELP MEASURES

Various self-help measures have been shown to enhance cervical ripening of a thick, unripe cervix or to induce labor if the cervix is ripe. A few such measures are as follows:

1. *Herbal preparations.* Blue cohosh, black cohosh, PN-6, or another safe herbal preparation taken orally may promote prostaglandin or oxytocin production (Hunter, Chern-Hughes, 1996; Woolven, 1997). The dosage of blue cohosh tincture is 3 to 8 drops in a glass of warm water or tea; it may be repeated every ½ hour for several hours until regular contractions occur (Hunter, Chern-Hughes, 1996).

2. *Orgasm.* Associated oxytocin or prostaglandin release stimulates uterine contractions.

3. *Sexual intercourse.* Semen contains prostaglandin, which may hasten cervical ripening.

4. *Bowel stimulation.* Stimulation of the bowel increases prostaglandin production, which may facilitate cervical ripening.

NURSING PROCESS

NURSING DIAGNOSES/COLLABORATIVE PROBLEMS AND INTERVENTIONS

- **POTENTIAL COMPLICATION: FETAL COMPROMISE** related to cord prolapse, uterine hyperstimulation, or maternal hypotension.

  DESIRED OUTCOMES: Fetal compromise will be minimized and managed as measured by an FHR maintained at a baseline between 110 and 160 beats/min with normal variability, reactivity, and absence of nonreassuring decelerations during the induction. Maternal uterine contractions will be less than four every 10 minutes and last less than 70 to 90 seconds, with a return to a resting tone below 20 mm Hg for at least 1 minute.

  INTERVENTIONS
  Amniotomy
  1. Assess the state of the cervix, and obtain a Bishop score.
  2. Assess FHR before and immediately following artificial rupture of membranes (AROM).
  3. Assess and describe the color of amniotic fluid.
  4. Compare progress of labor with the normal labor curve following AROM.
  5. If fetal compromise develops from a prolapsed cord, apply and maintain pressure to the presenting part; with other hand, push abdomen up; call for help; instruct help to put bed in a Trendelenburg position; evaluate FHR; start oxygen by

mask at 10 L/min; and start an IV line with an 18-gauge intracatheter if not present.

6. If fetal compromise develops and cord prolapse is not identified as the cause, reposition patient and administer oxygen by mask at 10 L/min; increase IV fluid rate.

7. Notify physician of cord prolapse or signs of fetal compromise, such as periodic late or nonreassuring variable decelerations, change in baseline, and meconium- or blood-stained amniotic fluid.

Prostaglandins, oxytocin, or breast stimulation induction

1. Obtain baseline FHR and uterine activity pattern readings for 15 to 20 minutes before starting the induction.

2. Obtain baseline maternal blood pressure and pulse readings.

3. Conduct induction according to already stated respective protocol.

4. Monitor uterine contractions and FHR continuously or according to hospital protocol.

5. Evaluate and chart uterine contraction pattern and FHR every 15 minutes during the induction.

6. Assess maternal blood pressure and pulse during oxytocin induction every time the oxytocin dosage is increased.

7. Monitor patient's response to induction by palpating contractions and performing vaginal examinations for labor progress. Evaluate progress of labor by graphing dilation and station on the normal labor curve.

8. Discontinue induction and notify physician if signs of fetal compromise develop; hypertonic contractions develop, such as contractions more than four every 10 minutes, lasting longer than 70 to 90 seconds, or a resting tone greater than 20 mm Hg; or a nonreassuring FHR pattern develops, such as late or severe variable decelerations, tachycardia, bradycardia, or decreased variability.

- **RISK FOR INFECTION** related to rupture of membranes or prolonged labor.

  DESIRED OUTCOME: The patient will remain infection free during intrapartum and postpartum periods as indicated by her temperature remaining below 38° C, absence of foul-smelling vaginal discharge, and a white blood cell count between 4500 and 10,000/mm^3.

  INTERVENTIONS

  1. Assess for indicators of infection by checking temperature every 2 hours after ROM and assessing vaginal discharge for a foul odor.

2. Monitor laboratory data, especially white blood cell count.
3. Maintain patient's bed dry and clean of amniotic fluid.
4. Notify physician if temperature is greater than 38° C or if foul-smelling vaginal discharge develops.

- **FEAR** related to knowledge deficit of the induction procedure and discomfort caused by induced uterine contractions.
  DESIRED OUTCOME: The patient and her family will communicate their concerns openly and participate in the decisions concerning induction.
  INTERVENTIONS
  1. Assess knowledge regarding the induction process and concerns related to the induction.
  2. Provide information as needed regarding the induction process and what to expect.
  3. Assess knowledge regarding breathing and relaxation techniques.
  4. Assess level of discomfort throughout induction.
  5. Instruct and support patient and coach with use of distraction and relaxation tools as needed.
  6. Administer pain medication during active phase of labor according to patient's request and written orders.
  7. Notify physician if discomfort is greater than patient's tolerance.

- **POTENTIAL COMPLICATION OF OXYTOCIN: FLUID OVERLOAD** related to the antidiuretic effect of oxytocin.
  DESIRED OUTCOME: Signs and symptoms of fluid overload will be minimized and managed as measured by a urinary output greater than 30 ml/hr or 120 ml/4 hr with clear breath sounds and no signs of increased edema.
  INTERVENTIONS
  1. Assess for signs of fluid retention such as decreased urine output, bounding pulse, peripheral edema, increasing blood pressure, shortness of breath, or rales.
  2. Keep an accurate intake and output record.
  3. Notify physician if urinary output is less than 120 ml/4 hr.

CONCLUSION

The use of labor stimulants enables many patients to have a vaginal delivery. However, risks are associated with their use. The primary role of the nurse is to monitor closely the labor progress, the uterine contraction pattern, and fetal well-being. Developing complications can then be recognized early so that the labor stimulant can be stopped before a negative development occurs. A labor stimulant should never be used just to speed up a labor or to initiate a labor for convenience.

BIBLIOGRAPHY

Oxytocin Induction

Ahner R and others: Fetal fibronectin as a selection criterion for induction of term labor, *Am J Obstet Gynecol* 173:1513-1517, 1995.

American College of Obstetricians and Gynecologists (ACOG): Dystocia and the augmentation of labor, *ACOG Techn Bull,* no. 218, 1995a.

American College of Obstetricians and Gynecologists (ACOG): Induction of labor, *ACOG Techn Bull,* no. 217, 1995b.

Association of Women's Health, Obstetric, and Neonatal Nurses (AWHONN): *Cervical ripening and induction and augmentation of labor: practice resource,* Washington, DC, 1993, The Author.

Bishop E: Pelvic scoring for elective induction, *Obstet Gynecol* 24:266, 1964.

Blakemore K, Petrie R: Oxytocin for the induction of labor, *Obstet Gynecol Clin North Am* 15(2):339-353, 1988.

Blakemore K and others: A prospective comparison of hourly and quarter-hourly oxytocin dose increase intervals for the induction of labor at term, *Obstet Gynecol* 75:757-761, 1990.

Blanch G, Olah K, Walkinshaw S: The presence of fetal fibronectin in the cervicovaginal secretions of women at term: its role in the assessment of women before labor induction and the investigation of the physiologic mechanisms of labor, *Am J Obstet Gynecol* 174(1):262-266, 1996.

Brindley B, Sokol R: Induction and augmentation of labor: basis and methods for current practice, *Obstet Gynecol Surv* 43(12):730-743, 1988.

Brodsky P, Pelzar E: Rationale for the revision of oxytocin administration protocols, *Obstet Gynecol Neonatal Nurs* 20(6):440-444, 1991.

Carsten M, Miller J: A new look at uterine muscle contraction, *Am J Obstet Gynecol* 157:1303-1315, 1987.

Casey M, MacDonald P: Biomolecular processes in the initiation of parturition: decidual activation, *Clin Obstet Gynecol* 31(3):533-552, 1988.

Chez R: Cervical ripening and labor induction after previous cesarean delivery, *Clin Obstet Gynecol* 38(2):287-292, 1995.

Chua S and others: Augmentation of labour: does internal tocography result in better obstetric outcome than external tocography? *Obstet Gynecol* 76:164-167, 1990.

Cunningham F and others: *Williams' obstetrics,* ed 20, Stamford, Conn, 1997, Appleton & Lange.

Dawood M: Evolving concepts of oxytocin for induction of labor, *Am J Perinatol* 6(2):167-172, 1989.

Frigoletto F and others: A clinical trial of active management of labor, *N Engl J Med* 333:745-750, 1995.

Fuentes A, Williams M: Cervical assessment, *Clin Obstet Gynecol* 38(2):224-231, 1995.

Goff K: Initiation of parturition, *MCH* 18(suppl):7-13, 1993.

Huszar G, Walsh M: Relationship between myometrial and cervical functions in pregnancy and labor, *Semin Perinatol* 15(2):97-117, 1991.

Leppert P: Anatomy and physiology of cervical ripening, *Clin Obstet Gynecol* 38(2):267-279, 1995.

Lopez-Zeno J and others: A controlled trial of a program for the active management of labor, *N Engl J Med* 326:450-454, 1992.

MacKenzie L and others: Prostacyclin biosynthesis by cultured human myometrial smooth muscle cells: dependency on arachidonic or linoleic acid in the culture medium, *Am J Obstet Gynecol* 159:1365-1372, 1988.

Mercer B, Pilgrim P, Sibai B: Labor induction with continuous low-dose oxytocin infusion: a randomized trial, *Obstet Gynecol* 77:659-663, 1991.

Muller P, Stubbs T, Laurent S: A prospective randomized clinical trial comparing two oxytocin induction protocols, *Am J Obstet Gynecol* 167:373-381, 1992.

O'Driscoll K, Foley M, MacDonald D: Active management of labor as an alternative to cesarean section for dystocia, *Obstet Gynecol* 63:485-490, 1984.

O'Driscoll K, Meagher D, Boylan P: *Active management of labor,* ed 3, St Louis, 1993, Mosby.

Peaceman A, Socol M: Active management of labor, *Am J Obstet Gynecol* 175(2):363-368, 1996.

Perry R and others: The pharmacokinetics of oxytocin as they apply to labor induction, *Am J Obstet Gynecol* 174:1590-1593, 1996.

Satin A, Hankins G, Yeomans E: A prospective study of two dosing regimens of oxytocin for the induction of labor in patients with unfavorable cervices, *Am J Obstet Gynecol* 165:980-984, 1991.

Satin A and others: High versus low-dose oxytocin for labor stimulation, *Obstet Gynecol* 80:111-116, 1992.

Satin A and others: High-dose oxytocin: 20- versus 40-minute dosage interval, *Obstet Gynecol* 83:234, 1994.

Seitchik J, Amico J, Castillo M: Oxytocin augmentation of dysfunctional labor. V. An alternative oxytocin regimen, *Am J Obstet Gynecol* 151:757-761, 1985.

Seitchik J, Castillo M: Oxytocin augmentation of dysfunctional labor. I. Clinical data, *Am J Obstet Gynecol* 144:899-905, 1982.

Seitchik J and others: Oxytocin augmentation of dysfunctional labor. IV. Oxytocin pharmacokinetics, *Am J Obstet Gynecol* 150(3):225-228, 1984.

Shyken J, Petrie R: Oxytocin to induce labor, *Clin Obstet Gynecol* 38(2):232-245, 1995.

Simkin P: Active management of labor, *Childbirth Instructor Magazine* 5(4):6-12, 46-47, 1995.

Thornton J, Lilford R: Active management of labour: current knowledge and research issues, *Br Med J* 309:366-369, Aug 6, 1994.

Ventura S and others: Advance report of final mortality statistics, 1993. National Center for Health Statistics, *Monthly Vital Statistics Rep* 44(suppl), 1995.

Wein P: Efficacy of different starting doses of oxytocin for induction of labor, *Obstet Gynecol* 74:863-868, 1989.

Willcourt R and others: Induction of labor with pulsatile oxytocin by a computer-controlled pump, *Am J Obstet Gynecol* 170:603-608, 1994.

Xenakis E and others: Low-dose versus high-dose oxytocin augmentation of labor—a randomized trial, *Am J Obstet Gynecol* 173:1874-1878, 1995.

Prostaglandins

American College of Obstetricians and Gyncologists (ACOG): Induction of labor, *ACOG Techn Bull,* no. 217, 1995.

Association of Women's Health, Obstetric, and Neonatal Nurses (AWHONN): *Cervical ripening and induction and augmentation of labor: practice resource,* Washington, DC, 1993, The Author.

Bernstein P: Prostaglandin E$_2$ gel for cervical ripening and labour induction: a multicentre placebo-controlled trial, *Can Med Assoc J* 145:1249, 1991.

Chatterjee M and others: Prostaglandin E$_2$ vaginal gel for cervical ripening, *Eur J Obstet Gynecol Reprod Biol* 38(3):197-202, 1991.

Chuck F, Huffaker B: Labor induction with intravaginal misoprostol versus intracervical prostaglandin E$_2$ gel (Prepidil gel): randomized comparison, *Am J Obstet Gynecol* 173:1137-1142, 1995.

Cunningham F and others: *Williams' obstetrics,* ed 20, Stamford, Conn, 1997, Appleton & Lange.

Husslein P: Use of prostaglandins for induction of labor, *Semin Perinatol* 15(2):173-181, 1991.

Iriye B, Freeman R: Induction of labor. In Queenan J, Hobbins J, editors: *Protocols for high-risk pregnancies,* ed 3, Cambridge, Mass, 1996, Blackwell Science.

Keirse M: Prostaglandins in preinduction cervical ripening: metaanalysis of worldwide clinical experience, *J Reprod Med* 38:89, 1993.

Miller A, Lorkovic M: Prostaglandin E$_2$ for cervical ripening, *MCN Am J Matern Child Nurs* 18(suppl):7-13, 1993.

Mundle W, Young D: Vaginal misoprostol for induction of labor: a randomized controlled trial, *Obstet Gynecol* 88:521-525, 1996.

Pollnow D, Broekhuizen F: Randomized, double-blind trial of prostaglandin E$_2$ gel versus low-dose oxytocin for cervical ripening before induction of labor, *Am J Obstet Gynecol* 174(6):1910-1915, 1996.

Rayburn W: Prostaglandin E$_2$ gel for cervical ripening and induction of labor: a critical analysis, *Am J Obstet Gynecol* 160:529-534, 1989.

Rayburn W and others: An intravaginal controlled-release prostaglandin E$_2$ pessary for cervical ripening and initiation of labor at term, *Obstet Gynecol* 79:374-379, 1992.

Rayburn W and others: A model for investigating microscopic changes induced by prostaglandin E$_2$ in the term cervix, *J Mat Fet Invest* 4:137, 1994.

Wing D, Paul R: A comparison of differing dosing regimens of vaginally administered misoprostil for preinduction cervical ripening and labor induction, *Am J Obstet Gynecol* 175(1):158-164, 1996.

Zatuchni G, Slupik R: *Obstetrics and gynecology drug handbook,* ed 2, St Louis, 1996, Mosby.

Other

American College of Obstetricians and Gynecologists (ACOG): Induction of labor, *ACOG Techn Bull,* no. 217, 1995.

Association of Women's Health, Obstetric, and Neonatal Nurses (AWHONN): *Cervical ripening and induction and augmentation of labor: practice resource,* Washington, DC, 1993, The Author.

Berkus M, Laufe L, Castillo M: Lamicel for induction of labor, *J Reprod Med* 35(3):219-221, 1990.

Blumenthal P, Ramanauskas R: Randomized trial of dilapan and laminaria as cervical ripening agents before induction of labor, *Obstet Gynecol* 75:365-368, 1990.

Busowski J, Parsons M: Amniotomy to induce labor, *Clin Obstet Gynecol* 38(2):246-258, 1995.

Chayen B, Tejani N, Verma U: Induction of labor with an electric breast pump, *J Reprod Med* 31:116-118, 1986.

El-Torkey M, Grant J: Sweeping of the membranes is an effective method of induction of labour in prolonged pregnancy: a report of a randomized trial, *Br J Obstet Gynaecol* 99:455-458, 1992.

Fraser W and others: Effect of early amniotomy on the risk of dystocia in nulliparous women, *N Engl J Med* 328:1145, 1993.

Garite T and others: The influence of elective amniotomy on fetal heart rate patterns and the course of labor in term patients: a randomized study, *Am J Obstet Gynecol* 168:1827, 1993.

Hunter L, Chern-Hughes B: Management of prolonged latent phase labor, *J Nurse Midwifery* 41(5):383-388, 1996.

Krammer J, O'Brien W: Mechanical methods of cervical ripening, *Clin Obstet Gynecol* 38(2):280-286, 1995.

Krammer J and others: Pre-induction cervical ripening: a randomized comparison of two methods, *Obstet Gynecol* 85:614, 1995.

Mastrogiannis D, Knuppel R: Labor induced using methods that do not involve oxytocin, *Clin Obstet Gynecol* 38(2):259-266, 1995.

McColgin S and others: Stripping membranes at term: can it safely reduce the incidence of post-term pregnancies? *Obstet Gynecol* 76:678-680, 1990.

McColgin S and others: Parturitional factors associated with membrane stripping, *Am J Obstet Gynecol* 169:71-77, 1993.

Mercer B and others: Early versus late amniotomy for labor induction: a randomized trial, *Am J Obstet Gynecol* 173:1371, 1995.

Moenning R, Hill W: A randomized study comparing two methods of performing the breast stimulation stress test, *Obstet Gynecol Neonatal Nurs* 16(4):253-257, 1987.

Rouse D and others: Active-phase labor arrest: a randomized trial of chorioamnion management, *Obstet Gynecol* 83:937, 1994.

Salmon Y and others: Cervical ripening by breast stimulation, *Obstet Gynecol* 67(1):21-24, 1986.

Sanchez-Ramos L, Kaunitz A, Connor P: Hygroscopic cervical dilators and prostaglandin E_2 gel for preinduction cervical ripening: a randomized, prospective comparison, *J Reprod Med* 37:335, 1992.

Trofatter K: Cervical ripening, *Clin Obstet Gynecol* 35:476-486, 1992.

UK Amniotomy Group: A multicentre randomised trial of amniotomy in spontaneous first labour in term, *Br J Obstet Gynaecol* 101:307, 1994.

Woolven L: Alternative therapies for pregnancy, labor and delivery, *Childbirth Instructor Magazine* 7(2):40-42, 1997.

Young J, Poppe C: Breast pump stimulation to promote labor, *MCN Am J Matern Child Nurs* 12(2):124-126, 1987.

27

Dysfunctional Labor

Labor does not always progress within the normal labor curve. Conditions can exist or develop that interfere with normal progress. An abnormal or difficult labor is usually termed *dysfunctional labor* or *dystocia.*

INCIDENCE

Dysfunctional labor occurs in approximately 8% to 11% of all deliveries (ACOG, 1995). Uterine dystocia is the most common cause of a dysfunctional labor. Malpresentations are the second most common cause, with pelvic disproportion the least common cause (Cunningham and others, 1997).

ETIOLOGY

Dysfunctional labor is caused by three main factors: uterine dystocia, fetal dystocia, and pelvic dystocia. Uterine dystocia is related to ineffective uterine activity. Some of the causes that appear to increase one's risk for developing uterine dystocia are as follows:

- Thirty pounds or more overweight (Thomson, Hanley, 1988)
- Short stature (Thomson, Hanley, 1988)
- Infertility difficulties
- Following a version (Lau and others, 1997)
- Masculine characteristics

- A congenitally abnormal uterus, an overdistended uterus as in the case of a multiple pregnancy, or polyhydramnios
- Lack of reflex stimulation of the myometrium related to malpresentations such as posterior positions; face, brow, or breech presentations; or transverse lie
- Fetopelvic disproportion; uterine activity usually slows if the pelvis is too small for fetal descent
- Overstimulation of the uterus with oxytocin
- Extreme maternal fear or exhaustion causing the adrenal medulla to secrete catecholamines that interfere with uterine contractility (Kennell and others, 1991)
- Dehydration
- Electrolyte imbalance
- Administration of an analgesic too early in labor
- Use of continuous epidural analgesia (Morton and others, 1994; Ramin and others, 1995; Thorp and others, 1993)

Fetal dystocia is usually related to one of the following:

- An abnormal fetal presentation or position, such as face, brow, or breech; posterior occiput presentation; or transverse lie
- Fetal anomalies, such as hydrocephalus, abdominal enlargement, tumors, or conjoined twins
- Excessive fetal size, usually greater than 4000 g (9 pounds) (Bruner, 1991)

Pelvic dystocia is usually related to one of the following conditions:

- A small pelvic inlet, midpelvis, or pelvic outlet as the result of heredity, previous pelvic fracture, or disease
- Pelvic tumors

NORMAL PHYSIOLOGY

Normal uterine contractions have a contraction (systole) and relaxation (diastole) phase. The contraction phase is initiated by a pacemaker situated at the uterine end of the right fallopian tube. The contraction, like a wave, moves downward to the cervix and upward to the fundus of the uterus. At the acme (peak) of the contraction the entire uterus is contracting, with the greatest intensity in the fundal area. The relaxation phase follows and occurs simultaneously in all parts of the uterus. The round ligaments contain muscle and are stimulated to contract as the uterus contracts, thereby anchoring the uterus and promoting a downward force on the presenting part.

Uterine contractions of an intensity of 30 mm Hg or greater

initiate cervical dilation. During active labor the intensity usually reaches 50 to 80 mm Hg. During the second stage of labor the intensity can peak at 100 mm Hg. Resting tone is normally between 5 and 10 mm Hg in early labor and between 12 and 18 mm Hg in active labor.

Normal labor usually begins with a latent phase, which is characterized by the cervix slowly dilating to about 4 cm. The average duration of this phase for the nullipara is 6½ hours, and for the multipara it is 5 hours. An active phase follows and is identified as the time when dilation takes place more rapidly. It is characterized by a period of acceleration and then a period of maximum slope followed by a period of deceleration (Fig. 27-1).

The deceleration phase, often referred to as *transition,* is not associated with decreased uterine activity, but during this phase the cervix is being retracted around the fetal presenting part. The normal rate of cervical dilation during the active phase should be at least 1.2 cm/hr in nulliparas and 1.5 cm/hr in multiparas (Friedman, 1989). Except for prelabor engagement, fetal descent generally does not begin until the active phase of dilation and starts

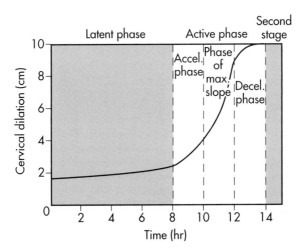

FIG. 27-1 Average dilation curve. Composite of average dilation curves for nulliparous labor based on analysis of data derived from patterns traced by large, nearly consecutive series of primigravidas. First stage is divided into relatively flat latent phase and rapidly progressive active phase. Active phase has three identifiable components: acceleration phase, linear phase of maximum slope, and deceleration phase.

From Friedman EA: *Labor: clinical evaluation and management,* ed 2, New York, 1978, Appleton-Century-Crofts.

to reach its maximum slope during the deceleration phase of active labor, which continues throughout the second stage of labor. The normal rate of descent is at least 1 cm/hr in nulliparas and 2 cm/hr in multiparas (Friedman, 1989).

PATHOPHYSIOLOGY
Uterine Dystocia

Two types of abnormal uterine activity lead to uterine dystocia. First, there is hypotonic uterine activity, in which the rise in uterine pressure during a contraction is insufficient (less than 25 mm Hg) to promote cervical effacement and dilation. The force provided by voluntary contractions of the abdominal musculature, facilitated by the urge to push, may be insufficient to facilitate fetal descent and delivery. Second, there is hypertonic or uncoordinated uterine activity, in which the contractions are frequent and painfully strong but ineffective in promoting effacement and dilation. They can be ineffective because the uterine pacemakers arise in other areas of the uterus. This causes the myometrium to contract spasmodically and frequently but ineffectively, and the presenting part is not forced downward.

Fetal Dystocia

The fetus can move through the birth canal with the greatest ease when the head is sharply flexed so that the chin rests on the thorax and the occipital area of the skull (vertex) is presenting anterior to the mother's pelvis. Thus the smallest diameter of the fetal head enters the mother's pelvis, and the most flexible part of the fetal body, the back of the neck, adapts to the curve of the birth canal. At times the fetus will assume other presentations, making labor difficult or impossible. These presentations are discussed in the following sections.

Occiput Posterior Presentation

Occiput posterior presentation occurs in approximately 10% to 25% of labors (Scott and others, 1990). The occiput of the fetus is in the posterior portion of the pelvis instead of in the anterior portion (Fig. 27-2). As the fetus moves through the birth canal, the occiput bone presses on the mother's sacrum. Severe back pain usually results from this presentation. The occiput must also rotate 135 degrees. This rotation can occur during fetal descent, causing slow progress in the active phase or a persistent anterior cervical lip. Most often it does not occur until the occiput reaches the pelvic floor. Therefore the second stage of labor is usually prolonged.

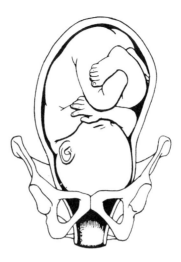

FIG. 27-2 Occiput posterior presentation.
From *The normal female pelvis: clinical education aid no. 8,* Columbus, Ohio, Ross Laboratories.

Face Presentation

Face presentation, or mentum, occurs approximately once in every 500 deliveries (Bowes, 1994) when the fetal head is in extension instead of flexion as it enters the pelvic inlet (Fig. 27-3). If the mentum is in an anterior position, the labor usually progresses very close to normal and vaginal delivery results without much difficulty. This is because the widest diameter of the presenting part is similar in size to an occiput presentation and the neck can glide around the short symphysis pubis with ease. When the mentum is in a posterior position, approximately 70% of the time it will rotate to an anterior face presentation, making vaginal delivery possible but causing the labor to be prolonged. If the posterior position persists, cesarean delivery will be necessary because the neck is too short to stretch the long distance of the sacrum.

Brow Presentation

A brow presentation occurs approximately once in every 500 deliveries (Bowes, 1994) when the fetal head presents in a position midway between full flexion and extreme extension (Fig. 27-4). This causes the largest diameter of the fetal head to engage. Vaginal delivery depends on the successful conversion to an occiput or a face presentation by varying degrees of flexion or extension, which occurs in 70% to 90% of the cases. A brow presentation may be

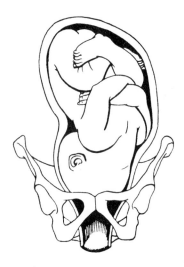

FIG. 27-3 Face presentation.
From *The normal female pelvis: clinical education aid no. 8,* Columbus, Ohio, Ross Laboratories.

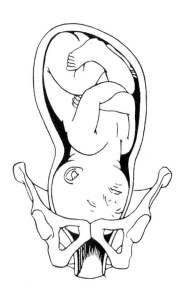

FIG. 27-4 Brow presentation.
From *The normal female pelvis: clinical education aid no. 8,* Columbus, Ohio, Ross Laboratories.

present when descent of the presenting part is prolonged or a long second-stage labor develops.

Shoulder Presentation

Shoulder presentation occurs approximately once in every 300 deliveries (Bowes, 1994) when the fetal spine is lying vertical to the mother's spine (Fig. 27-5). Because of the high mortality risk from prolapsed cord, cesarean delivery is usually the best management. However, if placenta previa and fetopelvic disproportion (FPD) are not present, external cephalic version has been successful in very controlled circumstances.

Compound Presentation

Compound presentation occurs approximately once in every 1000 deliveries (Bowes, 1994) when one or more of the fetal extremities accompany the presenting part. An arm with the head is the most common compound presentation. Vaginal delivery is usually possible unless cord prolapse occurs or labor fails to progress. Then an emergency cesarean delivery is done. Attempts should not be made to replace the prolapsed fetal part.

Breech Presentation

Breech presentation occurs in approximately 2.8% of all deliveries (Bowes, 1994) when the buttocks of the fetus present. The breech can present in three different attitudes. It is termed a *frank breech* when the thighs are flexed and the legs lie alongside the fetal body;

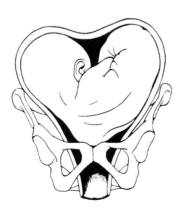

FIG. 27-5 Shoulder presentation.
From *The normal female pelvis: clinical education aid no. 8,* Columbus, Ohio, Ross Laboratories.

a *complete breech* when the legs are flexed at the thighs allowing the feet to present with the buttocks; and a *footling breech* when one foot (single footling) or both feet (double footling) present before the buttocks (Fig. 27-6).

Prematurity is the main cause of breech presentation (Lee, 1989). Other causes are uterine relaxation associated with parity greater than 5 and decreased fetal capability to move within the uterus associated with diminished muscle tone of the fetus, neuromuscular disorders, or decreased uterine space. Infrequent causes are placenta previa, polyhydramnios, and hydrocephalus.

A breech presentation is considered high risk for the following reasons:

1. Prolapse of the cord is more likely to occur, especially in a footling breech, because the buttocks do not fit as snugly into the cervix as does the fetal head.
2. Dysfunctional labor is much more likely to result because the buttocks are soft and make a poor dilating wedge against the cervix.
3. Birth trauma is more likely to occur because the head does not have time to mold and it must pass through the birth canal quickly. The fetus who is premature is even more prone to birth trauma from an incompletely dilated cervix.

For these reasons many obstetricians have elected in the past to deliver most breeches by cesarean. Today's trend is to attempt external version between 36 and 38 weeks of gestation. If the version is unsuccessful, an experienced obstetrician will attempt a vaginal delivery if it is a frank breech with adequate neck flexion, symmetric fetal body proportions, and an estimated fetal weight between 2500 and 3800 g (Scorza, 1996).

Pelvic Dystocia

Pelvic dystocia is related to a contraction of one or more of the three planes of the pelvis.

Inlet Contraction

The pelvic inlet is considered contracted when the widest part of the brim, the transverse diameter, is less than 11.5 cm and the anteroposterior diameter is less than 10 cm (Compton, 1987). The anteroposterior diameter can be approximated by measuring the diagonal conjugate, the distance from the lower portion of the symphysis pubis to the middle of the promontory of the sacrum, and subtracting 1.5 to 2 cm. The transverse diameter can be measured radiologically or with ultrasound.

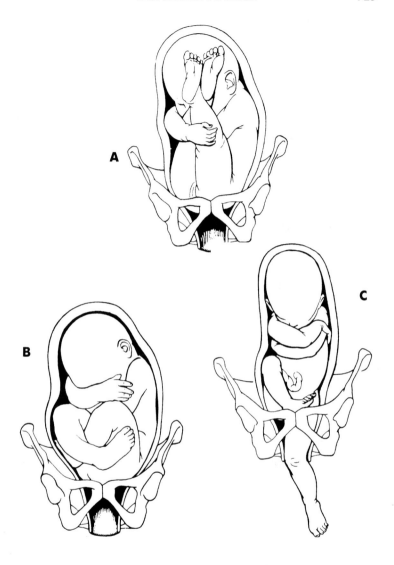

FIG. 27-6 Breech presentation. **A,** Frank breech. **B,** Complete breech. **C,** Single footling breech.
From *The normal female pelvis: clinical education aid no. 8,* Columbus, Ohio, Ross Laboratories.

No matter what the pelvic size measures, most obstetricians will allow the patient to go into labor. Descent and engagement of the fetal head would indicate an adequate pelvic inlet.

Midpelvis Contraction

Contraction of the midpelvis is more common than an inlet contraction and often causes an arrest of descent. It is more difficult to determine manually. Possible indicators are (1) prominent ischial spines, (2) convergent pelvic side walls, and (3) a narrow sacrosciatic notch.

Outlet Contraction

The outlet of the pelvis can be estimated by measuring the transverse diameter—the distance between the inner aspects of the ischial tuberosities. If it is 8 cm or less, the outlet is considered contracted. With the use of a Thoms retractor, the anteroposterior diameter can also be approximated by measuring from the middle of the lower margin of the symphysis pubis to the tip of the sacrum, not the coccyx; the fetal head can usually push the coccyx back. Normally, the anteroposterior diameter is 14 cm.

• • •

The final outcome of any labor depends on the interrelation of the size and shape of the pelvis; the size, presentation, and position of the fetus; and the quality of uterine contractions. Therefore dystocia can rarely be diagnosed until labor has progressed for a time. If the fetus is too large to pass through the pelvis or the pelvis is too small for the fetus to pass through, the condition is usually referred to as *fetopelvic disproportion* (FPD) or *cephalopelvic disproportion* (CPD).

SIGNS AND SYMPTOMS

Cervical dilation, effacement, and fetal descent should occur progressively during labor. In an abnormal labor (1) contractions slow or fail to advance in frequency, duration, or intensity; (2) the cervix fails to respond to the uterine contractions by dilating and effacing; or (3) the fetus fails to move downward. Thus labor does not progress normally.

MATERNAL EFFECTS

Any time the birth canal is too small to accommodate the presentation of the fetus, uterine rupture can result. This can lead to maternal death related to hemorrhage. However, the incidence is rare; an obstructed labor is not usually allowed to continue. The greatest risk to the mother with a dysfunctional labor is associated with maternal exhaustion and a cesarean delivery; 30% of all cesarean deliveries are the result of dysfunctional labor (Clarke, Taffel, 1996). Cesarean birth is associated with four times more maternal risks than is vaginal birth. These risks include postoperative complications of hemorrhage, endomyometrial and incision infections, urinary tract infection, aspiration pneumonitis, amniotic fluid embolism, thrombophlebitis, and bowel and bladder trauma (Depp, 1996; Enkin and others, 1992). Approximately one third to one half of maternal deaths of cesarean patients are related to the procedure itself (Depp, 1996). In a subsequent pregnancy following a cesarean birth, the risk of placenta previa is increased 50% (Taylor and others, 1994). In the presence of a placenta previa, the risk of accreta, increta, or percreta is 35 times higher in those with a uterine scar from a prior cesarean than in those with an unscarred uterus (Leung, 1995).

FETAL AND NEONATAL EFFECTS

Fetal and infant mortality are usually related to hypoxia or birth trauma. Hypoxia is often the result of intense, uterine contractions that lead to uteroplacental insufficiency or cord prolapse related to malpresentation. A malpresentation can also cause such birth traumas as cranial or neck compression; fracture of the trachea, larynx, or shoulder; and spinal cord injury during an attempted vaginal delivery. The various interventions to facilitate delivery also increase the risk to the fetus of hypoxia and trauma.

According to an extensive review of literature, increased cesarean rate has not decreased the rate of neurologic disorders or cerebral palsy (Scheller, Nelson, 1994). Further, continuous electronic fetal monitoring does not provide an advantage over periodic auscultation (ACOG, 1995; refer to Chapter 3).

DIAGNOSTIC TESTING

During the prenatal period the health care provider will determine general pelvic size and configuration and fetal position and presentation. This is done by abdominal palpation and vaginal examination. The Leopold maneuver is an effective method of screening for a fetal malpresentation (Lydon-Rochelle and others, 1993).

Diagnostic prediction of the outcome of labor is rarely possible before labor. This is because it depends not only on the size and shape of the pelvis but also on the size, presentation, and position of the fetus and the quality of uterine contractions. Therefore dystocia can rarely be diagnosed until labor has progressed for a time. The diagnosis is then based on such clinical findings during labor as the uterine contraction pattern or the progression of labor as indicated by cervical dilation and effacement and fetal descent. Labor progress historically has been evaluated according to Friedman normal labor curves or the labor line of active labor. These evaluation tools provide a visual picture of some basic labor patterns, but they fail to address extrinsic factors, such as the emotional and sensory reality of birth. Therefore the Friedman labor curve and the labor line of active labor should be used with this limitation in mind.

Labor Line of Active Labor

The labor line of active labor is based on the assumption that after 4 cm dilation, a woman in active labor normally dilates at a rate of 1 cm/hr or more. Therefore, for this method, the vertical side of square-ruled graph paper should be numbered from 1 to 10 in ascending order to indicate centimeters of dilation. Horizontally across the bottom, it is numbered from 0 to 10 to indicate hours in labor. The labor line is then drawn diagonally from the lower left corner to the upper right corner (Fig. 27-7). The admission time is

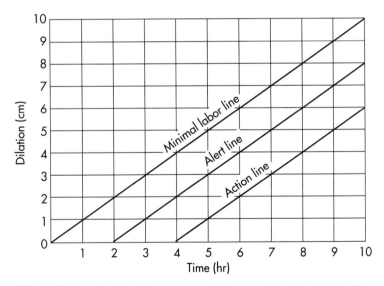

FIG. 27-7 Method of charting progress of labor against minimal labor line. Modified from O'Driscoll K, Meagher D: *Active management of labor,* ed 3, Philadelphia, 1993, Saunders; World Health Organization: *Lancet* 343:139, 1994.

the first interval entered on the graph so the cervical dilation at admission is marked on the vertical axis that corresponds with zero hour. Each time a vaginal examination is performed, the dilation is recorded on the corresponding hour's vertical axis on the graph. According to O'Driscoll and Meagher (1993), the labor line indicates the slowest rate of progress necessary to achieve delivery. If the patient's pattern of dilation falls below the labor line, a dysfunctional labor is diagnosed and oxytocin is initiated.

Some obstetricians have modified the minimal labor line by drawing alert and action lines 2 and 4 hours to the right, respectively (see Fig. 27-7). If the patient's progress is slow and crosses the alert line, the health team should be alerted to the possibility of an abnormal labor. If the labor progress is slowed enough to cross the action line, definitive measures of oxytocin or cesarean delivery should be taken (WHO, 1994).

Labor Curve

If the labor curve is chosen as the method of assessment, the amount of dilation and the fetal station found on examination should be graphed on the normal labor curve. This evaluation tool was developed by Friedman (1989) after graphically plotting the relationship of time to station and dilation of many patients in labor. He developed a normal labor curve for nulliparas and one for multiparas (Fig. 27-8).

The labor curve method of evaluation can be instituted using square-ruled graph paper. Across the top, number the hours the patient is in labor from left to right using hourly intervals. The vertical side should be numbered from 1 to 10 in ascending order to indicate dilation in centimeters and from -1 to $+5$ in descending order to indicate station. Dilation is usually indicated by small circles and station by small x's, each connected with a straight line (Friedman, 1989). The normal labor curve for a nullipara and a multipara should appear on the graph for easy comparison (Fig. 27-9). On admission the patient is asked when regular contractions began, and this time is the first interval entered on the graph. Each time a vaginal examination is performed, the dilation and station are recorded under that hour on the graph.

The various deviations from the normal labor curve are classified by Friedman (1989) as follows:

1. Prolonged latent-phase disorders (Fig. 27-10)
2. Protraction disorders, which include protracted active-phase dilation and protracted descent disorders (Fig. 27-11)

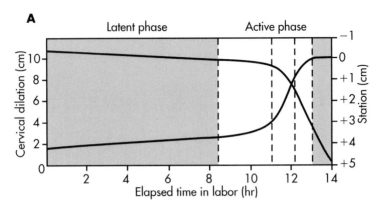

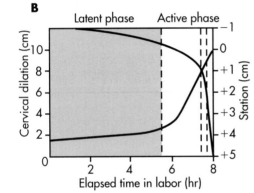

FIG. 27-8 Normal labor patterns. **A,** Normal labor pattern for nullipara. **B,** Normal labor pattern for multipara.
From Friedman E: *Hosp Pract* 5(7):82, 1970; artist: Albert Miller.

3. Arrest disorders, which include secondary arrest of dilation, arrest of descent, and failure of descent disorders (Fig. 27-12)
4. Precipitous labor disorders (Fig. 27-13)

USUAL MEDICAL TREATMENT

Cesarean delivery should be the last option. In 1994 in the United States 22% of all deliveries were by cesarean (Clarke, Taffel, 1996). Dysfunctional labor accounted for 30% of all cesarean deliveries, repeat cesarean birth for 25%, and malpresentations for 15%. Only 9% of cesarean births were done for fetal compromise (Gabay, Wolfe, 1994; Paul, Miller, 1995). Because of the increased maternal and fetal risks and the much lower cesarean delivery rate

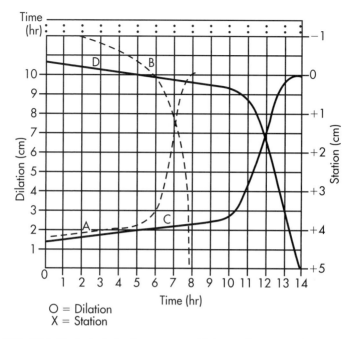

FIG. 27-9 Method of charting progress of labor against normal labor curves. *A,* Normal dilation for multigravida. *B,* Normal fetal descent for multigravida. *C,* Normal dilation for primigravida. *D,* Normal fetal descent for primigravida. Modified from Friedman E: *Hosp Pract* 5(7):82, 1970.

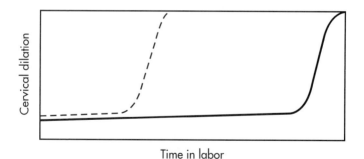

FIG. 27-10 Prolonged latent-phase pattern *(solid line)* is only disorder thus far objectively diagnosable in preparatory division of labor. It is an abnormality characterized by latent-phase duration exceeding established critical limits, shown with typical elongation of lower initial arm of sigmoid curve of cervical dilation. It is followed by a normal active phase here, as is usually the case. Average dilation curve for nulliparas *(broken line)* is shown for comparison. From Friedman EA: *Labor: clinical evaluation and management,* ed 2, New York, 1978, Appleton-Century-Crofts.

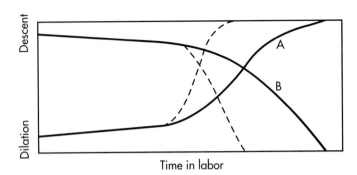

FIG. 27-11 Protraction disorders of labor. *A,* Protracted active-phase dilation pattern with abnormally slow maximum slope of dilation. *B,* Protracted descent pattern with maximum slope of descent less than prescribed critical limits of normal. These labor aberrations are similar to each other in many ways and frequently occur together in same patient. They are clearly different from average normal dilation and descent patterns *(broken lines).*
From Friedman EA: *Labor: clinical evaluation and management,* ed 2, New York, 1978, Appleton-Century-Crofts.

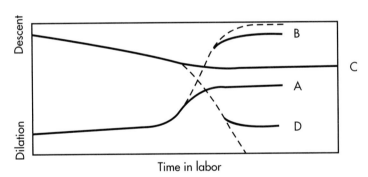

FIG. 27-12 Arrest disorders of labor. *A,* Secondary arrest of dilation pattern with documented cessation of progression in active phase. *B,* Prolonged deceleration-phase pattern with deceleration-phase duration greater than normal limits. *C,* Failure of descent in deceleration phase and second stage. *D,* Arrest of descent characterized by halted advancement of fetal station in second stage. These four abnormalities are similar in etiology, response to treatment, and prognosis, being readily differentiated from normal dilation and descent curves *(broken lines).*
From Friedman EA: *Labor: clinical evaluation and management,* ed 2, New York, 1978, Appleton-Century-Crofts.

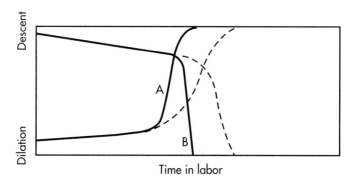

FIG. 27-13 Precipitate labor patterns. *A,* Precipitate dilation and, *B,* precipitate descent are defined by their excessively rapid rates of progressive cervical dilation and fetal descent, respectively, which distinguish them from course of normal labor *(broken lines).*

From Friedman EA: *Labor: clinical evaluation and management,* ed 2, New York, 1978, Appleton-Century-Crofts.

with no increased adverse effect on maternal and perinatal outcomes in many other countries, the goal for the year 2000 is to lower the cesarean birth rate to 15% (U.S. Public Health Service, 1991). In this attempt, ways to reduce the primary cesarean birth rate and decrease labor dystocia are being emphasized (Paul, Miller, 1995), such as the following:

1. Alternatives for a breech presentation, such as external version and possible vaginal delivery for breech presentations
2. Careful use of forceps or vacuum delivery when appropriate
3. A more aggressive use of oxytocin in the presence of a dysfunctional labor (Lopez-Zeno and others, 1992; O'Driscoll, Meagher, 1993; Peaceman, Socol, 1996; Satin and others, 1992; Xenakis and others, 1995)
4. Revision of the 2-hour limit for stage two of labor (ACOG, 1995), thus allowing the second stage of labor to continue as long as there is progress in descent without fetal compromise
5. Routine use of an epidural: being questioned because of its effect on labor progress (Morton and others, 1994; Thorp and others, 1993)
6. One-to-one labor support, which has been shown by research to decrease the rate of cesarean for a nulliparous low risk woman by 50% (Kennell and others, 1991)

To reduce the repeat cesarean birth rate, the goal is to increase the number of vaginal births after cesarean (VBAC) from 29.7% to 65% (U.S. Public Health Service, 1991). The American College of Obstetricians and Gynecologists (ACOG, 1994) recommends that repeat cesarean be done only if there is a specific indication and not because of patient choice. Therefore the current trend is to give almost all patients a trial of labor to determine if a vaginal delivery will be possible and safe for the fetus and minimize obstetric interventions. This has been demonstrated to improve maternal and perinatal outcome (Haire, Elsberry, 1991).

Dysfunctional Labor Disorders

Progress during the trial of labor should be evaluated as outlined under the signs and symptoms section of this chapter. Significant slowing of any phase of labor should be treated according to the cause of the disorder. Table 27-1 summarizes the types, possible causes, and possible management plans for each dysfunctional labor pattern.

Fetal Malpresentations

The manner in which the fetus presents also influences the outcome and manner of treatment. Table 27-2 outlines the various fetal malpresentations and the appropriate treatment.

NURSING PROCESS

PREVENTION

The nurse can have a significant influence on the progress and outcome of labor as shown in a research study by Radin and others (1993). In their research some patients of certain nurses had a low cesarean birth rate and patients of other nurses had a high rate. The nurse's use of a variety of therapeutic techniques to facilitate labor and the ability to instill confidence in the laboring patient can make a significant difference.

■ **CONTINUOUS EMOTIONAL SUPPORT**

Continuous emotional support has been demonstrated by many researchers (Gagnon, Waghorn, 1996; Hodnett, 1996; Kennell and others, 1991; Klaus and others, 1993; Wolman and others, 1993) to reduce the cesarean birth rate, the rate of forceps deliveries, the use of epidural anesthesia, and the need for oxytocin and to decrease the length of labor. Ongoing support includes emotional support for the patient and her significant others, providing comfort

Text continued on p. 742

TABLE 27-1 Summary of abnormal labor patterns

Type	Definition	Etiology	Management
Prolonged latent phase	Nullipara: latent phase of labor continues for longer than 20 hr (Friedman, 1989) Multipara: latent phase of labor continues for longer than 14 hr (Friedman, 1989) Diagnosis: after 6-8 hr of little progress, assessment can be made	Inhibitory effect of early administration of narcotic, analgesic, or sedatives Unripe cervix at onset of labor—thick, uneffaced, rigid cervix Anxiety or fear False labor Early administration of regional anesthesia Abnormal position of fetus Fetopelvic disproportion	*Expectant management* Therapeutic rest attempted with warm bath or shower and administration of large doses of narcotic analgesic such as morphine narcotic agonist-antagonist such as Nubain, or muscle relaxant such as Vistaril to inhibit contractions and provide rest period of 4-6 hr Assess for high stress and decreased fluid intake since they may cause irritable uterus If patient was in false labor or overly anxious, when she awakens her contractions will be gone; otherwise, she will usually awaken in active labor Only 5%-10% awaken to original problem and may benefit from oxytocin (Cohen, Brennan, 1995) If anesthetic has been used, let it wear off

Continued

TABLE 27-1 Summary of abnormal labor patterns—cont'd

Type	Definition	Etiology	Management
Protraction disorders Protracted active-phase dilation Protracted descent	Nullipara: rate of dilation in active phase less than 1.2 cm/hr or rate of descent less than 2.0 cm/hr (Friedman, 1989) Multipara: rate of dilation in active phase less than 1.5 cm/hr or rate of descent less than 2.0 cm/hr (Friedman, 1989)	Fetopelvic disproportion Excessive sedation Fetal malpresentation Early conduction anesthesia Rupture of membranes before onset of labor Inadequate nutrition Dehydration Maternal exhaustion Extreme anxiety	Amniotomy Administer labor stimulant *Active management* When cervical dilation falls 1-2 hr behind expected rate of progress, membranes are ruptured and trial of oxytocin augmentation is utilized in treatment of all patients (Cardozo, Pearce, 1990; O'Driscoll, Meagher, 1993; Sanchez-Ramos and others, 1990) *Expectant management* Rule out obvious FPD If FPD, patient will deliver by cesarean Initiate or continue following nursing interventions Monitoring continuously labor progress and fetal well-being Continuing to inform patient of progress and reassuring regarding possible reasons for slow progress

Encouraging patient to keep bladder empty

Providing physical and emotional support: letting her know you are there for her and that you have confidence in her ability

Keeping patient informed and allaying anxiety

Encouraging ambulation, position change

Assessing fluid and electrolyte needs and administering intravenous (IV) fluid as ordered

Augmentation with breast stimulation or oxytocin if contractions are ineffective because of myometrial dysfunction (Friedman, 1989)

Medicate if patient unable to relax between contractions; however, use of excessive sedation or conduction anesthesia can inhibit or arrest labor further (Friedman, 1989)

Continued

FPD, Fetopelvic disproportion.

TABLE 27-1 Summary of abnormal labor patterns—cont'd

Type	Definition	Etiology	Management
			Prognosis usually good if no signs of fetal compromise develop; cesarean birth necessary if non-reassuring FHR pattern develops
			Following protracted labor, increased rise of shoulder dystocia and postpartum hemorrhage
Arrest disorders			
Secondary arrest of dilation	Progressive dilation during active labor stops before full dilation occurs and continues for 2 hr or longer (Friedman, 1989)	Fetopelvic disproportion (most common cause; Cohen, Brennan, 1995)	*Active management*
		Excessive sedation	At first signs of lack of cervical change, membranes are ruptured and trial of oxytocin augmentation is used (Cardozo, Pearce, 1990)
Arrest of descent	Progressive descent stops during second stage of labor for longer than 1 hr in multipara and longer than 2 hr in nullipara	Fetal malpresentation (persistent occiput, face, and brow)	If arrest persists or fetal distress develops, delivery must be by cesarean; 11% required cesarean delivery (Cardozo, Pearce, 1990)
		Conduction anesthesia	
		Exhausted uterus	*Expectant management*
Failure of descent	Onset of descent fails to occur during deceleration phase of labor	Distended bladder	Assess for obvious FPD and fetal malpresentation
		Extreme anxiety	If obvious FPD, delivery will be cesarean
		Maternal exhaustion	
		Inadequate nutrition	

			If obvious FPD not indicated, labor stimulant will be used; postarrest slope should be monitored closely; if FPD not present, postarrest slope should be as great or greater than prearrest slope (Friedman, 1989) Continue or implement same nursing interventions as outlined for protracted disorders If arrest persists or nonreassuring FHR pattern develops, delivery must be by cesarean; 15%-20% will require cesarean birth (Bottoms and others, 1987; Friedman, 1989)
Precipitous labor	Nullipara: cervix dilates faster than 5 cm/hr or descent faster than 1 cm/12 min Multipara: cervix dilates faster than 10 cm/hr or descent faster than 1 cm/6 min	Abnormally low cervical resistance Abnormally strong uterine or abdominal muscular contractions	Tocolytic agents, such as magnesium sulfate or ritodrine/terbutaline, may be used in attempt to slow down progress of labor Magnesium sulfate bolus for 20 min followed by continuous infusion is beneficial (Valenzuela, Foster, 1990)

FHR, Fetal heart rate.

TABLE 27-2 Fetal malpresentations

	Occiput posterior	Face	Brow
Definition	Fetal occiput lies in either right or left posterior quadrant of mother's pelvis	Presenting head completely extended	Presenting head mid-way be-tween full flexion and extreme extension
Presenting part	Occiput	Chin (mentum)	Brow
Incidence	10%-25%	0.2%	0.2%
Diagnosis			
Leopold maneuver	Patient will often complain of severe back or suprapubic pain; differentiation by Leopold maneuver is difficult	Absence of smooth, flexed spine; prominent extremities and head	No differen-tiation
Vaginal ex-amination	Anterior fontanel can be felt in anterior quad-rant of mother's pelvis and pos-terior fontanel in posterior quadrant	Nose, eyes, and mouth can be felt	Anterior fon-tanel can be felt in center of cervical opening with eyes on one side

Shoulder	Compound presentation	Breech
Fetal spine lies vertical to mother's spine	One or more fetal extremities accompany presenting part	Buttocks of fetus present in one of three attitudes: Frank: thighs flexed and legs lie alongside fetal body Complete: legs flexed at thighs, allowing feet to present with buttocks Footing: one or both thighs extended and present before buttocks
Scapula		Sacrum
0.33%	0.01%	4%
Abdomen may look wider than long; head can be palpated on one side of mother's abdomen and buttocks on other	No differentiation	Fetal heart tones heard best above umbilicus; fetal head palpated in upper part of uterus
Scapula can be felt or no presenting part reached since it is often high	Fetal extremity felt alongside presenting part	Soft presenting part felt

Continued

TABLE 27-2 Fetal malpresentations—cont'd

	Occiput posterior	Face	Brow
Treatment	Almost all fetuses rotate spontaneously to anterior position and are delivered vaginally; in 10% that do not rotate completely, rotation usually done with forceps	Vaginal delivery if anterior rotation of chin occurs	Vaginal delivery if brow presentation converts by flexion to occiput presentation or extension to face presentation
	If posterior position persists without progress, cesarean delivery is done	Cesarean delivery done if chin is directed posterior and progress stops	Cesarean delivery if brow presentation persists

FPD, Fetopelvic disproportion.

measures, keeping the patient and her significant others informed, and being an advocate when needed.

■ **MOVEMENT**

Experimental studies clearly show that position and frequency of position change have a profound effect on uterine activity and efficiency. For specifics refer to the nursing interventions for activity/position pattern under the *enhancement of labor progress* nursing diagnosis.

■ **EMPTY BLADDER**

A full bladder interferes with fetal descent and may lead to a dysfunctional labor pattern.

Shoulder	Compound presentation	Breech
Cesarean delivery is best management; external cephalic version can be attempted under very controlled circumstances if placenta previa or FPD not present	Vaginal delivery unless cord prolapses or labor fails to progress	External version may be attempted between 36 and 38 wk of gestation Vaginal delivery in frank or complete breech, with adequate neck flexion, gestational age greater than 36 wk, and estimated fetal weight between 2000 and 4000 g
	Immediate cesarean delivery if prolapsed cord develops or progress stops	Cesarean delivery for all others because of increased risk of cord prolapse, entrapment by cervix caused by small trunk/head ratio in premature or small-for-gestational-age infant, and FPD in fetus over 4000 g

■ **NUTRITION**

According to Hodnett (1996) and Keirse's review of research (1989), simple measures such as encouraging movement and allowing women to eat and drink as desired may be as effective as oxytocin for a sizable portion of laboring women considered to be in need of labor augmentation. However, because of the rare but possibly devastating consequences of gastric aspiration in the event of general anesthesia, many labor and delivery units have a policy that the laboring patient should take nothing by mouth except sips of water or ice chips. Because the routine policy of giving the laboring patient nothing to eat or drink has not been scientifically substantiated and may affect her progress in labor, this policy should be seriously evaluated by labor and delivery medical personnel. This statement is based on the following:

- The policy of giving nothing by mouth (NPO) or ice chips only came into practice because of anecdotal reports of aspiration related to general anesthesia (McKay, Mahan, 1988; Roberts, Ludka, 1994).
- The risk of aspiration is almost entirely associated with general anesthesia (Johnson and others, 1989).
- Gastric emptying time is rarely delayed in early labor. Large volume of intake and fat slow gastric emptying time (Roberts, Ludka, 1994), as do narcotic medications (Keppler, 1988; McKay, Mahan, 1988).
- Fasting does not ensure an empty stomach or lowered gastric acidity (Johnson and others, 1989). According to Crawford (1986), aspiration-related maternal deaths rose after the dietary restriction in labor was implemented.
- The major reason for aspiration of gastric contents causing maternal mortality is improper anesthetic techniques. This has been shown repeatedly through research (Johnson and others, 1989; McKay, Mahan, 1988).
- The key factor in preventing aspiration deaths is proper administration of general anesthesia by an anesthesiologist or nurse anesthetist trained in perinatal anesthesiology. This includes application of cricoid pressure, in which the cricoid cartilage is pushed against the esophagus by a trained assistant. Next a cuffed endotracheal tube is correctly placed to seal the airway. Then proper placement of the endotracheal tube should be checked before releasing the cricoid pressure (Douglas, 1988; Johnson and others, 1989; McKay, Mahan, 1988).
- Research indicates that when low risk women are allowed to eat and drink during labor, 85.5% will choose to eat more in early labor and taper off during active labor. Women who were allowed to eat required less pain medication and less oxytocin, and their labors were shorter (Roberts, Ludka, 1994).
- Restricting food and fluid during labor can cause dehydration and ketosis.
- Water-soluble vitamins, such as vitamin C and B complex, are quickly excreted from the body when the woman is given nothing to eat. Vitamin B_1 is very important for the metabolism of carbohydrates used by the contracting uterine muscle (Newton and others, 1988).

- Enforced hunger and routine intravenous (IV) insertion can be very stressful for the laboring woman (Newton and others, 1988; Simkin, 1986a,b). An IV apparatus can interfere with movement as well.
- Routinely enforcing an NPO status, starting IV fluids, and placing a laboring mother in bed psychologically imply sickness, which can interfere with the normal progress of labor and set the mother up for labor augmentation or failure to progress (Broach, Newton, 1988).

NURSING DIAGNOSES/COLLABORATIVE PROBLEMS AND INTERVENTIONS

- **ENHANCEMENT OF LABOR PROGRESS THROUGH EACH OF THE 11 FUNCTIONAL HEALTH PATTERNS** to decrease risk of dystocia, epidural anesthesia, and instrumental delivery.

  DESIRED OUTCOME: The labor will progress according to the normal labor pattern without signs of fetal compromise.

  INTERVENTIONS

  Health-perception/health-management pattern
  1. Assess the woman's risk for dystocia.
  2. Assess the woman's progress in labor.
  3. Ask the patient and her coach about their birth plan. Parents have varying needs and expectations of care. As long as it does not affect the health of the mother or baby, to promote and carry out the plan would be therapeutic. Birth plans can decrease the family's anxiety and increase their feeling of control while facilitating communication with the health care team (Springer, 1996). However, during the prenatal care, families must be instructed that although a birth plan is a manner in which they sort out what will make their birth experience satisfying, it must be open to change when unexpected events develop (Jannke, 1995).

  Nutritional/metabolic pattern (preconception)
  1. Educate women about the importance of attaining an appropriate body weight before conception.
  2. Educate underweight women about the importance of eating appropriate nutritional foods in each of the food groups and avoiding empty-calorie foods, high in fat and refined sugar, before and during pregnancy. (Being underweight increases the risk of a small-for-gestational-age fetus and preterm labor, which increases the risk for a breech presentation and cesarean delivery.)
  3. Educate women who are overweight before conception

about the importance of a nutritious, weight-control, life-style diet change as opposed to an extreme quick weight loss program that usually leads to a return in weight gain and depletes the nutritional stores needed for a healthy pregnancy. Weight reduction is contraindicated during pregnancy. (Being overweight is related to an increased risk of gestational diabetes and large-for-gestational-age infants that increases the risk of cesarean birth.)

4. Educate diabetics about the importance of achieving normal blood sugar levels before conception and maintaining this control throughout conception with diet, exercise, insulin if needed, and self-monitoring of blood glucose. This will decrease the risk of congenital anomalies and a large-for-gestational-age or small-for-gestational-age fetus, which would increase the risk of a cesarean delivery.

Nutritional/metabolic pattern (intrapartum)

1. During early labor, unless there is a medical or obstetric contraindication, encourage the patient to eat high-carbohydrate, low-fat foods (e.g., frozen yogurt, lightly cooked eggs, crisp toast, canned fruit) and drink fluids with electrolytes (e.g., Gatorade, fruit juices, tea with honey, clear broth). During active labor, encourage electrolyte fluids only.

2. If medication becomes necessary, the patient is at high risk for a general anesthesia, or she is experiencing gastric upset, allow clear fluids only. IV fluids may then be therapeutic.

3. Question a labor policy that states routine use of IV fluids. IV dextrose during labor has been shown to increase the risk of hypoglycemia in the newborn (Hazle, 1986; Keppler, 1988). Lactated Ringer's solution has been shown to cause fewer problems if used when IV fluids are indicated during labor (ACOG, 1988).

4. If IV fluids are ordered only to keep a vein open, determine if a heparin lock could be used instead.

Elimination pattern

1. Encourage the patient to void every 2 hours. A full bladder interferes with fetal descent, and the sense of a full bladder is depressed related to pressure by the fetus.

2. Assess when the patient had her last bowel movement and whether she has been experiencing the natural diarrhea that

frequently precedes labor. Enemas are not needed unless the natural diarrhea did not occur. An enema is contraindicated if membranes are ruptured and during the second stage of labor.

Activity/position pattern
Antepartum
1. Educate pregnant women as to the benefits of a consistent, low-impact exercise program, such as walking, swimming, bicycling, or low-impact aerobics. Fitness during pregnancy reduces such pregnancy discomforts as back pain and fatigue and fosters a more normal labor and delivery (Clapp, 1990; Wong, McKenzie, 1987). Varrassi and others (1989) found that plasma beta-endorphin levels are elevated in women who exercise during pregnancy as compared with expectant women who do not exercise. A higher endorphin level means a higher pain threshold.

Intrapartum: stage one
1. During labor, provide opportunities for position changes every 30 minutes and encourage position changes. Choice of position change should be based on maternal preference, safety, comfort, effective progress, and knowledge of hemodynamics (Fenwick, Simkin, 1987; Romond, Baker, 1985; Rossi, Lindell, 1986). Malpresentations are frequently associated with increased pain. Allowing the mother to obtain a position of more comfort will frequently facilitate a favorable fetal rotation by altering the alignment of the presenting part with the pelvis. As the mother continues to change position based on comfort, the optimum presentation will be maintained (Fenwick, Simkin, 1987).
2. Supine positions should be avoided since they cause compression of the vena cava and decrease blood return to the heart.
3. Encourage the laboring woman to ambulate (Fig. 27-14, *A*). Ambulation facilitates weight-bearing and pelvic changes, which encourage rotation and descent of the fetus (Fenwick, Simkin, 1987).
4. During stage one of labor, the lateral recumbent and upright positions (see Fig. 27-14, *B, C, E,* and *F*) increase uterine intensity, decrease frequency, and decrease vena caval compression (McKay, Roberts, 1989; Roberts and others, 1983). Therefore the uterine contractions are more effective

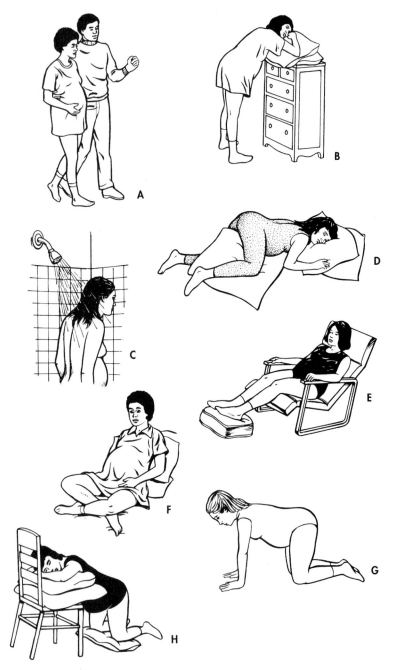

FIG. 27-14 Various maternal positions during first-stage labor.

because the upright position permits relaxation of the abdominal wall, allowing the fundus to fall forward. This facilitates the engagement of the fetal head and descent. As the fetal head is pushed against the cervix, the uterus receives increased stimulation to contract (McKay, Roberts, 1989). The supine and sitting positions increase the vena caval compression and decrease uterine intensity and frequency (Chen and others, 1987; McKay, Roberts, 1989; Roberts and others, 1983). Therefore uterine contractions are not as effective. These positions may cause poor alignment of the fetal presenting part to the pelvic inlet as well (Fenwick, Simkin, 1987).

Intrapartum: occiput posterior presentation

1. Assess for signs of an occiput posterior presentation, such as (a) complaint of suprapubic pain or back pain, (b) feeling the urge to push before full dilation, (c) abdominal contour showing a depression around the umbilical area, (d) early decelerations during latent phase labor, and (e) arrest of active labor (Biancuzzo, 1993).

2. When the fetus is in an occiput posterior presentation, having the woman obtain an "all fours" position or a kneeling (see Fig. 27-14, *G*) and leaning-forward position (see Fig. 27-14, *H*) may promote rotation to an anterior presentation. Pelvic rock and lateral abdominal stroking may further facilitate head rotation. The abdominal stroking should be performed in the direction toward which the fetal head should rotate. For rest periods the woman should be encouraged to assume a side-lying position on the side toward which the baby should turn (Biancuzzo, 1993; Hodnett, 1996; Roberts, Woolley, 1996).

Intrapartum: stage two

1. Provide care for second-stage labor based on understanding of the three phases of second stage of labor: (a) latent phase, a time to rest when there is a lull in the contractions; (b) active phase, when fetal descent takes place facilitated by maternal pushing; and (c) transition or perineal phase, which just precedes birth and in which the mother needs active support to relax and let the birth occur (Aderhold, Roberts, 1991; Roberts, Woolley, 1996). This phase is frequently characterized by a burning perineal pain as the head stretches the perineum if no anesthetic has been given.

2. The upright, slightly curled forward position (Fig. 27-15) decreases the length of second-stage labor, fetal heart rate (FHR) abnormalities, instrumental births, and pain perception because of decreased release of stress-related hormones (McKay, Roberts, 1989; Shannahan, Cottrell, 1989). Chen and others (1987) found the curled-forward, sitting position during the second stage of labor to increase the bearing-down sensation and increase the release of oxytocin, thereby enhancing effective pushing and shortening this phase of labor. The reclining-back, sitting position puts pressure on the sacrum, restricting posterior movement and reducing the pelvic size (Fenwick, Simkin, 1987).

3. Avoid the supine position during the second stage of labor since gravity works against the woman's pushing efforts (Fenwick, Simkin, 1987) and it has been shown to decrease fetal artery pH (Johnstone and others, 1987).

4. It may be advantageous for women to push in response to their body's urge rather than to sustain bearing-down efforts while holding their breath unless there is an obstetric indication to facilitate an immediate delivery (Held, 1994; Liu, 1989; McKay and others, 1990). This type of pushing initiated by the woman in response to an irresistible sensation is usually accompanied by expiratory grunting or vocalization and is less fatiguing to the mother and has less effect on umbilical cord blood gases (Cosner and deJong, 1993; Fuller and others, 1993; Parnell and others, 1993). Sustained, breath-holding bearing down can impose a hypoxic environment for the fetus and may conflict with the patient's own body sensations and increase the risk of perineal trauma (Aderhold, Roberts, 1991; McKay and others, 1990; Paine, Tinker, 1992; Parnell and others, 1993; Thomson, 1993).

5. Manage the "urge to push before full dilation" by assessing if (a) cervix is dilated 8 to 9 cm, (b) cervix is soft and retracting with contractions, (c) fetal head is rotating to transverse or anterior position, and (d) station is at least +1. Then allow patient to push at the peak of the contraction if she is experiencing an irresistible urge to push (Roberts, Woolley, 1996).

6. Manage "complete dilation and no urge to push" by (a) first assessing the fetal position, fetal station, and FHR and (b) then encouraging the mother to rest until she feels the urge to push, which is the result of the presenting part

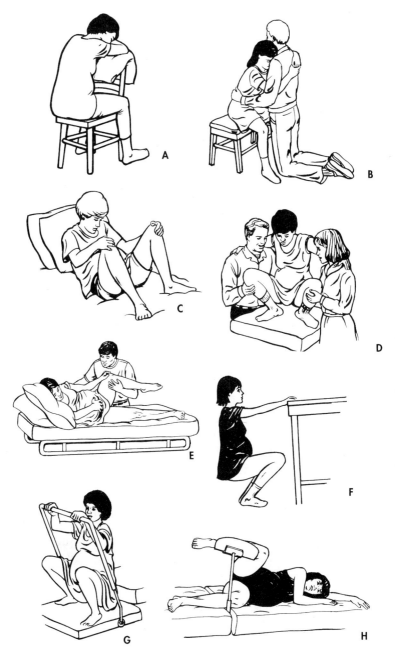

FIG. 27-15 Various maternal positions during second-stage labor.

stimulating the stretch receptors of the pelvic floor (Roberts, Woolley, 1996).

7. If second-stage labor is not progressing because of a large fetus in relationship to the size of the mother's pelvis, squatting (see Fig. 27-15, *D, F,* and *G*) may increase the pelvis size 0.5 to 2 cm (Fenwick, Simkin, 1987; Golay and others, 1993). Squatting may increase the bearing-down sensation and enhance effective pushing as well (Kurokawa, Zilkoski, 1985). Therefore it has been shown to shorten second-stage labor, lessen the need of oxytocin, decrease the need for mechanical-assisted deliveries, and decrease the need for an episiotomy (Golay and others, 1993; Roberts, Woolley, 1996). NOTE: Squatting is con-traindicated for patients with epidural analgesia.

8. Lateral recumbent position may be beneficial during the transitional phase of stage two labor when less bearing-down force is needed, to help control the speed of the delivery and decrease the risk of perineal lacerations (Golay and others, 1993; Roberts, Woolley, 1996).

Rest/relaxation pattern

1. Encourage use of visualization, patterned breathing, attention focusing, and music. These stimuli affect the thalamus part of the brain and influence the limbic system, which governs emotional responses as well as inhibition of pain transmission (Di Franco, 1988; Simkin, 1987). The limbic system has been shown to increase pain tolerance by reducing anxiety, decreasing catecholamine response, and decreasing muscle tension. It enhances blood flow to the uterus as well (Lowe, 1996).

Cognitive pattern

1. If involved with childbirth education, provide not only information about the birth process but also activities that will instill confidence to control pain and deal with childbirth-related fears (Crowe, von Baeyer, 1989).

2. Assess the patient's and her coach's understanding of labor, delivery, and effective tools. Determine which childbirth education method the couple plans to use, if any.

3. Assess the woman's level of confidence in her and her coach's ability to use the techniques they learned in their childbirth class. Increased confidence and decreased labor pain are related (Lowe, 1991).

4. Fill in the patient's and coach's knowledge gaps between contractions.

5. Teach the patient and coach to pace themselves, like in a race, and not to use all their tools at first.
6. Keep the patient and her coach informed of the progress.

Perceptual pattern

1. Assess patient's level of pain, location, and the degree of distress it is causing her (Lowe, 1996). A 10-point scale is an effective tool to use (1 = no pain or distress, and 10 = the worst pain or distress imaginable).
2. Assess for leg cramps.
3. Assess for back discomfort.
4. Assess how the patient and her coach feel they should respond to pain because of any cultural or personal values.
5. Encourage appropriate comfort measures.
   a. Back rubs and counterpressure for back labor
   b. Cool washcloth on the forehead if feeling hot or nauseated
   c. Hydrotherapy through baths and showers (activates bodywide tactile receptors, which transport pleasant stimuli over the pathways that pain stimuli must travel, thus closing the gate to pain and reversing the fight-or-flight responses that frequently occur during labor while increasing uterine activity [Simkin, 1995b])
   d. Whirlpool bath (decreases analgesia needs and instrumental rate while enhancing maternal satisfaction and confidence with no increased risk of infection [Rush and others, 1996]); contraindicated in the presence of thick meconium, oxytocin infusion, bleeding, or heavy bloody show [Rush and others, 1996])
   e. Superficial heat and cold with packs (activates local tactile receptors, thus closing the gate to some pain stimuli)
   f. Touch and massage (facilitates relaxation and bombards the brain with another stimulus, decreasing the amount of pain sensation being perceived)
   g. Position change and motion such as rocking or walking (Lowe, 1996)
   h. Double hip squeeze (decreases back pain [Simkin, 1995b])
   i. Moaning (decreases pain and medication need by releasing endorphins [Threlfall-Mase, 1997])
   j. Provide Chap Stick for dry lips, and keep the linen clean and dry, thus decreasing extraneous uncomfortable sensations and thereby the total amount of pain experienced

    k. Effleurage to abdomen (promotes relaxation of the abdominal muscle, allowing the uterine muscle to be unrestrained)

    l. Alleviation of leg cramps by stretching the cramping muscle instead of massaging

6. Value the doula if present as an important member of the health team.

7. Keep the patient clean and dry to promote comfort and decrease infection risk.

8. Portray to her a deep sense of empathy and caring that transmits confidence so she is enabled to trust her own body and relax more completely (Lowe, 1991).

9. Aid the woman to utilize appropriate techniques so her need for anesthesia or analgesia will be less. An epidural analgesia may increase the incidence of cesarean birth for dystocia, especially in the nulliparous woman (Morton and others, 1994; Thorp, Breedlove, 1996; Thorp and others, 1993) or increase the need of a forceps or vacuum delivery (Kaminski and others, 1987).

10. Know when pharmacologic interventions are needed and use them effectively.

    a. Narcotic analgesic, narcotic agonist-antagonist, or analgesic potentiators should be administered during the peak of a contraction and titrated to desired effects—not to a specific dose.

    b. Epidural analgesia is the most effective method of providing pain relief, but as with all procedures, there are accompanying risks that should be discussed with the expectant mother, ideally during a prenatal visit. Refer to the later section in this chapter on epidural anesthesia.

    c. Intrathecal narcotics (injection of narcotics in the subarachnoid space) is another form of pain management during labor (Manning, 1996).

Self-perception/self-concept pattern

1. Assess attitude toward pregnancy, labor, and delivery.

2. Provide ongoing labor support. Continuous labor support decreases the cesarean birth rate by 50%, decreases the length of labor, and significantly decreases the mother's need for pain medication (Hofmeyr and others, 1991; Kennell and others, 1991; Klaus and others, 1993; Wolman and others, 1993).

3. Ensure modesty at all times throughout the birth experience.

4. Facilitate a positive body image by helping the laboring woman maintain body control. This can be promoted if the nurse understands the laboring woman's behaviors and provides appropriate nursing interventions (Richardson, 1984).

   a. During the latent phase of labor the woman is usually excited, anxious, and very distractible. This is an ideal time to gather an assessment and educate as indicated.

   b. During the accelerated and maximum-slope dilation phases of active labor, the laboring woman has a need to focus because of the increasing inner body tension. The woman should not be distracted during a contraction but encouraged to focus on previously learned patterned breathing, utilizing mind focusing, relaxation, and diminished verbal and gross motor activities. Between contractions, questions, instructions, and socializing are distracting and appropriate.

   c. During the deceleration phase of active labor (transition), the laboring woman is very vulnerable. Because of the pain intensity, focusing is no longer effective. Rhythmic and repetitive verbal and gross motor activities are more effective in displacing tension. The woman may moan, chant, rock her body, or pedal her feet to maintain body control. Soft, repetitive, encouraging verbal contact from the coach or nurse can be helpful. Tactile intrusiveness or verbal demands only increase tension. Between contractions the woman frequently desires rest instead of social interaction.

Role relationship pattern

1. Assess role expectations of all participants during the birth process.
2. Assess economic needs and concerns.
3. Assess cultural practices that influence the various roles of the participants.
4. Promote family members' involvement, according to their birth plan, if possible.
5. Provide therapeutic interventions for the support person or persons by evaluating their comfort in the labor situation, orienting them to the environment and equipment being used, asking if they have any special requests, acknowledging their physical and psychologic needs, providing times for nutritional snacks, encouraging them to actively participate, and providing a welcome environment.

Coping/stress tolerance pattern

1. Assess the patient's and coach's fears and concerns.
2. Assess level of emotional tension with level of effective coping. Maintain an equilibrium, if possible, with comfort measures, effective labor support, and appropriate use of medications. Some anxiety is therapeutic for the birth process because increased catecholamines prepare the body for action, facilitate the oxygen conservation of the fetus, stimulate the adsorption of fluid from the newborn's lungs, facilitate neonatal respiratory function by stimulating surfactant release, and promote alertness in the neonate for the first 30 to 60 minutes of life (Copper, Goldenberg, 1990). Excessive catecholamines are not therapeutic and can decrease efficiency of uterine contractions, causing dystocia, decreasing uteroplacental blood flow, and increasing the possibility of poor neonatal adjustment (Simkin, 1986).
3. Offer ongoing encouragement, and avoid comments that may worry the patient.
4. Minimize common stressors of labor such as restriction of activity, vaginal examinations, and IV fluids.
5. Teach the family how to deal with unexpected changes in their birth plan through empowerment.
   a. Ask whether this is an emergency or there is time to discuss the situation.
   b. If it is not an emergency, ask questions that help them understand the situation.
   c. Ask questions to learn the risks and benefits of the suggested intervention.
   d. Ask questions to determine alternatives to the suggested intervention.

- **ALTERATION IN THE LABOR PROCESS**
  DESIRED OUTCOME: Labor progress will continue within normal limits without fetal compromise.
  INTERVENTIONS
  1. Determine onset of true labor.
  2. Evaluate the uterine contraction pattern every 30 to 60 minutes, or more often if needed, for frequency, duration, intensity, and resting tone.
  3. Assess state of cervix as to soft or hard, effaced or long, dilatable or resistant, and amount of dilation as indicated (depending on phase of labor). Use the Bishop system or a comparable scoring system.

4. Assess fetal position, station, and status of the presenting part.

5. Assess for a malpresentation by doing the Leopold maneuver to facilitate decision making as to maternal positioning.

6. Plot and compare the patient's labor using the Friedman labor graph or the labor line of active labor.

7. Assess for discomfort and tension.

8. Assess for signs of dehydration and electrolyte imbalance.

9. Assess for signs of hypoglycemia. A prolonged difficult labor depletes the mother's energy and glucose stores.

10. Encourage patient to void every 1 to 2 hours.

11. Catheterize for distended bladder if unable to void.

12. Encourage patient to verbalize anxieties and fears.

13. Encourage patient to try various position changes to facilitate labor progress (see Figs. 27-14 and 27-15).

14. Monitor for effective use of breathing and relaxation techniques.

15. Provide continuous emotional support. Be supportive of coping methods, and provide help with new ones as needed.

16. Provide support to the labor coach.

17. Encourage rest between contractions.

18. If labor begins to progress slower than normal, encourage ambulation and alternative positioning if not contraindicated.

19. Be prepared to administer a labor stimulant as ordered (see Chapter 26).

20. If it is necessary to withhold analgesia or anesthesia, explain the need to the patient and her coach.

21. Keep the attending physician informed of labor progress.

22. If a dysfunctional labor pattern develops, outline the treatment plan so that the patient and her coach will be prepared for what might occur. Stress the normalcy of patient's physiologic response to labor.

■ **RISK FOR INFECTION** related to prolonged labor and prolonged rupture of membranes.

DESIRED OUTCOME: The patient will remain infection free as indicated by her temperature remaining below 38° C (100° F), absence of foul-smelling vaginal discharge, and a white blood cell count between 4500 and 10,000/mm^3.

INTERVENTIONS

1. Assess temperature every 2 hours following rupture of membranes.
2. Assess amniotic fluid for foul odor.
3. Refer to such laboratory data as white blood cell count.
4. Change linen as needed.
5. Keep patient clean and dry.
6. Notify the physician if temperature above 38° C (100° F) develops, amniotic fluid develops a foul odor, or white blood cell counts are greater than 16,000/mm^3.

- **RISK FOR IMPAIRED FETAL GAS EXCHANGE** related to hypertonic uterine contractions preventing the intervillous spaces from filling adequately with oxygenated blood and cord prolapse caused by a fetal malpresentation.

  DESIRED OUTCOME: The fetus will remain active, and its heart rate will remain between 110 and 160 beats/min with present variability.

  INTERVENTIONS

  1. If the laboring woman develops a dysfunctional labor, monitor the FHR continuously (see Chapter 3).
  2. Assess color of the amniotic fluid. The passage of meconium may indicate fetal stress except in the presence of a breech presentation when pressure on the buttocks may cause the anal sphincter to relax.
  3. Assess FHR immediately following rupture of membranes to assess for cord prolapse or entanglement.
  4. Notify physician of the development of any signs of a nonreassuring FHR pattern, such as late or severe variable decelerations, increase or decrease in FHR baseline, or loss of variability.

- **POTENTIAL COMPLICATION OF FAILURE TO PROGRESS: SHOULDER DYSTOCIA**

  DESIRED OUTCOME: Shoulder dystocia will not develop, or if it occurs, no injury will result.

  INTERVENTIONS

  1. Be familiar with the major risk factors for shoulder dystocia, which according to the acronym *ADOPE* are as follows: A—**A**dvanced maternal age, D—**D**iabetes, O—**O**besity, P—**P**ostterm pregnancy or prior large-for-gestational-age infant, and E—**E**xcessive maternal weight gain (O'Leary, 1992). Other significant factors are mac-

rosomic fetus, enlarging caput succedaneum, or a dysfunctional labor pattern (Kochenour, Clark, 1994).

2. Assess labor progress closely, and use the squatting method when appropriate to increase pelvic capacity (Golay and others, 1993).

3. An early indication of shoulder dystocia is when the fetal head retracts against the mother's perineum as soon as the head is delivered (Hall, 1997).

4. When shoulder dystocia is diagnosed, the nurse can be prepared to assist by calling for added assistance, an anesthesiologist or nurse anesthetist, and a pediatrician or intensive care nursing team.

5. Be prepared to catheterize the patient to ensure a completely emptied bladder.

6. Be prepared to assist in the recommended shoulder dystocia manipulations as the health care provider instructs. Refer to Table 27-3 for various sequential maneuvers.

7. Following the delivery, assess the baby's Moro reflex, check for a fractured clavicle or humerus, and, if ordered, obtain cord blood for pH. (A complete symmetric Moro response usually indicates no brachial plexus injury, which is the most common serious resulting injury [Benedetti, 1991; Nocon, 1991].) Increased intracranial pressure and hypoxia occur less often.

8. If an injury occurred, be prepared to discuss the possible outcomes with the parents after the pediatrician has told them about the outcomes. Eighty percent of these injuries will resolve and cause no permanent damage with appropriate treatment (Benedetti, 1989).

9. Assess for postpartum hemorrhage since this is the greatest risk to the mother from a shoulder dystocia. The hemorrhage is usually related to uterine atony or vaginal or cervical lacerations (Bowes, 1994; Hall, 1997). Other maternal trauma can include bladder injury, vaginal hematoma, uterine rupture, or endometritis.

10. Document appropriately on the fetal monitor strip such things as the emergence of the fetal head and attempted maneuvers.

■ **POTENTIAL COMPLICATIONS OF EXTERNAL VERSION: PLACENTAL ABRUPTION AND CORD ENTANGLEMENT**
DESIRED OUTCOME: In the event of an external version, no complication will result.

TABLE 27-3 Sequential shoulder dystocia maneuvers

Name	Benefits and risks	Maneuver
McRoberts maneuver (Fig. 27-16)	Noninvasive Safe Straightens sacrum and decreases angle of incline of symphysis pubis Dislodges impacted shoulder 90% of time (Gonik and others, 1989)	Assist by grasping mother's posterior thighs and flexing them against her abdomen Fundal pressure is usually inappropriate since it may further impact anterior shoulder against symphysis and increase risk of a brachial plexus injury (Hernandez, Wendel, 1990; O'Leary, Leonetti, 1990)
Suprapubic pressure (Figs. 27-17 and 27-18)	Noninvasive Second maneuver to be used since it may cause a clavicular fracture	Assist by exerting firm downward or oblique pressure on anterior shoulder just above symphysis pubis Instruct mother to push during this maneuver
Woods screw maneuver (Fig. 27-19)	Invasive technique Thought to attempt to unscrew fetus like a bolt is unscrewed from a nut (Horger, 1995)	Health care deliverer intravaginally applies pressure against posterior shoulder, rotating it to an anterior position Health care deliverer may request suprapubic pressure during maneuver to help keep anterior shoulder adducted (Naef, Martin, 1995)

Rubin rotational maneuver or reverse Woods screw maneuver (Fig. 27-20)	Invasive technique	Health care deliverer intravaginally applies pressure against scapula of anterior shoulder and rotates it forward 180 degrees. Health care deliverer may request suprapubic pressure during maneuver to help keep anterior shoulder adducted (O'Leary, 1992)
Delivery of posterior arm (Fig. 27-21)	Invasive. Requires a large episiotomy. Risk of humerus fracture	Health care deliverer intravaginally applies pressure at antecubital fossa, which causes fetal arm to flex, at which time it is grasped and drawn across chest and toward opposite side of fetal face
Cephalic replacement	Last resort	Health care deliverer returns fetal head to maternal pelvis, followed by an emergency cesarean birth

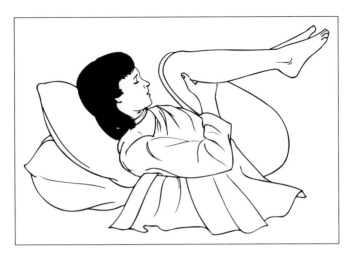

FIG. 27-16

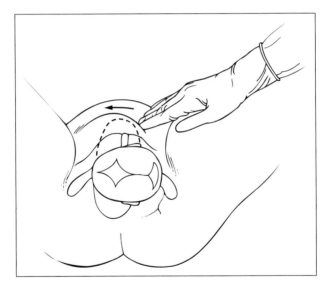

FIG. 27-17

INTERVENTIONS

Preprocedural

    1. Evaluate the patient's and her coach's understanding of the procedure. Approximately 65% of all attempted external versions are successful with a 2% reversion rate (Laros and others, 1995; Lau and others, 1997; Zhang and others, 1993).

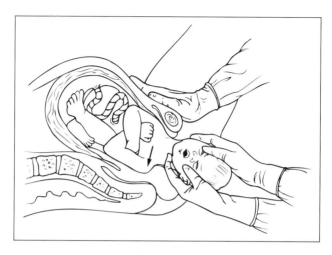

FIG. 27-18

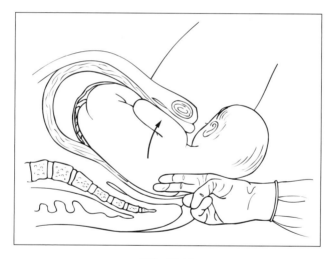

FIG. 27-19

2. Evaluate the patient's and her coach's understanding of the advantage and risks of version. Advantage is decreased cesarean birth rate (Cook, 1993). Potential risks include failed version, reversion, fetal stress, ruptured uterus, and abruptio placentae (Cook, 1993).

3. Evaluate the patient's and her family's understanding of alternatives to version. Postural exercises, visualization, and taped music or voices have been effectively used as an alternative to version. Postural exercises include the breech

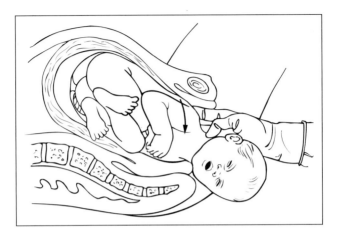

FIG. 27-20

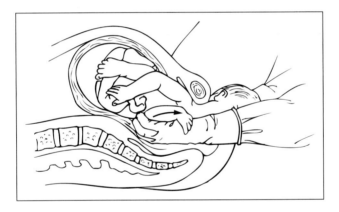

FIG. 27-21

tilt by raising the hips 12 inches with large solid pillows or cushions while knees are flexed three times per day for 10 to 15 minutes. Instruct the patient to relax during the exercise and visualize the baby turning. Music can be played on the lower abdomen to encourage the baby to turn. Chenia and Crowther (1987) in their randomized clinical trial found 41% of the fetuses rotated to and remained in a cephalic presentation with postural exercise.

Intraprocedural

1. Obtain a baseline FHR strip for 15 to 30 minutes before the procedure.

2. Assist with a preliminary ultrasound examination to locate placenta and fetal lie.

3. Start an IV infusion, as ordered, with an 18-gauge intracatheter.

4. Be prepared to administer piggyback a tocolytic agent before and continuously throughout the procedure. The solution will usually be prepared in the same manner and concentration as that used for tocolysis in premature labor (Marquette and others, 1996) (see Chapter 21).

5. Monitor the FHR every few minutes with a Doppler instrument during the procedure.

6. If fetal compromise develops, be prepared to assist with an emergency cesarean delivery.

Postprocedural

1. After the procedure, discontinue the tocolytic agent and reapply FHR and contraction monitors. Monitor FHR and uterine contraction pattern approximately 30 to 60 minutes after the version.

2. Be prepared to administer Rho (D) immune globulin (RhoGAM) (HypRho-D) following the procedure if the mother is D negative.

Intrapartum care

1. Consider the patient high risk and monitor carefully for dystocia following a version.

- ■ **POTENTIAL COMPLICATION OF VAGINAL BIRTH AFTER CESAREAN (VBAC): UTERINE RUPTURE**

   DESIRED OUTCOME: The patient's labor will progress according to the normal labor pattern with a continuous reassuring FHR and no uterine rupture.

   INTERVENTIONS

   Antepartum

   1. Encourage every pregnant woman who had a previous cesarean delivery to attempt a vaginal delivery with the current pregnancy unless she has a history of a classic vertical or unknown uterine incision or an absolute obstetric contraindication. A vaginal delivery is safer for the mother because of the increased risk of postpartum complications following a cesarean, such as a postpartum infection, postpartum hemorrhage, anesthesia complications, injury to other organs, and psychologic stress (Depp, 1996; Enkin and others, 1992). A vaginal birth is safer for the baby because of decreased respiratory distress, since active labor stimulates reabsorption of fetal lung fluid and

stimulates the release of stress hormones that help prepare the fetus for extrauterine life (DeMott, Sandmire, 1990; Flamm and others, 1994). There is only a 0.7% risk of the uterine scar completely separating following a low transverse cervical scar (Flamm and others, 1994; Hansell and others, 1990; Sufrin-Disler, 1990). Approximately 75% of all uterine ruptures occur in the unscarred uterus (Sufrin-Disler, 1990). The mortality following uterine rupture during an attempted VBAC is zero (Flamm and others, 1990). Dehiscence or a partial separation of the uterine scar that does not penetrate the uterine serosa, produce bleeding, or cause any problems occurs in 2% of VBAC patients. Symptoms are minimal or absent, and the dehiscences are usually left untreated without difficulty (Depp, 1996).

2. Educate the prior cesarean-delivered pregnant woman and her family early in the current pregnancy regarding the positive chances of a vaginal delivery. The overall success rate of a vaginal delivery after a cesarean delivery is approximately 60% to 80% (ACOG, 1995; Depp, 1996; Flamm and others, 1994).

3. Participate in the formation of support groups and childbirth classes for couples planning a VBAC.

4. Be involved with childbirth education training to increase childbirth educators' awareness and knowledge regarding VBAC, the importance of appropriate adequate nutrition, and the outcome of the pregnancy, labor, and delivery.

5. Educate the public in general to decrease a long-standing stigma of "once a cesarean, always a cesarean." If a repeat cesarean is scheduled, discuss with the practitioner the indication, risks, and benefits. Maternal morbidity from elective cesarean birth is 5% (Hood, Holubec, 1990). A repeat cesarean delivery is more difficult to do related to scar adhesions.

Intrapartum vaginal birth after a cesarean—trial of labor (VBAC-TOL)

1. VBAC-TOL standards are the same as for all obstetric clinical practice, which include capacity to respond to acute emergency by performing a cesarean within 30 minutes (ACOG, 1994, 1995).

2. Individualize the management of care based on a family assessment of physical and psychologic factors.

3. Determine the family's birth plan for vaginal delivery and a contingency plan in the event complications arise.

4. Use effective physiologic techniques for promoting labor.
5. Use effective psychologic techniques for promoting labor. Determine first what is the family's perception of the previous cesarean birth experience, their concerns, and their expectations. Determine if their expectations of themselves are realistic. It is important to prevent the patient from feeling like she failed or is less of a woman if she is unable to deliver vaginally.
6. Evaluate the terminology used, such as "successful VBAC" or "failed trial of labor," when talking to the patient and her family.
7. Assess FHR according to ACOG's standard of practice for a normal labor patient (refer to Chapter 3).
8. Assess for signs of scar separation. The most common sign is a prolonged FHR deceleration (Farmer and others, 1991). Other less common signs are hematuria, vaginal bleeding, alterations in uterine contractions, and abdominal pain. (Epidural anesthesia is generally believed to be safe since abdominal pain is an unreliable sign of rupture [Depp, 1996].)
9. Notify the attending physician immediately of any signs of fetal compromise or uterine scar separation.
10. If there is an obstetric indication for oxytocin during labor, it is not contraindicated, as once thought, in the patient attempting a VBAC. Close monitoring, however, is important to prevent hyperstimulation (Flamm, 1991), which can increase the risk of uterine rupture (Jones and others, 1991).
11. As a patient advocate, the nurse may be the spokesperson for women experiencing a VBAC. For example, routine manual exploration of the uterus following a VBAC delivery is usually painful, it may increase the risk of a postpartum infection, and its routine benefit has not been demonstrated by research (Enkin and others, 1992).

- **FEAR** related to the use of forceps or a vacuum extractor.
  DESIRED OUTCOME: The patient and her coach will communicate their fears and concerns openly.
  INTERVENTIONS
  1. Promote preventive nursing management during labor by encouraging upright positions during second-stage labor (see Fig. 27-15).
  2. Provide supportive techniques in labor to decrease the need for epidural anesthesia. Epidural anesthesia increases the

frequency of instrumental delivery (Thorp, Breedlove, 1996).

3. When delayed progress in second stage or decreased head rotation is noted, the nurse should (a) encourage the patient to try various positions such as on all fours or squatting, (b) check for maternal hydration, (c) check for a full bladder, and (d) assess pushing techniques, to decrease the need for forceps or vacuum use or if necessary make the procedure easier (Roberts, Woolley, 1996).

4. Provide educational opportunities for expectant parents to learn about the technique of forceps or vacuum extraction and reasons for their use to decrease anxiety in the event either is needed. The most common reasons for use are delayed progress in second stage or a nonreassuring FHR pattern in late second-stage labor.

5. Provide supportive care in the event it is needed by encouraging the mother to remain active in the birth process by continuing to push with each contraction unless there is a medical contraindication.

6. Encourage the patient to continue to feel in control by verbally reassuring her that she is continuing to facilitate the delivery by her pushing efforts.

7. Following the delivery, encourage parents to express their feelings about the procedure to resolve any negative feelings.

8. Following forceps delivery, observe the infant for facial nerve trauma and forceps marks. Discuss with the parents that these are only temporary effects and when they can expect them to disappear. Observe the mother for soft tissue trauma (Williams, 1995).

9. Following a vacuum delivery, assess the infant for caput succedaneum or cephalhematoma. If either is present, reassure the parents that it usually disappears in 3 to 5 days. Following a cephalhematoma, teach the parents to observe their infant for hyperbilirubinemia, signs of infection, and cerebral irritation and to report any signs to their pediatrician. Signs of cerebral irritation to be discussed are listlessness, vomiting, high-pitched cry, and neck and spine rigidity.

10. If the neonate is sleepy and sucks poorly, explain to the parents that this is a normal response following a difficult delivery and does not indicate any problem.

- **POTENTIAL COMPLICATION OF AN INTRAPARTUM EPIDURAL: HYPOTENSION, RESPIRATORY ARREST** if the medication is incorrectly administered into the spinal space, **DYSTOCIA,** and **INCREASED CESAREAN BIRTH RATE**

  DESIRED OUTCOMES: The signs and symptoms of epidural analgesia will be minimized and managed as measured by a stable blood pressure and respiratory rate, labor progressing within the normal limits, and no signs of fetal compromise.

  INTERVENTIONS

  Preprocedural

  1. Ensure information is provided, preferably before labor, regarding the procedural steps of epidural administration, maternal and fetal risks and benefits, alternative methods of pain relief, financial costs, and the expected restrictions in movement related to the epidural. Epidural anesthesia is a highly effective method of pain relief for labor and delivery, and minimal medication is transferred across the placenta to the fetus because the medication binds to maternal plasma protein and has a lower affinity for fetal plasma protein. A prolonged labor caused by anxiety may be speeded up. Hypotension is the most common side effect of an epidural and is nearly always preventable with a fluid load. However, an epidural may increase the length of first and second stages of a normal labor (Ramin and others, 1995; Thorp, Breedlove, 1996). It may also decrease the bearing-down reflex, thereby increasing the need for forceps (Ramin and others, 1995; Shyken and others, 1990; Thorp, Breedlove, 1996). Several randomized controlled prospective trials have shown an increase in the likelihood of a cesarean birth primarily related to uterine dystocia (Philipsen, Jensen, 1989; Ramin and others, 1995; Thorp and others, 1993). Other potential risks are shivering, IV injection, an inadvertent dural puncture, and postpartum backache from injection bruising (Liu, Luxton, 1991; MacArthur and others, 1990; Thorp, Breedlove, 1996). There is an increased incidence of maternal fever as well (Vinson and others, 1993; Ploeckinger and others, 1995). Such undesired effects on the newborn as irritability, inconsolability, uncoordinated suck, and decreased responsiveness have been observed (Simkin, 1991).

  2. Provide information regarding other medical interventions that often accompany use of an epidural. Those that are

always necessary include IV therapy, continuous FHR monitoring, and frequent blood pressure monitoring. Medical interventions that are frequently needed are oxytocin to augment labor contractions and urinary catheterization (Bennett and others, 1987).

3. Facilitate utilization of other methods of pain relief by the laboring woman.

4. Recognize when an epidural analgesia is needed by the patient. Become very familiar with alternative techniques such as low dose or ambulatory epidural analgesia or a patient-controlled epidural (Youngstrom and others, 1996).

5. Start an IV infusion, and administer a preload of 500 to 1000 ml of fluid as ordered to decrease the risk of hypotension (ACOG, 1996).

6. Obtain baseline maternal vital signs and an FHR tracing.

7. Have patient empty her bladder just before the procedure.

8. Prepare emergency equipment at the bedside, such as oxygen and suction equipment.

9. Make sure that resuscitation bag and mask and resuscitation drugs are readily available (ACOG, 1996).

Procedure

1. Position the patient in either a lateral decubitus or a sitting position with head and hips flexed and shoulders and hips squared to facilitate the insertion by a licensed anesthesia provider (AWHONN, 1996).

2. Provide ongoing emotional support and information to the patient.

Postinjection

1. Position patient on her side with head of bed elevated 30 degrees.

2. Continuously monitor FHR.

3. Check for signs of respiratory depression related to accidental administration of the medication into the spinal space. (Similar medications are used for spinal anesthesia, but much smaller doses are used.)

4. Check blood pressure every 15 minutes following an epidural, until delivery, because maternal hypotension can occur resulting from vasodilation.

5. If hypotension develops, turn patient on left side, elevate her legs, increase the IV fluid, administer oxygen, notify the anesthesiologist or nurse anesthetist, and be prepared to administer ephedrine if ordered.

6. Keep an accurate intake and output record. Encourage the

laboring patient to void every 2 to 4 hours. (Epidural anesthesia blocks sensations of a full bladder.)

- **POTENTIAL COMPLICATION OF POSTPARTUM EPIDURAL ANALGESIA: RESPIRATORY DEPRESSION, PRURITUS, NAUSEA/VOMITING, AND URINARY RETENTION**

  DESIRED OUTCOME: The signs and symptoms of epidural analgesia will be minimized and managed as measured by stable respiratory rate greater than 12 breaths/min, no itching, no nausea or vomiting, and sufficient urinary output quantity.

  INTERVENTIONS

  Preprocedural

  1. Evaluate patient's understanding of epidural analgesia if it is to be used in the event of a cesarean birth or fourth-degree laceration during vaginal delivery. Usual procedure is 4 or 5 mg of morphine analgesic injected through the epidural catheter at the close of the surgical repair. Maternal benefits include prolonged pain relief for 24 hours, ambulation, interaction with infant with minimal discomfort, and earlier recovery. Some patients experience side effects of respiratory depression, itching, nausea, vomiting, or urinary retention, but these side effects are generally mild (Inturrisi and others, 1988; Wright, 1991).
  2. Assist in obtaining an informed consent.

  Postprocedural

  1. Assess respiratory rate often. A typical assessment routine may be every 15 minutes for 2 hours, every 30 minutes for 6 hours (total of 8 hours after injection), and every 1 hour for 16 hours (total of 24 hours after injection).
  2. Assess for itching and nausea or vomiting per observational check while patient is awake.
  3. Keep accurate intake and output record.
  4. If a Foley catheter is present, do not remove for 14 to 16 hours after delivery. If urinary retention occurs, it usually develops early and is resolved by 14 to 16 hours after administration of medication (Inturrisi and others, 1988).
  5. Be prepared to administer naloxone (Narcan), 0.04 to 0.4 mg, as ordered, if side effects develop.
  6. A low naloxone dose of 0.04 mg will frequently alleviate mild side effects and not diminish the analgesic effect.
  7. Notify physician of the development of side effects and responsiveness to ordered treatment.

- **POTENTIAL COMPLICATION OF CESAREAN BIRTH: INFECTIONS SUCH AS ENDOMYOMETRITIS, PNEUMONIA, URINARY TRACT INFECTIONS, AND INCISION; THROMBOEMBOLIC DISEASE; HEMORRHAGE; BOWEL AND BLADDER INJURY; OR AN ILEUS**
DESIRED OUTCOME: No surgical complications will develop, or if they develop, the signs and symptoms will be minimized and managed as measured by temperature below 38° C, urination without pain, incision approximating without redness or swelling, stable vital signs, active bowel signs, and patient report of passing flatus.

INTERVENTIONS
Preoperative
1. Decrease the incidence of cesarean delivery by maintaining a positive attitude toward the laboring woman, supporting normal physiologic processes of labor, and implementing a variety of nontechnologic nursing interventions. (See nursing diagnosis on enhancement of labor progress.)
2. If cesarean delivery becomes medically or obstetrically necessary, assess the couple's understanding of the reason for the cesarean.
3. Emphasize it is an "alternative birth method," and encourage "family-centered options" where still possible.
4. Start an IV infusion with an 18-gauge intracatheter.
5. Shave the abdomen from the xiphoid process to about 5 cm (2 inches) below the pubic hairline.
6. Insert a Foley catheter, and connect it to continuous drainage to decrease the risk of bladder trauma during the surgery. This frequently can be inserted after the administration of the anesthetic to decrease the discomfort of the procedure.
7. Check to see if laboratory work has been done such as complete blood count, blood typed and cross matched for two units, and urinalysis.
8. Antacids are rarely used today since evidence is limited as to their effectiveness. In fact, because of the 30-ml volume, they may increase the risk of aspiration (Roberts, Ludka, 1994).

Postoperative
1. Be prepared to administer prophylactic antibiotics. They are frequently started just after the clamping of the umbilical cord. Endomyometritis is the most common complication following a cesarean delivery, occurring in 35% to 40% of cases; prophylactic antibiotics reduce the risk to approximately 5% (Depp, 1996).

2. Keep in mind that the patient is foremost a new mother. Help her find success in her mothering role within postsurgical limits.

3. Assess for signs of hemorrhage by recording blood pressure, pulse, and respirations according to protocol. A typical assessment routine may be every 15 minutes for eight times, every 30 minutes for two times, every 4 hours for two times, and then routinely. Check firmness of uterus and vaginal flow with each vital signs check. Keep a pad count.

4. Manually massage a relaxed, boggy fundus very gently until firm, and maintain oxytocics and IV fluids as ordered.

5. Assess for signs of an infection by checking temperature every 4 hours for 48 hours; if greater than 38° C (100.4° F), check every 2 hours. Check lochia every shift for odor.

6. Encourage abdominal tightening exercises and early ambulation to decrease the risk of gas pains.

7. Give patient nothing to eat or drink until bowel sounds are present. Then give patient full liquids until she passes flatus. Then a soft or regular diet can be given.

8. Encourage coughing and deep breathing to decrease the risk of respiratory infection.

9. Measure the first two voidings after the Foley catheter is removed. Assess for burning on urination and blood in the urine.

10. Notify physician if uterus fails to contract or stay contracted with massage, temperature is over 38° C, lochia develops an odor, the incision site shows signs of an infection, or the patient complains of burning on urination.

■ **RISK FOR SITUATIONAL LOW SELF-ESTEEM** related to cesarean delivery.
   DESIRED OUTCOME: The patient and her coach will verbalize a positive birth experience despite alternative birth process.
   INTERVENTIONS
   1. Involve the couple in as much of the decision-making process as possible to increase feeling of control.

   2. Continuously keep the couple informed of the laboring woman's progress. In the event a cesarean is necessary, help them to understand the reason.

   3. Support the coach in being able to provide support during the cesarean delivery.

   4. During the woman's postpartum hospital stay, encourage the couple to verbalize their feelings about the cesarean

delivery. The mother who experiences an unexpected cesarean delivery often relates a feeling of guilt or failure if she is unable to achieve a vaginal delivery (Fawcett and others, 1994).

5. Reassure the couple they did not fail, and reiterate the reason for the alternative birth.

6. If the couple expresses extreme failure, refer to a local cesarean birth support group or to therapy.

CONCLUSION

The ultimate goal for any patient during labor is progression of labor within the normal labor curve with absence of nonreassuring fetal responses. The nurse can have a significant influence on the progress of labor by imparting confidence in the patient's ability to deliver vaginally and by the use of a variety of therapeutic, nontechnologic techniques to facilitate labor (Radin and others, 1993). Other factors, however, can impede labor that the nurse cannot control. These the nurse must assess and report to the attending health care provider immediately. The medical team should then work together to facilitate the labor and delivery for the best maternal and neonatal outcome.

BIBLIOGRAPHY

Cesarean Delivery

Clarke S, Taffel S: Rates of cesarean and VBAC delivery, United States, 1994, *Birth* 23(3):166-168, 1996.

Cunningham F, MacDonald P, Gant N: *Williams' obstetrics,* ed 20, Norwalk, Conn, 1997, Appleton & Lange.

Ehrenkranz N and others: Infections complicating low risk cesarean sections in community hospitals: efficacy of antimicrobial prophylaxis, *Am J Obstet Gynecol* 162:337-343, 1990.

Fawcett J and others: Expectations about cesarean birth, *IJCE* 9(4):12-17, 1994.

Paul R, Miller D: Cesarean birth: how to reduce the rate, *Am J Obstet Gynecol* 172:1903-1911, 1995.

Radin T, Harmon J, Hanson D: Nurses' care during labor: its effect on the cesarean birth rate of healthy, nulliparous women, *Birth* 20(1):14-21, 1993.

Scheller J, Nelson K: Does cesarean delivery prevent cerebral palsy or other neurologic problems of childhood? *Obstet Gynecol* 83:624-630, 1994.

Thorp J and others: The effect of continuous epidural analgesia on cesarean section for dystocia in nulliparous women, *Am J Obstet Gynecol* 161:670-675, 1989.

Thorp J and others: The effect of intrapartum epidural analgesia on nulliparous labor: a randomized, controlled, prospective trial, *Am J Obstet Gynecol* 169:851-858, 1993.

Xenakis E and others: Low-dose versus high-dose oxytocin augmentation of labor—a randomized trial, *Am J Obstet Gynecol* 173:1874-1878, 1995.

Dysfunctional Labor

American College of Obstetricians and Gynecologists (ACOG): Dystocia and the augmentation of labor, *ACOG Techn Bull,* no. 218, 1995.

Bottoms S, Hirsch V, Sokol R: Medical management of arrest disorders of labor: a current overview, *Am J Obstet Gynecol* 156:935-939, 1987.

Bowes W: Clinical aspects of normal and abnormal labor. In Creasy R, Resnik R, editors: *Maternal-fetal medicine: principles and practice,* ed 3, Philadelphia, 1994, Saunders.

Bruner J: Routine C/S for macrosomic fetuses, *Contemp OB/GYN* 36(special issue):51-55, 1991.

Cardozo L, Pearce J: Oxytocin in active phase abnormalities of labor: a randomized study, *Obstet Gynecol* 75:152-157, 1990.

Clarke S, Taffel S: Rates of cesarean and VBAC delivery, United States, 1994, *Birth* 23(3):166-168, 1996.

Cohen G and others: A prospective randomized study of the aggressive management of early labor, *Am J Obstet Gynecol* 157:1174-1177, 1987.

Cohen W, Brennan J: Using and archiving the labor curves, *Clin Perinatol* 22(4):855-874, 1995.

Compton A: Soft tissue and pelvic dystocia, *Clin Obstet Gynecol* 30(1):69-76, 1987.

Cunningham F, MacDonald P, Gant N: *Williams' obstetrics,* ed 20, Norwalk, Conn, 1997, Appleton & Lange.

Depp R: Cesarean delivery. In Gabbe S, Niebyl J, Simpson J, editors: *Obstetrics: normal and problem pregnancies,* ed 3, New York, 1996, Churchill Livingstone.

Friedman E: Failure to progress during labor, *Contemp OB/GYN* 34(6):42-52, 1989.

Frigoletto F and others: A clinical trial of active management of labor, *N Engl J Med* 333(12):745-750, 1995.

Gabay M, Wolfe S: *Unnecessary cesarean sections: curing a national epidemic,* Washington, DC, 1994, Public Citizen's Health Research Group.

Haire D, Elsberry C: Maternity care and outcomes in a high risk service: the North Central Bronx Hospital experience, *Birth* 18(1):33-39, 1991.

Hofmeyr G: Breech presentation and abnormal lie in late pregnancy. In Chalmers I, Enkin M, Keirse M, editors: *Effective care in pregnancy and childbirth,* Oxford, England, 1989, Oxford University Press.

Hunter L, Chern-Hughes B: Management of prolonged latent phase labor, *J Nurse Midwifery* 41(5):383-388, 1996.

Kennell J and others: Continuous emotional support during labor in a US hospital, *JAMA* 265:2197-2201, 1991.

Lee W: Risk management of breech pregnancies, *Contemp OB/GYN* 33(special issue):195-208, 1989.

Leung W: Placenta previa and previous cesarean section, *Int J Gynaecol Obstet* 51(1):25-31, 1995.

Lopez-Zeno J and others: A controlled trial of a program for the active management of labor, *N Engl J Med* 326:450-454, 1992.

Lydon-Rochelle M and others: Accuracy of Leopold maneuvers in screening for malpresentation: a prospective study, *Birth* 20(3):132-135, 1993.

Morton S, William M, Keeler E: Effect of epidural analgesia for labor on the cesarean delivery rate, *Obstet Gynecol* 83:1045-1052, 1994.

Nageotte M: How we can lower the C/S rate, *Contemp OB/GYN* 35(special issue):63-74, 1990.

O'Driscoll K, Meagher D: *Active management of labour,* ed 3, Philadelphia, 1993, Saunders.

Peaceman A, Socol M: Active management of labor, *Am J Obstet Gynecol* 175(2):363-368, 1996.

Perkins R: Fetal dystocia, *Clin Obstet Gynecol* 30(1):56-68, 1987.

Ramin S and others: Randomized trial of epidural versus intravenous analgesia during labor, *Obstet Gynecol* 86(5):783-789, 1995.

Sanchez-Ramos L and others: Reducing cesarean sections at a teaching hospital, *Am J Obstet Gynecol* 163:1081-1088, 1990.

Satin A and others: High- versus low-dose oxytocin for labor stimulation, *Obstet Gynecol* 80:111-116, 1992.

Scorza W: Intrapartum management of breech presentation, *Clin Perinatol* 23(1):31-49, 1996.

Scott J and others, editors: *Danforth's obstetrics and gynecology,* ed 6, Philadelphia, 1990, Lippincott.

Taylor V and others: Placenta previa and prior cesarean delivery: How strong is the association? *Obstet Gynecol* 84:55-58, 1994.

Thomson M, Hanley J: Factors predisposing to difficult labor in primiparas, *Am J Obstet Gynecol* 158:1074-1078, 1988.

Thorp J and others: The effect of intrapartum epidural analgesia on nulliparous labor: a randomized, controlled, prospective trial, *Am J Obstet Gynecol* 169:851-858, 1993.

Valenzuela G, Foster T: Use of magnesium sulfate to treat hyperstimulation in term labor, *Obstet Gynecol* 75:762-764, 1990.

World Health Organization (WHO): Partographic management of labour, *Lancet* 343:1399, 1994.

Xenakis E and others: Low-dose versus high-dose oxytocin augmentation of labor—a randomized trial, *Am J Obstet Gynecol* 173:1874-1878, 1995.

Epidural Analgesia and Anesthesia: Intrapartum Management

American College of Obstetricians and Gynecologists (ACOG): Obstetric analgesia and anesthesia, *ACOG Techn Bull,* no. 225, 1996.

Association of Women's Health, Obstetric, and Neonatal Nurses (AWHONN): *Obstetric epidural analgesia and the role of the professional registered nurse: clinical commentary,* Washington, DC, 1996, The Author.

Bennett A, Lumley J, Bartlett D: Review article: the use of epidural bupivacaine for the relief of childbirth pain, *Aust Paediatr J* 23:13-19, 1987.

Culp R, Osofsky H: Effects of cesarean delivery on parental depression, marital adjustment, and mother-infant interaction, *Birth* 16(2):53-57, 1989.

Kaminski H, Stafl A, Aiman J: The effect of epidural analgesia on the frequency of instrumental obstetric delivery, *Obstet Gynecol* 69(5):770-773, 1987.

Liu W, Luxton M: The effect of prophylactic fentanyl on shivering in elective cesarean section under epidural analgesia, *Anaesthesia* 46:344-348, 1991.

MacArthur C and others: Epidural anesthesia and long-term backache after childbirth, *Br Med J* 301(July 7):9-12, 1990.

Morton S, William M, Keeler E: Effect of epidural analgesia for labor on the cesarean delivery rate, *Obstet Gynecol* 83:1045-1052, 1994.

Philipsen T, Jensen N: Epidural block or parenteral pethidine as analgesic in labour: a randomized study concerning progress in labour and instrumental deliveries, *Eur J Obstet Gynecol Reprod Biol* 30(1):27-33, 1989.

Ploeckinger B and others: Epidural anesthesia in labour: influence on surgical delivery rates, intrapartum fever and blood loss, *Gynecol Obstet Invest* 39(1):24-27, 1995.

Ramin S and others: Randomized trial of epidural versus intravenous analgesia during labor, *Obstet Gynecol* 86(5):783-789, 1995.

Rayburn W and others: Comparison of patient controlled and nurse administered analgesia using intravenous fentanyl during labor, *Anesthesiol Rev* 18(1), 1991.

Rush J and others: The effects of whirlpool baths in labor: a randomized, controlled trial, *Birth* 23(3):136-143, 1996.

Shyken J and others: A comparison of the effect of epidural, general, and no anesthesia on funic acid-base values by stage of labor and type of delivery, *Am J Obstet Gynecol* 163:802-807, 1990.

Simkin P: Weighting the pros and cons of the epidural, *Childbirth Forum,* pp 1, 3-5, Fall 1991.

Stem K: *Managing pain: labor-delivery-postpartum: professional presentation,* 1995, Phoenix, Professional Education Center.

Thorp J, Breedlove G: Epidural analgesia in labor: an evaluation of risks and benefits, *Birth* 23(2):63-83, 1996.

Thorp J, McNitt J, Leppert P: Effects of epidural analgesia: some questions and answers, *Birth* 7(3):157-162, 1990.

Thorp J and others: The effect of continuous epidural analgesia on cesarean section for dystocia in nulliparous women, *Am J Obstet Gynecol* 161(3):670-675, 1989.

Thorp J and others: The effect of intrapartum epidural analgesia on nulliparous labor: a randomized, controlled, prospective trial, *Am J Obstet Gynecol* 169:851-858, 1993.

Vinson D, Thomas R, Kiser T: Association between epidural analgesia during labor and fever, *J Fam Pract* 36(6):617-622, 1993.

Youngstrom P, Baker S, Miller J: Epidural redefined in analgesia and anesthesia: a distinction with a difference, *J Obstet Gynecol Neonatal Nurs* 25(4):350-354, 1996.

Epidural Analgesia: Postpartum Management

Inturrisi M, Camenga C, Rosen M: Epidural morphine for relief of postpartum, postsurgical pain, *J Obstet Gynecol Neonatal Nurs* 17(4):238-243, 1988.

Wright W: Continuous epidural block for OB anesthesia, *Contemp OB/GYN* 38(5):89-98, 1991.

External Version

Chenia F, Crowther C: Does advice to assume the knee-chest position reduce the incidence of breech presentation at delivery? A randomized clinical trial, *Birth* 14(2):75-78, 1987.

Cook H: Experience with external cephalic version and selective vaginal breech delivery in private practice, *Am J Obstet Gynecol* 168:1886-1890, 1993.

Laros R, Flanagan T, Kilpatrick S: Management of term breech presentation: a protocol of external cephalic version and selective trial of labor, *Am J Obstet Gynecol* 172:1916, 1995.

Lau T, Lo, Rogers M: Pregnancy outcome after successful external cephalic version for breech presentation at term, *Am J Obstet Gynecol* 176:218-223, 1997.

Marquette G and others: Does the use of a tocolytic agent affect the success rate of external cephalic version? *Am J Obstet Gynecol* 175:859-861, 1996.

Scorza W: Intrapartum management of breech presentation, *Clin Perinatol* 23(1):31-49, 1996.

Zhang J, Bowes W, Fortney J: Efficacy of external cephalic version: a review, *Obstet Gynecol* 82:306, 1993.

Instrumental Delivery: Forceps and Vacuum

Kaminski H, Stafl A, Aiman J: The effect of epidural analgesia on the frequency of instrumental obstetric delivery, *Obstet Gynecol* 69(5):770-773, 1987.

O'Grady J: A role exists for vaginal instrumental delivery, *Contemp OB/GYN* 35(special issue):49-56, 1989.

Williams M: Vacuum assisted delivery, *Clin Perinatol* 22(4):933-952, 1995.

Nursing Interventions

Aderhold K, Roberts J: Phases of second stage labor, *J Nurse Midwifery* 36(5):267-275, 1991.

American College of Obstetricians and Gynecologists (ACOG): *Guidelines for perinatal care,* ed 2, Washington, DC, 1988, The College.

Biancuzzo M: The patient observer: does the hands and knees posture during labor help to rotate the occiput posterior fetus? *Birth* 18(1):40-47, 1991.

Biancuzzo M: How to recognize and rotate an occiput posterior fetus, *Am J Nurs* 93:38-91, 1993.

Bonica J: *Obstetric analgesia and anesthesia,* Amsterdam, 1990, World Federation of Societies of Anaesthesiologists.

Broach J, Newton M: Food and beverages in labor. II. The effects of cessation of oral intake during labor, *Birth* 15(2):88-92, 1988.

Bryanton J, Fraser-Davey H, Sullivan P: Women's perceptions of nursing support during labor, *J Obstet Gynecol Neonatal Nurs* 23(8):638-644, 1993.

Chen S and others: Effects of sitting position on uterine activity during labor, *Obstet Gynecol* 69:67-73, 1987.

Clapp J: The course of labor after endurance exercise during pregnancy, *Am J Obstet Gynecol* 163(6):1799-1805, 1990.

Clarke S, Taffel S: Rates of cesarean and VBAC delivery, United States, 1994, *Birth* 23(3):166-168, 1996.

Copper R, Goldenberg R: Catecholamine secretion in fetal adaptation to stress, *J Obstet Gynecol Neonatal Nurs* 19(3):223-226, 1990.

Cosner K, deJong E: Physiologic second stage labor, *MCN Am J Matern Child Nurs* 18:38-43, 1993.

Crawford J: Maternal mortality from Mendelson's syndrome, *Lancet* 1:920-921, 1986.

Creehan P: Ask the experts: hydrotherapy, *AWHONN Voice* 4(7):4, 1996.

Crowe K, von Baeyer C: Predictors of a positive childbirth experience, *Birth* 16(2):59-63, 1989.

Di Franco J: Music for childbirth, *Childbirth Educator,* pp 36-41, Fall 1988.

Douglas M: Commentary: the case against a more liberal food and fluid policy in labor, *Birth* 15(2):93, 1988.

Eggers P: Pain is not a four letter word, *IJCE* 10(4):4-5, 1995.

Fenwick L, Simkin P: Maternal positioning to prevent or alleviate dystocia in labor, *Clin Obstet Gynecol* 30(1):83-89, 1987.

Fuller B, Roberts J, McKay S: Acoustical analysis of maternal sounds during the second stage of labor, *Appl Nurs Res* 6:7-13, 1993.

Gagnon A, Waghorn K: Supportive care by maternity nurses: a work sampling study in an intrapartum unit, *Birth* 23(3):1-6, 1996.

Geden E and others: Effects of music and imagery on physiologic and self-report of analogued labor pain, *Nurs Res* 38(1):37-40, 1989.

Golay J, Vedam S, Sorger L: The squatting position for the second stage of labor: effects on labor and on maternal and fetal well-being, *Birth* 20:73-78, 1993.

Green J: Expectations and experiences of pain in labor: findings from a large prospective study, *Birth* 20(2):65-72, 1993.

Green J, Coupland V, Kitzinger J: Expectations, experience, and psychological outcomes of childbirth: a prospective study of 825 women, *Birth* 19(1):15-23, 1990.

Hazle N: Hydration in labor: routine intravenous hydration necessary? *J Nurse Midwifery* 31(4):171-175, 1986.

Held N: Myths about second stage labor, *Childbirth Instructor Magazine* 4(1):15-20, 1994.

Hodnett E: Nursing support of the laboring woman, *J Obstet Gynecol Neonatal Nurs* 25(3):258-264, 1996.

Hofmeyr G and others: Companionship to modify the clinical birth environment: effects on progress and perceptions of labour, and breastfeeding, *Br J Obstet Gynecol* 98:756-764, 1991.

Jannke S: Birth plans, *Childbirth Instructor Magazine* 5(3):26-29, 1995.

Johnson C and others: Nutrition and hydration in labour. In Chalmers I, Enkin M, Keirse M, editors: *Effective care in pregnancy and childbirth,* Oxford, England, 1989, Oxford University Press.

Johnstone F, Aboelmagd M, Harouny A: Maternal posture in second stage and fetal acid base status, *Br J Obstet Gynaecol* 94:753-757, 1987.

Keirse M: Augmentation of labour. In Chalmers I, Enkin M, Keirse M, editors: *Effective care in pregnancy and childbirth,* Oxford, England, 1989, Oxford University Press.

Kennell J and others: Continuous emotional support during labor in a US hospital, *JAMA* 265:2197-2201, 1991.

Keppler A: The use of intravenous fluids during labor, *Birth* 15(2):75-79, 1988.

Klaus M, Kennell J, Klaus P: *Mothering the mother,* Menlo Park, Calif, 1993, Addison-Wesley.

Kurokawa J, Zilkoski M: Adapting hospital obstetrics to birth in the squatting position, *Birth* 12:87-90, 1985.

Liu Y: The effects of the upright position during childbirth, *IMAGE J Nurs Sch* 21(1):14-18, 1989.

Lowe N: Maternal confidence in coping with labor: a self-efficacy concept, *J Obstet Gynecol Neonatal Nurs* 20(6):457-463, 1991.

Lowe N: The pain and discomfort of labor and birth, *J Obstet Gynecol Neonatal Nurs* 25(1):82-92, 1996.

Mallak J: P.A.I.N., *IJCE* 10(4):6-7, 1995.

Manning J: Intrathecal narcotics: new approach for labor analgesia, *J Obstet Gynecol Neonatal Nurs* 25(3):221-224, 1996.

McEwan E, Tier D: Birth planning: a reality-based script for building confidence, *J Nurse Midwifery* 34(3):111-114, 1989.

McKay S, Barrows T, Roberts J: Women's views of second stage labor as assessed by interviews and videotapes, *Birth* 17(4):192-198, 1990.

McKay S, Mahan C: Modifying the stomach contents of laboring women: why and how; success and risks, *Birth* 15(4):213-220, 1988.

McKay S, Roberts J: Maternal position during labor and birth: what have we learned? *IJCE* 13(2):9-30, 1989.

Morton S and others: Effect of epidural analgesia for labor on the cesarean delivery rate, *Obstet Gynecol* 83(6):1045-1052, 1994.

Newton N, Newton M, Broach J: Psychologic, physical, nutritional, and technologic aspects of intravenous infusion during labor, *Birth* 15(2):67-72, 1988.

Paine L, Tinker D: The effect of maternal bearing-down efforts on arterial umbilical cord pH and length of the second stage of labor, *J Nurse Midwifery* 37:61-63, 1992.

Parnell C and others: Pushing method in the expulsive phase of labor, *Acta Obstet Gynaecol Scand* 72:31-35, 1993.

Perez P: When a birth causes trauma, *Childbirth Forum,* pp 1-5, Summer 1996.

Piper J, Bolling D, Newton E: The second stage of labor: factors influencing duration, *Am J Obstet Gynecol* 165:976-979, 1991.

Radin T, Harmon J, Hanson D: Nurses' care during labor: its effect on the cesarean birth rate of healthy, nulliparous women, *Birth* 20(1):14-21, 1993.

Rayburn W and others: Comparison of patient controlled and nurse administered analgesia using intravenous fentanyl during labor, *Anesthesiol Rev* 18(1), 1991.

Richard L, Alada MO: Effect of delivery room routines on success of first breastfeeding, *Lancet* 336:1105-1107, 1990.

Richardson P: The body boundary experience of women in labor: a framework for care, *MCN Am J Matern Child Nurs* 13(2):91-101, 1984.

Roberts C, Ludka L: Food for thought: the debate over eating and drinking in labor, *Childbirth Instructor Magazine* 4(2):24-29, 1994.

Roberts J, Mendez-Bauer C, Wodell D: The effects of maternal position on uterine contractility and efficiency, *Birth* 10(4):243-249, 1983.

Roberts J, Woolley D: A second look at the second stage of labor, *J Obstet Gynecol Neonatal Nurs* 25:415-423, 1996.

Romond J, Baker I: Squatting in childbirth: a new look at an old tradition, *J Obstet Gynecol Neonatal Nurs* 14(5):406-412, 1985.

Rooney B and others: Is a twelve-percent cesarean section rate at a perinatal center safe? *J Perinatol* 16(3):215-218, 1996.

Rossi M, Lindell S: Maternal positions and pushing techniques in a nonprescriptive environment, *J Obstet Gynecol Neonatal Nurs* 15(3): 203-208, 1986.

Rush J and others: The effects of whirlpool baths in labor: a randomized, controlled trial, *Birth* 23(3):136-143, 1996.

Schorn N, McAllister J, Blanco J: Water immersion and the effect of labor, *J Nurse Midwifery* 38:336, 1993.

Shannahan M, Cottrell B: The effects of birth chair delivery on maternal perceptions, *J Obstet Gynecol Neonatal Nurs* 18(4):323-326, 1989.

Shearer E: Once a cesarean, always a scar, *Birth* 23(3):172-175, 1996.

Simkin P: Stress, pain, and catecholamines in labor: a review, *Birth* 13(4):227-240, 1986a.

Simkin P: Stress, pain, and catecholamines in labor. II. Stress associated with childbirth events: a pilot survey of new mothers, *Birth* 13:234-240, 1986b.

Simkin P: Comfort measures for labor and how they work, *IJCE* 11(1):5-7, 1987.

Simkin P: The labor support person: latest addition to the maternity care team, *IJCE* 16(1):19-28, 1992.

Simkin P: Active management of labor, *Childbirth Instructor Magazine* 5(4):8-12, 1995a.

Simkin P: Reducing pain and enhancing progress in labor: a guide to nonpharmacologic methods for maternity caregivers, *Birth* 22(3):161-170, 1995b.

Springer D: Birth plans: the effect on anxiety in pregnant women, *IJCE* 11(3):20-25, 1996.

Stem K: *Managing pain: labor-delivery-postpartum: professional presentation,* 1995, Phoenix, Professional Education Center.

Thomson A: Pushing techniques in the second stage of labour, *J Adv Nurs* 18:171-177, 1993.

Thorp J, Breedlove G: Epidural analgesia in labor: an evaluation of risks and benefits, *Birth* 23(2):63-83, 1996.

Thorp J and others: The effect of intrapartum epidural analgesia on nulliparous labor: a randomized, controlled, prospective trial, *Am J Obstet Gynecol* 169:851-858, 1993.

Threlfall-Mase A: The moaning option, *Childbirth Instructor Magazine* 7(2):43-45, 1997.

U.S. Public Health Service: *Healthy people 2000: national health promotion and disease prevention objectives—full report, with commentary* (DHHS pub no. 91-50212), Washington, DC, 1991, U.S. Department of Healthy and Human Services, Public Health Service.

Varrassi G, Bazzano C, Edwards W: Effects of physical activity on maternal plasma B-endorphin levels and perception of labor pain, *Am J Obstet Gynecol* 160:707-712, 1989.

Wolman W and others: Postpartum depression and companionship in the clinical birth environment: a randomized, controlled study, *Am J Obstet Gynecol* 168:1388-1393, 1993.

Wong S, McKenzie D: Cardiorespiratory fitness during pregnancy and its effect on outcome, *Int J Sports Med* 8(2):70-83, 1987.

Youngstrom P, Baker S, Miller J: Epidural redefined in analgesia and anesthesia: a distinction with a difference, *J Obstet Gynecol Neonatal Nurs* 25(4):350-354, 1996.

Shoulder Dystocia

Benedetti T: Added complications of shoulder dystocia, *Contemp OB/GYN* 33(special issue):150-161, 1989.

Benedetti T: Dystocia: causes, consequences, correct response, *Contemp OB/GYN* 36(special issue):37-48, 1991.

Bowes W: Clinical aspects of normal and abnormal labor. In Creasy R, Resnik R, editors: *Maternal-fetal medicine: principles and practice,* ed 3, Philadelphia, 1994, Saunders.

Gonik B, Allen R, Sorab J: Objective evaluation of the shoulder dystocia phenomenon: effect of maternal pelvic orientation on force reduction, *Obstet Gynecol* 74:44-48, 1989.

Hall S: The nurse's role in the identification of risks and treatment of shoulder dystocia, *J Obstet Gynecol Neonatal Nurs* 26(1):25-32, 1997.

Hernandez C, Wendel G: Shoulder dystocia, *Clin Obstet Gynecol* 33(3):526-534, 1990.

Horger E: Shoulder dystocia, *Female Patient* 20(12):12-58, 1995.

Kochenour N, Clark S: OB emergencies: shoulder dystocia, *Contemp OB/GYN* 39(1):9-12, 1994.

Naef R, Martin J: Emergent management of shoulder dystocia, *Obstet Gynecol Clin North Am* 22(2):247-259, 1995.

Nocon J: Shoulder dystocia: managing risk to avoid negligence, *Contemp OB/GYN* 36(special issue):15-23, 1991.

O'Leary J: *Shoulder dystocia and birth injury: prevention and treatment,* New York, 1992, McGraw-Hill.

O'Leary J, Leonetti H: Shoulder dystocia: prevention and treatment, *Am J Obstet Gynecol* 162:5-9, 1990.

Penney D, Perlis D: Shoulder dystocia: when to use suprapubic or fundal pressure, *MCN Am J Matern Child Nurs* 17(1):34-36, 1992.

Vaginal Birth After Cesarean (VBAC)

American College of Obstetricians and Gynecologists (ACOG): *Vaginal delivery after previous cesarean birth: ACOG committee opinion no. 143,* Washington, DC, 1994, The College.

American College of Obstetricians and Gynecologists (ACOG): Dystocia and the augmentation of labor, *ACOG Techn Bull,* no. 218, 1995.

Cunningham F, MacDonald P, Gant N: *Williams' obstetrics,* ed 20, Norwalk, Conn, 1997, Appleton & Lange.

DeMott R, Sandmire H: The physician factor as a determinant of cesarean birth rates, *Am J Obstet Gynecol* 162:593-602, 1990.

Enkin M, Keirse M, Chalmers I, editors: *A guide to effective care in pregnancy and childbirth,* Oxford, England, 1992, Oxford University Press.

Farmer R and others: Uterine rupture during trial of labor after previous cesarean section, *Am J Obstet Gynecol* 165:996-1001, 1991.

Flamm B: VBAC: low risk, not no risk, *Contemp OB/GYN* 36(10):24-32, 1991.

Flamm B and others: Vaginal birth after cesarean section: results of a multicenter study, *Am J Obstet Gynecol* 158(5):1079-1084, 1988.

Flamm B and others: Vaginal birth after cesarean delivery: results of a 5 year multicenter collaborative study, *Obstet Gynecol* 76:750-753, 1990.

Flamm B and others: Elective repeat cesarean delivery versus trial of labor: a prospective multicenter study, *Obstet Gynecol* 83:927-932, 1994.

Hangsleben K, Taylor M, Lynn N: VBAC program in a nurse-midwifery service: five years of experience, *J Nurse Midwifery* 34(4):79-84, 1989.

Hansell R, McMurray K, Huey G: Vaginal birth after two or more cesarean sections: a five year experience, *Birth* 17(3):46-50, 1990.

Hood D, Holubec D: Elective repeat cesarean section: effect of anesthesia type on blood loss, *J Reprod Med* 35(4):368-372, 1990.

Jones R and others: Rupture of low transverse cesarean scars during trial of labor, *Obstet Gynecol* 77:815, 1991.

Sufrin-Disler C: Vaginal birth after cesarean, *IJCE* 14(3):21-32, 1990.

28

Postterm Pregnancy

Postterm or *prolonged pregnancy* is one that has a gestational period of 42 weeks or more from the first day of the last menses if the menstrual cycle is 28 days. *Postmaturity* refers to the abnormal condition of the fetus or newborn resulting from a postterm pregnancy.

INCIDENCE

The incidence of postterm pregnancy is approximately 10% (Cunningham and others, 1997). However, others have found the incidence to be 7.5% when a reliable menstrual history was used (Wood, 1994).

ETIOLOGY

The actual physiologic cause of postterm pregnancy is still obscure. There is some evidence that a placental estrogen deficiency may be a possible cause. When there is insufficient estrogen, there is decreased production and storage of prostaglandin precursors and decreased stimulation to form oxytocin receptors in the myometrium. These physiologic processes are very important in the initiation of labor. (Refer to the normal physiology section of Chapter 21.) The reason for the estrogen deficiency is unknown.

Fetal Cause

Occasionally, estrogen deficiency can result from fetal pituitary or adrenal insufficiency. Lack of secretion of the precursor hormone *dehydroisoandrosterone sulfate,* which is necessary for the placenta to produce increasing amounts of estriol, may also partially explain the fetal contribution to causing postterm pregnancy.

Maternal Cause

When the woman has had one pregnancy that continued postterm, there is a 50% risk of recurrence in subsequent pregnancies (Ahn, Phelan, 1989). The maternal reason for repeated prolongation of pregnancies is unknown at this time.

NORMAL PHYSIOLOGY
Amniotic Fluid

The normal physiology of amniotic fluid (its volume and functions) is relevant to understanding the pathologic complications in postterm pregnancy.

Volume

Amniotic fluid is derived from the following sources:
- Maternal circulation, primarily from placental sufficiency
- Amniotic membrane
- Fetal plasma

The volume changes in quantity because of (1) the fetal contribution through excretion of urine and (2) fetal use of the fluid for nourishment by swallowing the fluid and sending it into the gastrointestinal tract.

The volume of amniotic fluid gradually increases until it reaches its maximal level at approximately 38 weeks of gestation, at which time it begins to decrease normally. By 40 weeks the level is approximately 800 ml. In contrast, by 42 and 43 weeks the levels are 400 and 300 ml, respectively (Resnik, 1994).

Functions

The following functions of amniotic fluid are relevant to postterm pregnancy:
- Cushions the fetus and umbilical cord from direct pressure and injury
- Allows the fetus to move and exercise freely
- Assists the fetus in respiratory efforts
- Facilitates fetal lung development and surfactant production

Placenta

Exchange

The placenta provides a large surface area through which materials can be exchanged across the placental membrane between the fetal and maternal circulations. From the maternal blood the fetus obtains nutrients and oxygen. Waste products formed by the fetus are transferred back across the placental membrane into the intervillous space.

Function

The placenta has an optimal functional period of about 40 to 42 weeks. There appear to be no significant morphologic changes in the postterm placenta until about 42 weeks (Nahum and others, 1995). After 43 to 44 weeks it begins aging by depositing calcium and fibrin within its tissue (McLean and others, 1991).

PATHOPHYSIOLOGY

Amniotic Fluid

Decreased Amniotic Fluid

Decreased amniotic fluid, or oligohydramnios, is the factor most frequently associated with postterm pregnancy (Cunningham and others, 1997; Veille and others, 1993). Decreased amniotic fluid below 400 ml can reduce the cushioning effect of the fluid. As a result it becomes far more likely that the fetus will entrap or compress its own cord, shutting off blood flow to and from itself for intermittent intervals.

Meconium Contamination

Meconium in the amniotic fluid occurs in postterm pregnancies 25% to 30% of the time (Freeman, Lagrew, 1996), as compared with 19% of all deliveries (van Heijst and others, 1995). When the fetus is postterm, the expulsion of meconium into the already diminished volume of amniotic fluid causes the meconium to thicken, inhibits the normal antibacterial properties of the amniotic fluid, and pulls fluid from Wharton jelly, promoting stiffening of the cord.

Placenta and Umbilical Cord

Placental Dysfunction

When the placenta ages, depositing fibrin and calcium, intervillous hemorrhagic infarcts occur and the basal membrane of the placental blood vessels thickens and degenerates, affecting diffusion of oxygen. These changes have been noted in the postterm placenta. Whether these placental changes affect the fetal outcome in the postterm pregnancy is unknown at this time since most fetuses continue to grow (Harris and others, 1991a; McLean and others, 1991). This type of placental deprivation may be primarily hypoxic, not nutritional, unless maternal vascular disease is also causing further placental deprivation (Smith, 1990). Therefore, in some prolonged pregnancy cases, suboptimal placental function may be the cause of decreased amniotic fluid but the fetus may continue to grow (Katz, Bowes, 1992; Phelan, 1989; Silver and others, 1988).

Decreased Wharton Jelly

As aging takes place, water content is lost from the Wharton jelly encasing the umbilical cord, decreasing the amount of Wharton jelly. As the amount of Wharton jelly decreases, the cord stiffens and becomes firm rather than flexible and pliable.

Decreased Umbilical Cord Blood Flow

As a result of umbilical cord stiffening, susceptibility to pressure on the cord and to bending of the cord is increased. If the cord bends or kinks, much like a sun-baked garden hose, increased resistance to fetal blood flow can result in serious neurologic damage or sudden intrauterine fetal death.

SIGNS AND SYMPTOMS

A number of obstetric warning signs in conjunction with a pregnancy continuing past the estimated due date (EDD), including the following, can alert caregivers to potential problems.

Maternal Weight Loss

In the last weeks of pregnancy a weight loss in excess of 3 pounds/wk, caused by a decreased amount of amniotic fluid, may warn of a postterm pregnancy.

Decreased Uterine Size

Decreased amniotic fluid (less than 400 ml) frequently correlates with maternal weight loss and with a decrease in uterine size.

Meconium-stained Amniotic Fluid

Meconium in the amniotic fluid can represent a normal physiologic event in the maturation of the fetal gastrointestinal tract, can be the result of vagal stimulation from transient umbilical cord compression that results in increased peristalsis, or can be the direct result of fetal hypoxia (Nathan and others, 1994).

Advanced Bone Maturation

Advanced bone maturation can be detected by palpation of an excessively hard fetal head. It can lead to a lack of cephalic molding and a high arrest of the fetal head with potential for failure to progress, prolongation of the active phase of labor, and failure to complete the transitional phase of labor.

Prolonged Labor

Prolonged labor can be caused by a macrosomic fetus or failure of cephalic molding.

MATERNAL EFFECTS
Physical Exhaustion

Many women report extreme fatigue if their pregnancy is prolonged.

Psychologic Depression

Women express a great deal of frustration with the prolongation of the pregnancy and a feeling of total lack of personal control in effecting an end to the pregnancy (Campbell, 1986). Feelings of inadequacy emerge because of their inability to complete the process of the pregnancy "like everyone else." Women often blame themselves for prolonging the pregnancy by working too hard, working too long into the pregnancy, or not seeking adequate help with everyday tasks.

Relationships with those people closest to them become strained. Resentment is expressed because friends and relatives repeatedly check on the woman's progress and condition. Physical discomfort becomes an intolerable burden, which in turn decreases the ability to continue caring for the home and other family members in the accustomed manner. Women describe feeling awkward, big, and ugly. They comment that they have lost their "glow" and feel generally unattractive. A woman's negative feelings about herself may be projected as feelings of resentment toward the baby for not cooperating or for being a "stubborn" child.

Realistic fears are commonly shared about the continued well-being of the baby. Women report fears that the baby is "stuck" and will somehow be harmed or that something is very wrong and that the baby has decided not to be born.

Other Maternal Risks

Most other risks are related to the increase cesarean delivery risk.

FETAL AND NEONATAL EFFECTS

When 42 weeks of gestation is exceeded, intrapartum perinatal risk is increased (Cunningham and others, 1997). This is related to a wide range of features.

Macrosomia

Macrosomia is defined as a birth weight greater than 4000 to 4500 g (ACOG, 1995). Macrosomia occurs in approximately 25% of postterm fetuses (Harris and others, 1991a). It develops because the fetus has a longer time to grow in the uterus (Sims, Walther, 1989). Macrosomia poses a risk to the postdate fetus because it can lead to shoulder dystocia and birth trauma.

Dysmaturity Syndrome

Dysmaturity syndrome occurs in approximately 1% to 2% of postdate fetuses (Wood, 1994) because of a compromised environment. This syndrome is characterized by degrees of skin change with or without loss of subcutaneous fat and muscle mass and meconium staining dependent on severity of cord compression and placental dysfunction. Dysmaturity syndrome was initially classified by Clifford (1954) and was later revised by Vorherr (1975). However, most of these infants regain their weight quickly and exhibit few long-term neurologic problems (Freeman, Lagrew, 1996).

First Stage

In the first stage of dysmaturity syndrome the skin becomes desquamated. It is characterized by a dry, cracked, parchment-like peeling, with or without loss of subcutaneous fat and muscle mass.

Second Stage

The second stage of dysmaturity syndrome includes first-stage characteristics and also green meconium–stained fetal skin and umbilical cord.

Third Stage

The third stage of dysmaturity syndrome includes the first two stages plus yellow staining of the skin and the umbilical cord. This yellow staining is related to meconium being passed several days before. The bile in the meconium, as it breaks down, turns the fluid yellow.

Fetal Hypoxia

Fetal hypoxia can be caused by placental deprivation or decreased amniotic fluid that leads to cord compression (Smith, 1990).

Meconium Aspiration Syndrome

Five to ten percent of infants with meconium below the vocal cords develop meconium aspiration syndrome (Katz, Bowes, 1992). Meconium-stained amniotic fluid is present in 25% to 30% of all postterm deliveries (Freeman, Lagrew, 1996). The fetus normally moves fluids into and out of the lungs in utero by two breathing patterns. Shallow, regular breathing comprises 90% of fetal respirations, and deep, irregular breathing comprises the other 10%. An abnormal pattern of breathing may be stimulated in the presence of hypoxia, which is characterized by compensatory gasping respirations. Aspiration of meconium from the amniotic fluid into the lungs occurs if gasping respirations are stimulated by asphyxia, and a small amount may occur during the normal deep respiration breathing (Katz, Bowes, 1992). If meconium aspiration occurs, it is normally cleared through the pulmonary circulation in the same manner as amniotic fluid is normally cleared from the lungs. If pulmonary vascular damage has occurred because of asphyxia, the mechanism of clearing the lung fields of fluid is affected and meconium aspiration syndrome results (Katz, Bowes, 1992).

Hypoglycemia

Acute episodes of hypoxia related to cord compression result in anaerobic glycolysis, which exhausts carbohydrate reserves. Placental deterioration can lead to chronic fetal nutritional deficiency and further depletion of the carbohydrate reserves (Sims, Walther, 1989).

Polycythemia

The fetus increases production of red blood cells as a compensatory response to hypoxia. The polycythemia can be a significant problem in the newborn period, contributing to hyperbilirubinemia from destruction of no longer needed red blood cells.

Birth Injury

Shoulder dystocia and birth trauma are injuries that are directly related to fetal macrosomia.

DIAGNOSTIC TESTING

When a pregnancy extends beyond 7 days past the EDD, the prenatal chart should be reviewed for confirmation of the due date. Parameters for review include the following aspects.

Gestational Length Variables

Based on the Nägele rule, the length of gestation is 280 days. However, the length of gestation has been shown to vary among women. Parity may influence gestational length. One study has shown that 287 days is the mean gestation for the primigravida and 281 days is the mean for the multigravida (Nichols, 1985). Other studies have shown that there may be ethnic variances (Mittendorf and others, 1990). White primiparas' average length of gestation is 288 days; for white multiparas it is 283 days; for Japanese women it is 278 days; and for African-American women it is 277½ days.

Menstrual Cycle Length

If the woman has a prolonged preovulatory phase, the EDD should be appropriately adjusted to a later date.

Contraceptive Use

Oral contraceptives may delay ovulation.

Quickening

Pregnant women should be asked prospectively to note the date they felt their fetus move for the first time (quickening). For the primigravida this should occur when the fetus is approximately 18 to 20 weeks of gestational age. For the multigravida it usually occurs around 16 to 18 weeks.

Audible Fetal Heart Sounds

The fetal heart sounds can be heard with the Doppler ultrasound at around 10 to 12 weeks of gestation and with the fetoscope at 16 to 18 weeks.

Fundal Growth

Between 20 and 32 weeks of gestation, fundal height measurement, assessed with the mother's bladder empty, from the symphysis pubis to the top of the fundus should approximate gestational age within 2 weeks.

Diagnostic Ultrasound Findings

For accurate dating, ultrasound measurements should be done before 20 weeks of gestation. An early crown-ramp length, between 4 and 10 weeks of gestation (Nichols, 1987; Silva and others, 1990), offers the most accurate means. By averaging the biparietal diameter, head circumference, abdominal circumference, and femur length between 14 and 20 weeks, diagnostic ultrasound is 90% accurate in determining the EDD within ±2 weeks (Warsof, Abramowicz, 1990). After 26 weeks, and particularly during the last 10 weeks of gestation, accuracy of estimating gestational age is progressively limited. For these reasons, in the presence of a questionable last menstrual period (LMP), ultrasound should be used as early as possible and preferably before 20 weeks to prevent confusion regarding diagnosis of postterm pregnancy once the EDD is past. Weeks 10 to 13 should be avoided because during the uncurling of the fetus the crown-rump length is too variable and the biparietal diameter is not yet reliable (Nichols, 1987).

Fetal Fibronectin

Fetal fibronectin (FFN) enters into vaginal secretions when light uterine contractions cause movement of chorion against the decidual layer of the uterus (Ahner and others, 1995a, 1995b). Low concentrations of vaginal FFN may predict an increased risk of having a postdate infant. Lockwood and others (1994) found that 92% of women with a gestation of 39 weeks and a vaginal FFN value greater than 60 ng/ml would deliver in 10 days. Only 57% would deliver in 10 days if the FFN was lower than 60 ng/ml.

USUAL MEDICAL MANAGEMENT AND PROTOCOLS FOR NURSE PRACTITIONERS

The antepartum intervention of a postterm pregnancy is still controversial. The first major issue is when to initiate intervention, at 41 or 42 weeks of gestation. The second issue is what intervention should be implemented: labor induction or expectant management using antepartum fetal testing.

The American clinical trial by NICHHD (1994) concluded that either management protocol was acceptable with no cost difference (Gardner and others, 1996). The Canadian clinical trial (Hannah and others, 1992) concluded that induction of labor once the woman reached 41 weeks of gestation decreases cesarean birth rate with no difference in the incidence of perinatal mortality. In the Canadian study, in the expectant managed group, 66% went into labor spontaneously and the cesarean birth rate increased if an induction was required. However, prostaglandins were used less frequently if an induction was indicated in the expectant group as compared with the routine induction group (Hannah and others, 1992). Grant (1994) concluded from a meta-analysis of 11 clinical trial studies that routine induction had a lower rate of perinatal mortality, cesarean delivery, and meconium staining.

According to ACOG recommendations (1995), at 42 or more weeks of gestation, if the cervix is ripe, an induction is advocated; however if the cervix is unfavorable, fetal surveillance or cervical ripening can be implemented. Therefore without a defined protocol, women should be informed of the benefits and risks of induction of labor and expectant management. The woman's preferences should be considered in the plan of management. Individualize the plan of care with the goal of not pushing nature too soon, but do not allow variables to develop that will decrease tolerance to labor, such as decreased, meconium-stained amniotic fluid, a hard fetal head, and macrosomia.

Induction of Labor

Any of the interventions of labor stimulation outlined in Chapter 26 can be used to induce a postterm pregnancy. Stripping fetal membranes has been shown to decrease the incidence of postdate gestations without increasing complications (El-Torkey, Grant, 1992; Krammer, O'Brien, 1995). Cervical ripening, with a cervical ripening agent, is usually attempted before oxytocin induction is started. If the cervix is ripe, with a Bishop score of 5 or greater for a multigravida or 9 or greater for a primigravida, labor induction with oxytocin is usually initiated.

Expectant Management With Fetal Surveillance

Daily fetal movement counts may be started around term. In the United States a baseline fetal surveillance with a nonstress test (NST) and/or an amniotic fluid index (AFI) is usually obtained between 40 and 41 weeks. Continuous fetal surveillance is initiated during the forty-first week of pregnancy (Freeman, Lagrew, 1996). These studies will continue until the cervix becomes ripe, spontaneous labor is started, an antepartum fetal test becomes abnormal, or induction is done at the completion of 42 weeks (Cunningham and others, 1997).

A single means of fetal surveillance or a combination of two studies may be used. Usually twice weekly AFI is used as one of two methods of fetal surveillance when twice weekly NSTs or weekly contraction stress tests (CSTs) are used as the principal means of evaluating fetal well-being. Biophysical profile may be used, but it is more costly. For a complete discussion of methods, procedures, interpretation, and management, see Chapter 3.

NURSING PROCESS

NURSING DIAGNOSES/COLLABORATIVE PROBLEMS AND INTERVENTIONS

- **POTENTIAL COMPLICATION: ALTERATION IN THE LABOR PROCESS** related to advanced skull maturation, decreased ability to mold, and therefore decreased descent and less wedge pressure on the cervix.

  DESIRED OUTCOME: Labor progress will continue within normal limits without fetal compromise.

  INTERVENTION
    1. Facilitate a normal labor progression as outlined in Chapter 27 under enhancement of labor progress through each of the functional health patterns.

- **FEAR** related to potential problems because the pregnancy did not end when expected.

  DESIRED OUTCOME: The patient and her family will be able to express their feelings and fears about the prolonged pregnancy and maintain open communication among themselves.

  INTERVENTIONS
    1. Encourage the patient and her family to openly express their anger, frustrations, feelings regarding the extreme fatigue and unattractiveness, and fears related to fetal well-being with professional health care providers and each other.
    2. Discuss the meaning of the EDD with the patient and her family. The EDD is merely a midpoint in a 1-month range during which 90% of women will deliver (Nichols, 1987).
    3. Provide opportunities for the patient to listen to the fetal heart rate (FHR) and see evidence of FHR reactivity during fetal surveillance studies.
    4. Assist in planning alternative arrangements for help in the home for the present and postpartum periods because of fatigue.
    5. Discuss the importance of obtaining fetal surveillance studies and the findings from them with the patient and her family, if present.
    6. Acknowledge expressed feelings as important, and discuss measures that might be helpful in relieving them.

7. Encourage self-advocacy if responses to fears are inadequate. Reassure about relevancy of fears to potential fetal compromise.

8. Refer to available and appropriate support services, such as social service, high risk pregnancy support group, home health aides, visiting nurse, and church or other supportive community resource.

■ **RISK FOR IMPAIRED FETAL GAS EXCHANGE** related to decreased amniotic fluid or hypoxic type of placental deprivation.

DESIRED OUTCOMES: The fetus will remain active, and its heart rate will be maintained at a baseline between 110 and 160 beats/min with normal variability, normal reactivity, and no nonreassuring decelerations. The biophysical profile will continue to be greater than 6. The AFI will be greater than 8 with at least one pocket of amniotic fluid greater than 2 cm and amniotic fluid throughout the uterine cavity. The amniotic fluid will be free of meconium. The 1- and 5-minute Apgar scores will be 7 or more.

INTERVENTIONS

Antepartum

1. Instruct the patient about the importance of and how to assess for daily fetal activity.

2. Prepare the patient and her family so they understand the reason for the proposed medical plan of care.

3. Assess for signs of fetal compromise by carrying out the ordered fetal surveillance studies.

4. Prepare the patient for the reason for weekly cervical examinations to determine cervical ripening.

5. Prepare the patient for potential medical interventions, such as an induction of labor, delivery aided by forceps, or cesarean birth.

Intrapartum

1. Admit patient when she is in early labor or for an induction.

2. Use pain medications and sedatives very cautiously and only after other alternative methods of coping have been determined to be inadequate alone.

3. Use continuous fetal monitoring to recognize early evidence of a nonreassuring FHR change.

4. Manage the labor in a facility that can provide a cesarean birth or forceps delivery if either of these becomes necessary and where personnel qualified for infant resuscitation can be immediately summoned.

5. When rupture of membranes occurs, assess FHR and note

the amount and color of amniotic fluid. (Minimal amniotic fluid on amniotomy is predictive of meconium 50% of the time, even if obvious meconium is not immediately observed [Druzin, Adams, 1990].)

6. Be prepared to assist with fetal scalp blood gas analysis if desired before delivery. Be prepared to collect cord pH sample from umbilical artery immediately after delivery.

7. Be prepared to manage a saline amnioinfusion if multiple variable decelerations occur related to decreased amniotic fluid or combined with thick meconium on rupture of membranes (Owen and others, 1990; Ogundipe and others, 1994; Wallerstedt and others, 1994).

8. Notify the physician at the first signs of a nonreassuring FHR change.

■ **POTENTIAL COMPLICATIONS OF AMNIOINFUSION: ABRUPTIO PLACENTAE AND AMNIOTIC FLUID EMBOLISM** related to over-distention of the uterus with saline or a rising uterine resting tone; umbilical cord prolapse related to a gush of amniotic fluid; and fetal bradycardia related to infusing cold saline.

DESIRED OUTCOME: Nonreassuring variable decelerations will be minimized or eliminated as measured by a significant decline in frequency of variable FHR decelerations, presence of FHR baseline variability, and continued normal baseline rate.

INTERVENTIONS

1. Rule out cord prolapse.

2. Assess patient's understanding of the procedure.

3. Educate patient about the reasons for the procedure.

4. Assess baseline maternal vital signs, FHR, and uterine activity.

5. Obtain a 1000-ml bag of normal saline that has been stored in a heating unit or warmed in a microwave oven to 37° C.

6. Connect the warmed normal saline to the intrauterine pressure catheter by way of intravenous (IV) tubing.

7. Give an initial bolus of 300 to 500 ml and then 150 to 200 ml/hr. This rate can be accomplished without an infusion pump by hanging the saline bag 3 to 4 feet above the uterus, but it is preferable to use an infusion pump when available.

8. Continue infusion until the variable decelerations resolve and an additional 250 ml has been infused; or intolerable side effects develop, such as an increasing uterine resting tone, nonreassuring signs of fetal compromise, or uterine tenderness.

9. Monitor FHR and uterine activity continuously with a separate or solid, multiple-lumen intrauterine pressure catheter.

10. Check temperature every 2 hours.

11. Measure and mark fundal height and reassess every hour.

12. Keep the patient as dry as possible by changing the pads often.

13. Notify the physician if nonreassuring variable decelerations are not resolved with a total of 800 ml of warmed saline or when signs of maternal or fetal response are not reassuring (Strong, Phelan, 1991).

14. Document the amount of uterine input, amount and character of vaginal discharge, uterine activity including resting tone, FHR, and vital signs.

- ■ **POTENTIAL COMPLICATION OF POSTDATISM: FETAL INJURY AND MECONIUM ASPIRATION**

   DESIRED OUTCOMES: During labor, the FHR will be maintained at a baseline between 110 and 160 beats/min with normal variability, normal reactivity, and no nonreassuring decelerations. At delivery the neonate will be free of injury and of meconium-stained amniotic fluid below the vocal cords.

   INTERVENTIONS

   1. Assist with ultrasound to rule out macrosomia.

   2. Graph the labor against the normal labor curve to detect early signs of labor dystocia related to large-for-gestational-age fetus or advanced bone maturation of the fetal skull.

   3. Be prepared to manage an amnioinfusion during the labor to decrease the viscosity of meconium and decrease cord compression (Phelan, 1989). However, amnioinfusion used to thin meconium before delivery has not been shown to decrease the incidence of meconium aspiration syndrome (Folsom, 1997; Usta and others, 1995).

   4. Notify pediatric personnel for presence during delivery if meconium is noted in the amniotic fluid, so that prompt resuscitation and oxygenation can be administered as needed. Visualization of the vocal cords and deep suction of the trachea to clear the airway of meconium before the infant takes its first breath may be required.

   5. Confirm findings with the attending physician if meconium is noted on amniotomy. Also notify the physician if there is a nonreassuring change in the FHR baseline, nonreassuring decelerations are noted, or loss of variability

develops. In the presence of a nonreassuring FHR pattern, meconium in the amniotic fluid is a critically important sign. (It can signal an increased risk of meconium aspiration syndrome [Katz, Bowes, 1992].)

CONCLUSION

The etiology and pathophysiology of postterm pregnancy are not completely understood, but early and ongoing prenatal care is essential and the importance of assignment of an accurate EDD is clearly evident. When postterm pregnancy can be diagnosed without significant shades of doubt, the nurse can then collaborate with the other health care team members in developing an effective plan of care to prevent undue maternal anxiety, reduce sources of fears, and lower infant mortality and morbidity.

BIBLIOGRAPHY

Ahn M, Phelan J: Epidemiologic aspects of the postdate pregnancy, *Clin Obstet Gynecol* 32(2):228-234, 1989.

Ahner R and others: Fetal fibronectin as a marker to predict the onset of term labor and delivery, *Am J Obstet Gynecol* 172:134-137, 1995a.

Ahner R and others: Fetal fibronectin as a selection criterion for induction of term labor, *Am J Obstet Gynecol* 173:1513-1517, 1995b.

American College of Obstetricians and Gynecologists (ACOG): Fetal macrosomia, *ACOG Techn Bull,* no. 159, 1991.

American College of Obstetricians and Gynecologists (ACOG): *Quality, evaluation, and improvement in practice: postterm pregnancy. Committee on Quality Assessment.* Criteria set no. 10, Washington, DC, 1995, The Author.

Brace R: Amniotic fluid dynamics. In Creasy R, Resnik R, editors: *Maternal-fetal medicine: principles and practices,* ed 3, Philadelphia, 1994, Saunders.

Campbell B: Overdue delivery: its impact on mothers-to-be, *MCN Am J Matern Child Nurs* 11(3):170-172, 1986.

Clifford S: Postmaturity with placental dysfunction: clinical syndrome and pathologic findings, *J Pediatr* 44:1, 1954.

Cunningham F and others: *Williams' obstetrics,* ed 20, Stamford, Conn, 1997, Appleton & Lange.

Druzin M, Adams D: Significance of observing no fluid at anniotomy, *Am J Obstet Gynecol* 162:1006-1007, 1990.

El-Torkey M, Grant J: Sweeping of the membranes is an effective method of induction of labour in prolonged pregnancy: a report of a randomized trial, *Br J Obstet Gynaecol* 99:455-458, 1992.

Folsom M: Amnioinfusion for meconium, *MCH* 22(1):74-79, 1997.

Freeman R, Lagrew D: Postdate pregnancy. In Gabbe S, Niebyl J, Simpson J, editors: *Obstetrics: normal and problem pregnancies,* ed 3, New York, 1996, Churchill Livingstone.

Gardner M and others: NIH Maternal-Fetal Medicine Units Network: cost comparison of induction of labor at 41 weeks versus expectant management in the postterm pregnancy, *Am J Obstet Gynecol* 174: 351, 1996.

Goeree R, Hannah M, Hewson S: Cost-effectiveness of induction of labour versus serial antenatal monitoring in the Canadian Multicentre Postterm pregnancy trial, *Can Med Assoc J* 152:1445, 1995.

Grant J: Induction of labour confers benefits in prolonged pregnancy, *Br J Obstet Gynaecol* 101:99, 1994.

Guidetti D, Divon M, Langer O: Postdate fetal surveillance: is 4 weeks too early? *Am J Obstet Gynecol* 161:91-93, 1989.

Hannah M and others: Induction of labor vs antenatal monitoring in posterm pregnancy, *N Engl J Med* 326:1587, 1992.

Harris B and others: Prolonged pregnancy. I. Identifying the patient at risk, *Female Patient* 16(2):43-50, 1991a.

Harris B and others: Prolonged pregnancy. II. Monitoring and intervention, *Female Patient* 16(3):47-60, 1991b.

Haubrich K: Amnioinfusion: a technique for the relief of variable deceleration, *J Obstet Gynecol Neonatal Nurs* 19(4):299-303, 1990.

Katz V, Bowes W: Meconium aspiration syndrome: reflection of a murky subject, *Am J Obstet Gynecol* 166:171-183, 1992.

Knorr L: Relieving fetal distress with amnioinfusion, *MCN Am J Matern Child Nurs* 14(5):346-350, 1989.

Krammer J, O'Brien W: Mechanical methods of cervical ripening, *Clin Obstet Gynecol* 38(2):280-286, 1995.

Lockwood C and others: Low concentrations of vaginal fibronectin as a predictor of deliveries occurring after 41 weeks, *Am J Obstet Gynecol* 171:1-4, 1994.

McLean F and others: Postterm infants: too big or too small? *Am J Obstet Gynecol* 164:619-624, 1991.

Mittendorf R and others: The length of uncomplicated human gestation, *Obstet Gynecol* 75:929-932, 1990.

Nahum G, Stanislaw H, Huffaker B: Fetal weight gain at term: linear with minimal dependence on maternal obesity, *Am J Obstet Gynecol* 172:1387, 1995.

Nathan L and others: Meconium: a 1990s perspective on an old obstetric hazard, *Obstet Gynecol* 83:329-332, 1994.

NICHHD Network of Maternal-Fetal Medicine Units: A clinical trial of induction of labor versus expectant management in posterm pregnancy, *Am J Obstet Gynecol* 170:716, 1994.

Nichols C: The Yale nurse-midwifery practice: examining the outcomes, *J Nurse Midwifery* 30(3):159-165, 1985.

Nichols C: Dating pregnancy: gathering and using a reliable data base, *J Nurse Midwifery* 32(4):195-204, 1987.

Nurses Association of the American College of Obstetricians and Gynecologists (NAACOG): *NAACOG video series: critical concepts in EFM,* Washington, DC, 1990, The Association.

Ogundipe O, Spong C, Ross M: Prophylactic amnioinfusion for oligohydramnios: a reevaluation, *Obstet Gynecol* 84:544-548, 1994.

Owen J, Henson B, Hauth J: A prospective randomized study of saline solution amnioinfusion, *Am J Obstet Gynecol* 162:1146-1149, 1990.

Phelan J: The postdate pregnancy: an overview, *Clin Obstet Gynecol* 32(2):221-227, 1989.

Resnik R: Postterm pregnancy. In Creasy R, Resnik R, editors: *Maternal-fetal medicine: principles and practice,* ed 3, Philadelphia, 1994, Saunders.

Rodriguez H: Ultrasound evaluation of the postdate pregnancy, *Clin Obstet Gynecol* 32(2):257-261, 1989.

Silva P and others: Early crown-rump length: a good predictor of gestational age, *J Reprod Med* 35(6):641-644, 1990.

Silver R and others: Umbilical cord size and amniotic fluid volume in prolonged pregnancy, *Am J Obstet Gynecol* 157:716-720, 1987.

Silver R and others: Fetal acidosis in prolonged pregnancy cannot be attributed to cord compression alone, *Am J Obstet Gynecol* 159:666-669, 1988.

Sims M, Walther F: Neonatal morbidity and mortality and long term outcome of postdate infants, *Clin Obstet Gynecol* 32(2):285-293, 1989.

Smith C: Postterm pregnancy: monitoring vs intervention, *Female Patient* 15(7):19-32, 1990.

Strong T, Phelan J: Amnioinfusion for intrapartum management, *Contemp OB/GYN* 37(5):15-24, 1991.

Usta I and others: The impact of a policy of amnioinfusion for meconium-stained amniotic fluid, *Obstet Gynecol* 85:237-241, 1995.

van Heijst M, van Roosmalen J, Keirse M: Classifying meconium-stained liquor: Is it feasible? *Birth* 22(4):191-195, 1995.

Veille J, Penry M, Mueller-Heubach E: Fetal renal pulsed Doppler waveform in prolonged pregnancies, *Am J Obstet Gynecol* 169:882, 1993.

Vorherr H: Placental insufficiency in relation to postterm pregnancy and fetal postmaturity, *Am J Obstet Gynecol* 123(1):67-101, 1975.

Wallerstedt C and others: Amnioinfusion: an update, *J Obstet Gynecol Neonatal Nurs* 23(7):573, 1994.

Warsof S, Abramowicz J: Routine ultrasound in obstetric care, *Obstet Gynecol Rep* 2:114-127, 1990.

Wood C: Postdate pregnancy update, *J Nurse Midwifery* 39 (suppl 2):110s-122s, 1994.

INDEX